NURSING CARE OF THE CHILD WITH LONG-TERM ILLNESS

NURSING CARE OF THE CHILD WITH LONG-TERM ILLNESS

2nd Edition

EDITED BY
SHIRLEY STEELE, R.N., M.A., Ph.D.

CONTRIBUTIONS BY
DONNA JUENKER, R.N., M.Ed.
CAROL REN KNEISL, R.N., M.S.
MARY NORMA O'HARA, R.N., M.A.
JACQUELINE THOMPSON, R.N., M.Ed.

ILLUSTRATIONS BY
HELEN PTAK, R.N., M.A., Ph.D.

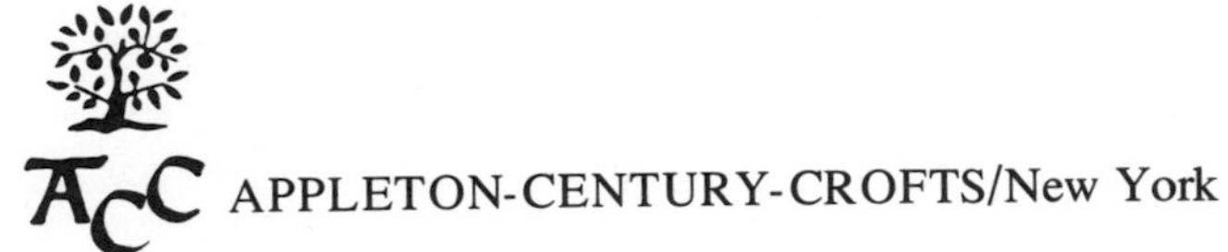
APPLETON-CENTURY-CROFTS/New York

Library of Congress Cataloging in Publication Data
Main entry under title:

Nursing care of the child with long-term illness, 2nd ed

Includes bibliographies and index.
1. Chronic diseases in children—Nursing. I. Steele, Shirley. II. Juenker, Donna M. [DNLM: 1. Long term care—In infancy and childhood. 2. Pediatric nursing. WY159 N968]
RJ380.N87 1977 610.73'62 77-24157
ISBN 0-8385-7017-8

77 78 79 80 81 / 10 9 8 7 6 5 4 3 2 1

Prentice-Hall International, Inc., London
Prentice-Hall of Australia, Pty. Ltd., Sydney
Prentice-Hall of India Private Limited, New Delhi
Prentice-Hall of Japan, Inc., Tokyo
Prentice-Hall of Southeast Asia (Pte.) Ltd., Singapore
Whitehall Books Ltd., Wellington, New Zealand

PRINTED IN THE UNITED STATES OF AMERICA

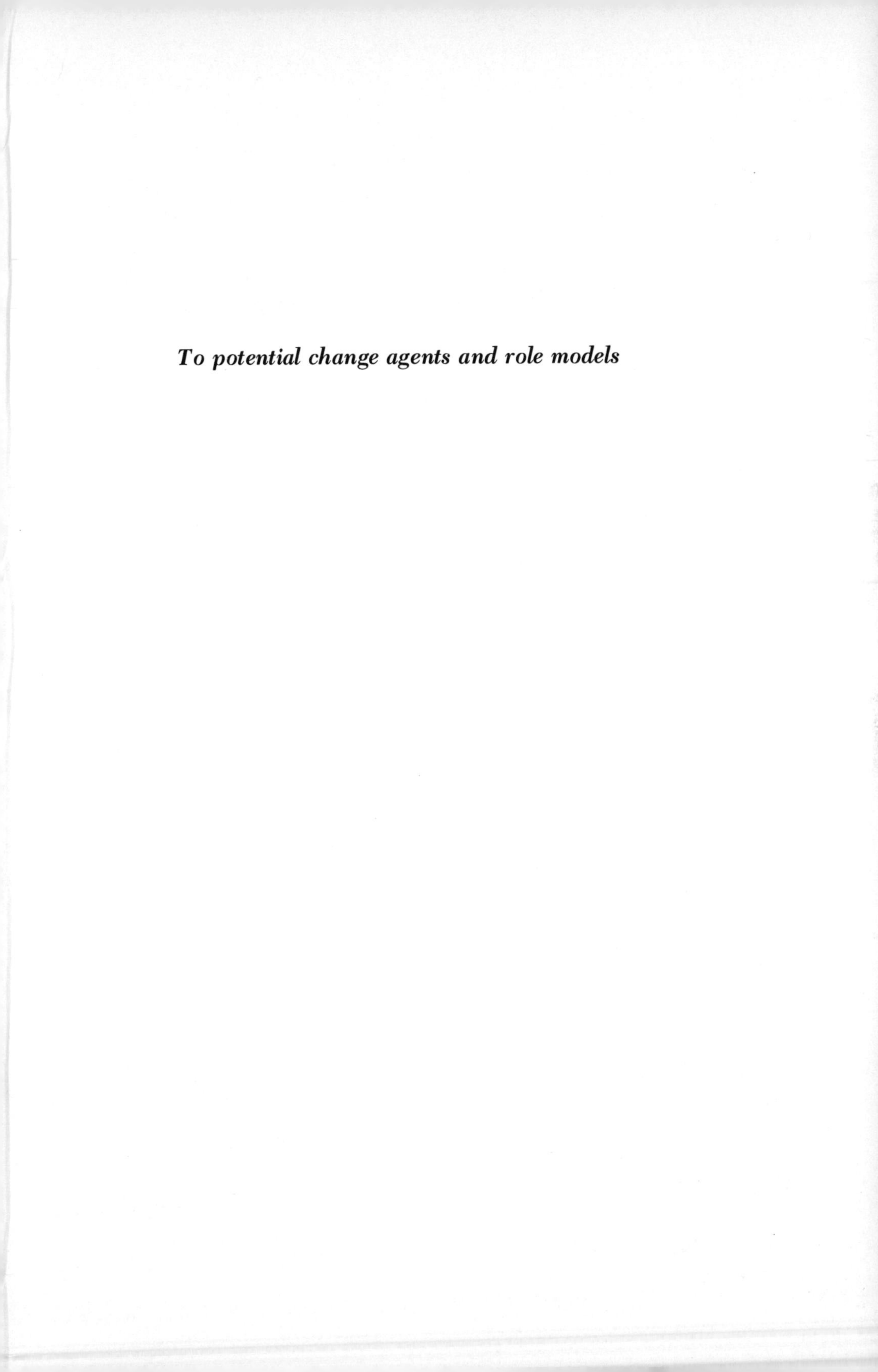

To potential change agents and role models

Contributors

Donna Juenker received her diploma in nursing from Sisters of Charity Hospital, Buffalo, New York. She completed her Baccalaureate degree at D'Youville College, Buffalo, and has a Master of Education degree from Teachers College, Columbia. She is an Associate Professor of Nursing at the State University of New York at Buffalo.

Carol Ren Kneisl received her diploma in nursing from Millard Fillmore Hospital, Buffalo, New York. She completed her Baccalaureate degree at the University of Buffalo. She has a Master of Science degree in Psychiatric Nursing from the University of California at San Francisco, and is a Doctoral candidate. She is an Associate Professor of Nursing at the State University of New York at Buffalo.

Mary Norma O'Hara received her diploma in nursing from the Charles S. Wilson Memorial Hospital, Johnson City, New York. She completed a Bachelor of Science degree at the Catholic University of America in Washington, D.C., and a Master of Arts degree from Teachers College, Columbia. She is an Associate Professor of Nursing at the State University of New York at Buffalo.

Shirley Steele received her diploma in nursing from the Waterbury Hospital, Waterbury, Connecticut. Her Baccalaureate and Master's degrees are from Teachers College, Columbia University, her doctoral degree is from the Ohio State University. She is a Professor of Nursing at Texas Woman's University, Houston, Texas.

Jacqueline Thompson received her R.N. and Bachelor of Science degree from the University of Minnesota. She spent two years at Purdue University in Child Development and Family Life. She received her Master of Education degree in Early Childhood Education from the State University of New York at Buffalo. She is an Associate Professor of Nursing at the State University of New York at Buffalo.

Contents

Preface

Since the publication of the first edition of this book, nursing has continued to expand its boundaries in many directions. Certainly one of its most significant areas is the expanded use of physical assessment in the nursing process. It was tempting to include chapters in this area in this edition. However, I decided not to do this. Three of our colleagues in the field, Mary Alexander, Marie Scott Brown, and Peggy Chinn have already produced excellent volumes covering this aspect of child care. After considerable thought I decided to keep this edition clearly focused on the special needs of the child with long-term illness. We have had very positive feed-back from nurses who felt that the first edition offered them excellent material to help them understand the challenges presented by these children and their families or significant others. Therefore, this edition continues to focus on many of the same areas as were presented in the first edition. However, the material is expanded or changed to reflect the advances which have taken place since the publication of the first edition.

I am hopeful that the reader will be able to use the material to creatively plan for the nursing care of these children and their significant others. The excitement surrounding a field which is so dynamic cannot be adequately captured on paper. However, the practitioner will soon find the self-satisfaction which evolves from being a part of the nurse-child-family triad. It is a privilege to be able to interact with these clients in a humanistic way and the authors of this volume are all indebted to the families who have given us the privilege of collecting clinical data while facilitating their health maintenance and restorative care needs. While the title of the book continues to specifically acknowledge the child, we view the child as an integral part of a social system, usually a family. This philosophical commitment underlies the reason we focus special attention on the significant others who interact with the child with a long-term illness. We also believe that the professionals who are responsible for the child's care are an important part of the child's social system and their ability and expertise in integrating cognitive, affective and psychomotor skills into on-going care plans will enhance the child's probability to achieve his highest potential.

The book continues to be a supplement to other child health nursing textbooks. The primary audience is the undergraduate student in nursing. However, nurses working in the field should find it a valuable resource volume. The editor has used her editing perogative to try to produce consistancy of terminology from one chapter to another.

We continue to owe many persons thank you's for their assistance. We again express our special appreciation to the nursing staff of the Children's Hospital of Buffalo under the leadership of Ms. Pauline Keefe. In addition, the editor wishes to acknowledge the cooperation of the nursing staff of the Hermann Hospital in Houston under the leadership of Ms. Carol Ann Consolvo. The editor also wishes to acknowledge the valuable assistance of Ms. Evelyn Bedard of the Jesse Jones Library in Houston, Texas who contributed a great deal to the updating of the library research by notifying me of new library acquisitions. Most importantly, we thank our colleagues in the field who continue to be our "sounding boards" for new ideas.

Introduction

The role of the nurse in the care of children is changing dramatically. Once a matter of baby sitting and diaper changing—a rather bland combination—it is now a position demanding the most critical of observations and actions. There are many reasons for the change in the nurse's role. The increase in the number of children is a factor, as are the advances in the field of medicine which result in the prolongation of life where life was previously not possible. The lack of qualified pediatricians is another. The more advanced preparation of nurses to assume increasingly complex roles is another. The spiraling costs of hospitalization also plays a part. The trend to ambulatory care is another reason. Perhaps the most outstanding reason is that nurses are demanding and getting the recognition they deserve for the health care services they render so competently.

The term "child health nurse" is all-encompassing. Therefore it will include the nurse in the newborn nursery, the nurse on the in-patient and out-patient services relating to child care, the nurse in the child health conferences, in home care of children, and in school health—in other words, nurses in a variety of settings who are concerned with the maintenance of health and prevention of disease of children.

The care of children is now satisfactorily strengthened by the use of the nurse practitioner. The child health nurse consults with practitioners in other specialty areas. The nurse practitioner has developed skill in physical and developmental assessment of children. She has increased expertise in the art of interviewing, history-taking and counseling. She is family-centered rather than child-centered. She is keenly aware of the family and attempts to plan and implement care which will strengthen this family unit.

The nurse practitioner is able to provide expert services to manage and monitor the majority of long-term illnesses of children. In cooperation with family members she plans for the long-term management of the chronic phases of the child's condition. She is astute at recognizing early signs of acute episodes and quickly and efficiently refers the child and family to the physician or clinic for acute care management.

The child health nurse is able to contribute both professionally and as a citizen to the needs of children with long-term illness. Her knowledge can be effectively used to help stimulate persons to provide needed programs in her community. With her expert knowledge she is able to provide information to her state and national leaders regarding the need for new legislation and programs to guarantee that her clients have the opportunity to develop to their maximum potential.

The authors of this book believe that nursing has "come of age" and that child health nurses have led the field in the trend towards promoting wellness and emphasizing the need for health education. The offerings in this book exemplify our beliefs.

It is with deep humility that we offer the material in this volume as a resource for the improvement of nursing care to the numerous children in our country who have a long-term illness.

BIBLIOGRAPHY

Alexander MM, Brown MS: Pediatric Physical Diagnosis for Nurses. New York, McGraw-Hill, 1974

Chinn P: Child Health Maintenance. St. Louis, C.V. Mosby, 1974

Erikson F: The need for a specialist in modern pediatric nursing. Nurs Forum 4:24–31, 1965

Ford LC, Silver HK: The expanded role of the nurse in child care. Nurs Outlook, 15:43–45, Sept. 1967

Rudick E: Nursing and the new pediatrics. Nurs Clinics NA (Philadelphia, Saunders) 1966, pp 75–81

NURSING CARE OF THE CHILD WITH LONG-TERM ILLNESS

PART 1
Background Information

JACQUELINE THOMPSON

1 *Human Growth and Development: A Basis for Nursing Assessment*

Can knowledge of normal human growth and development be used as a basis for nursing assessment? Obviously, the answer is *yes* and has been since the beginning of organized baccalaureate nursing education. But commitment to a strong developmental background has been as varied as are the schools of nursing and the individual nursing faculties who teach in them. It has always seemed logical to conclude that the nurse cannot fully assess the abnormal without a knowledge of the normal. However, the nursing curriculum has either only lightly covered or omitted a great deal of normal developmental information on the assumption that past life experiences is an adequate exposure for students. Many nursing faculties have felt that since the students are exposed to normative information in their prerequisite anatomy, chemistry, psychology, and physiology courses, they will be able to integrate these scattered pieces of information and to produce for themselves a composite referent man, woman, or child. I contend that it is unrealistic to assume that the student will independently integrate this piecemeal presentation of developmental information, and yet such an integration is clearly a necessary foundation for working with clients who have abnormal findings. The integration of information about normal growth and development in the nursing curriculum, as well as its implementation in the nursing process, is the subject of this chapter.

I believe that the solution to the problem of making normative developmental information clearly relevant to the nursing process lies in the construction of a conceptual framework, a developmental framework that will guide the student and the nurse in assessment, planning implementation, and evaluation of each client's total needs. The problems met with in today's practice seem to arise from both a lack of commitment to a strong developmental background and to an absent, inadequate, or personally irrelevant conceptual framework. If nursing practice is to be based upon present research from both our own and other disciplines, the practitioner must have some mental construct in which to place this new information. Unfortunately, research into both normal and abnormal development does not come neatly packaged in an existing framework. I have often been startled when discussing new research with students and practicing nurses to find that pieces of information remain isolated, rather than being clearly integrated into a meaningful cognitive structure. Indeed, one finds thread upon thread of developmental information illogically connected, more often than not, and therefore of little use without a framework of the whole to guide the practitioner to new levels of functioning.

Thus, a conceptual framework of development is essential to give the nursing process direction, and a structure is necessary for the systematic assessment of the child's total needs. It is from such a holistic view that both immediate and long term goals can be made, and a plan for the redirection of the abnormal development that brought the child into the protective environment of the hospital can be devised. Realistic goals of wherein nursing can be influential during the hospitalization and after the child has been discharged, when he is under the direction of his parents and follow-up professionals, can be formulated. Thus, the child and his family will leave our sphere of influence with a sense of knowing what has happened, what is happening, and what may be done to return the child back to the highest level of health and normal growth and development possible. This is indeed a difficult task, but, well within the realm of nursing care. This kind of comprehensive care presupposes that the nurse has a strong commitment to knowledge of normal developmental ranges *and* to the development of a clear and personally meaningful framework capable of assessment and integration of current and future developmental information.

As for the structure or design of the developmental framework, numerous constructs are possible, so long as it tolerates the dynamic nature of development information. It must be possible for all developmental information to fit within its borders; thus, the structural categories must be widely inclusive. In other words, the categories must be of a sufficiently high order of abstraction that current as well as future information is not only easily integrated but quickly retrieved. Additionally, the dynamic nature of developmental information also implies the need for a certain amount of flexibility.

The conceptual developmental framework, with its inherent concreteness must be (1) sufficiently abstract to give form but not rigidity, (2) structured so as to give security without being so concrete and confining as to make it impossible to incorporate valid new understandings, and (3) broad enough that the vast range of development can be considered as each client's behavior is assessed. This personally relevant developmental framework, with broad categories containing readily available normative information, is essential to initial nursing care. All too often the nurse must interact with the client without a complete analysis of his total developmental needs. With the developmental framework, the inadequacies of the initial assessment will be glaring enough to compel, even the most hurried nurse, to continue to develop a full and comprehensive data base, and yet allow the practitioner to feel secure in the soundness of his/her first tentative assumptions. It seems only logical that this basic structure will lead to better initial nursing planning with fewer destructive interactions. The framework's dynamic and concrete features will also be useful as a tool for daily reassessments, planning, implementation, and evaluation.

TOWARD A CONCEPTUAL FRAMEWORK OF GROWTH AND DEVELOPMENT

In this chapter, I will discuss the development of a conceptual framework for human growth and development. Before the details of a possible conceptual framework can be considered, several underlying assumptions about the character of the professional nurses' commitment to the collection of a comprehensive data base must be explored. It is assumed that it is a goal of nursing to meet the total needs of the client, insofar as it is possible within a given set of circumstances. It is also assumed that meaningful child-nurse interactions can take place only so long as they are based upon the unique expression of each child's development. This point of view, that of developing a plan of care which includes all aspects of the individual's development, is labeled the *holistic view of human growth and development*. This concept is basic to comprehensive nursing care. All of the preceeding assumptions are secondary to the primary assumption that even though the nurse may have responsibility for the care of many clients, each client's plan of care is individually determined. For example, nurses generally do not plan for the care of juvenile diabetics, but they plan for the care of each particular individual juvenile whose problem list includes diabetes mellitus.

Principles of Human Growth and Development

Besides assumptions related to the nursing process, the practitioner must be cognizant of the principles underlying human development. These principles must be considered as the nurse develops a conceptual framework.

Principle I. *Human growth and development proceeds in an orderly manner.* This principle of order allows the nursing practitioner to assess the meaningfulness of the child's behavior. (Here, the term *behavior* denotes the functioning levels of both the psychologic and biologic developmental spheres.) The emerging abilities of many children follow a general pattern that researchers have been able to document. Noteworthy has been the work in motor development of Gesell and Thompson (1941) and McGraw (1963) and the longitudinal work of Shirley (1933) in which developing children were followed into adulthood. From their work the nurse has a basis for judging any individual child's motor development within the context of a phylogenetic pattern. In other words, the fact that every aspect of human development—whether it is, for example, motor development or the development of blood pressure—has an inherent pattern of order to its emergence.

Within the context of the principle of orderliness we find that development preceeds in specific directions. This subprinciple of developmental direction has given much guidance to the nurse as immediate and long-term goals are being developed. This principle of developmental direction includes both cephalocaudal (head to foot) and proximodistal (from the center of the body to its periphery) directions. Neurologic development may be the clearest example of this principle. The brain develops to 90 percent of its adult size during the first 4 years of life, while the development of peripheral nervous system of the lower extremities must wait upon the end of somatic growth—an obvious head to foot directional movement. The brain is also an excellent example of the proximodistal developmental direction, with the early embryologic development of the midbrain followed by development of the cortex. In another example of neurologic functioning, we see almost total lower center functioning during the first few weeks of life followed by cortical development (slowly developing over approximately the next 15 years) (Piaget, 1963); postnatal vegetative functions, such as eating and sleeping, are reflexive during this time and reflect the capacities of the spinal cord and hypothalmus (Peiper, 1964).

While the nurse has historically been more comfortable discussing development in terms of the physical findings, a more comprehensive conceptual framework of growth and development will encourage a stronger incorporation of language development, socialization, identification, and information into the nursing process. Examples of cephalocaudal developmental direction can be seen as the young infant discovers first his hand and later the rest of his body, until he finally acts with a knowledge of where his body is in space. He begins to know himself as separate from other creatures and objects (Piaget, 1954). The infant and child's world develops proximodistally as he moves from a self-perception where he is the center of all activity (or solitary play) to parallel play and later cliques and gangs (Hegethorn, 1968).

Principle II. *The basic rate of development is essentially constant.* This principle is highly influenced by the individual's environment. Both short- and long-term ill health may be accompanied by major interruptions of the individual's developmental rate, but in healthy, well-developed children a constant rate of development is seen. Its impact is most demonstrable in studies comparing normal children with children with developmental lags.

Principle III. *There are different developmental rates for different biologic and psychologic systems.* Research stimulated by this principle has reaped rich rewards. It is well known that the reproductive system lies dormant until stimulated during the prepubertal period. Precocious development of secondary sex characteristics is a red flag for an intense investigation into the cause of such a deviate developmental rate. The nurse who has in-depth knowledge of the normal rate of body system development will have a firm foundation for the assessment portion of the nursing process.

Principle IV. *All developmental aspects are interrelated.* Anyone who has cared for the child who has been hospitalized for an extended period will surely appreciate the import of this principle. Abnormality or chronic disease in any bodily system will have its impact on other systems not directly under stress. The impact of a congenital heart defect on motor, social, and identification development cannot be overlooked when nursing care is planned. Because bodily systems are interrelated, comprehensive nursing care is only possible from the holistic point of view.

Principle V. *Each individual has a unique pattern of emerging abilities.* For example, some children seem to spend only a little time practicing and new abilities appear to burst forth suddenly, while other children tend to practice endlessly before the new skill is mastered. Even after mastery, some children will revert to old motor patterns during occasions of stress or for no apparent reason. For example, deviation from the norm on a Denver developmental screening one day may be eradicated the following day. Thus, it is imperative to keep this principle in mind.

Before we delve any further into construction of a developmental framework, a word of caution about growth and developmental information seems necessary. Since most developmental information has been documented in terms of "norms" or "averages," the nurse must constantly question whether any particular piece of information correlates with a single client's unique pattern. In other words, one must ask the question, "How does the individual's normal pattern of emerging abilities fit into the overall range of normal growth and development for his age, genetic background, cultural and familial environment?" What may be normal for one individual may be abnormal for another; for example, a non–life-threatening illness —such as an allergy—may have vast implications for one client but be of lesser importance to another client because of their individual unique patterns of *normal* development.

In general, two research approaches have been used when studying human growth and development. They are the developmental crises, or "ages" and "stages," approach and the longitudinal approach. The developmental crises approach devises its norms by interrupting development at what the researcher believes to be a critical point and proceeds to enumerate the exhibited behavior. A critical point is defined as a point in the chronologic development of children when a large number of developmental areas are in disequilibrium or in change (Hurlock, 1956; Ericson, 1963). Many students of nursing have been exposed to this approach. Unfortunately, exposure to only this approach may result in confusion for the student, since it often leaves the student with a vague notion that the children with whom they interact should fit into what they remember of particular "normal" stages. This may happen even when the student is aware that "norms" are not sufficiently refined to apply to every single child. Additionally, these norms may or may not be remembered correctly, since they were taught in unwarranted concreteness and enormous detail.

I believe that the study of developmental crises should be used only as a rough cognitive stimulus for the professional nurse. This approach can help "place" the child in a broad category (eg, 2½ years of age equals the negativistic stage), but it tells us relatively little about how the individual child may express himself. For example, will he be verbally or physically negative? We can certainly see that if a particular child is *verbally* negative at this age and must have his jaw immobilized, it will cause a greater stress than if he is *physically* negative and must have his jaw immobilized.

The second approach to the study of growth and development places emphasis upon the longitudinal growth and upon individual developmental aspects. Various behavioral responses are studied in a general way to search out a basic trend or flow during the life span. The problem with this approach, however, is that one can get the feeling that the human being has been sectioned into numerous responses, never to meet again. Nonetheless, it does give us some valuable insight into where the child has been and what we may expect of his behavior in the future; and its categories are often useful in the construction of the developmental conceptual framework.

In nursing we work with individuals with their own unique heredity and distinctive internal and external environments, and many times we find that these generalizations do not lead us in precisely the right direction. I believe that the best answer is an exposure to both approaches, with a strong emphasis upon observing the *facts* and accounting for the interaction of the various behavioral responses with the major influences of heredity and internal and external environments. The teaching strategy will accentuate the development of this holistic developmental point of view.

How can the holistic point of view work to our advantage when we are assisting the child who will be hospitalized for an extended period? The expression of an individual human's growth and development is stimulated and directed by the troika: heredity, internal envirnoment, and external environment. We can see examples of this interaction by observing the newborn's activity level. The newborn infants in any given nursery vary in their degree of general activity and vary in their sensitivity to stimuli. After all, each child has been developing at his own unique rate since conception, when the hereditary basis for the expression of his development was programmed (Breckenridge et al, 1958, Breckenridge and Vincent, 1966; Carmichael, 1966).

The infant begins his cognitive development (Piaget, 1932) with the satisfaction of basic needs, of which feeding is an example. As he is fed there is a reduction of an internal need, hunger. He begins to attach a vague conceptual meaning to either the bottle or breast by which he is fed. His feeling of satisfaction will depend upon his individual needs (ie, the rate of growth determined by his genetic programming and the amount of milk offered by the environment). The infant will begin his development of language as he hears the cooing and verbal communication of those close to him. The character of his language development depends, in part, upon the intactness of his auditory system (internal environment), which in turn largely depends upon genetic programming. Thus, we see that the troika of hereditary, internal environment, and external environment enters into the expression of each piece of behavior exhibited by the infant. These examples depict the interweaving of developmental stimuli as they work together to stimulate the expression of the various psychologic and biologic aspects of growth.

The interactions between the psychologic and biologic aspects of an individual's development has been explored for many years (Piaget, 1932, 1954, 1963; Gesell and Thompson, 1941). We know that these aspects of the child's behavior correlate positively. If this troika interacts harmoniously or works together ideally, the growth and development of the individual will be maximal. Obviously, since there is a high probability that the countless facets may interact in less than an ideal manner, we can see that the end results rarely reach an optimal state.

The child cannot be physically ill without the illness interfering in some way with his psychologic functioning; similarly, the child cannot be mentally ill without the illness interfering with his biologic functioning. To some extent, his whole life will be changed or modulated by a long-term illness, his subsequent hospitalization, and his recovery. Our role in nursing is to interfere with a series of abnormal environments, both internal and external, in such a way that the greatest degree of normality can be achieved. Subsequent chapters will detail a variety of these interventions as they pertain to particular abnormalities.

What follows then is a discussion of a sample developmental conceptual framework from a holistic point of view. There are many ways of breaking down the kinds of biologic and psychologic behavior seen throughout life. The following seems to me to be a reasonable one for persons working with children in the intense manner necessary when the child will be hospitalized for long periods. But again let me state that each nurse must work with and develop a personal framework into which he/she can categorize new ideas, research, readings, etc., as he/she is exposed to them.

The following categories will be used:

Body Structure and Functional Responses
Habitual Responses
Motor Behavior
Development of Reality
  Sensory responses
  Cognitive processes
  Language behavior
Identification Behavior
Emotional Behavior
Social Behavior

These aspects not only influence each other as they develop but are also influenced by heredity and the internal and external environments. These biologic and psychologic aspects change through the processes of growth, maturation, and learning. These dynamic relationships interact throughout all of life, but it is during the period from birth through adolescence—that time in an individual's life when he develops his *individual reality*—that the most remarkable changes occur. It is this critical period that concerns the nurse working in the child health area. Human growth and development can be visualized as an intricate web of interrelating parts.

Body Structure and Functional Responses

We can define body structure as the conglomerate of the various tissue structures: bone tissue, skin, internal organs, and so forth. Most nurses are well aware of the normally defined body and it is one of the first observations of gross growth and development made when the child is admitted to the hospital. Body function is also of immediate concern to the nursing staff since hospitalization is often precipitated by abnormal functioning of a body system.

Since many schools of nursing are beginning to teach the extended physical assessment skills as well as use a history form which includes a review of biologic systems, this type of protocol fits well into the author's concept of body structure and function. Other protocols are satisfactory, so long as they include all body units.

The inquiry to be made is, of course, what is the nature of the structure, how does it function, and are these consistent with the normal *range*. Range is the key word because there is some normal deviation in all systems because of the uniqueness of each human being. Much of the individual information concerning this area will come from tests, physicians' reports, discussion with the patient and family, and from old records. Who collects the information is quite unimportant so long as it is accurate and detailed. It is most likely within this area that our first information concerning the patient's growth and development will be found. The obvious goal for this area when caring for the child with a long-term illness is interrupting the imbalanced cycle (administration of prescribed drugs, diet, some therapy, and so forth) and bringing the body system back in equilibrium. While it is true that all growth and development are accompanied by varying degrees of stress and system imbalance, the body normally compensates for them until it can readjust itself. For example, when the pre-adolescent growth increase occurs, the child has a tendency to ingest more food and need more sleep. It is a time when the body seems to concentrate on the physical aspect of development. It is only when something goes wrong with the internal programming (eg, giantism) or external environment (eg, malnutrition) that the disequilibrium becomes too much for the body and it becomes overwhelmed. We should remember when we are thinking of the general overall interrelationship of the developmental areas that more often than not we will see the child in the hospital for long-term care during one of these disequilibrium phases (Nelson, 1948; Williams, 1956; Anderson, 1957).

Habitual Responses

The second area—habitual responses—can be rather open-ended or contain only material pertaining to such things as sleeping, eating, elimination, dressing, and other daily care. These areas are biologically straightforward enough, but more often than not they are so interwoven with emotional behavior that they can cause distress not only for the child but also for the nurse. Habit in the functional sense denotes routine sameness. Of course, immediately upon the patient's entering into a new environment, such as the hospital, old habitual responses must be modified. To say that this is stressful to the child is putting it mildly. Of course, how much distress ensues also depends upon the age, general life style of the child, and the nursing staff's tolerance of behavioral variance.

Perhaps the second most important information (sometimes it is the first) we gather about the child's behavior is the manifestation of his habitual responses. For our part we do not concern ourselves immediately in the area of norms but only in the area of what exists. Our first concern is for the child's feelings of security and comfort and this is one area where we can usually close some of the gaps between the home reality and the hospital reality. The child should know that every effort is being made to adapt the *hospital* to his habitual responses. I cannot maximize the importance of having information about and being highly sensitive to habitual behavior during the first few days in the hospital. The extra work will reap benefits beyond your wildest imagination.

What about later on in the hospitalization? There are, of course, suggested norms for all behavior during hospitalization. Our goals for the end of the child's hospitalization will certainly include these norms as we help the child to progress in this area of development. Sometimes these later goals can be carried out in a straightforward, uncomplicated manner. For example: The toddler learning to eat with a spoon or becoming toilet trained while hospitalized (Brazelton, 1962).

Please remember this word of caution! Find out the habitual response goal of the mother before you go too far. After all, the child is going back into his home following hospitalization, and this readjustment is easier without the undue strain of alienation from the family mores. In other words, the nurse must have an awareness of the habitual behavior of the child, his family culture, and his social group in order to set developmental goals for the hospital stay. Of course, with the parents' understanding and backing, it is possible to make some minor deviations in goals. It really becomes a major concern when the child's illness interferes with the goals of the family in this area, such as special diets, unusual elimination needs, and so forth. A great deal of time can then be spent with patient and family bringing back into equilibrium or assimilating these new habits so that they do not interfere with other areas of growth and development or the family's life style.

Motor Behavior

The development of motor behavior for the well child seems to take place somewhat automatically and while hospitalization can indeed distort the pattern, there is some research to reassure us that the child can make up the differences later (Sandler and Torpie, 1968; Shirley, 1933; Chamberlin, 1966). Collecting data concerning the motor development of the child *prior* to his illness is essential. At this time it is important to look for developmental rates. For example, if the child has been developing at a slow rate, we can expect this rate of development to continue after the child is well. Obviously our goals for this child's motor development would be much different from those for a child who had been developing at an average or rapid rate. The setting of these kinds of goals is relatively straightforward; any developmental book will give approximate normal ranges (Bee, 1975; Medinnus and Johnson, 1976; Smart and Smart, 1967).

It is more difficult to set goals when: (1) the child has been ill all of his life and, therefore, not exhibiting his hereditary program of motor developmental patterns; (2) the child's illness will continue to interfere with his natural or hereditary programming of motor development; and (3) the child's illness has caused motor delay, but repair of system function will now allow the re-establishment of genetic control. In these cases goals must be very tentative; one has to play it by ear. It is doubly important to know in detail exactly what the child has been doing, thus permitting some understanding of the level of motor development.

If you can satisfy yourself that you have enough information concerning the child's currently exhibited motor behavior and if you have explored with the parents their expectations and goals for the child (expectations and goals in the motor area are often sex-oriented with ill boys coming off second best), you can then initiate appropriate stimulation (stimulation possibilities are discussed in the chapter on play). Only by trial-and-error and listening and observing the child carefully can you time advances in stimulation toward succeedingly more complex motor behavior. After a number of weeks you may be able to set a realistic goal (Cratty, 1970; McGraw, 1963).

Development of Reality

This next category could be a very inclusive one. All of the subcategories—sensory responses, cognitive processes, and language behavior—are based on the child's experiences with reality, as are some phases of identification, emotional, and social behavior, but to include the latter here would be too cumbersome.

Later on in the chapter we will discuss ways of determining the difference between hospital and outside, or consensus, reality. These differences will cause some consternation to both patient and nurse. Included will be a short discussion of nonconsensus and consensus reality and our commitment and responsibility to both.

Church (1961) speaks of a nonconsensus or individual reality as made up of one's wishes, daydreams, inner thoughts, and of an outer or consensus reality as one which any defined group will hold in common. For example: a four-year-old patient may call the nurse at night to tell a frightening tale of a large bear entering her room. Outer reality or consensus reality would tell us that the child could not have seen a large bear in her hospital room for a number of obvious reasons. It is not within our adult consensus reality. It is also not within the child's consensus reality which they can come to understand if we take the time to explain to them about the difference between the two. It is the *individual* or *nonconsensus reality* that makes us different from each other. I make this point because we often confuse the expression of inner reality with negative things such as lying. The large bear should be brought into the open and talked about. The key to any discussion of the fantasies of inner reality is whether another human could also have seen it. Sometimes we are the only ones who see something and it will not fit into a reality which everyone will acknowledge. We are very understanding and sympathetic of ourselves when we have an inner thought which is so revealing and comprehensible. Of course, it may become another matter when we try to explain our wonderful concept to another individual. This is where it becomes uncomfortable and long conversations with others become necessary. Let us try to think of the large bear within this context and work with the child to grow in the knowledge of his inner or nonconsensus reality and consensus reality. I have often seen little tolerance for the child's inner reality; perhaps it is because we have been negatively reinforced for our own inner realities. Building a rich understanding of inner and consensus reality will help the child grow and understand himself, as well as others. So much for reality or realities, since in the specific they vary from day to day, year to year, and person to person, making our culture chaotic without our elaborate system of symbols: language. It is through language that we attempt to communicate our world (inner reality) to each other and we must be satisfied with something less than perfect interpretations (consensus reality).

To put it simply, the child uses his senses to gather material from his environment and as he gathers data he stores them. His use of the data available to him is, to a great measure, determined by his cognitive process—which develops slowly through the years from rather concrete related interests and manipulation of objects, to abstract thinking in which the child can rely on reason to understand the world around him (Piaget, 1954; Baldwin, 1955; Akutaguwa and Benoir, 1959; Flavell, 1963; Bruner, 1966).

Obviously, the behavior which assists the child in his discovery by organizing and labeling is language (Brown, 1973; Church, 1961). Language helps him manipulate his totally symbolic thoughts into new concepts. In a real sense language is the integrating force that acts between the child and his senses and the external environment. Language is the tool which differentiates humankind from other creatures. Language function can be viewed as being superimposed upon the physical structure of the human being. The senses have specified physical structures to carry out their functions (eg, eyes for seeing), but language must use physical structures whose primary functions are unrelated to it (eg, lungs for breathing).

Language is not a concrete, tangible entity, but only a symbol for something in reality; or, more precisely, some concept in the child's reality. Some kinds of words have meanings which are rather well accepted and very useful in discussion with others, but not nearly so many as one would expect.

Language is, in many respects, a reflection of our internal and external environment and the one area of development most damaged by long periods of institutionalization or hospitalization (Chamberlin, 1966; Sandler

ment of the child's identification with his parents is a difficult one. It takes a great deal of ingenuity plus a real sense of commitment to the necessity of continuing some semblance of the old relationship on the part of parents and the staff. It means reinforcing in the child's mind the existence of an absent parent even when the nurse feels angry that the parent is not visiting as much as might be desirable. It means helping the parent to feel less guilty about the child's illness. It means helping the parents to participate, in a meaningful way, in the recovery of the child. This does not necessarily mean giving physical care, but it certainly means interacting in the areas of language, motor, and reality developments. In other words, it is making sure that the child understands that all the important people in his present and past environment are harmoniously working toward the day he can be discharged. It also means stimulating the child to identify himself as an individual, apart from the things in his environment, and increasing his sense of self-integrity. A disappointing aspect of assisting the child to develop an identification or a concept of self is that we may never see any results and therefore cannot measure our effectiveness.

Emotional Behavior

The development of emotions is closely related to family and general culture, the age of the child, the functioning of the internal environment, general maturation, and the extent to which reality is understood. For example, the four-year-old has many unwarranted fears as a result of his expanding awareness of the environment and his cognitive level (Prugh, 1973; Sutterley and Donnelly, 1973).

We must remember that children's emotions differ from those of the adult in the following ways (Hurlock, 1956):

1. Children's emotions are short-lived.
2. Children's emotions are more intense (ie, to children the sun is either shining brightly or there is a downpour).
3. Children's emotions come as quickly as they go. We can elicit a drastic change in behavior by the introduction of some new toy or idea.
4. Children have more emotional outbursts than adults, who frequently try to hide their emotions.
5. Children's emotional behavior can be a sign of their general feeling of well-being. If a child's reality does not meet his expectation he may develop nervous mannerisms, frequent hysterical outbursts, tension, restlessness, etc.
6. Children's emotions are individual.

It is our task to set up the environment of the hospitalized child in a way that will foster good emotional tone. Examples of environmental ingredients which foster good emotional tone are the following (Lee and Lee, 1958):

1. The child must have a feeling of confidence in himself.
2. The child must have some success in the tasks he attempts.
3. The child must recognize reality.
4. The child must have recognition of his efforts.
5. The child must have status from his peers.
6. The child must be accepted as he is, with respect.
7. The child must have empathetic understanding.
8. The child must have love and affection.

Social Behavior

Social development is often severely curtailed in the hospital situation where the child is somewhat isolated from normal peer situations. When the child is very ill, little socialization goes on except between the adults in the situation and the individual child. Later on, as the child recovers, he will come in contact with other children in the sheltered envrionment of the nursing unit's playroom. When there is intermingling of children of all ages, a reasonable facsimile of normal neighborhood socialization can take place, that is, with a range of ages. This heterogeneous age grouping is more beneficial to the advancement of growth and development than grouping children of the same age (Sandler and Torpie, 1968).

Obviously this socialization should be carefully planned with regard to the child's age and his physical ability. Some children will need more help with socialization than others. A general rule of thumb applies here: the larger the number of children and the younger the age of the child the more the adult must assume responsibility for interpretation of goals and intentions in the setting. The larger the group of children assembled, the greater the number of activities and toys that must be available for use.

ASSESSING GROWTH AND DEVELOPMENT

With the foregoing information in mind we come to the task of growth and development assessment. There are numerous biologic and psychologic charts, lists, and descriptions of the various categories of behavioral response available to the practitioner. I will assume at this time that the reader has formulated a conceptual framework and filled it with growth and developmental information. I should now like to discuss developmental assessment and our responsibility and commitment to it. The role or task of developmental assessment is far more complicated and critical when we are dealing with children with long-term illness. This is true for a number of reasons.

First, since the infant or child may be hospitalized for long periods of time, the nursing team has a 24-hour-a-day influence and responsibility for him. This is in contrast to other professionals who also work with children but for lesser periods of time (for example, the teacher, the physician, the social worker, to name a few). During hospitalization, the child is taken out of his normal environment and placed in a relatively abnormal one.

Second, not only is this new external environment abnormal but the child's internal environment is also abnormal, sometimes through all or most of his stay. With this in mind our first assessment problem is to find out as much as he can about the child's previous pattern of development. The most reliable way of finding out this pattern is through communication with the family or significant others. All information concerning the child's previous responses to stimuli must be carefully considered. If you attempt to assess a child's development without consulting information gleaned from interviews (I emphasize the plural) with the persons involved in caring for the child previous to hospitalization, you are treading on dangerous ground not only for yourself as a professional, but also, and more importantly, for the child.

The second task in assessment is detailed observation of the child's behavior and the results of tests in areas which are not observable. It is important not to eliminate any of the aspects, since the key to adequate assessment is in an understanding of the total child. In this case the whole is often greater than the sum of its parts. Whenever a discussion of the child takes place it is important to find patterns in his growth and development and/or some clues to his unique developmental pattern. This will make his behavior more understandable. When the first two steps in assessment are thoroughly covered, the nursing staff can make its preliminary statement or initial assessment of the child's needs.

There should be some difference between the child's prehospitalized behavior as communicated by the concerned adults and the behavior seen during the first few days of hospitalization. With some children there will be differences throughout hospitalization, particularly for the child whose internal environment is substantially deviating from "average" or "normal." Regression to an earlier stage of average development in one or several areas may be seen. We may also see a general closure or minimalization of response behavior (eg, silence or nonresponsiveness) as a reaction to the added stress of an abnormal external environment, or occasionally the opposite, an increased response behavior to stimuli (eg, open aggression, increased attempts to manipulate the environment). This initial reaction should be expected and anticipated. It should be considered a normal aspect of the child attempting to come to grips with this new, very strange, and stressful reality. In fact, if the parent interviews are complete, some information about the child's normal manner of dealing with stress should be ascertained early in the hospitalization (ie, the first day or so).

With this is mind, the nurse can take some of the deviations from "normal" behavior in stride, without alarm or negative reactions. It will help the child to adjust to the new environment if this temporary initial crisis is taken at face value and the child reassured that support will be freely and nonpunitively given. The nursing staff must have confidence in themselves and understand the child who is weathering this period in order to establish a positive relationship.

The assessment of developmental behavior is something that may go on during the total stay of the child because of the dynamic nature of development. Goals may be adjusted numerous times as the web of the individual child's growth and development unfolds.

I suspect the reader may like to make some comments about the impossibility of this kind of assessment for every child. I am afraid I am rather unsympathetic of this point of view. I am particularly unsympathetic when it comes to children who will be in the nurses' care 24-hours-a-day over a long period of time. Remember, a week is a long time in the life of an infant, toddler, or preschooler.

Obviously, I believe that *great* care should be extended and much time spent with the child before any substantial problem list can be made. This includes team-written and personal-working-nonwritten problem lists. I believe there should be numerous insightful but nonwritten observations or perhaps brief notations made before the formal nursing assessment, since in order to interact and work with the child some kind of temporary assessment must be made. Please keep them just that—temporary and flexible. When you make both kinds of notes on observed behavior, make strong attempts to include facts rather than judgments concerning the child's developmental expressions; they will be more helpful to you. I do not see that the role of the nurse in this situation includes sophisticated developmental testing; that is the role of the psychologist. However, evaluations such as the Denver Developmental screening test, certainly may give valuable insight, particularly if they are carried out with parental input. Our gathered information should result in action on our part and hopefully change on the part of the patient.

For example, let us examine notations concerning a child's eating habits: Johnny ate his yellow carrot first, his bread second, his peaches third, and one-fifth of his meat after the nurse said he could eat his peaches. After we recorded a number of days' facts concerning food ingestion, we could gain some insight into the child's dietary pattern. When a pattern such as this continues, we should become concerned about his protein intake, and perhaps about calcium since no milk is mentioned and vitamins since there is no mention of green vegetables. This concern would be relayed to the nutritionist who would make the adjustment in menu content that seemed necessary. We would also be concerned that food may have been used as a usual bribe in the home. While food is sometiems used as a bribe with the "normal," "healthy" child, it is unfortunate if it is used excessively. It can be extremely harmful to the child who must adjust his food intake around some metabolic error. Of course, the bribe may not be in the food but in the personal attention a fuss in this area reinforces. Unfortunately, our society does have a tendency to connect food and love—or so it seems when we contemplate the statistics on obesity in the United States.

This kind of information is more useful than what we sometimes see written: "Johnny eats well with encouragement." The major team assessments will be constructed from looking at everyone's facts, not everyone's opinions. Hopefully there will be some observed fact in all gross categories of a team's conceptual framework for growth and development.

Here I should make some mention about possible differences between a personal conceptual framework and a team conceptual framework. Ideally, the team conceptual framework will be devised by the consensus of the team. In this way, the members have time to work out any differences between personal word-meanings and/or theoretical concepts. In other words, when they use a category—sensory development, for example—they will know just what will be found in the category. Are they going to include development of the five senses only or are they going to include the five senses plus kinesthetic development and vestibular development?

From the preceding discussion I hope that I have emphasized sufficiently the following points:

1. A conceptual framework for growth and development includes a gross structure which includes all aspects of human development.
2. Each professional nurse should develop her/his own framework with its own detailing material or find a standard one that she/he can live with in harmony.
3. A personal major nursing assessment plan is based upon inferences taken from the various categories of the conceptual framework and is devised from the facts collected.
4. A collection of all team members' observed facts is also one essential facet for a complete nursing assessment and plan of action.
5. Growth and development must be an understanding of both the developmental crises and longitudinal kinds of material.
6. All areas of development have traits unique to the area, but at the same time have traits or characteristics common to all.

THE INTERACTION

In this final portion of the chapter I wish to discuss the matter of the nurse's role as one part of the total environmental influence on the child who experiences either a long-term hospitalization or serial short-term hospitalizations.

When the child becomes hospitalized our influence upon his behavior becomes intensified as opposed to the nurse's role, say, in community-health, school-health, physician's-office or in independent practice. Much of the time during hospitalization the nurse is the center of the child's external environment, or he/she directs other persons who make it up. The nurse also greatly influences the internal environment. While other members of the health team prescribe or plan (eg, through the use of drugs or food, changes in the internal environment), their hoped-for and planned-for changes will not occur unless the drugs and food enter the child's internal environment.

From the above I am sure we can all see the vast areas of influence the nurse has as she/he interacts with the ill child and provides for the ingredients of his environment. I called this portion of the chapter The Interaction for a number of reasons. First, I believe that there must be an interaction between the professional nurse and his/her patient if satisfactory care is to be given. Without the nurse playing a dominant role in caring for and directing the care we cannot hope to achieve an integrated plan of action. Confusion will set in and an added stress will be placed upon the child who is already in stress because of his long-term illness and hospitalization. In order to have an interaction you must have the principal role players within the approximate physical environment. This means relatively low ratios of professional nurses to patients. If you are thinking this is impossible in your situation do not be surprised if the children show signs of the added stress. The little energy the child has will go into an often futile attempt to organize his environment into some semblance of order, a task essential to his understanding of and coping with the situation (Piaget, 1954). It is not the nurse, overworked and self-seen martyr, who bears the brunt of the ensuing stressful confusion but the ill child. Thus the physical and mental nearness of the nurse is a prime positive ingredient in the hospital life of the child.

Second, an interaction brings along with it some essential ingredients for the health and well-being of both nurse and patient. It is the interaction which fosters a feeling of shared control on the part of the nurse and patient. This sharing of control will help the child to maintain his body integrity. Through interacting with a patient we pick up those important clues to his growth and development needs—changes not only general in nature but the daily small changes which also need to be made in his environments (internal and external). Needless to say, the nurse should not be satisfied to have a child leave his/her care no better off than he entered it. After all, he and his family should have been under the influence of a professional child-care worker who should have created an atmosphere or environment for his unique growth and development. A positive interaction will also bring with it a feeling of worthwhileness. Infants and children seem to learn very early a sense of worth, importance, or a positive self-image. On the other hand, they also learn very early the feelings of worthlessness, unimportance, or negative self-image. We cannot overestimate the emphasis the child places upon his understanding of his importance to the external environment. He makes some of his estimate of his self-worth by how much time is spent on his behalf. An ongoing interaction will give the child a feeling of integration and worthwhileness—certainly an undisputed ingredient for becoming well (White, 1959; Smart and Smart, 1967; Mussen, et al, 1974).

The continuing interaction with a limited number of professionals will lend security and stability to the child's environment. There is also another not so recognizable benefit from continuous interaction. Because the interaction takes concerted effort on the part of both participants, some energy from the ill child's storehouse must be used with each new person. Obviously, the highly skilled child-care worker will use many means to determine the least traumatic approach for initial interactions and strive throughout the relationship to manage her role in such a manner that little strain will be placed upon the child (Prugh, 1973).

Because energy must be used by the child when he attempts to interact with each new adult, it is only rational for the staff to limit the number of new persons during any critical period or at any other time when the child is low on energy. It seems to me that staffing must necessarily be of a different routine on nursing units where children with long-term illnesses are cared for than on nursing units whose patients stay for short periods. The least that should be done is assigning the same nurses to the same patients. It not only reduces the stress of making new relationships but also gives the child a feeling of security—a feeling of knowing how this person reacts to his various behaviors (some children must find out how far they can go by behaving negatively with each new interacting adult). No matter how coordinated the staff, there always exists some variations in rule importance and tolerance for minor infractions.

This brings us to another benefit of continuous interaction with a small number of persons: that of consistency. Consistency is, of course, a basic ingredient for reducing the child's anxiety about the new situation. All adults in the situation should be playing the same music, reinforcing the same rules, and building a similar internal and external environment which is based on knowledge of the individual child's needs. Hospital environment definitely should be considered a managed therapeutic environment.

Throughout the preceding discussion, the nurse-child interaction has been nurturing and protecting in nature. Along with the positive interaction between the nurse and the child with long-term illness there should be an awareness expanding phase. The child with the long-term illness will be best assisted in his growth and development if he is helped to understand himself better as a person who is temporarily or permanently different from many other peers in the "real" or nonhospital world. The child should also be expanding in the various areas in his general growth and development.

The nurse-child interaction should have some demonstrable outcomes. There should be a sharing or a feeling of having a reasonable amount of control over one's own behavior and the behavior of others. Each interaction should bring with it new clues to the child's growth and development and a reinforcement on the child's part that his needs are being met by the nursing staff. He should gain feelings of worthwhileness, environmental security, and consistency.

I hope I have given the impression that the planning and interaction with an individual child is a complicated and difficult task, calling forth a great deal of general knowledge of growth and development plus restraint, control, and thought on the part of the professional nurse. I believe that the most difficult part of the job is the self-understanding and self-constraint that this kind of interaction demands of the adult. For these reasons I do not believe we can place nonprofessional personnel in the role of the interactor. It is too much to expect of them and the potential risk to the patient is too high. I also contend that this kind of interaction takes a great deal of planning. Nursing care of children with long-term illnesses, who require repeated long-term hospitalizations, is not a thing that can be turned on for 8 hours a day, five days a week, and then turned off. We must think in terms of quality of care and not quantity care on an ongoing basis.

PITFALLS TO CONSIDER

Interaction pitfalls are numerous, but with care many of them can be avoided or rendered harmless. In the preceding discussion of nursing assessment we talked about the child's initial reaction to the new abnormal environment. One important pitfall is that we become so accustomed to working in the abnormal environment of the hospital with children whose internal environments are abnormal that we lose track of the real world of consensus reality. We may lose our tolerance and understanding of this general reality. We are shocked by normal childhood reactions to illness and family separation, deeming it negatively abnormal. This is one place where our knowledge of the average or normal age behavior of the child we are interacting with assumes importance. We must keep in mind what children in the "real" world are like. I believe it is also a mentally healthy exercise to acknowledge to the child (and sometimes repeatedly to ourselves) that this environment is indeed abnormal. The child needs to know that while he is ill his needs are quite different than when he is well. Obviously, the extent to which this can be understood by the child will depend upon his age. If the child is too young for this kind of interpretation it can take place between the nurse and the parents or guardians.

In other words, the child and his parents should be introduced to hospitalization as if they were visitors from a foreign land. All the staff should be constantly reminded that even seemingly unimportant changes in reality may be very important and confusing to the child. If there is some question in your mind about the differences between hospital reality and outside reality perhaps a series of discussions among yourselves and perhaps some nonmedically oriented persons and, if possible, a developmentalist would sharpen your understanding of the problem.

Because of the first pitfall, that of losing track of consensus reality, there is a tendency to make hospital reality more discrepant than necessary. Hospitals lose insight of the individual's rights. Individual's rights are taken away often for the convenience of hospital "routine" and expediency. Having one's basic rights taken away is a very destructive act regardless of the age of the child. The question becomes: Who is on the child's side, who is protecting the child's rights? It seems obvious that it is the same profession that is also concerned with his total developmental needs—the nursing profession. We are indeed in the best position to bring about a closure between hospital reality and consensus reality since our contact hours are so extensive. How we can bring about this closure is the focus of comprehensive nursing care.

DISCIPLINE VS. INDIVIDUAL RIGHTS: A CASE OF MINE, YOURS, OURS

If you visit a nursing unit which has a number of patients who have been there for some time, you will more often than not find some children who feel and behave as if they had no rights or place to call their own and, on the other end of the continuum, children who seem to be "running" the unit, impinging on everyone's rights. Both of these behaviors are abnormal within the context of consensus reality. The question becomes: How can we clarify communication during our beginning interactions to place behavior less out of context with consensus reality? It is not normal for the child to feel he has no place, and I do not know of any child-health nurse who would not be shocked by the realization that she had communicated this idea. It is important for the child to have a specific place even if it is only his bed and dresser or room. In a real sense the area should be guarded as his haven, a place where he can be alone and where his possessions will not be disturbed without permission. The nurse and all personnel should understand that an invisible wall exists if a real one does not; and when you enter this area, it should be by permission—as if it were the child's home. To some this may sound a bit strange, but one of the first things one encounters in a hospital is a loss of normal courtesy and individual rights. While we cannot readjust some of the abnormalities in the hospital environment there is one important area we can readjust, that of private property.

Is it all that important? I contend that it is, for a number of reasons. First, it carries with it a feeling of control and possession on the part of the child. It increases the feeling of being an intact unit or strengthening the child's self-image, which may be rather confused and distorted by the illness. Second, and more important for the discussion of *yours, mine,* and *ours,* is that if we protect the child's area it is only fair that there may be areas which will belong to the other children and the nurses. The nursing staff also needs an area for their activities apart from the children —preferably a quiet place to plan and organize. It is only fair for everyone to have a protected area which is theirs. I believe the key to establishing a cooperative atmosphere is fairness. I do not think we need to go into what is fair and what is not fair, because it seems to change with the situation. This brings us to the ours portion of the nursing unit physical plant. The nursing staff will find that most of the nursing unit will be composed of ours space; space which may be used all the time by both nurse and patient. This space, with its rules, will have to be negotiated individually with each child. It is space in which there is some control by both parties. The rules of the space will be different from the mine space and yours space. In fact, the rules will obviously differ slightly depending upon the patient census, amount of disability, and general life style of the individual child.

Some of you will stop here and ask how the rules can be one thing for one child and another for the next. If so, you have forgotten we are not dealing with mass care. We are developing an environment to fit growth and developmental needs of individuals. The child and his parents will understand this and be reassured. Those of us who have worked with children know how very early they can understand that people are different from one another. I have seen it in children as young as two and three. They also can understand that if the adults in the situation carefully attend the needs of the child as an individual, when he has special needs they will also be attended to—for that is only fair. This, of course, is based upon communication; we must let the child know what is going on and our reasons for our actions. With the very young child we often have to articulate and interpret not only our actions but also the actions of his peers and sometimes his own actions. I hope I have given you the impression that there is a lot going on at one time because there should be and there will be. The question is whether we are going to manage the nursing unit environment or whether we are going to allow confusion and chaos to manage it, for someone or something must be the leader. In other words, we not only use ourselves through the interaction as therapy and as a stimulus for the growth and development of the children in our care, but we also use the nursing unit space to stimulate and promote understanding and growth. And I contend that the most growth-promoting areas will be those negotiable through the daily give-and-take of ours spaces.

Another common pitfall of the interaction are the elements of rigidity, routine, and rest. These three R's most often interfere with the mutual understanding of the nurse and patient. This is not to say there should be no structure because that does not work either. But the rules should be few in number. A good rule of thumb is that all rules should pertain to the health and safety of the child and that a child can be held responsible for remembering as many rules as he has had birthdays. If you now go over the rules you expect your patients to follow, you may find the source of much confusion and irritation. The second R, routine, is another hangup or pitfall most nursing units indulge themselves in. I am not questioning the fact that there are certain things that must be done during the day and that sometimes they must be done at a certain time. Many kinds of routines about the "what" and the "when" of nursing care cannot be changed, but we can be creative with the "how" and "who." It is in the areas of "how" and "who" that we can use acts which are routines as tools for the growth and development of the child. Rest, the third R, is a most important ingredient for healing the body and it needs to be encouraged. But not all children need the same amount at the same time. Some of them must fall asleep to rest while others rest when participating in quiet activities. An opportunity for individualization of the rest period is best accepted by the child. Again, while the routine activity is present each day, the expression of the activity is the choice of the child or the outcome is mediated by the adult if the child in unable to make a choice which leads to the goal.

Another interaction pitfall related to this area is how much interaction we can expect on the part of the ill child. We have said that the child's initial reaction to the abnormal environment may take many negative forms until he comes to understand and see that being in the hospital will make him feel better or fulfill some of his goals. For the very ill child the interaction takes place on a nonverbal plane. Even if the child seems not to be responding, or may be responding very subtly, you may still be building a positive relationship. As an aside, please remember that even normal healthy children do not play the same role when making new relationships. They normally differ in their approach to adults and our approach to them must necessarily be different. (Parent interviews will give many clues.) The standing rule should be that the professional nurse changes his/her approach to match the one that seems most comfortable to the child, not vice versa. Actually, if one tries to be flexible and uses, or at least tries to use, some of the current techniques of child management, the hospitalization of the child may be advantageous in many areas of growth and development.

The first question posed in this chapter was: Can knowledge of normal human growth and development be used as a basis for nursing assessment? I hope the content of the chapter has led you to believe that when we plan and assess the areas of needed nursing intervention we do so against our background of human growth and development. An assessment of individual growth and development needs is the articulation of needed nursing intervention.

BIBLIOGRAPHY

Akutaguwa D, Benoit EP: The effect of age and relative brightness on associative learning in children. Child Dev 30:229–38, 1958

Aldrich C, Anderson C, Aldrich MM: Babies Are Human Beings. New York, Macmillan, 1954

Allport GW: Pattern and Growth in Personality. New York, Holt Rinehart and Winston, 1961

Anderson J: Dynamics of development: system in process. In Harris D (ed): The Concept of Development. Minneapolis, University of Minnesota Press, 1957

Baldwin A: Behavior and Development in Childhood. New York, Dryden, 1955

Baruch DW: New Ways in Discipline. New York, McGraw-Hill, 1949

Beasley J: Slow to Talk. New York, Bureau of Publications, Teachers College, Columbia University, 1956

Bee H: The Developing Child. New York, Harper and Row, 1975

Bem SL: Fluffy Women and Chesty Men. Psychology Today, 5:10, Sept, 1975

Berelson B, Steiner GA: Human Behavior: An Inventory of Scientific Findings. New York, Harcourt, Brace & World, 1964

Bowlby J: Child Care and the Growth of Love, 2nd ed. Baltimore, Pelican, 1959

Brazelton BT: A child-oriented approach to toilet training. Pediatrics 29:121–28, 1962

Breckenridge M, Murphy M (eds): Rand, Sweeney, and Vincent's Growth and Development of the Young Child. Philadelphia, Saunders, 1958

———, Vincent EL: Child Development, Physical and Psychological Growth Through Adolescence, 5th ed. Philadelphia, Saunders, 1966

Breznitz S, Kugelmass S: Intentionality in moral judgment: developmental stages. Child Dev 38:469–79, 1967

Brown R: A First Language: The Early Stages. Cambridge, Mass., Harvard University Press, 1973

Bruner JS et al: Studies in Cognitive Growth. New York, Wiley, 1966

Burnshaw S: The body makes the mind: excerpt from the seamless web. The American Scholar, 38:25, 1968

Call JD: Lap and finger play in infancy, implications for ego development. Int J Psychoanal 49:375–78, 1968

Carmichael L: Manual of Child Psychology, 2nd ed. New York, Wiley, 1966

Chamberlin RW: Approaches to child rearing: their effects on child behavior. An analysis of reported surveys. Clin Pediatr 5:688–98, 1966

Christensen CM: Relationship between pupil achievement, pupil affect—need, teacher warmth, and teacher permissiveness. J Educ Psychol, 51:169–74, 1960

Church J: Language and the Discovery of Reality: The Development of Psychology Cognition. New York, Random House, 1961

Cratty B: Perceptual and Motor Development in Infants and Children. New York, Macmillan, 1970

Denenberg VH, Myers RD: Learning and hormone activity: I. Effects of thyroid levels upon the acquisition and extinction of an operant response. J Comp Physiol Psychol 51:213–19, 1958

Dennis W: Piaget's questions applied to a child of known environment. J Genet Psychol 60:307–20, 1942

Dollard J, Miller NM: Personality and Psychotherapy. New York, McGraw-Hill, 1950

Elkind D: Egocentrism in adolescence. Child Dev, 38:1025–34, 1967
Epstein R: Effects of commitment to social isolation on children's imitative behavior. J Pers Soc Psychol 9:90–95, 1968
Erikson EH: Childhood and Society, 2nd ed. New York, Norton, 1963
Gardner DB: Development in Early Childhood, 2nd ed. New York, Harper and Row, 1973
Gesell A, Thompson H: Twins T and C from infancy to adolescence. Genet Psychol Monogr 24:3, 1941
Greenson RR: Dis-identifying from mother: its special importance for the boy. Int J Psychoanal, 49:370–74, 1968
Harsh CM, Schrickel HG: Personality Development and Assessment. New York, Ronald, 1950
Hatrup W: Social behavior of children. Rev Educat Res 35:22, 1965
Hegethorn B: An elementary developmental stage and its significance for the etiology of psychoses. Acta Psychiatr Scand (Suppl) 203:189, 1968
Hurlock EB: Child Development, 3rd ed. New York, McGraw-Hill, 1956
Hymes JL Jr: Behavior and Misbehavior—A Teacher's Guide to Action. Englewood Cliffs, NJ, Prentice-Hall, 1955
Josselyn I: Psychosocial Development of Children. New York, Family Service Association of America, 1948
Kirkendall LA, Rubin I: Sexuality and the life cycle: a broad concept of sexuality. Siecus, July 1974
Krogman WM: The concept of maturity from a morphological viewpoint. Child Dev 21:25, 1950
Landreth C: The Psychology of Early Childhood. New York, Knopf, 1958
Lawrence FK: Individual Development. New York, Doubleday, 1955
Lee JM, Lee DM: The Child and His Development. New York, Appleton, 1958
Lewis MM: How Children Learn to Speak. London, Harran, 1957
Lidz T: The Person—His Development Throughout the Life Cycle. New York, Basic Books, 1968
Martin WE, Stendler CB: Child Behavior and Development. New York, Harcourt, Brace & World, 1959
McGraw MD: The Neuromuscular Maturation of the Human Infant. New York, Hafner, 1963
Mead M, MacGregor F: Growth and Culture. New York, Putnam, 1951
Medinnus GR: Child and Adolescent Psychology, 2nd ed. New York, Wiley, 1976
Missildine WH (ed): Feelings and their medical significance—the parent in the parent-child relationship. Columbus, Ohio, Ross Laboratories, 9:1, February, 1967
Murphy L: Personality in Young Children. New York, Basic Books, 1956
Mussen PH, Conger JJ, Kagan J: Child Development and Personality, 4th ed. New York, Harper and Row, 1974
Neilen P: Shirley's babies after fifteen years: a personality study. J Genet Psychol 73:175, 1948
Nelson WE. In Stuart H, Stevenson S (eds): Textbook of Pediatrics, 6th ed. Philadelphia, Saunders, 1957, pp 10–66
Oakes ME: Children's Explanations of Natural Phenomena. New York, Teachers College, Columbia University, 1946
Otto HA: New light on the human potential. Saturday Review 52:14, 1969
Patter MC, Levy EJ: Spatial enumeration without counting. Child Dev 39:265, 1968
Peiper A: Cerebral Function in Infancy and Childhood. New York, Plenum, 1964

Piaget J: Construction of Reality in the Child. New York, Basic Books, 1954
———: Language and Thought of the Child. New York, Harcourt, Brace & World, 1932
———: The Origins of Intelligence in Children, Cook M (trans). New York, Norton, 1963
Prugh DG: Emotional aspects of the hospitalization of children. Child & Family 12:19, 1973
Radin N, Kamil CK: The child-rearing attitudes of disadvantaged negro mothers and some educational implications. J Negro Educat 34:38, 1965
Rebble MA: The Personality of the Young Child. New York, Columbia University, 1955
Reichard S, Schneider M, Rappaport D: The development of concept formation in children. Am J Orthopsychiatry 14:156, 1944
Sandler L, Torpie B: Improvement of residential care of infants and children from birth to age 3. Arch Environ Health 17:80, 1968
Segal J, Luce GG: Now I lay me down to sleep. McCall's 88, October 1968
Shirley M: The First Two Years: A Study of Twenty-five Babies—Personality Manifestations, vol III, Institute of Child Welfare Monograph, University of Minnesota Press, 1933
Sigel IE: The need for conceptualization in research on child development. Child Dev 27:241, 1956
Smart M, Smart R: Children Development and Relationships. London, MacMillan, 1967
Sonis M: Implications for the child guidance clinic of current trends in mental health planning. Amer J Orthopsychiatry 38:515, 1968
Speil O: Discipline Without Punishment: An Account of a School in Action, Fitzgerald E (trans). London, Faber and Faber, 1962
Sutterley DC, Donnelly GF: Perspectives in Human Development: Nursing Throughout the Life Cycle. Philadelphia, Lippincott, 1973
Walters CE: Comparative development of negro and white infants. J Genet Psychol 110:251, 1967
Watson EH, Lowrey GH: Growth and Development of Children, 5th ed. Chicago, Year Book, 1967
White RW: Motivation reconsidered: the concept of competence. Psychol Rev 66:297, 1959
Williams R: Biochemical Individuality. New York, Wiley, 1956
Witmer R, Kotinsky R (eds): Personality in the Making, Fact Finding Report of Midcentury White House Conference on Children and Youth. New York, Harper and Row, 1953
Zigler E, Butterfield EC: Motivational aspects of changes in I.Q. test performance of culturally deprived nursery school children. Child Dev 39:1, 1969
Zubeck JP, Salberg PA: Human Development. New York, McGraw-Hill, 1954

DONNA JUENKER

2
Play as a Tool of the Nurse

Oh quench not the child's hope,
Oh do not repress one impulse of enthusiasm
FRANK LLOYD WRIGHT

A child at play is a source of delight. His evident joy in his discoveries and the intensity of his self-absorption underscore the importance of what play means to him. It is serious business—not a luxury. It is physical and it is fantasy. It can tell a child who he is or it can be a stage on which he acts out the role of the person he would like to be. Pickard (1965) significantly concludes that "as they play, the children are the ceaseless agents of their learning, about both the outer and the inner world". Certainly then, opportunities for play should abound for all children—those who are ill as well as those who are healthy.

In this chapter I will elaborate on the subject of play from several points of view with particular attention focused on children with long-term illnesses. After describing the meaning and value of play, I will explore the age factors that influence play behavior. An explanation of the nurse's role in establishing an environment that is conducive to play will be included along with a description of an assessment tool for identifying play needs. One section will include a delineation of the special play problems experienced by immobilized children. The chapter will conclude with the examination of the nurse-parent interaction in regard to play. Hopefully, the content will excite the reader to an enthusiastic response toward the recreational and therapeutic play needs of young patients.

MEANING AND VALUE OF PLAY

Play is a subject open to much speculation. The existance of play has never been disputed. Systematic investigations of why and how man plays, however, are products of relatively recent times. Do people play for gain or gamble? Do they play with gusto or grin? Philosophers, psychologists, and even theologians have provided a rich collection of definitions and rationales for play (Groos, 1901; Huizinga, 1950; Piaget, 1962; Rahner, 1967). Any description of play must point to origins in childhood since each individual's philosophy about play and his personal style of play result from a composite of experiences that begin in infancy.

Adults may consider play in a variety of ways. Some may view it as instinctive behavior pursued for its own sake. Some see it simply as a leisure-time activity. For others, it is a means of emotional escape—a catharsis for pent-up feelings. To the child, play is much more. It is a medium through which he views himself and his surroundings. Play is a stable enough concept to pervade all of childhood and yet dynamic enough to accommodate the child's changing needs as he grows to maturity.

How does play serve the child's needs? Groos (1901), who was one of the earliest to systematize the study of play, draws attention to instinct as the motivating factor in play. For example, it develops important elements of skill such as running and jumping. These initial impulses are then transferred to intellectual behaviors useful in adult living. In other words, play develops coordination and physical efficiency necessary for adult pursuits.

While not wholly supported, Schiller's (1875) surplus-energy theory of play does have some credibility. It is an obvious fact known to anyone who observes children that young people have boundless energy. They seem to have more muscular energy than they need. Consequently, the activity of play becomes a release. Spencer (1873) gave a physiologic rationale for the need to release energy based on the discharge potential of living nerve cells. If a physiologic need is forcing its expression, it is difficult if not impossible for the child to withhold his response. He needs outlets for these strong drives. Play experiences permit energy release in a manner acceptable to the child and to those around him.

There are psychologic considerations in play as well. Play is satisfying for its own sake. Pleasure, a dominant feature, is derived from the play stimulus itself as well as from the pleasant feelings it arouses. It is Groos' contention that this psychologic criterion is part of the essence of play.

The sociologic aspect of play should also be noted. As the child grows from infancy through childhood, his social radius widens beyond the family to include peers. This opens up a richly exciting world of play. Much of it focuses on social imitation. Play also affords good practice in communication and in the art of governing a group. It is an avenue through which social laws can be tested. Groos calls this the "cheering and humanizing effect of play."

In a more recent analysis of childhood play, Erikson (1963) describes it as an attempt to synchronize the bodily and social processes into a concept of self and as such defines it as necessary for the development of the ego. In this sense, childhood play becomes a preparation for mature behavior. Piaget

(1969) stresses its value when he comments that it is a process of assimilating reality to the self. In effect, play becomes the child and the child becomes the play. To view a child without considering his play is not to see the child at all.

These benefits, while described only in general terms thus far, give testimony to the value of play. The extent to which these outcomes can be realized depends upon two basic components of play. It must be free and it must be fun. In keeping with its nature, play is a voluntary activity—one without coercions. The child must be free to direct his play within the context of his own style, that is, free to react to his own spontaneity. A child who is made to play is not really playing. He is simply performing a task assigned by an adult.

The child should have a good time during play. The pleasure should come from the activity itself and not solely from the practical consequence the play activity may have. As a matter of fact, play often lacks a tangible outcome. It is the process of play that is important—the body movement, the fantasy, the spirit, the risk, and the excitement of mastery.

The freedom and pleasure of childhood play may seem to give it an exclusiveness requiring no adult participation. On the contrary, the child's play will not be free and pleasurable if the adult absents himself from the play world. There are several important things that the adult must do. In the first place, he must encourage what is good and useful about play. In this sense, he motivates play. He should respond with interest to the child's discoveries but must not overpower with discoveries of his own. The adult provides the materials for play, controlling elements of high risk or probable danger while at the same time opening up opportunities for experimentation. Adults must allow children to explore in a variety of settings, using as many modes of expression as age and imagination permit.

Adults vary widely in their approach to children's play. Some are obviously ill at ease with children. Some make it a practice to join in and play with the child. Others pride themselves by playing for the child. Some are content to give the child "something" to play with, and then there are those who dismiss "child's play" as a matter deserving little attention. There is danger in all of these approaches. The person who is ill at ease makes a sensitive child ill at ease, too. These individuals may have experienced some degree of play deprivation in their own youth and consequently lack important recollections that would permit them an entrée into the child's world of play. The child, if he is old enough to perceive the problem, is inadvertently placed in a position of trying to relieve the stress of the uncomfortable adult. Those who play with the child all the time fail to note that this creates an unnatural play environment. Children customarily play alone or with peers. Adult-child interaction is based upon a different set of "ground rules." Those who play for the child—the "let-me-show-you"–type—lack the capacity or

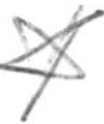

the insight to permit the child the joy of making his own discoveries. Perhaps this individual is too concerned about the outcome or product of the play experience and consequently makes the child play on adult terms. In this way, he insures that the child does not "color outside the lines" or make a lopsided treasure chest. Play suggestions, when offered, should be extensions of the child's own intent. Adults should not become impatient if the child's limited ideas do not correspond with the projected adult view based on many more years of experience. Those who do not enter the child's world at all stand to lose the most. They miss a youthful excitement and vitality that can awaken their own enthusiasm for living and learning.

Perhaps it is unfortunate that analysis of children's play has become the work of adults. Since adults are removed from the personal realities of childhood, some dimensions of play are lost simply by virtue of an experiential gap. Although, as nurses, we should recognize this fact, we ought not to be discouraged by it. It simply means that there is always something left to "discover" about children and how they play. Therein lies a key to success in working with children—that is, a willingness to be open to the various ways children express themselves and manifest their needs. By maximizing the play experiences of a child, nurses can expand the dimensions not only of the child's world but also their own.

Those of us caring for sick children are challenged to seek appropriate ways to help them enjoy the satisfactions of play in whatever circumstances they find themselves. To accomplish this, it would be helpful to explore some of the relationships between play and long-term illness.

Diagnosis and treatment of illness may require frequent and sometimes prolonged periods of hospitalization. As a result, a change in the life style of the child and his family may be observed. The extent of the change depends upon the type of illness and the capacity of the child and parents to cope with the existing stress and make realistic plans for the future. Nevertheless, if we accept the premise that growth and development is an ongoing process marked by maturational achievements of special significance at certain ages, it quickly becomes evident that the child and family may pass through some of these developmental steps during the course of an illness. Naturally, developmental progress may be modified. For example, the toddler who is confined because of a dislocated hip may not be able to practice his newly acquired skill of walking; the eight-year-old boy under treatment for rheumatic fever may be unable to enjoy the school activities with his friends; the teenage girl immobilized for treatment of scoliosis misses some of the important peer group activities characteristic for her age. By facilitating play experiences for these children, some of these deficits can be minimized. The toddler can experience some mobility through "action stories" and rides in a wagon. The eight-year-old can continue to keep up with his schoolmates through blackboard games and word games which will maintain his interest in printing and spelling. The teenager can be encouraged to keep in touch with her friends by letter exchanges and telephone calls. She can give expression to her feelings by writing to "Dear Diary" or she can "paint her feelings" on canvas to hang in her room. There are many avenues through which play can accommodate developmental needs.

Long-term illness is marked by repeated periods of dependency. The child must rely on persons outside the family circle for the treatment of his illness. This often happens at a time in his developmental continuum when he is struggling to achieve or maintain his own autonomy. He may have to relate to many members of the health team because of the complexity of his illness. Yet his capacity to absorb new persons into his reality may be inadequate. The child, under these circumstances, hardly welcomes the "helpers"—especially if they perform intrusive acts that are painful or in other ways appear to invade the integrity of the body. Added to his stress is the fact that these people occupy positions of power and exercise great control over his activities. Through play, the child can "act out" fearful experiences and reduce the level of anxiety. He can recreate past events and imaginatively project future happenings which will help him to more fully understand himself and others.

Elements of freedom are curtailed during periods of prolonged illness. Freedom of mobility is often affected, favorite foods may be restricted, and the type and quantity of social interaction is limited. The frustration of these circumstances is heightened by the anticipation of repeated episodes of illness and by prospects of a long period of treatment. Play behavior is also limited to a certain extent. However, because play is basically confined only by the limits of imagination, there remains a wide range of options. With so many other limits being imposed, play can well serve as a means of providing opportunities for self-chosen activities.

Discouragement is associated with long-term illness. Children become discouraged by the slow progress of their illness and the sameness of each day. Nurses, too, can become discouraged when the intensity of their care is not matched by a similarly dramatic improvement in their young patient's condition. Both the child and nurse can benefit in this instance from involvement in play activities. It helps the child to meet the demands of each day and gives him the satisfaction of achieving short-term goals. By watching the child in play and enjoying his accomplishments the nurse can see small gains and become more satisfied that some progress is being made.

In general, it could be said that many children with long-term illnesses will have to reorient themselves to a different set of lifetime goals. They will have to learn how to do things: adapt themselves to the environment and, when feasible, effectively change the environment to suit their own special needs. This adaptive capacity does not develop intuitively. It is learned over time and through a variety of satisfying experiences. Acceptance of long-term illness and adjustment to its many physical and psychologic demands will therefore require many talents on the part of the child and his family. It is in this regard that I believe that play can offer a child abundant support. I believe that one of the most significant outcomes of play is the creative behavior that such activity encourages.

Torrance (1965) suggests that creative children are stimulated by challenging problems. These children tend to probe for answers to difficult questions. Their accomplishments are self-initiated and reflect a wholehearted commitment to a task. They do not seem to be overly intimidated by their age-mates or adults who occupy positions of authority. In fact, even in relatively tense situations, they can maintain a sense of humor (Torrance, 1961). They seem better able to resist the conformity often demanded by pervading social and cultural conditions. The creative child is inclined to be independent and to aspire to long-range goals.

These qualities would well serve the needs of a child with a long-term illness. Certainly, a handicapped child would benefit by a development of a certain inner resourcefulness, a capacity for creativity that would make his satisfactions emerge from within himself. Freely selected play activities, pursued in a direction that the child elects, will give him a good feeling about himself, confidence in his ability to perform or achieve, and, most importantly, he will feel capable of controlling and modifying his environment. Therefore, given the stimulus of appropriate play, the child might better achieve his potential and more fully enjoy the process of accomplishing such an achievement.

THE INFANT

Many long-term illnesses have their origins at birth or in early infancy. Because of the nature of medical management, the infant often requires complicated treatments and may have to undergo periods of hospitalization. Because of significant stages in development occurring early in life, hospitalization can seriously affect the behavior of the infant.

While it is true that infants lack language skills and, therefore, symbolic function, it is evident that much learning takes place during the early months of life. Piaget and Inhelder (1969) emphasize that during the first 18 months the child constructs all of the cognitive substructures that are necessary for future perception and intellectual development.

This learning takes place at a sensorimotor level of function. These sensorimotor experiences emerge in the framework of infant play. A sensorimotor experience exists in relation to the environment—that is, it is aroused by persons and things that enter the child's reality as stimuli. In the process of reacting to stimuli, infants develop habits of play. Although initially based on reflexive behavior, these habits become very meaningful. Usually the habits are intimately related to satisfaction of basic needs such as the need for food, sleep, excretion, and care of the body. Once these habits are formed, the infant resists disruptive changes. Illness and hospitalization will certainly alter both the internal and external environment of the infant and may upset the infant's lifestyle. The infant who hides his face in a special blanket with a smooth binding as part of a satisfying sleeping pattern may have difficulty sleeping if he cannot repeat this behavior in the new setting.

An interruption in an expected sequence of events results in an expenditure of energy. For example, energy is used in longer periods of wakefulness in an attempt to locate anticipated events. It may take the form of fretful crying that indicates general uneasiness about the unexpected situation or, in some cases, energy output becomes an angry scream testifying to the infant's awareness of the magnitude of the change in his environment. The ill child, whose illness is accompanied by physiologic stress, needs to focus his body's reserve on trying to reestablish homeostasis. Therefore, anything that the nurse can introduce in the care plan that will relieve psychologic stress could have a real impact on the child's recovery. The nurse has three primary sets of clues readily available to guide the selection of stimuli for a particular infant: (1) history of meaningful play activities from the parents, (2) current and anticipated development achievements of the infant, and (3) type of illness and consequent limitations.

Knowledge of the kind of play activities experienced by an infant and his response to those stimuli helps the nurse provide play rituals that may help to stabilize his environment. (Further comment on the use of a play profile follows in another section of this chapter.) Very likely, the kind of play that an infant engages in reflects his abilities at a given point in time. If he is able to sit up and reach for and transfer objects, he is a more independent "player" than the infant who is not yet able to support himself in an upright position. If the infant's activities are limited because of the stress of lower-extremity immobilization, for example, his ordinary play needs will be frustrated and development achievements may be delayed. By redesigning play experiences, through provision for additional upper-extremity activity and upright positioning when possible, much of the loss can be compensated and energy redirected in a beneficial way.

What are some of the special play problems experienced by infants? Hospitalized infants often miss the consistent stimulation of an expressive face of another—a purposeful "locking of eyes." This very personal experience provides the infant with an explicit contact with reality. Infants can receive very good physical care that includes holding and feeding and still miss this stimulation. This may happen because the nurse shares her attention with many infants and also because she underestimates the importance of this kind of interaction. Eye-to-eye contact most often comes about

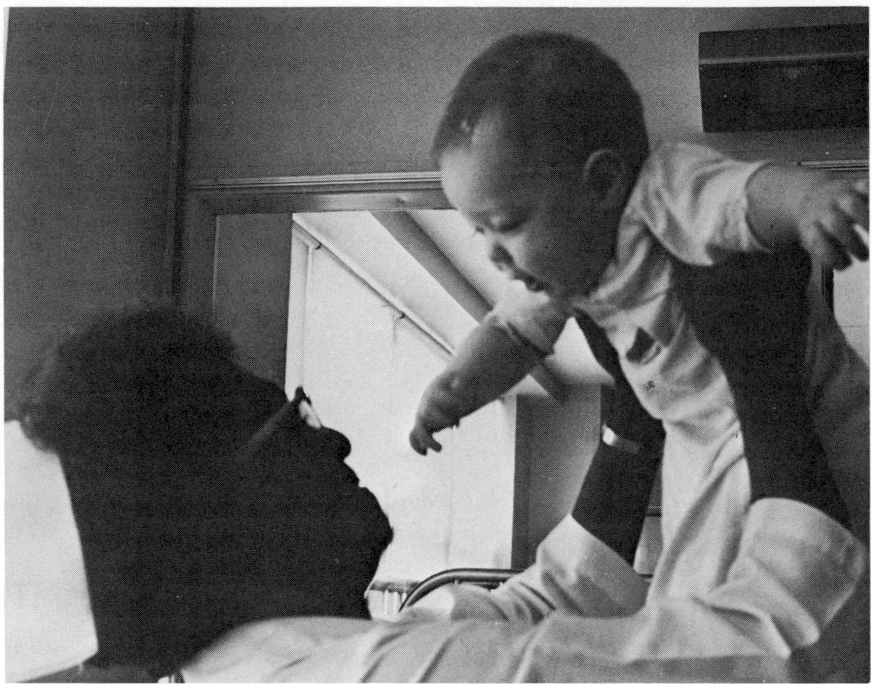

FIG. 1. This nurse and infant are having fun with a special kind of play—an infant "game."

through games. Games are simply styles of interaction that are usually the creation of mother and infant. Generally the game involves some manipulation of a part of the body, an accompanying verbal symbol, and an expressive face that responds to the mutual enjoyment felt by the adult and the infant (Fig. 1).

One classic example is the game of peek-a-boo. Maurer (1967) describes the significance of the game and connects specific learnings derived from it with later ego development. In fact, she states that peek-a-boo contributes to the development of self-confidence and an early sense of identity, and even helps to allay anxiety. "The game of peek-a-boo is a replay in safe circumstances of the frightening feeling of nonbeing followed by the joyous affirmation of aliveness in the recognition accorded the child by the intimacy of eye to eyeness" (Maurer, 1967, p 119). It is such a universal behavior that even in situations in which parents do not encourage the game, the child "invents" it himself. Other examples of early ego-supporting play include lap and finger play.

As previously mentioned, vocalization supports these games. Personally directed and intimate "conversations" with the infant are important, not only because the sound of the human voice can be soothing but also because it encourages the infant's own vocal response. In turn, the infant's own utterances are a rich source of amusement for him (Fig. 2).

How does one communicate with the very young infant? One of the best techniques the adult can use is to imitate the infant's actions and sounds —when he sighs or gurgles, you do the same. When he smacks his lips, you smack your lips. Since these sounds and actions are already in the behavioral repertoire of the infant, it is easy for him to imitate in response to your noises and gestures. Observations of parents interacting with their young infants reveal that the pitch of the adult voice increases and words are exaggerated in length and spoken more slowly. It seems to be a natural tendency and obviously appreciated by the infant, who, of course, is the only one for whom it matters. One should not feel silly or self-conscious "talking" to infants in this way. It is an important way to maintain meaningful contact with the infant.

When an infant is acutely ill, it must be remembered that his capacity to respond to new stimuli is limited. In contrast, familiar and loved items are cherished to an even greater extent than usual. The infant's "defenses" are down and he resorts to passive absorption of familiar sounds, feels, and

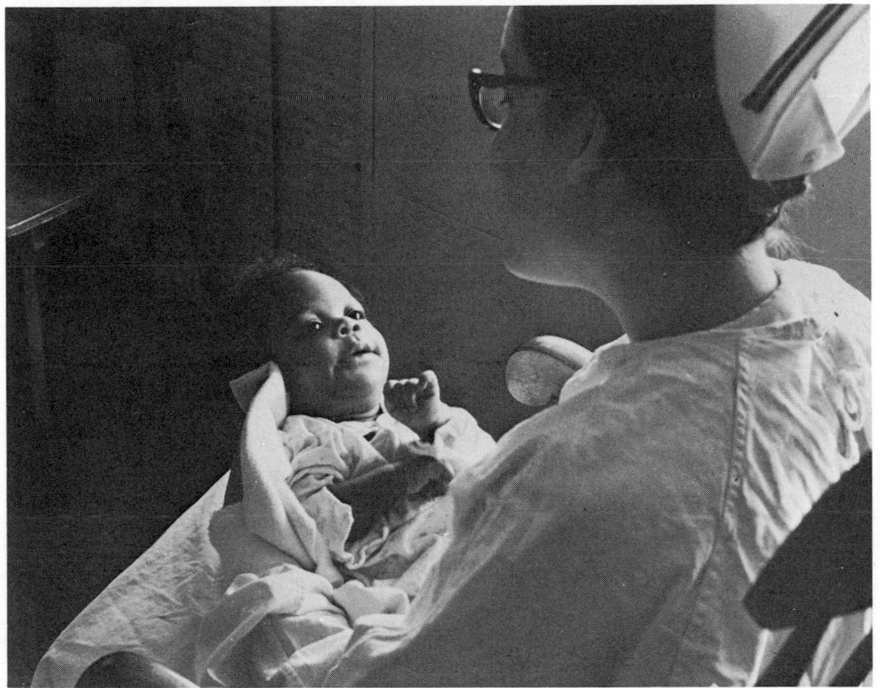

FIG. 2. This nurse and baby are enjoying an intimate "conversation."

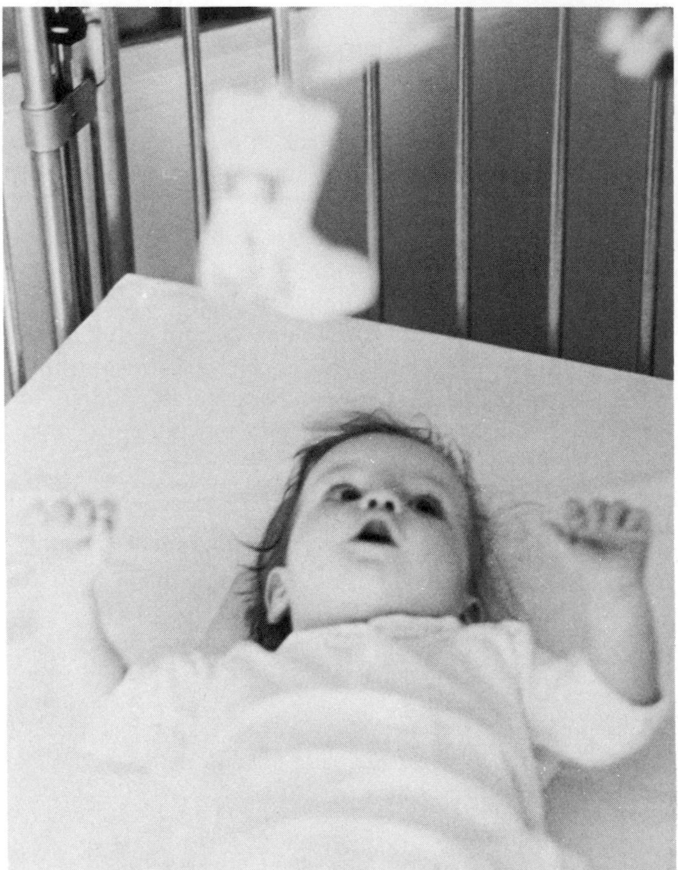

FIG. 3. This four-month-old infant is excited by the bright mobile. Her animated expression and body movements indicate responsiveness to her environment.

smells to help him tolerate the frustrations of the situation at hand. The use of transitional objects such as favorite blankets, special toys, and familiar feeding utensils becomes very important in his adjusting to the stress of illness.

When the infant becomes more aware of his external environment he can respond to new things with interest and enthusiasm. The games of "rock-a-bye baby," "pat-a-cake" and "this little pig" are familiar to all. The words themselves are not important but rather that they mark progress toward the climax of the game—the sensation of being dropped and caught, being poked in the stomach or tickled under the chin. The delighted laughter that accompanies these games should be enough to encourage their repetition. The color, shape, sound, feel, and movement of toys within the infant's field of vision and hand (and foot) space are internally satisfying. You have no doubt watched infants respond with evident delight as a bright mobile moved above their heads (Fig. 3). Of course, you cannot separate the "things" from the people who provide them—the toys offered are often loving extensions of the person and help the infant to develop trust in both people and things. Appropriate stimuli during convalescence can increase the infant's learning, rather than merely hold fast to the status quo. An infant who is ill for weeks or months will need assistance in achieving new tasks. However, the infant must be relatively tension-free before he can enjoy new sensorimotor and social activities.

The timing of play is a significant factor. An infant who is very ill or who has an overpowering physiologic need such as hunger must direct all his energy toward reducing this discomfort. He has little, if any, energy left for exploring his world. To play he must be capable of giving his individual attention to the matter at hand and to exercising some control over the part of the body involved in the play. When the infant is best able to play is a decision that the nurse makes in relation to the infant's overall needs. Call (1966) notes that most games in infancy are played after the feeding, when many infants have a wakeful period. At this time physiologic tension is at a minimum and the infant is especially alert to the external world. Play time for the older infant, which is much broader in scope, should keep pace with expanding abilities, increasing attention span, and widening social radius.

Bath time, whatever time of the day it might be, offers great potential for enjoyable play both for the infant and the nurse. It brings them into close personal contact. Water is a universally enjoyed play material. Splashing and kicking, unencumbered by restricting clothing, are delightful activities for the active youngster. Even for those less inclined to vigorous activity, the feel of warm water over the body creates a pleasant, relaxing sensation. The infant's own participation in the bath can be encouraged by the inclusion of bath toys such as small, brightly colored sponges. A tub bath is the best means for this kind of enjoyable play and should be much more widely used than is currently the custom. However, if the illness contraindicates a tub wash, some provision for water play can generally be provided even if it only consists of splashing the hands in the water basin.

The infant, especially the very young one, is handicapped in the sense that he is dependent on others for mobility. If he is left in the supine position, the ceiling and the sides of his crib become his world. Turning the infant to the prone position or putting him in an infant seat or playpen does much to alter a dull and narrow visual field and expand his awareness of surroundings.

While a finger has been pointed at the tendency toward understimulation, a word must be said about overstimulating experiences for the infant.

One sometimes forgets about the magnitude of stimulation in a hospital environment. There is considerable noise, both continuous and intermittent. How aware are we of the effects of the incubator motor or the sound of the mist tent? How disruptive is the noise of the page system, the voices of the doctors as they make rounds, or the clatter of dietary equipment? There are visual stimuli as well—bright lights on 24 hours a day, light reflected from metal equipment, distorted images viewed through glass partitions, and a disturbing eeriness in dim hours of twilight. Then, of course, there is the stimulus of people: people looking, people handling, people feeling, wrapping and wiping; people intruding on the privacy of the infant's world. We must tread more carefully to preserve the infant's right to integrate his experiences at his own rate. We must be persistent in our attempts to reduce overabundant and disruptive stimulation.

Most of the stimuli just referred to are peripheral stimuli—all around the infant but not directed to him. The nurse also needs to be concerned about bringing meaningful objects and people within the infant's spatial limits where he can see, hear, taste, touch, and smell. Giving a rattle to an infant is helpful only if the infant can hold it comfortably, transfer it, and retrieve it if it falls from his grasp. If the infant is not maturationally able to do these things, the nurse must be the active instrument in helping him enjoy and learn from the experience. A mobile or overbed toy that the infant can see and reach may be a good play tool during the nurse's absence (Fig. 4).

Although the infant delights in random body movements, his lack of control over them sometimes requires restraint in the interest of his safety and the efficacy of treatment. In cases where such restriction has to be imposed, the infant's play activity is often passive. However, this should not deemphasize its importance. The same visual, auditory, and tactile materials are used in this as in other circumstances of infant play. The difference lies in the fact that the nurse initiates the play, since the infant cannot bring objects or people into his real world through his own action. Singing to the infant, stroking his body, and gentle rocking are simple activities that will help to relieve tension. A snuggle toy next to the infant may be comforting when the nurse or parent is absent.

The nurse must exercise careful judgment about the effect that a particular play stimulus has on the infant. A restrained infant who is literally "beside himself" struggling to reach a suspended toy or a nearby nursing bottle shows the effects of indiscriminate stimulation.

Periods of supervised freedom from restraint are a "must" both for physiologic and psychologic reasons. Arm or hand restraints are particularly frustrating to an infant experiencing intense oral drives or to one who is in the stage of exploring his body and discovering through finger play that his hands are part of him. During the latter period of infancy when locomotion

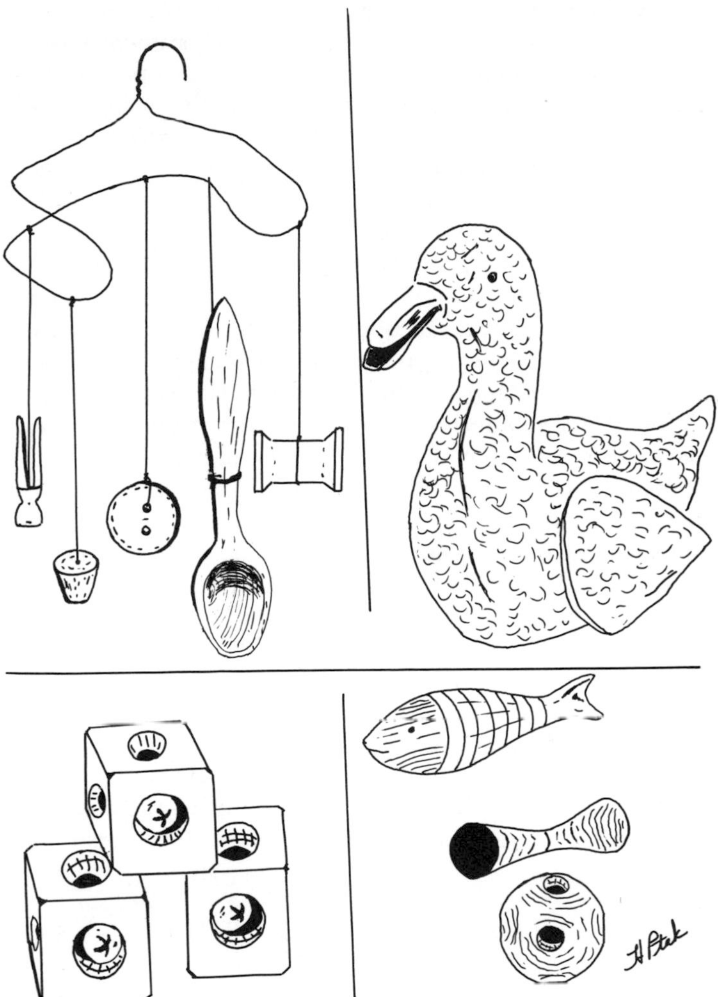

FIG. 4. This mobile can be constructed from ordinary household materials. An infant unit should have ample supply of toys like these to provide age-appropriate stimuli.

skills emerge, similar frustrations are aroused by restraint of the legs. It is not unusual to see an immediate expression of relief and contentment when the infant is permitted to suck his thumb, hold the edge of a favored blanket in his mouth, or explore a toy by chewing on it. The infant need not be denied such satisfactions because of prolonged restraint. Needless to say, the nurse should use only the minimum amount of restraint necessary to achieve desired physical results.

It should be noted that with repetition of any set of stimuli, an infant will become accustomed to a certain sequence of events which he will expect to experience. Even though the "restraint" stimulus is rightly viewed as frustrating, it is somewhat consoling to know that the infant can tolerate it if the limitation in activity does not cause actual discomfort (Dennis, 1940). Hence, if the restraint is gentle and if other tensions such as hunger and pain are reduced, negative reactions to confinement can be significantly decreased. Parents are grateful for this encouraging information.

Parents, too, need help in playing with their infant particularly during and after an illness. They are often frightened by the infant's condition and the kind of treatment required. Sometimes this fear manifests itself in diminished contact with the infant in terms of handling or other kinds of stimulation. Their hesitancy is quite understandable and should in no way diminish feelings of motherliness or fatherliness. Nurses working with the infant can interpret the infant's need for stimulation and offer the parents frequent opportunities to participate actively in the infant's play. This kind of interaction and support should occur throughout the hospitalization so that the parents will have the confidence to continue such stimulation at home. Infants who have visual or hearing handicaps or severe motor disturbances will need special kinds of stimulation. Therefore, parental guidance should not be overlooked.

Thus there are many avenues of play open to the infant who is ill. Of greatest importance is the intimate contact with a warm, expressive person whose "intimacy" touches every one of the infant's senses and sparks his awareness of surroundings and develops his capacity to trust. The "thing" world is significant, too—the mobiles, blocks, comfort items, and musical toys must always complement, but never replace, the "personal touch."

THE PRESCHOOL CHILD

The preschool period is exhilarating and exasperating for the child and for those who care for him. Play during this volatile age has many unique and interesting facets. A dramatic transition occurs as the child moves from the parallel play of the toddler toward the cooperative play of the six-year-old. Episodic, disconnected play gives way to coherent themes. Early in the preschool period the child struggles to achieve autonomy. He acquires a new and very important dimension to his self-concept—the meaning of "I" as separate from others. In the best of circumstances, this stage has its ups-and-downs. Even though a child has a long-term illness (superimposed on normally anticipated struggles), he still needs to develop independence. If one opportunity for independent pursuit is cut off by illness, other avenues have to be provided. The nurse must look at the total environment and the needs and abilities of the child in order to encourage autonomy. At the same time, she must realize that illness implies dependence.

The toddler is bent on discovery. The fact that he "discovers" in a hospital or while ill may not diminish the number of his discoveries.

Like the infant, the young preschooler continues to explore largely through sensorimotor activities. The primary differences between the infant and preschool child are the extent of mobility and the range of interpretation of new experiences. The child is no longer content with a narrow radius of interests. If he is able to be up and about at this critical stage of development, he has an obvious advantage. Unfortunately, the child who must be confined for reasons of illness does not always have a corresponding decrease

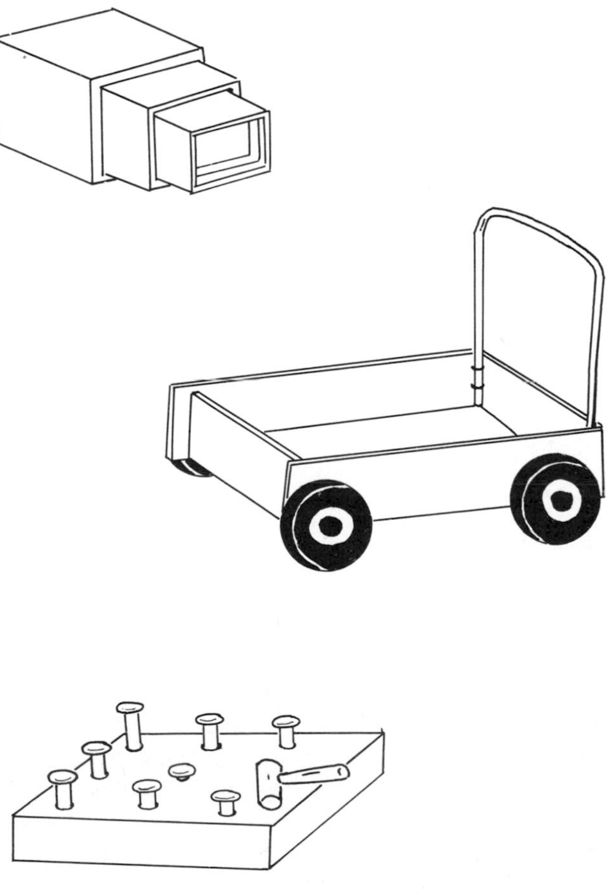

FIG. 5. These toys will interest the toddler since they encourage locomotion and hand skills.

in the intensity of his desire to roam about at will. This child challenges the nurse to find new and appropriate outlets for his boundless energy which will support feelings of independence. For example, the toddler confined to bed can enjoy vicarious locomotion activities through action stories in which he can make locomotion sounds like "swishing through the air" or running fast and "panting." Although such activities involve an admittedly limited amount of freedom, their expression does expand the child's inner resources to cope with his frustration.

Large muscle activity is the preschooler's forte. His muscles are growing rapidly and he is still testing his ability to control his body. Riding tricycles, pushing and pulling small wagons, and jumping off low stairs provide hours of satisfying activity (Fig. 5). Hospital corridors and playrooms as well as backyards should accommodate this equipment to a reasonable extent. If existing facilities are too cramped for such an expenditure of energy, or the child's illness does not permit such activity, one should not overlook the value derived simply from walking. It is a wonderful play activity in itself. Exploratory walks are rich with excitement even if the same path is traveled each day. The child's imagination permits him to view each trip from a different perspective.

An effort should also be made to provide outdoor play. As under normal conditions, the sick child benefits through an improved appetite and sound sleep if he can spend a portion of each day in the fresh air and sunshine.

Although the preschool child continues to enjoy "feeling" things, he is now more impressed with the shapes that he can form and the colors that he can blend. The hospital playroom needs simple but functional facilities for waterplay, sandbox activities, and finger painting. The hospital carpentry shop can easily construct a workable water table as illustrated in Figure 6. A similar arrangement for sand also works well, and a low table covered with oil cloth is good for finger painting.

Attention span in the early preschool period is very short. The intensity of play may be all-absorbing but short-lasting. Consequently, a variety of materials is necessary for this age group. However, the child is better able to fix attention if he is not overstimulated by too much, too fast. A toy-bag at the bedside may contain several interesting play tools but the child may only be able to handle two or three items at a time. He can then more fully experiment with all of the potentials for learning that a particular stimulus offers. I can recall a child of 2½ years hospitalized for treatment of nephrosis. The nurses became concerned because the child would not play; yet, his bed was literally covered with toys of every description. This, it seemed, was the problem. The toys were gathered up and stored in a paper bag at his bedside. A favorite stuffed animal and several bright plastic blocks were left in his bed. The boy propped the animal in a corner of his bed within his reach and vision and then turned his attention to the blocks. He lined them up,

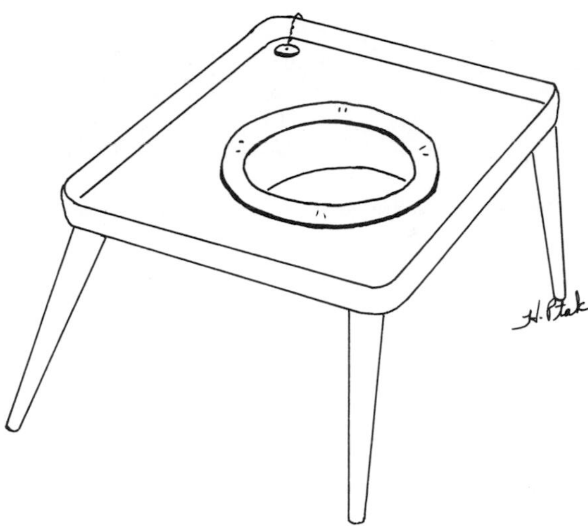

FIG. 6. Children can enjoy water play with simple equipment. This waist-high table is a comfortable height for busy preschoolers. A plastic basin on a chair works well, too.

stacked them, knocked them down, and experimented with them in a variety of ways. Intermittently, he reached out to the animal to adjust his position, pat him on the head or simply acknowledge his presence. The animal seemed to offer him enough security to permit him to explore the blocks. Too much stimulation had divided the child's attention to the point where he became so confused and fatigued that he protected himself by withdrawing.

The preschool child's increasing awareness of himself and his surroundings generally exceeds his ability to express his feelings verbally. Consequently, he often "acts out" his feelings in very physical and primitive ways. Play becomes an especially useful tool for the nurse at this time because the content of it reveals so well what the child is thinking. Enactment of family roles while the child is absent from the home environment may keep family relationships intact. Such play can also help the child to work out ambivalent feelings toward those he loves when the need to do so is most evident. He may also wish to express intense feelings of anger toward those who are caring for him. Aggressive play materials are useful in this regard because they permit the child to display his hostility in an acceptable manner without arousing guilt. It is important that the nurse or doctor carefully avoid any evidence of retaliatory behavior if they find themselves appearing in the child's fantasies. The child who "cuts up" his nurse is simply reacting to a fear about his own safety.

Regression is a common defense mechanism, especially during the early

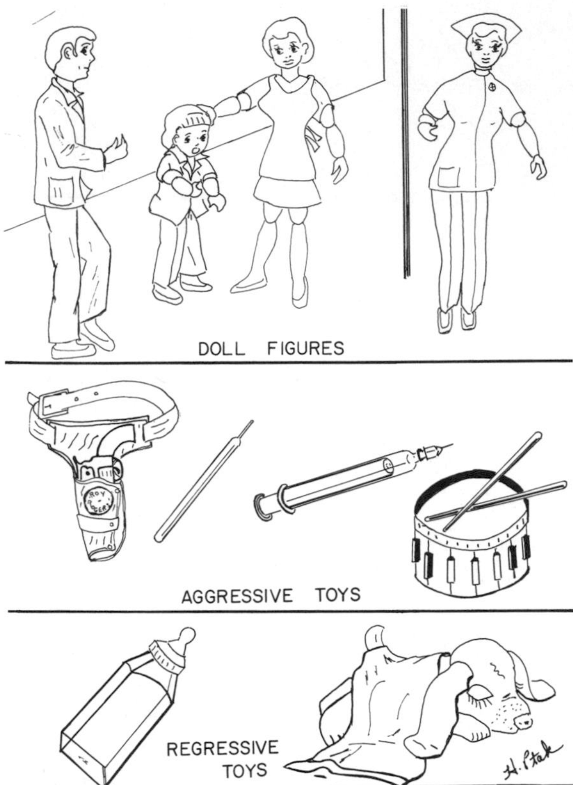

FIG. 7A. Preschool children can give expression to their strong feelings in dramatic play. These "props" will encourage them to work out conflicts, allowing for both aggressive and regressive responses.

preschool period. Newly acquired skills are not firmly consolidated as yet, so that under stress the child abandons them in order to resume more satisfying infantile modes of behavior. Regressive toys such as the nursing bottle are often favorite items in the dramatic play of the preschool child (Figs. 7A and B).

This age period is fraught with fears, expanding social expectations, and an inability to distinguish between reality and fantasy. The child who is ill may perceive his illness as a threat to his bodily integrity. Unable to give adequate verbal expression to his concerns, he works out his crisis by manipulating safe replicas of himself, by handling intrusive pieces of equipment, or by playing a role until it becomes manageable by use of his own resources. F. H. Erickson (1958) found that 19 of the 20 hospitalized preschool children in her study were able to dramatize or verbalize their feelings about the

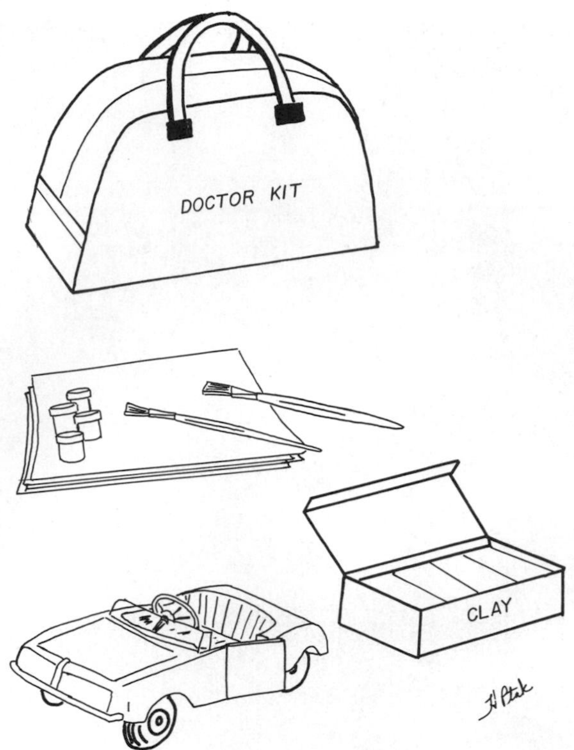

FIG. 7B. Brush painting and modeling with clay provide pleasant sensory experiences. The car and doctor kit are good tools as the child becomes involved in identification-imitation processes.

procedures that they had experienced. Their dramatizations involved the use of clinical equipment (such as hypodermic syringes, tongue blades, thermometers, and medicine bottles), doll figures, and a variety of small toys (such as beds, bathtubs, and guns). Erickson noted that most intrusive procedures (except those in the oral area) were perceived in a hostile context by the majority of the children. The play experiences obviously had much meaning for the children and she recommends that such play be encouraged as soon as possible after the hospital procedures have been performed (Fig. 8). Repetition characterizes these activities almost to the point of adult exasperation; yet the child's need to repeat an episode indicates that he has not yet worked out all of his feelings.

Miniature figures that represent both family members and hospital workers are often desired to recreate a wide range of meaningful situations. Room partitions enhance a child's imaginative doll play. The opportunity to have these props need not be restricted by the hospital situation. For the

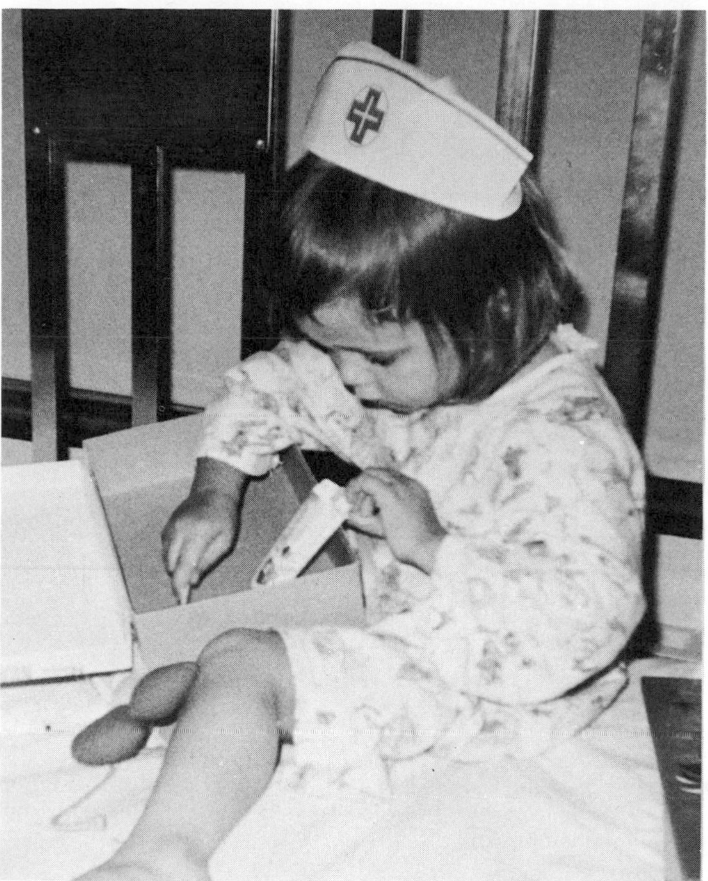

FIG. 8. This young lady is learning by doing. Playing out stressful situations relieves anxiety.

child confined to bed, a sectional piece of wood or sturdy cardboard that can be folded, as illustrated in Figure 9, works well. It can be rearranged as the child wishes in order to serve as a hallway, a large room, three small rooms, a fenced-in backyard, or the operating room.

Dress-up clothes, especially hats, are also helpful. Hats are very suitable for children confined to bed since they are easily handled, comfortable for the child, and highly visible—and, of course very symbolic. The nurse's "hat" takes its place with the hats of fireman and the policeman. Purses, large and small, are also good accompaniments to imaginative play. A place to keep "his things" is very important for the preschool child who is wrestling with elements of ownership. Children can likewise find many exciting uses for pieces of brightly colored cloths, either as adornments for them-

selves or for their dolls. A boxful of such easily collected materials should be available on every hospital unit for young children. Of course, not everything that the child enacts is truly representative of what the situation "played out" really is. Furthermore, not all feelings are tied up with hospitalization and illness; some of the playing is a reflection of normal developmental interests. Children of this age live in a rich fantasy world and their fabrications can be expressions of pure make-believe without any link with reality.

It is during the preschool period that children first develop the capacity to pretend. The boundaries between fact and fantasy become very flexible. Pretending affords the child an opportunity to explore the way things *might* be rather than the way they are. This is a source of great encouragement for the child. It develops a certain optimism and initiative since pretending suggests to the child that he himself can alter his world to suit his desires. Pretend play should be taken seriously and not ridiculed. It is especially important that ill children be supported in their pretend play. Because of the circumstances of their illness they may be especially aware of their smallness and powerlessness. Pretending can bolster their confidence.

Sometimes the preschooler, particularly around the age of four, will create imaginary companions. One early study (Ames and Learned, 1946) revealed that at least as many as 20 percent of children enjoy such companionship. Others feel the incidence is much greater. Usually imaginary playmates come into existence in response to a special need of the child—for a friend, a model, perhaps for a scapegoat! It seems best to accept the

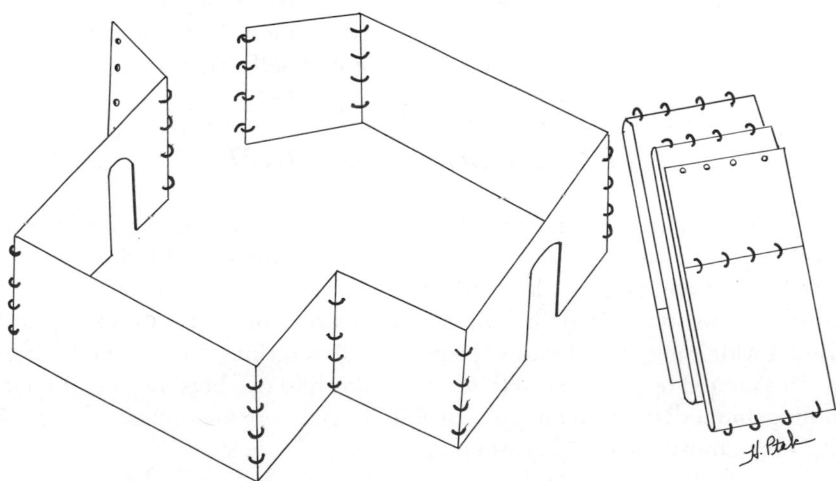

FIG. 9. Folding room partitions can be made from any firm material and held together with plastic rings.

and Torpie, 1968). The solution to eradication of the problem of language retardation lies with the amount of stimulation given the child. Language development begins with the coos and smiles of the mother (or substitute) during feeding times, with the imitative babble of the toddler, and with the serious discussion during the preschool years of, for instance, why there is a moon in the sky during the day. In other words, it is that part of our development which is directly stimulated by people rather than things in our environment. It is other humans who must interpret for the child what the world is all about. Language development must have human-to-human contact in a communication phase. This process will not be facilitated by talking to one's co-workers or to the wall while working with children. It will be facilitated by talking with the child about realities surrounding him. All our communication with the child and all the experiences we plan for him should be aimed at increasing his understanding of reality and his symbolization of it. This is one of the child's prime occupations throughout infancy, childhood, and adolescence.

When we are discussing the hospitalized child and our role as a nurse working in child health, we must remember that the hospital reality is not normal everyday reality. We must compensate for the experiences the child is missing during his hospital stay. Close attention must be given to the level of language development at the time preceding hospitalization and any signs of slowing of progress during hospitalization should be quickly noted and attempts made by the staff to compensate for them.

Identification Behavior

The exhibited behaviors of identification (emotional or social responses) are closely interrelated with each other and are greatly influenced by the external environment. Identification or self-identity is a learned response. In a real sense we are who we are by the reaction of others to our being. This is not totally true, but the developing individual is very flexible and can change behavior that has met with negative reactions of others into behavior that will elicit a positive response. All the communication which occurs between the infant and the mother (verbal or nonverbal) builds identification behavior. The games and attention shown the child by his mother all help the child distinguish himself from his environment. This identification development continues throughout childhood and adolescence. It usually centers around those who continuously care for the child (Call, 1968; Epstein, 1968; Greenson, 1968; Sonis, 1968; Kirkendall and Rubin, 1974; Bee, 1975). There are, of course, major differences in the development of identification as there are in emotional and social responses (Elkind, 1967; Greenson, 1968; Gardner, 1973; Mussen, Conger, and Kagan, 1974; Bee, 1975).

The question of how nursing care can foster the continuing develop-

playmate who has all the solid characteristics of a real object and accommodate the child's desires. Most often it will leave as quietly as it appeared, the child having no further need for it.

The preschool years, particularly in the later stages, marks the period of children-to-children social play. Watching others, imitating them, and sharing with them becomes more and more frequent. The pleasure of this kind of activity is sometimes limited during illness. The thoughtful nurse, however, will be aware of this important need to engage in social play and will encourage it whenever possible in hospital or home. Much learning occurs during this type of play. We are judged later by our ability to manage social behavior and it is in these early stages of development that we learn how to take turns, how to compromise, and how to let the other person be the central person. It teaches the concept of reciprocation. Every child likes to be the boss, but through social play with peers he comes to believe in the efficacy of cooperation as well.

Lowenfeld (1967) reminds us that every play object is likely to have three meanings—the obvious one; the correct or incorrect knowledge possessed by the child about the object; and the significance that the object itself has for the child. Consequently, interpretation of a play episode should not be too hasty.

Play, then, for the preschool child, is a composite of many activities rich with emotional meaning. Foremost among its characteristics are the child's excursions into the world of fantasy. Through symbolic, make-believe play the child stores sensations and perceptions that he will apply to the interpretation of future experiences. He does this in a most pragmatic way. As the preschooler delights in his play discoveries, he leaves physical and verbal imprints on the people and things in his environment. They, in turn, reinforce the child's desire to continue his pursuit of self-mastery.

THE SCHOOL-AGE CHILD

The hospitalized school-age child has several things going for him in regard to play. Erikson (1963) stresses that this is the age of industry—the time when the child is busy doing things. Physically, the school-age child has matured to the point where fine motor coordination and large muscle control permit a wide range of activities. Piaget (1969) describes this stage as that of concrete mental operations—a time when the child can become absorbed in handling immediate and tangible problems and can manipulate them by using elementary logic and reasoning.

Using these general guidelines, the nurse can call upon the traditional collection of games that have delighted children for decades. Games of chance and skill should be employed as the child desires them. Craft skills and hobbies may also occupy a good portion of the child's time. Since these things involve use of small muscles and fairly long attention spans, a hospital environment may not be too restricting (Fig. 10).

However, a word of caution ought to be introduced when one considers using such games. Energy consumption varies with the meaning that a child attaches to a particular activity. A competitive game requiring considerable skill may be quite exhausting and border on overstimulation, especially for a child who always needs to win. The circumstances under which a game is played are also important. A child who is coming to grips with a changed body image or who is getting accustomed to a restriction in his activities needs an opportunity to experience a few successes. School-age children have very high expectations for themselves and can be devastated by failure, even if it is only a game of checkers that is lost. A reasonable hope for achievement must exist in any play activity. However, children rightfully resent it if you "let them win;" they do not want reality altered. What I am emphasizing is the value of selecting the right activity at the right time.

Children of this age enjoy a culture of their own. The process of growing to maturity necessarily involves participation in sustaining this culture. Adults are relatively uninformed about the characteristics of this way of life because it is nearly impossible to penetrate the peer world of the school-age child. In fact, much of the pleasure of the age comes from the fact that adults do not know the intimate details of this existence.

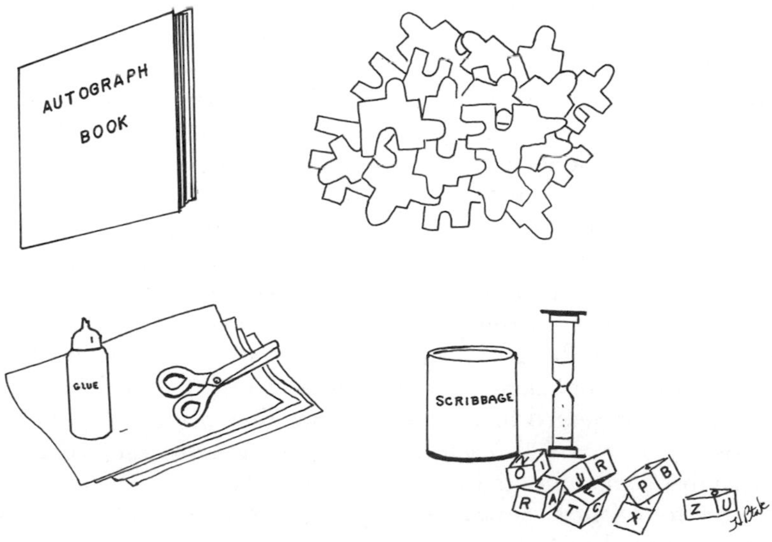

FIG. 10. These simple materials provide the school-age child with opportunities for creative expression and for development of intellectual and manipulative skills.

Nevertheless, we do know that these children are their own best entertainers. The rhymes, riddles, puns, and songs that dance on their lips are evidence of their adherence to rituals. They have a special language all their own that spoofs reality and transmits meanings impossible to express in a conventional way. It becomes a secret code of entry into the child's world. According to Opie and Opie (1959), rhymes and riddles capture the children's views of friendship, authority, truthfulness, and humor in a unique way. A child who seeks the answer to a riddle enjoys interrogating, and probably feels superior in knowing the answer. Adults can facilitate this enjoyment by helping children make up riddles and then joining in the fun by acknowledging the joke—no matter how corny it is. One way of starting is to think of words with double meanings and make them into a riddle. Everyone knows the familiar riddle, "What is black and white and read all over?" And its answer, "The newspaper." This is an example of similar sounding words having different spellings and different meanings. Searching out this kind of thing can be much fun.

Often the satisfaction enjoyed through peer-group activities is derived from the group's ability to test adult authority. Rhymes are often directed at persons in authority. Word tricks can be used to express legitimate aggression. Teachers are especially vulnerable to this kind of play, but anyone who controls the child's environment and prescribes certain kinds of activities on a consistent basis is open to them. Nurses fall into this category, and should expect to receive a goodly amount of normal discrimination. Mimicking, making faces, and giving nicknames are all important experiences for children. The exclusiveness of play at this age should also be noted with interest. The quick act of hiding something when you enter the room, or the silly, self-conscious giggles that follow a "clique" conversation are not so much directed against the nurse as they are directed at preserving the special flavor of middle-childhood fun. Children of this age cherish privacy to an extent not often appreciated by the adult.

Hospitalization, of course, places many limits on this kind of activity. There are too many adults in the environment and there is generally too much space between children and too wide an age variation. Hopefully these factors can be modified. I believe that we sometimes overdo the necessity for close supervision of the school-age children's activities. In reality, even in play, they are seldom alone long enough to "do their own thing." This is certainly a peer-oriented time, so efforts should be made to bring children into closer proximity with each other by moving beds, carts, chairs, and tables so that communication is facilitated (Fig. 11).

The role of fantasy in the developmental expression of the preschool child has already been alluded to. Fantasies are expressed quite spontaneously by young children. The older child, however, is not quite so free. Because the child is older, he is more affected by the constraints of the

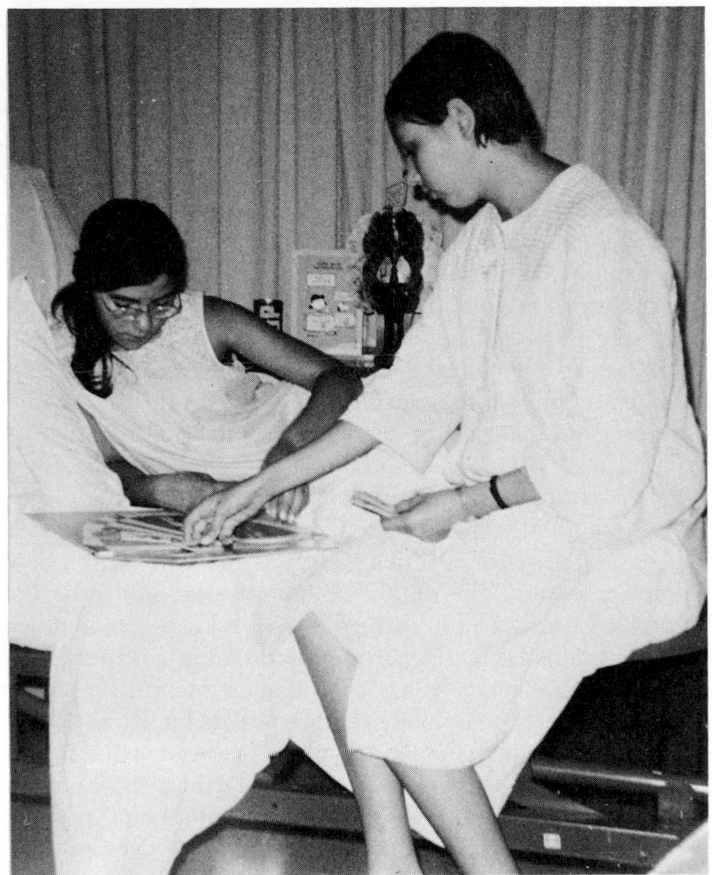

FIG. 11. The closer the better for these "pals." Peer group solidarity in the school years.

"realities" of life and has a more elaborate collection of defense mechanisms. He is more inclined toward the conventional and competitive activities than toward the kind of play that might risk self-revelation.

It seems reasonable to expect that school-age children who have long-term illnesses might harbor more fears and unsettling feelings about themselves than would be experienced by healthy children. Helping the child find ways that might encourage expression of emotions without the attendant risk of losing face can become an important nursing function. Marcus (1966) successfully used the costume technique as one way of encouraging dramatic play among school-age children. He noted that these children respond better if the enactment of their fantasy is supported by props—materials related to real-life situations. Although Marcus describes the technique in relation to psychotherapy, I think that it would be a decidedly useful play stimulus for children whose age discourages their spontaneous expression.

Hand puppets and marionettes are also good tools for this purpose. Puppets objectify the play situation and serve as a mask to cover up the child's sensitive self. In support of this method, Green (1975) describes her experiences in working with an 8½-year-old chronically ill boy who withdrew from social interaction with staff and peers and acted out negatively against the treatment regime. Using nondirective therapeutic play techniques involving puppet figures, she was able to help the child openly confront his anxieties and work through his problems. By speaking through the puppets he was able to reveal his own true feelings. The nurse responded through the "nurse" puppet, thereby reducing his own psychologic risk taking. Therapeutic puppet play may require much time and patience because the child's readiness must be carefully assessed and the progress of the play experiences must be paced according to the child's capacity for growth.

Thus far I have referred primarily to manipulative and verbal activities for the school-age child. Not to be underestimated is the importance of acquiring a sense of physical well-being and adequacy through involvement in gross motor activities. The middle-childhood years do focus upon the learning of a wide variety of highly valued physical skills—running, jumping, balancing, and playing of games requiring coordination and speed. Illness, at its best, limits the opportunity to test and demonstrate this physical competence; at its worst, it may completely remove outlets for activity by isolation and superimposed restraint. (Reference will be made later in this chapter to specific ways that children can be helped to adapt to restrictions of illness without completely sacrificing their need for action-oriented pastimes.)

The school-age child is particularly vulnerable to what might be called the hospital culture. The activities of this age involve many significant aspects of development—developing conscience, inner control, and cooperation; learning how to think and make judgments; learning the role expectations of male and female; understanding the limitations of social class. All, in effect, move the child toward increasing independence. All of these are explored through the medium of play. Some have been described already. I should like to direct particular emphasis to the area of social class.

It is a fact that hospital clothing, room arrangements, and services tend to disguise social and economic class differences. Yet the child himself operates within the context of his past experiences. By the time he is in eighth grade, the child perceives social class in about the same way that adults do. Depending on the social class in which he was raised, certain kinds of behaviors are reinforced while others are discouraged. The hospital environment may create conflict. This is especially noticeable during long hospitalizations. Two sets of circumstances may prevail, each with its own dangers. If the child's adherence to the behavior of his social class is strong and prevails over the mores of the staff, conflicts may emerge which can be psychologically and physically disruptive. On the other hand, the child may be captivated by the hospital mores and change his behavior in order to conform and receive the system's rewards. If this pattern of response spans a considerable time period, the child may incorporate these behavioral expectations into his lifestyle, and then the problems emerge at the time of discharge from the hospital. The child experiences a conflict between his new goals and those of his family and neighborhood. Such seeds of conflict may lay the groundwork for a troubled readjustment to his environment. I can well remember a young girl from a city slum who was hospitalized for more than a year with rheumatic heart disease. During the period of hospitalization, she became the "favorite" of many nurses. She visited their suburban homes, enjoyed many gifts for her birthday and holidays, and began a strong identification with middle-class mores to the exclusion of values held by a disrupted family. Old enough to take an active role in decision-making, she obviously resented a return to her family. She was dissatisfied with what they could materially provide for her and she became acutely aware of her own limited resources in providing the "luxuries" for herself. She obviously needed help to blend both value systems and to retain the best of each.

How can play be helpful in this regard? If the child comes from a situation characterized by economic hardship, the use of play materials that do not involve a large monetary expenditure should be encouraged. Focus should be directed on the child's resourcefulness rather than on the material itself. Activity should be based on the child's interest. It is likely that if his social class and that of the nurse differ markedly the nurse may not understand the relevance of the activities he describes. Encourage him to teach you the games and the corresponding vocabulary or jargon. This shows respect for his idea of a good and productive use of his time and also places him in the important position of making decisions about his own activities. It also will provide indirect clues about what motivates this child's behavior. This knowledge becomes valuable in helping him adjust to his illness.

I can recall receiving from a 12-year-old patient a thorough education about the dance crazes that were popular among the youngsters in a black community. Agility in performance of these dances was a mark of social acceptance within her neighborhood youth groups. The fact that some of this skill could be lost during the hospitalization was of more concern to the girl than was the fact that she was to undergo surgery for treatment of osteomyelitis. She was able to keep her interest alive and her peer position relatively secure by resorting to pop records and frequent visits from her friends. And, quite importantly, she derived much pleasure from teaching me about her "special thing."

As one can see, play during the school years is better organized than that during the preschool period, though it still retains imagination and inventiveness. It has an excitement of its own. The period is marked by strict adherence to rules and high expectations for one's performance. Leadership qualities emerge as the youngsters experiment with group interaction and begin to learn the meaning of altruism. Within the context of school-age play, the nurse holds a position of importance—not in the sense of becoming an active player but rather serving as a model of behavior. The child still looks to the adult for guidelines in choosing satisfying and acceptable modes of conduct. Sutton-Smith (1974) says that "as children get older, we have to play with them less, but we have to understand them more" (p 232).

THE ADOLESCENT

Havighurst (1952) lists no less than ten important developmental tasks that characterize physical and emotional maturing during adolescence. Acceptance of one's physique, involvement in satisfying heterosexual relationships, emancipation from parents, and some assumption of economic independence are among the important achievements of this age. Stone and Church (1962) sum up the central theme of teenagers' strivings as finding one's self. In more contemporary terms, adolescents are looking for answers to questions posed by sex, money, education, justice, conservation, peace, and war. These have been the concerns of young adults for a long time, but more and more these topics find their way into the conversations of high-school children.

Many of these learnings presuppose a certain level of physical and mental well-being and, obviously, most of them are learned in the context of a social setting. Consequently, there is no age when illness is more threatening than during adolescence. Not only is it a threat to personal integrity, but it is maddeningly inconvenient to be ill during adolescence when there are so many things to do. If the illness is of long duration, involves a reorientation of life goals, or results in disfigurement of a part of the body, the threat may be temporarily immobilizing.

It is natural for hospitalized adolescents to be angry, distrustful, and annoyed. With their idealistic points of view, they cannot readily accept an unplanned interruption at this point in their life. The question "Why me?" is a common one. Adjustment to illness and hospitalization can be eased by implementation of a thoughtfully conceived and relevant program of activity.

Peer-group activities are all-absorbing at this age. The adolescent values his ability to choose his friends and the type, scope, and duration of the activities they experience together. Hospitalization will limit this freedom, but not nearly to the extent ordinarily supposed. There are many ways to encourage friendships. The spontaneity of the social encounter is important.

The nurse's role is one that provides opportunities for young people to meet under natural circumstances rather than one that forces social contacts.

It is best to proceed slowly in this regard. While the adolescent may feel confident and at ease with his reference group outside of the hospital, it may take some time before he can safely open himself to a new roommate or hospital group. Pushing a relationship too enthusiastically may actually retard a meaningful social experience. Teenagers are quick to be suspicious and resent situations where they feel that they are losing control. I can recall an experience involving two 15-year-old boys. One had had surgery to treat Meckel's diverticulum; the other was hospitalized with ulcerative colitis. They were the only teens on the unit and their rooms were at opposite ends of the corridor. The nurse who was caring for one of the boys decided to promote some social interaction, so she introduced them and suggested that they meet for craft work. The boys dutifully complied but it was a strained experience for both of them. They plodded along with the task but there was little enthusiastic communication between them. After two days of this arrangement both boys found excuses to avoid the meeting. The next day both boys coincidentally found themselves sharing the game room. Left completely to their own resources, they became interested in each other's activities. One boy was a talented cartoon artist; the other was very proficient at playing pool. Each felt a certain competence in his special skill and, on this common ground, they shared their experiences. They respected each other's individuality and their friendship grew strong during the hospitalization and continued after they went home.

One way to encourage spontaneous interaction is to set up a teen "lounge" (not a playroom, please!, adolescents are extremely sensitive about childish labels). Ideally, it should be equipped with a record player, radio, and simple musical instruments (guitars and bongo drums are popular). Board games of chance and skill, playing cards, a typewriter, writing paper, and magazines are also of interest to young people. A small pantry for snacks is always a good added feature. With these supportive props, teenagers can be as open to interaction as their emotional or physical state permits (Fig. 12).

The adolescent confined to bed can benefit from some communication network that keeps him socially "in tune." This can take the form of a tape-recorded conversation passed between two patients or between himself and his classmates at school or members of his family. A weekly gossip sheet can be great fun as a group activity. A sullen, withdrawn teenager can come alive as the "star reporter." The sheet can contain hospital news, "feature" articles by the adolescents themselves, announcement of coming events such as teenage luncheons or an evening "social," and birthday and graduation congratulations. A challenging crossword puzzle or a "thought for the

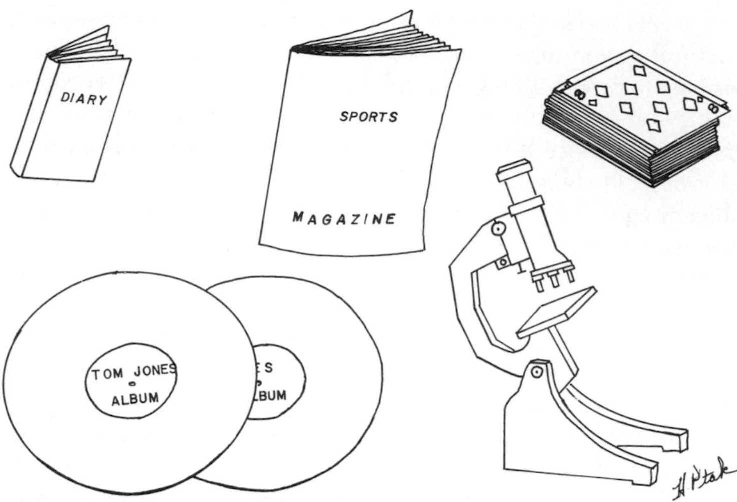

FIG. 12. The adolescent is approaching adult interests. These common materials serve a wide range of abilities and help to bridge the gap between childhood play and adult recreation.

week" might go far to relieve a little boredom and spark some animated conversation. Telephone and letter contacts both in and out of the hospital setting are other ways of preserving social awareness. Visits from other patients and school friends, while it seems almost too obvious to mention, should also be encouraged.

In planning adolescent activities, it is important to remember that young people come from a media-filled world. Stereo and radio are as important to teenagers as food and water. School experiences are enriched by a variety of audiovisual techniques. Social gathering spots are accented by revolving lights and the penetrating sound of the "beat." A world full of vicarious experiences comes to them through television. Consequently, it should not surprise us that many adolescents suffer acutely from restless boredom. The sensory deprivation of the hospitalized adolescent ought to come under closer scrutiny. Television certainly has its place in any adolescent activity program. In settings in which new audiovisual facilities are being proposed, consider closed circuit television. Its potential for teaching and entertainment is great. Use of movies, film-strips, and cartridge tapes are also well received if the content is relevant to adolescent interests.

One very important need for most adolescents (both boys and girls) is maintenance of physical strength, agility, and excellence in sports. A long illness will affect these abilities to some extent. However, in many situations, atrophy of muscles and diminished skill are needless accompaniments of illness. Weightlifting, muscle setting exercises, workouts in physical therapy, or use of an overhead trapeze or a punching bag can help to maintain a level of skill that compliments the child's image of himself. For example, I cared for a 16-year-old boy with diabetes who was hospitalized for treatment of a skin infection. He was trying out for the track team at school and was worried that his training progam would suffer. After discussing the situation with the physician and the physical therapist, arrangements were made for him to go to physical therapy to "work out." I later learned that he did make the team.

It is often presumed that adolescents disregard school performance as completely irrelevant. For some of these young people this is indeed a fact. However, it is unwise to make this assumption for all. Adolescents understand well the stereotyped expectation that they "ought to" reject authority. Consequently, those who are interested in school achievement are reluctant to admit it. Therefore, it is important to provide matter-of-fact opportunities to do school work without forcing the adolescent to say that they love it, or otherwise draw unnecessary attention to it. On the other hand, if an adolescent's interests are not scholastic, he should not be criticized. His illness probably undermines his self-confidence enough without adding another dimension—that is, failure to measure up to the nurse's expectations.

Every adolescent has some talent. Finding it might be a challenge for the nurse. When the talent is too obscure, it might be because the adolescent does not feel that his interest is acceptable enough to the nurse to bring it out in the open. Whatever the talent might be—crafts, art, poetry, music, mechanics, whittling, sports, farming, or simply hanging around with the gang, he should be given every opportunity to continue to develop it if his illness permits. It will establish his identity in the hospital and maintain his level of proficiency when he returns to home and school.

Adolescence is a time for much soul-searching, which requires taking an inward look into the self. Consequently, solitary recreation constitutes a vital part of adolescent activity. We must respect the adolescent's right to do nothing. Time for daydreaming, thinking, and mirror-gazing is necessary for all adolescents. It is even more significant if he is also struggling to accept an illness. Sometimes we overdo the tendency to keep adolescents busy. We feel compelled to keep their minds active so they won't become preoccupied with their illness. If there is no time to ponder new ideas or make sense out of the day's events, worries and fears may be so diffuse that they enter into all of the adolescent's activities—diminishing his capacity to enjoy anything.

The adolescent's room should reflect his interests. Closets and cupboards are in demand to hold the various and sundry items that adolescents cannot live without. Cork boards should be hung in prominent places so that such things as newspaper clippings, cards, art work, and cartoons can be viewed at their pleasure. Mirrors are important to accommodate the adolescent's preoccupation with his body and grooming. Bright contemporary colors should predominate in room decor. (The pastels of most children's units are more appealing to adults than to children.) Bedside units with telephones and radios are also appreciated by adolescents.

While these environmental enticements do make hospitalization more pleasant, perhaps the most important part of an adolescent activity program is the role assumed by the nurse. The adolescent is really anxious to respect adults but he fears deception. He is extremely sensitive to a lack of sincerity or superficial attention to his concerns. Consequently, he is cautious about opening new relationships.

There is no doubt that an experiential gap exists between the nurse and the adolescent patient. Dress, language, and interests may differ, but these things are relatively unimportant if there is a desire to help the young person think well of himself. The nurse who cares for adolescents must be someone who is convinced that adolescents are competent and can act responsibly.

Adolescents love to shock and taunt persons in authority. The nurse should expect his/her share of this behavior. However, he/she must not retaliate by trying to "put something over on this fresh kid." Once the adolescent feels manipulated, all further attempts at meaningful interaction are jeopardized. Most of all adolescents appreciate a good listener who judiciously refrains from giving pat advice.

In spite of the obvious experiential differences between nurse and patient, the nurse should strive for a congruent orientation with adolescent goals. She/he must not be in conflict with what he wants to achieve; nor should she/he feel threatened if her/his reasoning meets resistance. The "says-who" attitude is an understandable response from a disillusioned 16-year-old who is newly diagnosed as having diabetes. The optimum benefit from the activities and facilities that I have mentioned depends upon the existence of a nurse-patient relationship that is based on mutual respect.

ENVIRONMENT FOR PLAY

The resourcefulness and energy that a child brings to his play comes from within, but the richness of the experience does depend in large measure on external stimuli. A suitable environment for play must be established whether the child is sick at home or in the hospital, confined to bed or visiting the ambulatory care facility. Certain environmental elements should be considered when one plans satisfying play experiences.

Space

The first of the environmental elements that a child needs is space. Ordinarily, space is defined as boundlessness or extension in all directions. Obviously, a child's play space must have some fixed dimensions, and the sick child's world is even more confined. I prefer to think of space not so much in terms of physical dimensions but rather in terms of "feeling." A relatively small area can be made to appear open and airy if walls and curtains are bright, the lighting is good, the bed has at least two open sides, and windows are low enough to "bring in the outdoors." Drab colors, poor lighting, obstructive screens, and high windows create a barrier from the real world and tone down the excitement of play. Objects that do not interest the child, such as linen and unnecessary pieces of equipment, should be elsewhere.

Spatial needs can also be considered from other points of view. Certain kinds of play activity require certain spatial characteristics. Riding a tricycle demands enough space to build up at least some sensation of speed and, of course, requires a turn-around area. Building blocks are excellent materials for creative play. However, the preschool child often delights in saving his elaborate masterpiece until his mother or father sees it or until he himself is ready to destroy it. This takes not only space, but also respect for the products of the child's own ingenuity.

Bed space is also important. Games that require delicate balance may prove frustrating on an already tilted bed; board games that require an intricate layout of materials may present difficulties for a child who has a limited reaching span. Part of the excitement and pleasure of a game is to play according to the rules. Improvisation has its place but only when used at the right time. Lightweight, folding cardboard bases can be easily constructed to spread on the bed so that play materials can be level.

Independence is encouraged when the child has control over his play materials. Assemble the items of special interest in a reachable spot so that the child can determine the focus of his play and change it at will whether or not adults are available to assist him. This encourages his creativity by permitting a combination of materials in new play experiments. A toy bag, a small suitcase, or a sturdy box attached to the bed can contain enough "raw material" to keep an inventive mind well stimulated for a long time (Fig. 13).

The child's personal space is another consideration. This is the area that he understands as his own. Both in the hospital and at home, a child needs to know what is his—that is, how far his domain extends. It becomes a source of self-satisfaction as well as an element of power and control . Furthermore, it supports his wish for freedom in that the child can change his things to suit his needs and interests.

If a child knows the limits of his space he can confidently speak (or fight) for what he knows is his. The hospital situation often presents elements of a community where objects are shared by everyone. Sometimes the aggressive child captures the most cherished items. By knowing what is his, the child does not have to become anxious about having to give up his possessions. Young children can become very upset when "mommy's chair" is

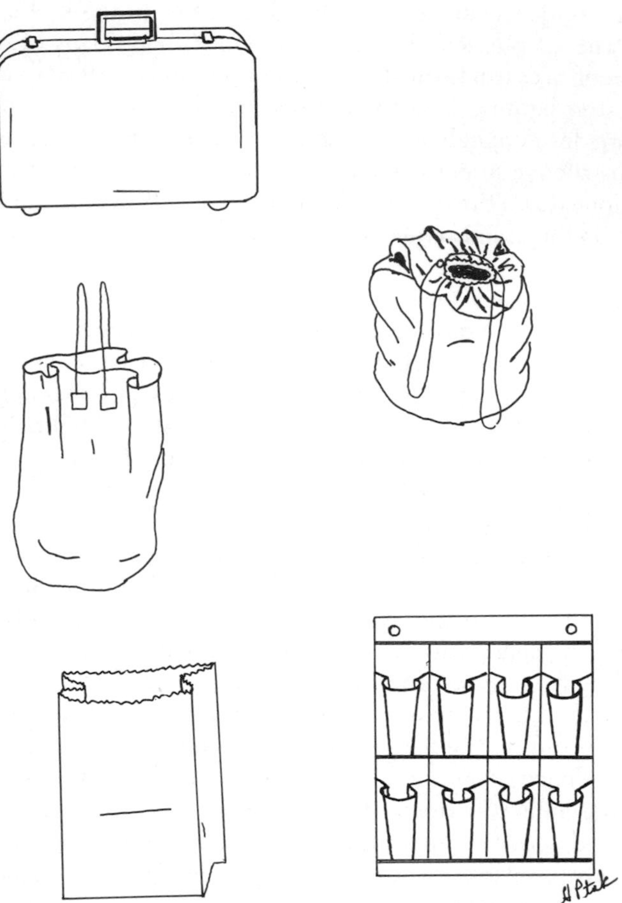

FIG. 13. Toy storage is an easy matter when these containers are used. If kept within the child's reach, they provide much independence in selecting play materials. Besides, it is fun just to "put things in and take them out."

suddenly whisked away for someone else, or when their favorite toy is passed on to another child. Realistically, many hospital toys are community property and will not go home with the child. Of course, children must be helped to accept this limitation. Understanding this reality will be less disturbing if the child knows the limits of his personal space.

Time

The child also needs time to play. We must respect his interest in his own activities. Nurses sometimes find it difficult to take play seriously. How many times is the child interrupted in the middle of a play period to have a treatment performed, to eat, or take a bath? I do not recommend that the child's care plan revolve solely around his play needs, but I do plead that careful consideration be given to the child's own timetable of events whenever possible.

The child also needs time to develop competence in his play. When suggesting an activity, one must keep a reasonable completion time in mind. If the activity such as craft or art work involves a fair amount of preparation time, be sure that enough time is allowed for some enjoyment of the activity itself before the materials have to be put away. Accomplishment is one of the outcomes of play. A child who continually gets things half done never has a chance to see himself as a successful doer.

Also important is time to terminate play. If play is afforded the respect that it deserves, we can readily understand the child's reluctance to refocus his attention on something the adult considers more essential to his care. As a matter of fact, the child may find it difficult to reassemble his resources for a new experience, particularly if he has been fully absorbed in a re-creation of a meaningful or stressful event. However, he can adjust to limitations if he is aware of them. It is important to give a child reasonable notice about an upcoming treatment or change in routine before it occurs so that he can terminate his play partially on his own terms.

The last consideration about time is often overlooked. Every child needs time not to play. Judicious timing of play periods should offer opportunities to rest, daydream, plan the day's events, enjoy a pleasant view, or simply retreat to the confines of one's inner resources for refreshment and strength to face new challenges.

Feasibility

Another factor to consider in building an environment for play is the feasibility of play—from the standpoint of both the player and the play material. Several questions may be posed to illustrate this point. Is the player able to perform the activity without undue fatigue? Will the time required to enjoy the activity match the time available for it? Will the materials function appropriately where they will be used? Are all essential parts of the material available for use? Let us suppose that a right-handed child has his left hand restrained while receiving a blood transfusion. In looking for a pleasant activity to occupy the time, paper and crayons are offered. It sounds reasonable since the child is right-handed. However, the activity will lead to frustration if some method is not devised to keep the paper from moving on the overbed table. The solution may be simply a large clipboard or a clamp that might fit over the edge of the table. A child is quick to lose interest and is easily frustrated when things do not work for him. A four-legged animal needs four legs and something to stand on. Because of the young child's concrete way of dealing with things, he has a difficult time seeing a reproduction-type of toy outside of its intended function. Crayons that keep rolling out of reach could be stored in a box or bag that will give the child much better control of the situation. The pockets of a shoe bag suspended on the side of the crib or bed will easily keep a variety of small toys within the child's reach.

Given space, time, and feasibility, two important ingredients remain: the availability of people and things. There is no doubt that the child is the player, but the nurse creates the atmosphere conducive to enjoyable play. This happens only when the nurse understands the value that play has for his/her young patients and has the interest, ability, and time to encourage it through his/her own ingenuity and by consultation and collaboration with recreational and occupational therapists and volunteer play-helpers. The nurse and therapist working together can assess such factors as the meaning that a particular activity has for a child, the existence of fatigue, and the length of attention spans. The nurse can also point out the restrictions imposed by the illness and identify specific kinds of activities that may enhance a particular treatment plan. For example, a child with upper-extremity contractures from burns might well enjoy using a loom supported on a frame, suspended in front of her. She can experience the pleasure of a productive activity and also prevent the untoward development of further contractures. The therapist can assess the child's interest and skill, and supply materials to match them and the know-how to use them creatively.

Often, the source of failure of many enthusiastically initiated play programs is a lack of materials. This can wear ingenuity to the point where it is too thin to be effective. Donated materials are, of course, encouraged but they cannot be expected to fulfill all play needs. Hospital and health agency budgets must include funds for play materials. The initial cost of durable, safe materials may be significant but, over time, the monies will have been well spent. However, many resources are available at minimal cost. Hospital carpentry shops can assemble simple yet serviceable equipment—work tables, benches, stools, stairs, bulletin boards, toy boxes, and easels—by using scrap wood left from other construction jobs. Volunteer organizations are also very helpful in this regard. Parents, too, are ready to lend a hand. One father of a five-year-old girl constructed a special dolly to improve locomotion possibilities for his young daughter; he drew up a set of directions based on his design and the hospital carpenters have used it in many similar situations (Fig. 14A and B).

Obsolete hospital equipment can be adapted to serve as play materials. A good look should be taken at what disposable equipment is replacing so that useful items are not inadvertently discarded. Also, observe the "disposables" themselves. Looking at them from different points of view, you might

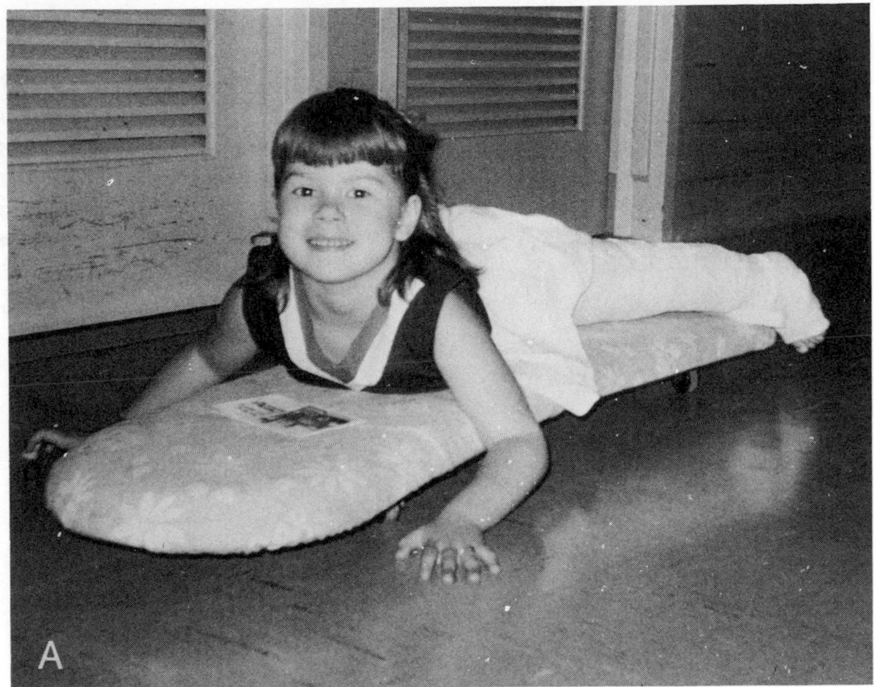

FIG. 14A. This five-year-old really "gets around." A dolly like this permits her to participate actively in family affairs and play groups. **B.** If not available commercially, a dolly can be easily constructed as illustrated.

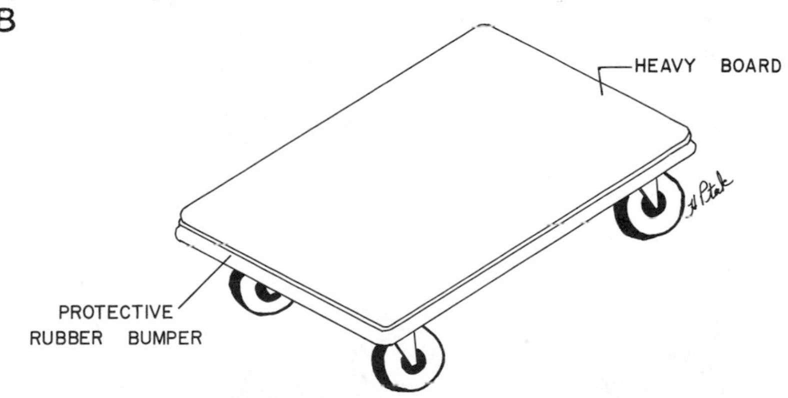

see them as containers for crayons or paints or as small toys such as hats, drums, or cooking utensils. Old bedside tables make delightful refrigerators for little mothers, with an added shelf or two and some bright paint. Unused venetian blind slats make interesting tracks for automobile racers.

Playroom

One important aspect of the environment for play is the playroom itself. Every agency offering services for children should have a play area. The setting need not be elaborate but the equipment assembled must reflect the interests of the children. Otherwise, the area will not receive maximum use. Before space and equipment are selected, identify the characteristics of the children to be served. Their age and health problems are two primary factors for consideration. Previous sections in this chapter alluded to the significance of age in determining patterns of play. The nature of the health problem is important, too. For example, if many of the children have orthopedic

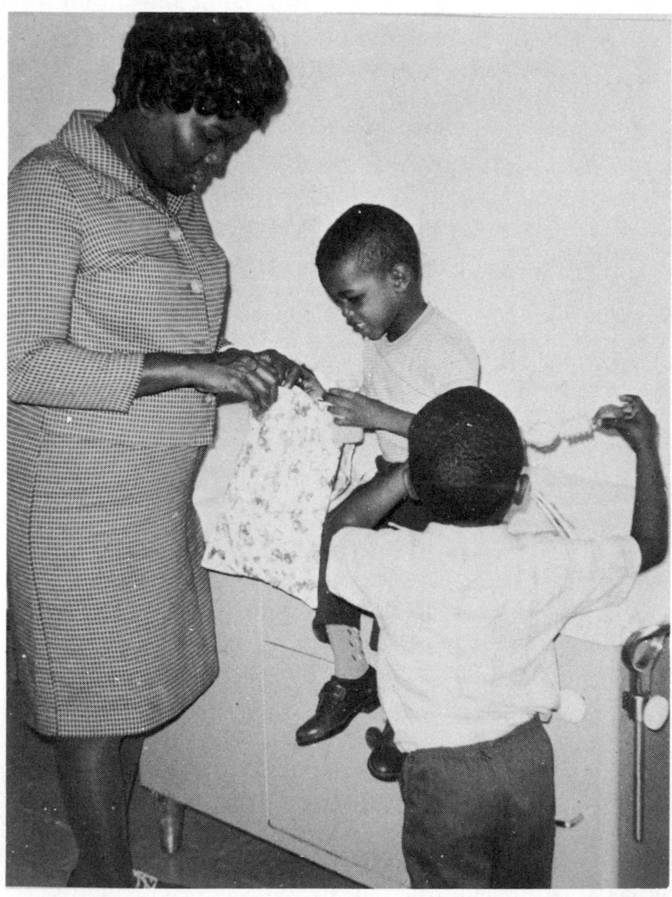

FIG. 15. This little boy is fascinated by his exploration into the toy bag that his grandmother is holding. While they wait for the doctor, learning is taking place.

problems, provision must be made to accommodate carts, beds, and traction apparatus. The height of the tables may need adjustment for children in wheelchairs. On the other hand, if the playroom is being planned in an ambulatory care facility, different considerations will be in order. A larger number of adults will be present with the children. There should be a reasonable proximity between the playroom and the waiting area so that parents can be free to participate in the child's activity whenever desirable. Because of the transient nature of the ambulatory visit, toys should not be too elaborate or require a long attention span on the part of the child.

In a clinic service, children frequently spend considerable time waiting in examining rooms. (Hopefully, with new approaches to health care delivery, this time is being shortened.) The playroom concept should be broadened to extend into these areas as well. A small toy box or bag in each room can make the waiting time seem short, especially for the parent whose patience is being tested by a restless child (Fig. 15). Also, the doctor will find that the toys make good conversation openers and pleasant distractions during an uncomfortable examination.

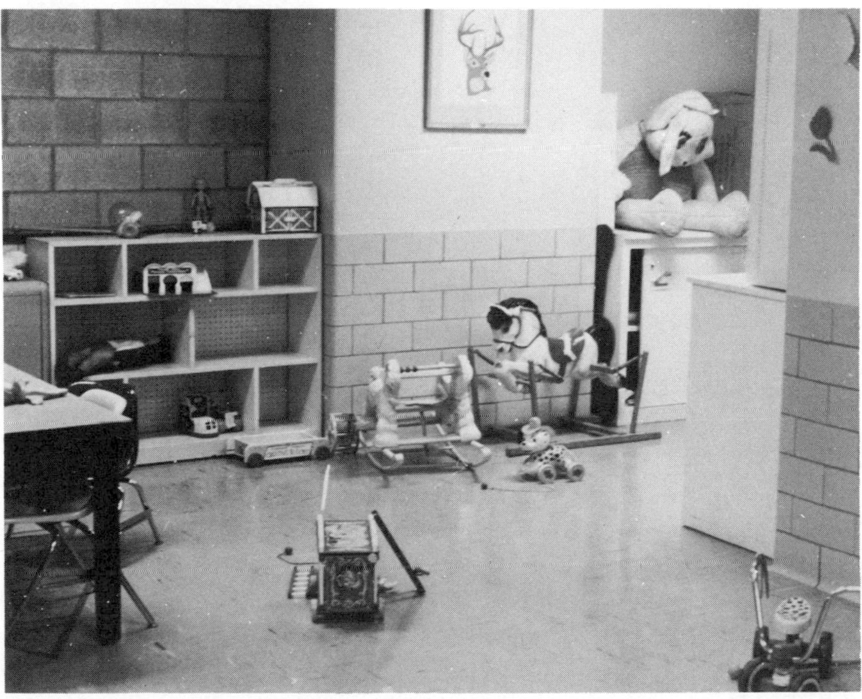

FIG. 16. This playroom is equipped for the toddler. Note the push-pull toys, rocking horse, low shelves, and plenty of space to move about. (Courtesy of Children's Hospital of Buffalo, New York)

If the hospital population consists entirely of children, a logical way of organizing play facilities may already exist. Patients may be grouped according to age and type of illness. In these cases, the play area on each unit can be highly individualized. An infant unit may not require separate recreational facilities, but the patient rooms should be large enough to accommodate playpens, infant swings, walkers, highchairs, and rocking chairs for use by mothers and nurses. On the other hand, recreational and play areas are extremely important on preschool units. When facility planning can focus on one age group, play materials can be scaled to the child's height and reflect his special needs (Figs. 16 and 17). Homogeneous units also ease the work of supervising adults since they can concentrate their efforts on the need of a particular age.

In most situations, however, the pediatric unit is a conglomerate of ages and illnesses. Thus the playroom will have to be very adaptable. To accommodate all, assess available space and select the largest area in the interest of flexibility. A collapsible dividing wall can make two separate play areas. One section can be enjoyed by preschool children and the other made to accom-

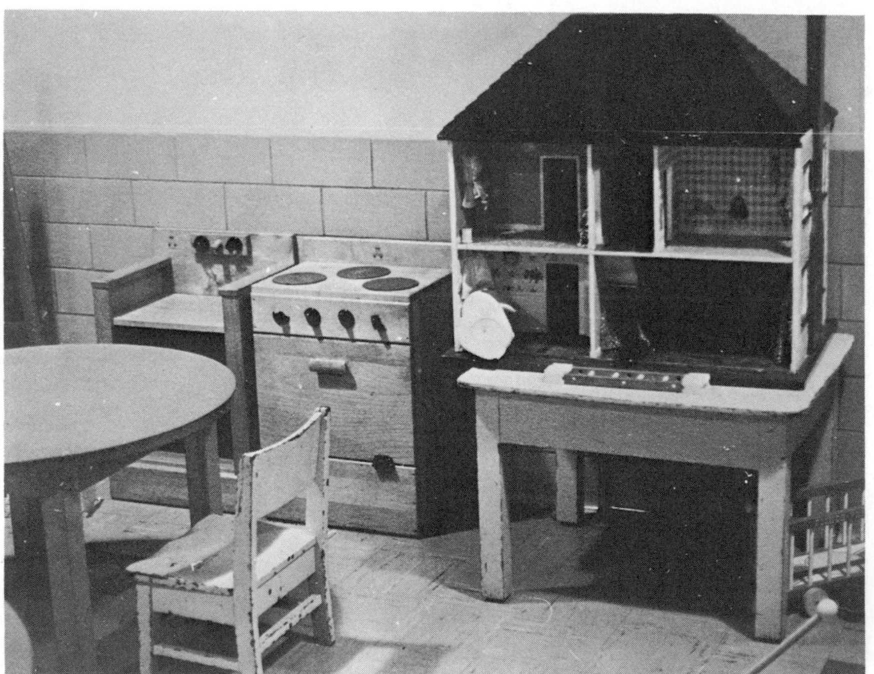

FIG. 17. The three- to six-year-old enjoys these materials. House play is readily stimulated by sturdy replicas of household furnishings. The doll house is another favorite as the child explores new roles. (Courtesy of Children's Hospital of Buffalo, New York)

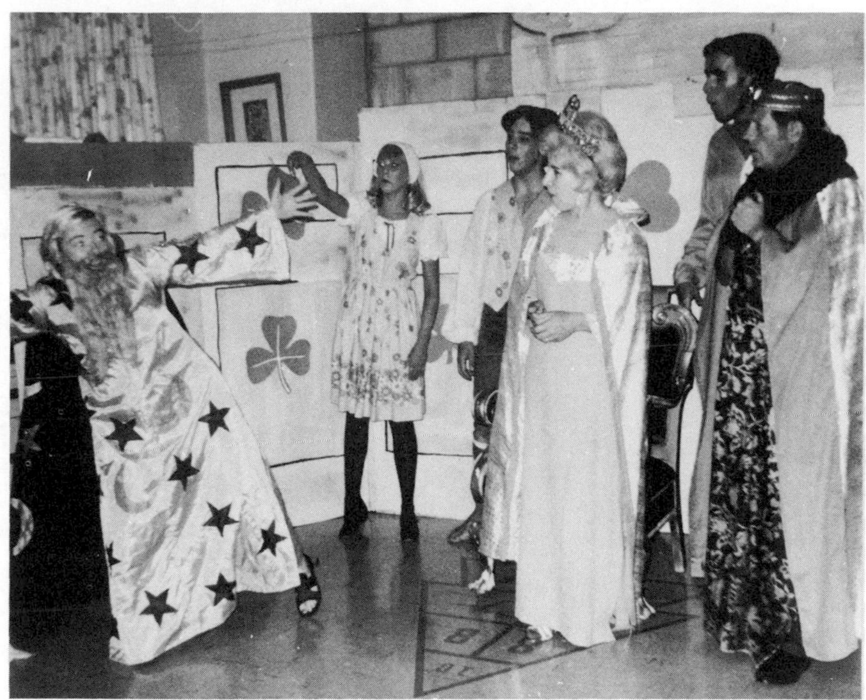

FIG. 18. A group of excited children are watching this theater troupe perform. (Hamburg Children's Theater, Hamburg, New York)

modate the older boys and girls. When necessary, the retractable wall can expand the size of the room to allow exercise of large muscles or to permit group attendance at special programs (eg, holiday parties, circus acts, or musical programs; see Figure 18).

Age of the child should be kept in mind when one is arranging the room furnishings. A possible suggestion would be to group preschool equipment on one side of the play area. The following play materials should be included: house corner (simple but sturdy wooden replicas of a stove and refrigerator, shelves, crib, small table, and chairs); a low sink or basin for water play; a stand-up sand box; a dress-up corner (with full-length mirror); a large, low table for drawing, painting, working puzzles, or other manipulative tasks; a low-hung blackboard and bulletin board; and wall easels. On the other side of the room (for the older children) arrange the following kinds of equipment: game and craft tables; a tilted table for art work; cupboards containing craft and graphic materials; record player; books and magazines; puzzles; pool table with folding removable top; comfortable lounge chairs; and cork boards. A retractable movie screen is a good addition if visual programs are likely to be planned. Recessed shelves, cupboards, and drawers make stor-

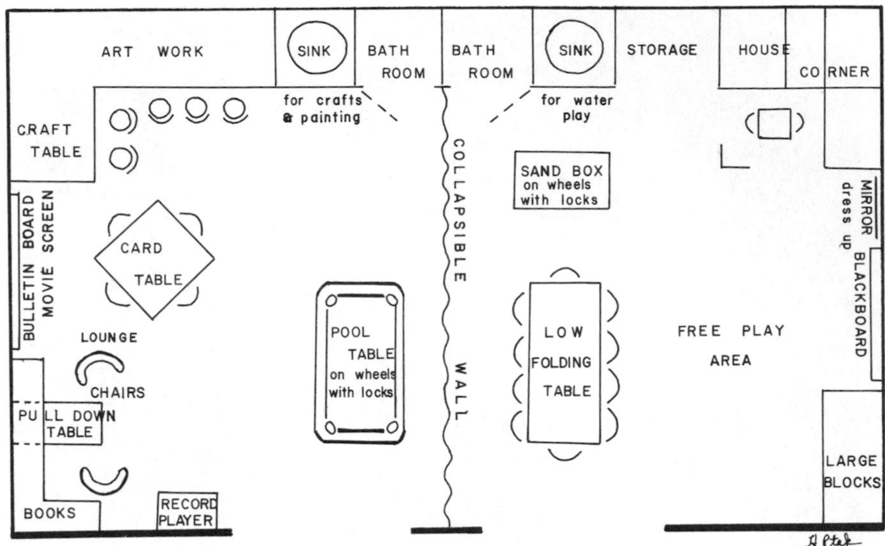

FIG. 19. Playroom designed for flexibility.

age of materials easy and keep them readily available. Running water and toilet facilities should be included in the play area. All "middle-of-the-room" equipment should be on wheels or casters with locks so that their positions can be easily rearranged to accommodate beds or carts or some special activity. Of course, doorways should be wide enough to allow passage of beds. Figure 19 illustrates how such a playroom could be arranged.

An outdoor play area, either in a courtyard or on a porch, is a great asset and every attempt should be made to plan for it. The fresh air, sunshine, and freedom of movement that outdoor play provides cannot be duplicated in any other way. Safety and comfort factors must receive proper consideration. Fencing might be in order if street traffic poses a threat; shading from the sun is also necessary especially around sand boxes and swings where children are likely to be absorbed in play for long periods.

The presence of play facilities in an agency that serves children is evidence that the administration is client-centered. It indicates to parents that the staff is concerned about the whole child. For the child with long-term illness, enjoyable play experiences may also mean that the inevitable return to the hospital or clinic may be less unpleasant (Fig. 20A and B).

ASSESSMENT OF PLAY BEHAVIOR

Part of the nurse's initial and on-going assessment of her/his patient's status should include an assessment of play behavior—a play profile. The purpose of such an assessment is to determine the kinds of play experience

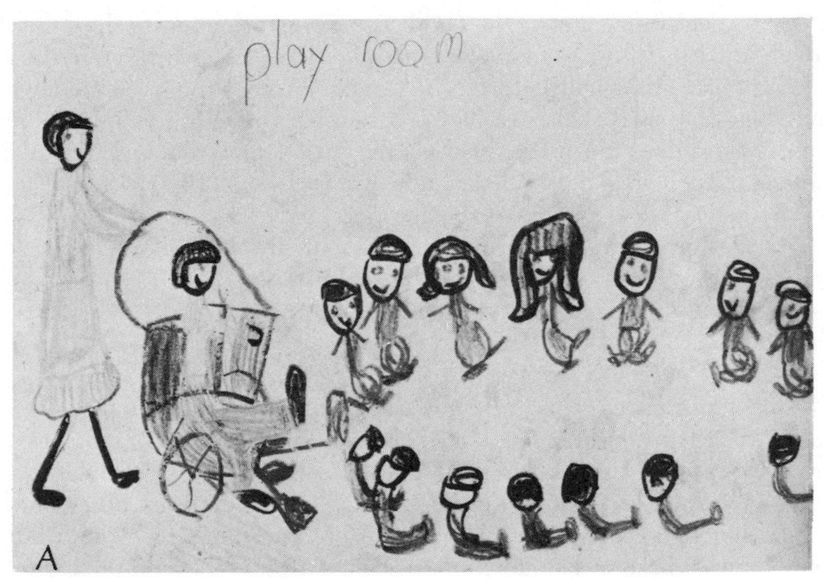

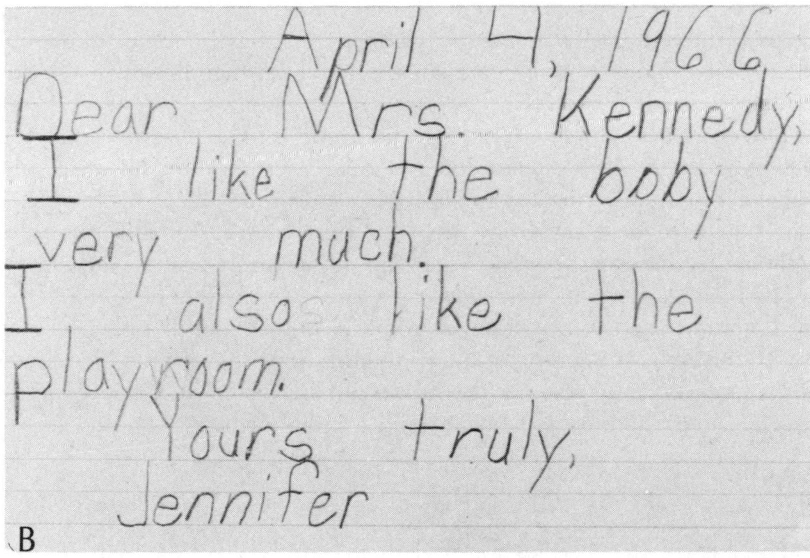

April 4, 1966
Dear Mrs. Kennedy,
I like the boby very much.
I also like the playroom.
Yours truly,
Jennifer

FIG. 20. The hospital playroom certainly impressed a six-year-old visitor. Her drawing, A, and her letter, B, reflect pleasant memories of her trip. (Courtesy of Children's Hospital of Buffalo, New York)

that have special meaning to the child. By calling attention to these needs through the use of an assessment tool, play is more clearly viewed as a significant part of the child's care. The profile becomes the basic framework around which to plan a balanced play program. A profile, of course, is merely an outline—it does not prescribe a course of action. Individual judgment, based on the collected data, must personalize each situation. Nevertheless, a good framework does provide a starting point.

What should the profile include? Essentially, the classic questions should be posed: Who, what, where, when, and how?

Who?

This question refers to the significant people in the child's play world. The answer to this question depends partly on the child's social radius. One can safely assume that the infant's play is solitary and oriented toward "taking-in" activities with the caretaker as the most significant other. However, as the child grows older, assumptions are not so reliable. The child of three or four, whose social radius still has not expanded beyond the parents, will have a play style that is quite different from the child who has a neighborhood or nursery-school reference group. Presuming that the former child will comfortably enjoy an active playroom setting may be unfair to the child and introduce more stimulation than the child can handle given the additional stress of his illness.

The child who plays with one special friend is likely to experience some separation anxiety. If the separation is a long one, something like grief might occur. I can remember talking to eight-year-old Jimmy about his friends. He said, "I hate to be away from my very best friend. We did everything together." His downcast eyes and sad expression amply conveyed the loss he felt. His feelings were intensified because the last time that he and his friend were together, the chum sustained an injury to his hand in a play accident. Now, confused by the timing of the hospitalization, Jimmy imagined himself partly responsible for the accident. He felt punished and also expressed concern about whether his friend would remember him.

What?

The answer to this question reveals the kinds of play activity and play material the child prefers. There are stages in development when children enjoy representational objects. Materials that invite sensory exploration and body movement—such as water, sand, clay, and paint—are preferred at other times. Table games become important when the child is able to think abstractly and develop his own strategies.

Comfort toys are important to maintain a feeling of security away from home. The loved teddy bear or blanket may be overlooked in the confused circumstances that attend illness. Queries about the existence of such things will assure that the child who needs these supports will have them. Knowing the materials that the child enjoys and handles with ease does not operate against the positive outcomes derived from new experiences. It seems logical that a familiar play activity, particularly as an initial experience in the hospital, would eliminate the need for the child to struggle with new problems right away. His energies are more properly directed toward resolution of problems related to his illness. Much time remains for developing new interests and skills.

There is interesting evidence, however, that contradicts this view. Gilmore (1966) studied a group of 18 children between the ages of five and nine who were hospitalized for tonsillectomy and matched them with 18 control subjects. He found that the children experiencing the anxiety of hospitalization preferred novel toys over simple ones and especially those novel toys —such as a doctor's kit, toy syringe, and stethoscope—that were relevant to the hospitalization. It appears from his study that anxious children wish to become familiar with the source of the anxiety. In additional studies to substantiate these results, Gilmore raises questions about the significance of the intensity of the anxiety. His findings suggest that a high level of anxiety does indeed cause disruption of play. Under circumstances of extreme anxiety children selected play materials that were not relevant to the source of anxiety. Perhaps, as a consequence of this study, both relevant and nonrelevant toys ought to be available from which the child can make a choice. Careful assessment of anxiety level will provide additional clues to the child's play needs.

When the child's interest in an offered play material is not immediately evident, it should not necessarily be abandoned. A so-called boring toy can become very interesting at another time or under different circumstances. Sometimes adults are disappointed about the child's response to a toy that they have presented. In an attempt to arouse interest, adults often talk to the child about what the toy can do and how the child could play with it. Trying to get interest in this way may have just the opposite effect. Zivin (1974) studied a group of five- to seven-year-olds and found that encouragement of contemplation and talk about the toy actually tended to dampen exploration of it. It seemed wiser to let the child determine his own active exploration without outside suggestions. Individual judgment in this regard must be made, however, for some children do respond favorably to adult suggestions about their play. A sensitive, balanced approach is desirable.

It is quite conceivable that the thing that a child cherishes most is a pet. He may feel so responsible for its care that he fears for the animal's well-being in his absence. If the animal is a dog or cat or other large animal it is generally not feasible to house the pet in the hospital. (I know of some exceptions to this rule—so do not overlook it as a solution to a grave separation problem.) However, when the pet is a turtle, fish, or hamster, the child may be able to continue to care for it. On the other hand, children who do not have pets at home can really enjoy an introduction to pet care. They enjoy the responsibility and it directs them away from total preoccupation with themselves. (Hospital research laboratories can be resources for interesting pets.) Whenever animals become part of the child's care, be sure that you know how to care for them in the hospital setting. Have the parents write down food, air, and water requirements or consult with a local pet shop. There is little to be gained from complicating the situation by a high rate of animal mortality!

Where?

Where the child customarily plays is an important consideration, too. If the illness or hospitalization is preceded by play activities that are expansive outdoor experiences, the child can be expected to have more difficulty in adjusting to the confinements of a hospital room than a child who generally plays indoors in a small apartment. How much a child is permitted to do in bed at home is another factor not often considered. The bed is frequently off-limits for eating and playing certain kinds of games. A child who seems restrained in his play may simply be reflecting his discomfort over interpretation of his mother's command at home, "Don't use paints on the bed." Such inadvertent conflicts are important to many children but especially those who are accustomed to strict limits at home. The child has no experience by which to judge his mother's response if she should find him painting in the hospital bed.

When?

The child organizes his play periods into a schedule that is satisfying for him. His routine is a reflection of many things—the arrangement of activities of daily living in his home, availability of facilities for play, and his own physical need for a balance between rest and activity. The daily morning trip to the neighborhood playground may be sorely missed. A trip in the wheelchair to see the day-by-day changes in a window box flower garden can be an exciting adventure for such a child. Certainly, the parents and the nurse ought to be keenly aware of the child's view of important routines.

The young child times his activities according to tangible events —things happen after breakfast, before dinner, when daddy comes home, or when it gets dark outside. He is not ordered by the clock. The hospital rest period may not coincide with his plan. His after-lunch activity may consist of a romp outdoors, so that he is not inclined to settle in to a new routine without some restlessness and anger.

Bedtime play rituals are also a meaningful part of the child's day. Sleep ends the day's events and the child approaches nighttime either excited by the good things that happened to him or worried and puzzled by events that had unfavorable outcomes. Loneliness overcomes some children and they often have exaggerated responses to strange noises, shadows, and even the sound of their own heartbeats. As a result there may be a reluctance to leave the state of wakefulness. Illness and the strange environment of the hospital compound and intensify feelings at the hour of sleep. Unfortunately, many hospitals require that parents leave at this time. Consequently, not only does the child have to cope with bedtime problems, but he often has to cope with them alone. Parents should be encouraged to stay with their young children until they are sleeping, but care must be taken to avoid deluding the child that parents will remain all night. The nurse must be careful to find out from the parents whether the child expressed special concerns so that she can be better prepared to help him cope. I have found that the nurse's attention to a child at bedtime is well spent. She can help the child give

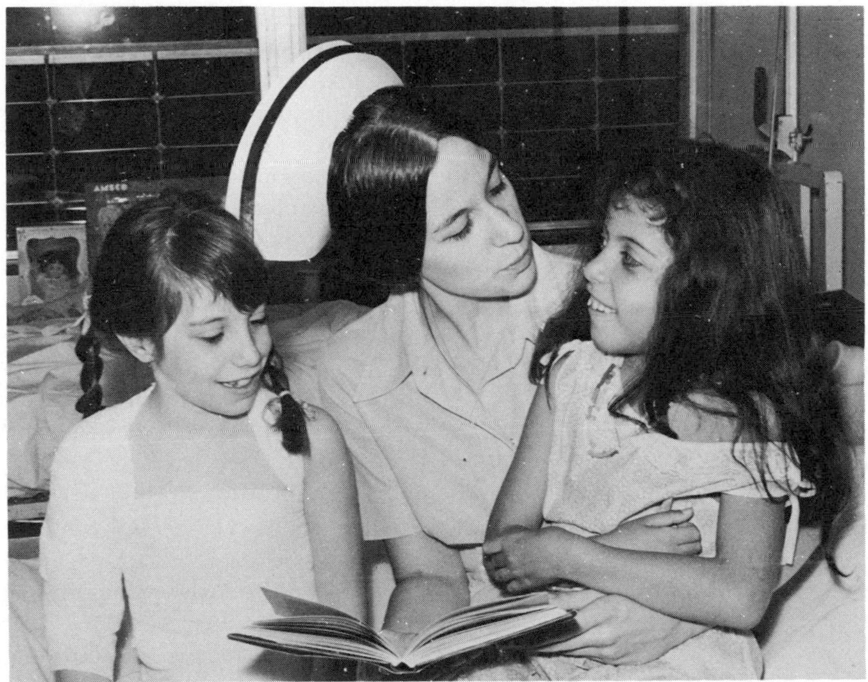

FIG. 21. A bedtime story is a good close to a busy day. These girls felt a special "closeness" to their nurse for she had just prepared them for surgery scheduled the next day. They appreciated the warmth of her attention. (Incidentally, this nurse's uniform is especially appealing to her young patients—it is bright orange!)

expression to his concerns. Children seem to be psychologically more vulnerable and open at night than during the daytime. Since there are fewer external distractions the child turns inward and fantasies and worries are reawakened. The understanding nurse who tucks the child in, listens to his prayers, reads a good-night story, or sings a lullaby is in a good position to uncover fears and answer sensitive questions (Fig. 21). A teenage girl that I cared for reversed the usual circumstances and sang to me at bedtime. She had a very pleasing voice but was self-conscious about displaying her talent in front of a group. At night as I was readying her for bed, she would relax and sing. Her songs were rich with meaning. She composed many of the lyrics herself and set them to popular folk tunes. For her it was an important expressive outlet. Then, after her song she would always ask, "Do you know why I sang that?" and would launch us into a conversation about a wide variety of topics. Among other things, we discussed the meaning of love, her maturing body, and her great fascination with horses.

How?

Every child has his own style of play. Some children have a rich imagination. Their minds are so fertile with their own ideas that they are completely absorbed and cannot include other children until they have worked out their thoughts. Often these children move from one activity to another because one stimulus quickly sparks an idea for a new project. Other children perceive more slowly and can derive satisfaction from repetitive use of simple materials. They may approach new situations with timidity and thus may not take much initiative in determining their own play activities. These youngsters may need considerable support and direct approval of their activities until they feel confident enough to fully enjoy them.

Temperament is certainly a factor in style of play. For some children emotional arousal comes easy; these youngsters are often quick to react and to show aggressive behavior. They may show impatience with their inability to implement all of their ideas and express anger toward themselves and others.

Children explore their environment in many ways. A child may approach it visually first; then after the situation is surveyed carefully and he feels competent to explore more directly he might reach out to touch the people or objects. On the other hand, there are children who rush headlong into the situation only to find through trial and error that they may have acted too hastily. The first child needs encouragement and warm approval so that he can better "discover" himself and his surroundings; the other child needs help in limit setting so that he can delay his gratification in the interest of his own safety. In any event, these styles must be reckoned with so that wasteful effort will not be expended trying to fit a round peg into a square hole.

Use of a Play Profile

A play profile can be employed as an assessment tool at all stages of the child's illness—at the time of admission to the hospital, periodically throughout the hospital stay, at the time of discharge, and during convalescence. The profile obtained at time of admission resembles a history of information about play behavior at home as described by parents and the child. It is important to remember that this history provides only baseline data and therefore should not give a sense of finality to expected play behavior. The admission play profile is a guide for initial nursing intervention.

After the profile is determined, a plan for play is developed jointly by the parents, child, and nurse. The plan is implemented and the child's response to it is recorded. Observation of the child's behavior may validate the nurse's expectations or it may indicate that the play program needs modification.

It is a well-known fact that play behavior will change as the child's condition either improves or deteriorates. Change in play may result from the child's increasing maturation as he grows older. This is particularly significant when children are hospitalized for a period of months. Play behavior may also reflect everyday experiences as well as special hospital events such as surgery or transfer to another unit. Consequently, the play profile should be reassessed periodically during the hospitalization. The revised profile is not derived from a history-taking process, but from the nurse's own observations of the child at play. Others who have participated in the child's play add their contributions as well. The nurse then compares the new observations with the previous profile. He/she may find that a child who manifested aggressive behavior at the time of admission is now tending to withdraw from social contacts. The circumstances surrounding this behavior will need careful interpretation and play stimuli may need to be altered to encourage more free expression. A reassessment of an infant's play experience might reveal that an infant hospitalized for one month has gained sufficient eye-hand skill to benefit from block play. The profile in many such instances can become a tool that draws attention to the subtle clues that indicate learning readiness.

While the child is in the hospital, the profile should be available to all who care for him. Persons (including the parents) who have significant information about the child's play should be encouraged to make notations. Productive ideas can be lost through ineffective communication. Someone's good idea can generate many new ways of approaching a particular problem. However, to avoid a hodgepodge of information, some one person—such as the team leader—should oversee the plan and coordinate activities. It should be her/his special responsibility to see that play becomes a meaningful part of nursing care. Realistically, this nurse cannot note the play behavior of all of his/her young patients. It is not necessary that he/she do so. If members of the nursing team are knowledgeable about how to encourage ordinary play and what to observe about it, the team leader can direct attention to those high-risk children who are more likely to have potential play problems. These youngsters could be categorized into four major groups.

In the first group are those children who have a developmental lag or are mentally superior. The nature and quantity of stimuli will be quite different for these children since they must keep pace with the child's maturational readiness rather than chronological age. A second group would consist of children who demonstrate psychosocial limitations in the style of their play. These children will benefit from carefully selected play materials that specifically encourage energy release as well as interpersonal contacts that reflect awareness of the child's defense mechanisms. Children who have had or who are about to experience stressful situations comprise the third group. Play can serve as an excellent tool to prepare a child for an unpleasant event and, of course, the content of play afterwards may reveal feelings about the experience that cannot be expressed in other ways. A fourth high-risk group are those children with kinds of physical disabilities that could be improved through the judicious use of play. For example, the spastic hands of an infant with cerebral palsy might open more easily if the infant can support his weight in a prone position. Placing toys within reach or hanging a jingly mobile in his view will add to his enjoyment and encourage him to sustain the prone position.

Since these children have such special play needs, the nurse must rely on other members of the health team for guidance in selecting effective methods of stimulation. The occupational, physical, and recreational therapists are important consultants. In unusual circumstances in which the child's behavior reveals a deep-seated conflict, a psychiatric consultant becomes necessary. A reciprocal relationship among the team members is essential if the child is to benefit from these people's individual talents. A meshing of goals will assure that the child will be looked at as a totality. A consistent approach must be used 24 hours a day—not just during the hours that the therapist is present.

When the child is about to leave the hospital, the play profile becomes part of the discharge plan. The content of the profile can provide practical guidelines to parents as they anticipate convalescent play. The nurse can use the tool to illustrate how the child can be expected to behave at home. (More specific ways that the nurse can assist parents will follow in another section of this chapter.)

The discharge profile should not be discarded. It should become part of the child's record so that it can be used in a comparative manner when the child visits the clinic or is readmitted to the hospital.

Significant information from the play profile should be included when referral is made to the community health nurse so that she/he can provide

NAME Karen E. (Kari) AGE $3\frac{1}{2}$ yrs. DIAGNOSIS Congenital Dislocation Right Hip - Cystitis

PROFILE 6/1	PLAN 6/1	RESPONSE 6/2
MATERIALS - wagon, play furniture, turtle, sunglasses, rag doll *, dress-up hat	LIMITATIONS DUE TO ILLNESS bed rest, blood drawn each morning, fatigues easily, spica cast	Sunglasses in view on bedside stand. Wears hat during all dramatic play. In doll play, child doll frequently punished by doctor doll - only verbally. Very absorbed in this play.
PARTNERS - parents, occasional contact with same age cousins	Father to bring in sunglasses and hat	
PLAY AREA - backyard, kitchen, bedroom (restricted in other areas of house)	Wooden blocks and miniature doll play (while prone) - use doctor, nurse, child figures	Dabbed in paints with finger tips wanted painting saved for mother
STYLE - timid, watches others, not an easy joiner, long attention span, solitary play	Finger painting Play with one agemate (Linda)	Parallel play with Linda - no verbal communication
SCHEDULE - plays midmorning, early afternoon, 2 hr. nap between 2 and 4 P.M., needs quiet time before meals	Water play during bath (plastic cover for cast) Rest period in AM Story or puzzle before meals	Loves *Magic Bunny* story
BEDTIME - prayers, rag doll in bed, sleeps in prone position (head of bed elevated)	Bedtime prayers Rag doll in easy reach	Wants nurse to pray with her - 'Now I Lay Me Down to Sleep' Goes to sleep quickly - mother not present
MISC.		
* CHILD HAS ITEM IN HOSPITAL		
ADMISSION PLAY PROFILE	INITIAL PLAN FOR PLAY	RESPONSE TO PLAY

FIG. 22. See text for explanation.

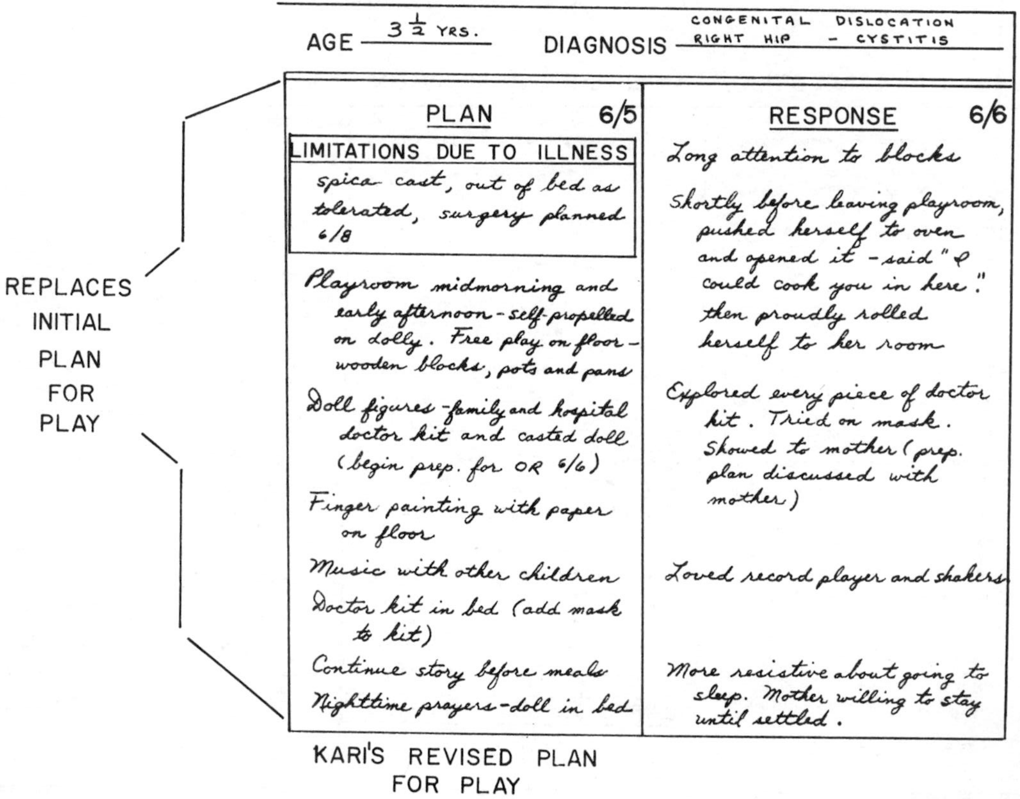

AGE 3 ½ YRS.   DIAGNOSIS CONGENITAL DISLOCATION RIGHT HIP – CYSTITIS

PLAN 6/5	RESPONSE 6/6
LIMITATIONS DUE TO ILLNESS: spica cast, out of bed as tolerated, surgery planned 6/8	Long attention to blocks
Playroom midmorning and early afternoon – self-propelled on dolly. Free play on floor – wooden blocks, pots and pans	Shortly before leaving playroom, pushed herself to oven and opened it – said "I could cook you in here." then proudly rolled herself to her room
Doll figures – family and hospital doctor kit and casted doll (begin prep. for OR 6/6)	Explored every piece of doctor kit. Tried on mask. Showed to mother (prep. plan discussed with mother)
Finger painting with paper on floor	
Music with other children	Loved record player and shakers.
Doctor kit in bed (add mask to kit)	
Continue story before meals	More resistive about going to sleep. Mother willing to stay until settled.
Nighttime prayers – doll in bed	

REPLACES INITIAL PLAN FOR PLAY

KARI'S REVISED PLAN FOR PLAY

FIG. 23. See text for explanation.

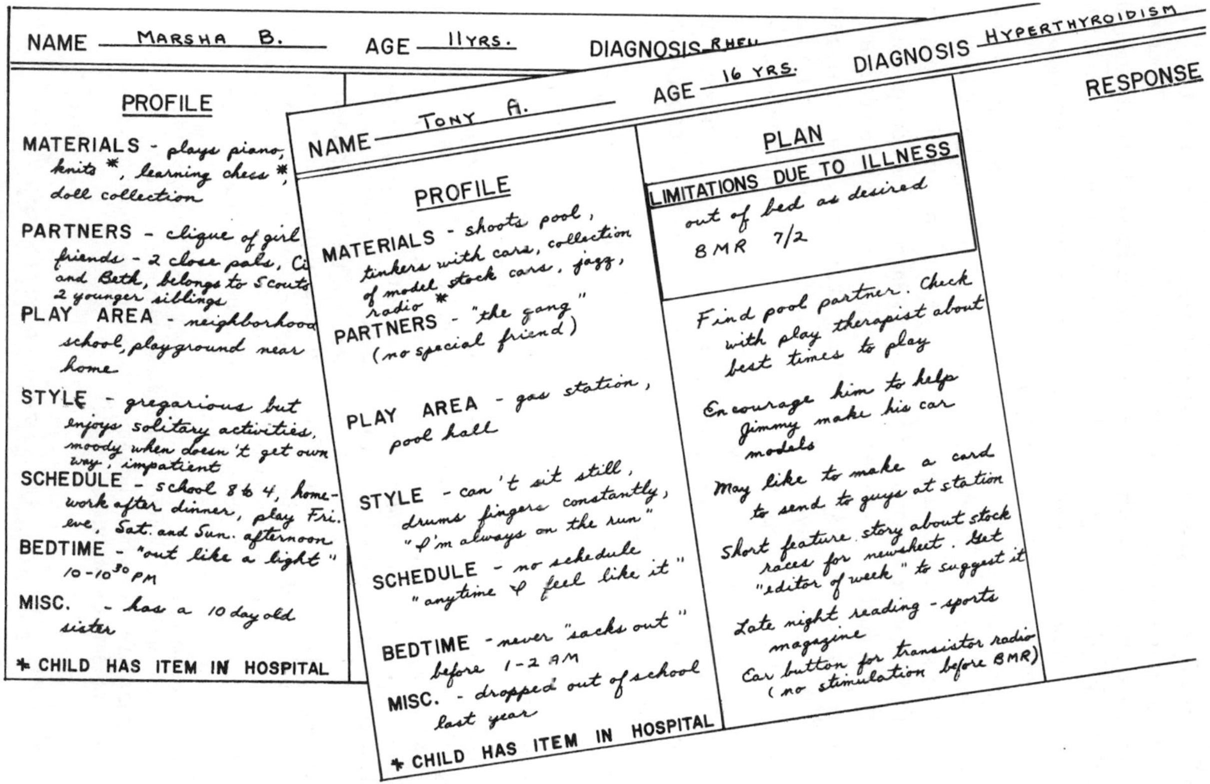

NAME MARSHA B. AGE 11 YRS. DIAGNOSIS RHEU…

PROFILE

MATERIALS - plays piano, knits *, learning chess *, doll collection

PARTNERS - clique of girl friends - 2 close pals, C… and Beth, belongs to Scouts, 2 younger siblings

PLAY AREA - neighborhood school, playground near home

STYLE - gregarious but enjoys solitary activities, moody when doesn't get own way, impatient

SCHEDULE - school 8 to 4, homework after dinner, play Fri. eve, Sat. and Sun. afternoon

BEDTIME - "out like a light" 10-10^{30} PM

MISC. - has a 10 day old sister

* CHILD HAS ITEM IN HOSPITAL

NAME TONY A. AGE 16 YRS. DIAGNOSIS HYPERTHYROIDISM

PROFILE

MATERIALS - shoots pool, tinkers with cars, collection of model stock cars, jazz, radio *

PARTNERS - "the gang" (no special friend)

PLAY AREA - gas station, pool hall

STYLE - can't sit still, drums fingers constantly, "I'm always on the run"

SCHEDULE - no schedule "anytime I feel like it"

BEDTIME - never "sacks out" before 1-2 AM

MISC. - dropped out of school last year

* CHILD HAS ITEM IN HOSPITAL

PLAN

LIMITATIONS DUE TO ILLNESS

out of bed as desired

BMR 7/2

Find pool partner. Check with play therapist about best times to play

Encourage him to help Jimmy make his car models

May like to make a card to send to guys at station

Short feature story about stock races for newsheet. Get "editor of week" to suggest it

Late night reading - sports magazine

Car button for transistor radio (no stimulation before BMR)

RESPONSE

FIG. 24. See text for explanation.

continuity in the constructive use of play for a particular child. The community health nurse is in the enviable position of seeing the child in the home environment, where she/he can assess resources and suggest reasonable improvisations. She/he can encourage the parents, and the child if he is old enough, to compile their own profile periodically. If the whole family takes a purposeful look at play activities, their collective creativity will certainly enrich the sick child's experiences. If and when the child returns to the hospital for continued treatment, the community health nurse offers input to the admission profile—in effect, the cycle repeats itself.

The precise format of the assessment tool is not essential to its success. Many different styles can be effectively used. The nursing staff should develop a tool to suit their own needs, the needs of the specific pediatric population that they are serving, and the needs of their particular agency. The format that is devised, however, should reflect consideration of conciseness in recording and an easy way of making changes in plans whenever necessary. If the tool is highly complicated or too time-consuming for practical use, its benefits are not appreciated. And, of course, experience dictates that when an idea fails it takes doubly long to generate enthusiasm to revive it. Assessment and planning of play experiences can easily be incorporated within the general admission assessment process as well as becoming part of the ongoing revision in the plan for care.

For purposes of illustration, consider the following situation:

Karen E., better known as Kari, was admitted to the pediatric unit for an open reduction of a congenitally dislocated hip that had responded poorly to conservative treatment. This 3½-year-old girl had been in a double-leg cast for three months prior to the admission. On the day following her arrival in the hospital, Kari developed symptoms of cystitis. The anticipated surgery was delayed until recovery from the urinary tract infection was complete. Kari was an only child who lived with her parents in an isolated rural area. Her mother stayed in a nearby motel to be with her during the hospitalization. Her favored play materials at the time of admission were a rag doll that she brought with her and a pair of green sunglasses that her grandmother had given her the week before. Unfortunately, the glasses were forgotten in the excitement of coming to the hospital. Her father brought along the low, wheeled platform that he had constructed so that Kari could scoot easily around the house. Figure 22 is the admission play profile, the initial plan for play, and Kari's response. The revised plan based on the same profile but reflecting her changing needs is illustrated in Figure 23. (Figure 24 shows how the same basic format can be adapted to suit the needs of children of different ages.)

PROBLEMS OF IMMOBILITY

Some restriction in normal activity is witnessed during the treatment of many long-term illnesses in childhood. For some children, restriction may be minimal, requiring only additional rest periods. Other boys and girls

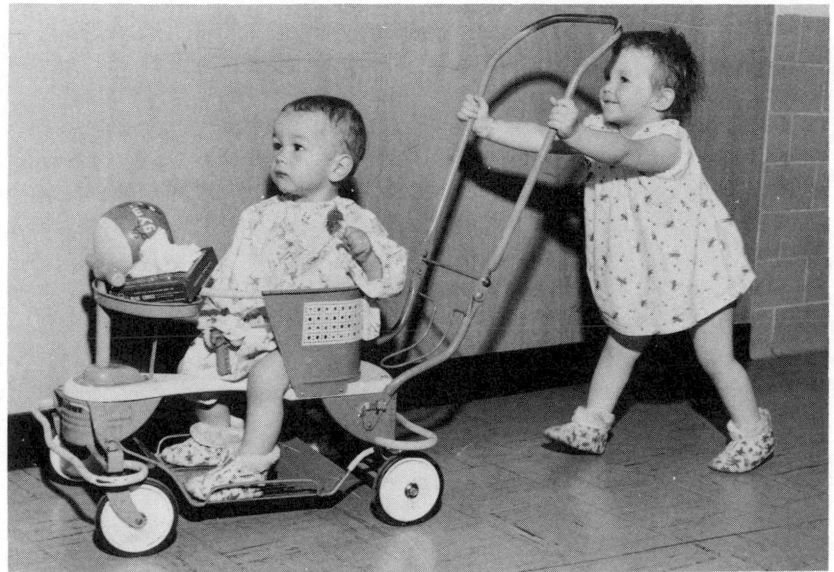

FIG. 25. The expression on this toddler's face reveals the excitement that freedom of mobility arouses. (Courtesy of Children's Hospital of Buffalo, New York)

experience complete change from the customary way of living due to prolonged periods of bed rest or complete immobilization of part of the body.

Freedom of body movement has special significance during every stage of childhood. The infant responds to internal stirrings by random but satisfying body movements. It is a great achievement for the toddler to assume an upright posture (Fig. 25). The preschool child uses his body as a primary mode of expressing his feelings. The school-age child concentrates on precision and skill in manipulation and locomotion activities through which he gains acceptance in his peer group. The adolescent heartily applauds competitive sports which demand speed and agility. Thus many measures of personal achievement and self-satisfaction are derived from one's ability to move about without constraint.

Curtailment of activity introduces a high degree of frustration. Feelings of helplessness and rage are common accompaniments. The thwarting of the biologic urge for activity is a highly charged situation from an emotional point of view. Several factors contribute to this emotional upheaval.

Physical constraint brings with it enforced dependency. The child's feelings may be quite ambivalent. Since he is ill, he knows that his own resources are inadequate to meet his needs, yet he will fight vigorously to retain his autonomy. The threat of regression heightens anxiety and the whole cycle perpetuates itself. The child worries about this dependency. The specific worry varies a great deal from one child to another. Some children may be concerned about not being able to play; others worry about such practical matters as who will bring their food. I can recall several older children confined in body casts who expressed sophisticated concern about their safety. They queried, "What will happen to me if this place burns down? How can I get out?"

The child who is immobilized is in a very vulnerable position. He cannot remove himself to a more protected environment. At times he may be able to do no more than turn his face toward the wall. He cannot fight to retain what he thinks is his. Indeed, he is in a precarious spot. The significant elements of power and self-control that mobility brings are notably undermined by restraint.

One primary function of movement is self-expression, and for the child who is immobilized this avenue of expression is limited. Physical activity is often an acceptable and satisfying way of "letting off steam." The "jumping for joy" phenomenon is well known. Curtailed from this kind of expression, the child who is immobilized must rely on language to express strong emotions. Depending on the child's age, this might be a rather inefficient system of communication. For example, the preschool child finds himself in a special predicament because his language skills are not well developed. Under ordinary circumstances the child in the preverbal stage helps himself by reverting to physical forms of acting out his frustrations—he stomps, bites, and kicks. He is simply not sophisticated enough to express strong emotions verbally. Consequently, not only does the immobilization impose a physical restriction on him but there are verbal restraints as well.

Immobility may be accompanied by social isolation. Social experiences differ in kind and duration. These children have greater difficulty seeking out friends and are restricted in the degree to which they are physically able to participate in group activities. Their social contacts are often limited to those who take the initiative to visit them. The duration of their friendships is subject to chance. Discharge from the hospital, transfer to other units, and occasionally death may intervene to sever social ties.

These are just a few of many reasons why play is an essential aspect of care for these youngsters. Play for these children should aim to satisfy their need for an expressive outlet. In this section, I will explore use of art, music, and storytelling—all of which can be enjoyed by children whose physical mobility is limited. Of course, any child may find these activities stimulating and fulfilling.

Art

Art is an excellent method of widening the range of human experiences and, at the same time, it demands exercise of a motor skill. Children's art is being studied with increasing interest—both in terms of its form and its content (Alschuler and Hattwick, 1947; Dennis, 1966; Kellog, 1967; Di Leo, 1970). Although the artistic endeavors of children can be quite revealing, accurate interpretation of symbolic content is a complex matter requiring specialized educational preparation. I wish to emphasize the "feeling" outcomes derived from the process of painting.

Painting and drawing require only the simplest of materials, but the use of them brings rich rewards. An observer of a child engaged in some form of art will note expressions of joy, rhythm, vitality, and relaxation. In addition to these emotional outcomes, the colors, textures, and shapes that characterize the child's work all contribute to perceptual development. Painting with sponges, string, or cotton swabs teaches the child that there are many ways to apply paint. Forming images in the three-dimensional medium of wet, water-based clay is another avenue through which the child can shape an idea. In any event, the child derives much learning and much pleasure in shaping his piece of art.

For the very young child, the crayons, paint, plain paper, and brushes are objects to explore and nothing more. It is fun to try out new experiences. 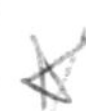 Di Leo (1970) calls this the kinesthetic stage. It is the muscular element that predominates in the scribbling done by the young child. The scribbler is not trying to give us insight into his conflicts, but rather is interested in transferring body movements to paper. That is why the nurse should expect the young child to paint his hands and apron as well as the paper or repeatedly to stab the brush into the paint just to make a splash. The very young child is not able to draw a representational object. He is helplessly confused and discouraged by the nurse whose first question is: "What is that?" The child is not being coy by refusing to answer; he doesn't know what it is either! By rewarding only drawings that conform to adult standards of excellence, the nurse is imposing a mental restriction just as confining as the immobilization itself.

Later, in the preschool period, a child's painting may reflect emotions that cannot yet be translated into words. Painting can provide emotional release without weakening defenses. It is not unusual for a shy, inhibited child to show much more expression during painting sessions than is evident during other activities. The child who is angry or resentful about his confinement can use art as a means of expressing his discontent. Art serves as a good catharsis and permits him to advance to more mature forms of behavior (Fig. 26A and B).

Not every child will respond to the media in the same way. Take finger painting as an example. As you well know, some children literally put their whole selves into the art. Other children are anxious to wash their "dirty" hands. It is conceivable that such a difference in response may not reflect a deep-seated psychologic problem on the part of the more inhibited child, but rather may simply be a function of the child's social environment. Reac-

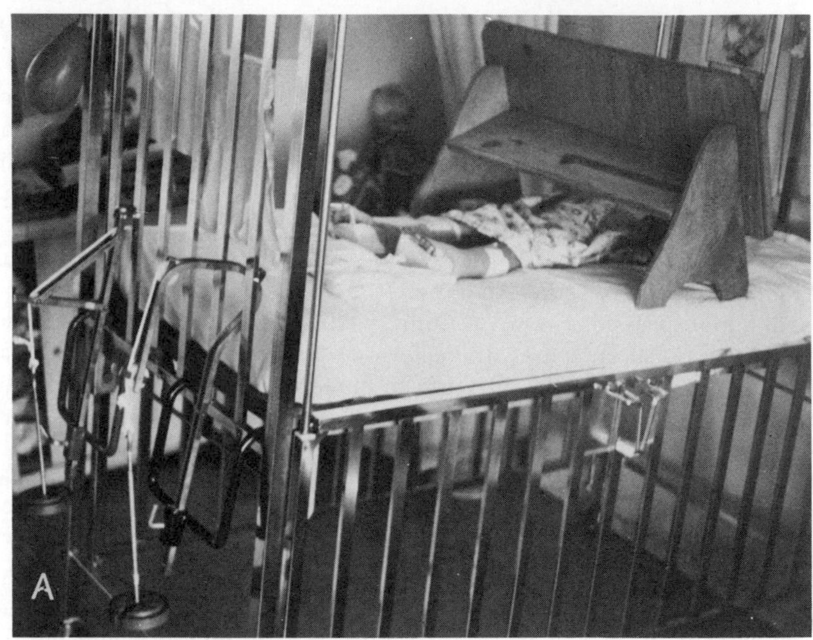

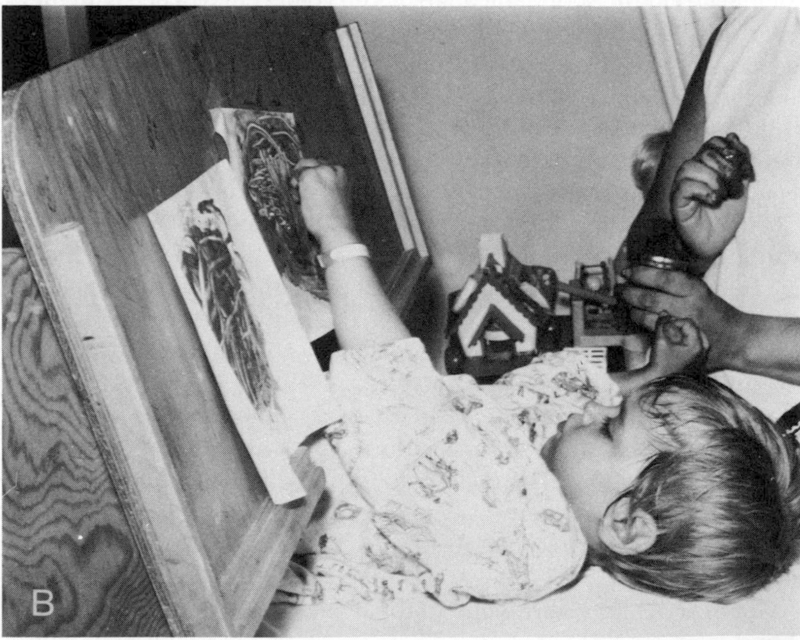

FIG. 26A. This child is hiding behind a tilted table that provides a convenient play surface for an immobilized child. **B.** On the other side of this table, an artist is at work. Still clutching her mother's finger with one hand, she is gradually "moving out" to express herself in green paint.

tion to finger painting was studied in a small sample of middle- and lower-class children (Alper, 1955). The middle-class children showed a lower tolerance for getting dirty, for staying dirty, and for products they produced while they were dirty. They took a longer time to select colors of paint and to begin painting and tended to mutilate their paintings more than did the group of lower-class children. This study reminds us to be aware that not all children have the same degree of enthusiasm about commonly used play materials. Some children will need a longer warm-up period before they can utilize the media's full potential. If the child is hesitant to dip his fingers into paint, he can be encouraged to spread his paint with a brush at first. The greater distance between the child and the paint may permit him to become accustomed to the messy paint more gradually.

The school-age child has special characteristics that favor the use of graphic materials. He is capable of concentrated effort and has good mastery of the media (Fig. 27). Yet, since defenses are not fully established, painting may reveal conflicts as the children tell their stories. Often, however, the children are self-protective enough to describe their stories in disguised forms. Since the older child has a better understanding of the use of a variety

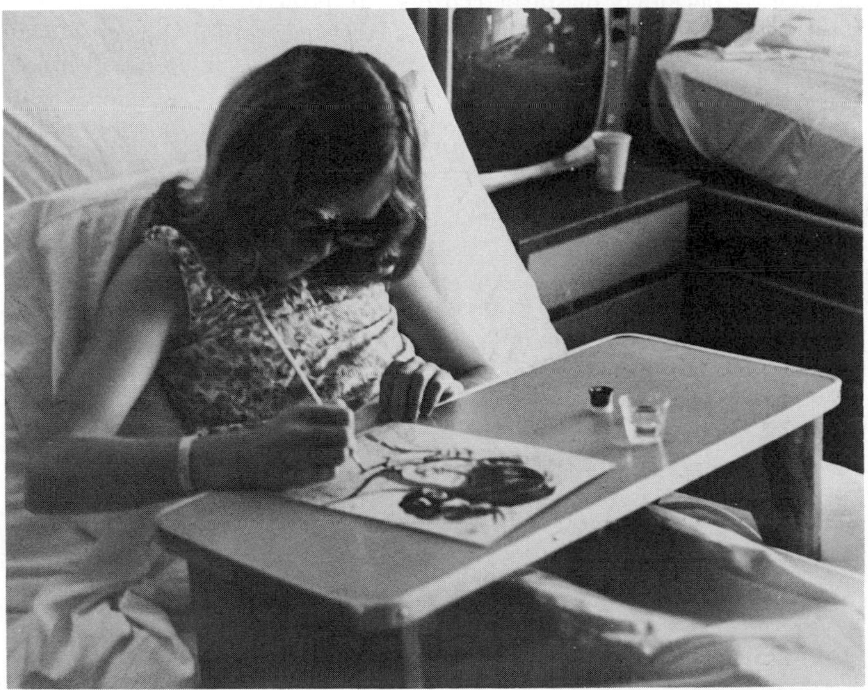

FIG. 27. The art of concentration. The fine detail of her work is satisfying to this adolescent who places a high premium on the quality of the finished product.

of materials, he should be encouraged to try more sophisticated graphic techniques such as collage and papier maché.

Art can be a good medium for social interaction. Children have a feel for each other's art and, when painting together, they can express their understanding verbally and nonverbally. Preschool children thoroughly enjoy painting with each other. They will often pause in their work to intently watch the actions of other "artists." Putting an easel on a cart between two beds stimulates verbal as well as motor activity.

Regardless of a child's age, one should remember that the child is not limited to painting what is actually visible. He can paint what he sees, but he can also draw what he feels or knows. Try to help the child go beyond mere copying of another image. Conformity stifles creativity.

The environment for art should convey the freedom intended by the media itself. There should be ample time to allow for sufficient exploration. Many materials should be available to reflect the child's uniqueness and encourage his inventive potential. A wide variety of paint colors is not necessary for the very young child, but, with advancing age, selection of colors and experimentation with mixing them is part of the fun. A large cardboard box with a few modifications makes a lightweight but sturdy easel (Fig. 28). Inexpensive oilcloth or plastic bed covers and aprons or bibs will serve nicely as adequate protection against the "mess" that may result. Of course, some limits must be set but if they are known in advance, children will usually respect them.

The nurse should make every effort to include the art medium in play

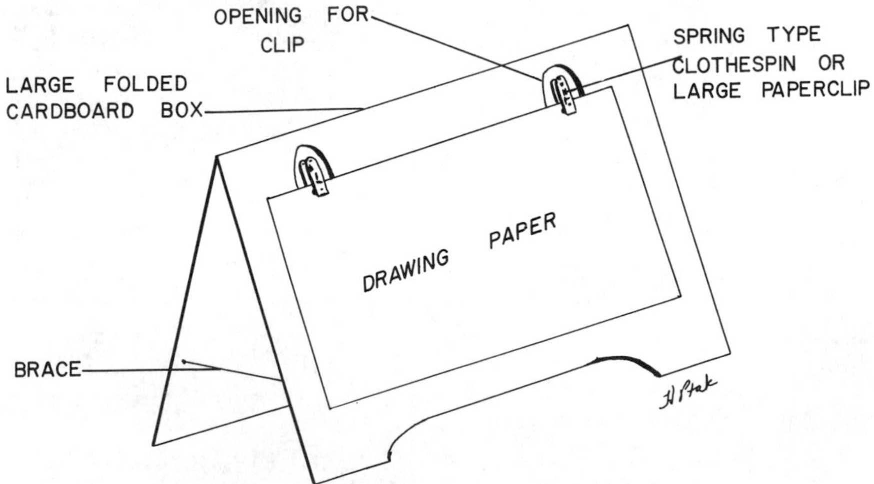

FIG. 28. This easel is so simple to construct that a pediatric unit should never be without one.

since it might be the only way that a particular child can express his feelings. Furthermore, it is a way children can acquire a sense of their own value. And besides, above all, painting is *fun!*

Music

Children who are immobilized have a special need for musical experiences; these activities, too, stimulate expansive body movements. The child can enjoy listening to music as well as making it. It has long been known that music induces relaxation in tense children and also has a beneficial effect on unhappy children. Since sick, confined children are both anxious and unhappy, this should be reason enough to provide music for them. However, there are additional benefits. Music awakens the imagination. In response to exciting band music, for instance, children can mentally move to its rhythm. If the feet or legs are immobilized, "marching arms" can be very expressive. A lilting melody can be accompanied by sweeping arm movements that simulate birds in flight. The child can add to his enjoyment by waving brightly colored silk scarves to the rhythm of the music. He not only enjoys the music, but also the tactile pleasure of the silky scarf as it flows across his face and over his body. With the stimulus of appropriate musical accompaniment, children enjoy acting like trucks, planes, and animals and, in the process, benefit from exercise, body control, and movement. Finger play like "Thumbolina" or "Inccy, Wincey Spider" are also more exciting when done to music. For the child who cannot participate in such an active way, conversational records or those with simple lyrics can be listened to with great enjoyment.

An adolescent can hardly be expected to tolerate immobilization without the aid of a stereo or radio. Keeping tempo with the beat by snapping fingers, shaking the shoulders, or wiggling the toes is a far cry from the optimum, but goes a long way toward making a bad situation somewhat manageable. Adolescents like their music loud. Unfortunately a hospital environment demands some restrictions on noise. Head sets for stereos and ear buttons for transistor radios do help this problem, but one should also consider the possibility of a music room in addition to a playroom or simply soundproofing the playroom. Even if it can accommodate only a few children it would be worthwhile. Its arrangement can be flexible enough to encompass a wide variety of uses when young musicians are not occupying it.

Music is a good stimulus for group interaction. If one patient can play an instrument, he can be the focus of a musical experience that many can enjoy. Today, a guitar is a passport anywhere. Music breaks down barriers to communication because everyone can participate in the activity in some way even if it is only to hum the melody (Fig. 29).

Musical instruments can be constructed easily. Drums and shakers can

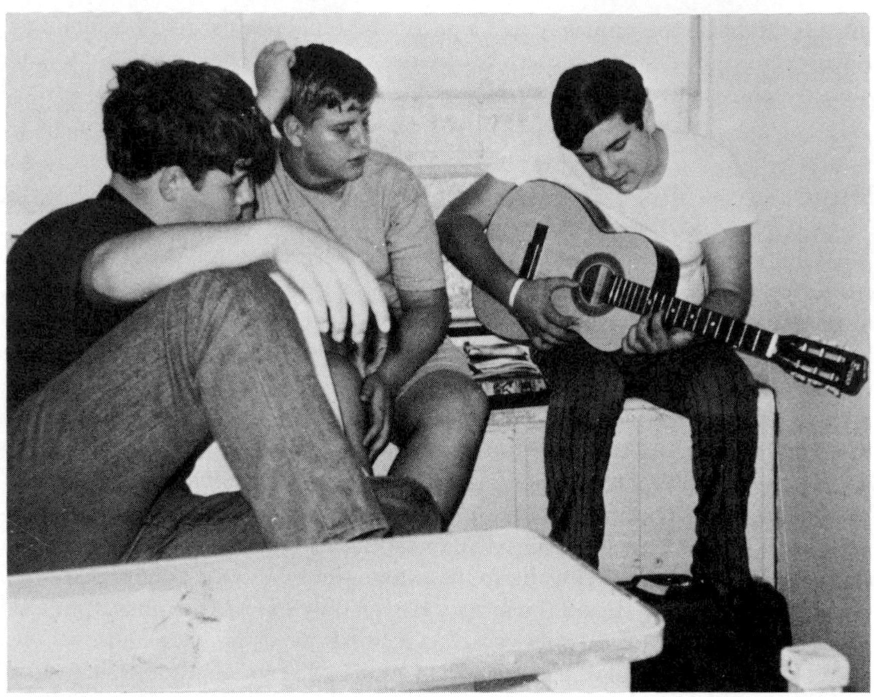

FIG. 29. These boys take their music seriously. Folk tunes can be good expressive outlets for youthful ideals and concerns.

be made out of accessible materials such as tin cans and plastic bottles. Horseshoes suspended on a cord make good cymbals. Glasses filled with varying amounts of water produce interesting sounds and teach a science lesson at the same time. Having a modest collection of "real" but inexpensive instruments may provide an opportunity for a child who has not been initiated to the world of music to find a new interest. The record collection should be varied enough to satisfy the interests that a wide range of ages will demand. Young children enjoy band music and strong rhythms with full-bodied sounds. Repetitious lyrics and melodies encourage them to join in singing. The adolescent is the pop, rock, and country and folk fan, and the library also should include a collection of these albums. Of course, most adolescents have their own collection which they can be encouraged to share with their hospital age-mates.

Give the child freedom to respond to the music in a way that seems natural for him. Occasionally some direction may be necessary, but generally most children will select a mode of expression that is peculiarly their own. They may even assume regressed but comfortable body postures and infantile activities like rocking and sucking. What is important is that the child respond in his own style.

In addition to providing the stimulus, the nurse can assist the child in another way—by her/his own active participation with the child. The child will be comfortable and more likely to throw himself into the activity if the nurse's spontaneity is evident. If she/he assumes the role of spectator, it places a restraint on the child's activity. Involvement is a key to the successful use of music.

While the points that I have mentioned have special relevance for children who are immoblized all sick children should have opportunities to enjoy experiences with art and music. A further comment about the value of these media relates to their usefulness for non-English-speaking children. These children often feel frustrated when they cannot make their needs understood. In a sense, art and music are universal languages through which they can express themselves in a manner similar to their peers. Both the nurses and the children may feel comfortable communicating via these media when the spoken word arouses confusion and anxiety.

Storytelling

One of the most enjoyable experiences of childhood is listening to stories. For the child who is ill and unable to participate fully in the usual activities of childhood, listening to stories can have special significance. It puts the child in touch with another person and encourages the child to draw upon the resources of his own imagination. The child is constantly organizing his experiences and transforming them into his concept of the world. Storytelling enhances these processes because it fosters listening, drama, and writing—all important ways of communicating human experience. The vivid, concrete imagery in a story arouses in both the reader and the listener a deeper appreciation of the world.

Storytelling also develops interest in good books, increases word recognition and understanding, and offers opportunity for oral expression. Not to be overlooked is the powerful influence stories have in molding a child's character. It is natural for children of all ages to be seeking answers to who they are. A sense of self comes from many sources—from parents, schoolmates, teachers, people in the neighborhood. Another important source is from characters in stories. When illness or disability is superimposed on normal developmental needs, much additional understanding and support are needed to give the child a sense of his own unity. Well-selected stories can do much in these situations to dispel disquieting thoughts about physical and psychologic integrity. The world of make-believe is one where the child is strong, bold, courageous, and, above all, always loved. Through stories a child can grow in his understanding of how children can feel—lonely, afraid, happy, powerful. He can come to appreciate that he is a very special person and this can be a source of great comfort to him.

Selecting the Story. If one can agree that stories are worthwhile, the next question is "How does one go about selecting good stories?" First of all, you, the reader, must really like the story. If it is something that does not appeal to you, it is very difficult to make it appealing to the listener. Assuming you like the story, the next step is to determine whether it is of interest to the child. Your understanding of the child's personal characteristics, developmental needs, and life experiences should guide the choice. Some general suggestions can be made, but it is well to remember that needs of each child are unique.

The preschool child is very much occupied with the process of self-discovery. Therefore, books that show distinction between people and animals or inanimate things are helpful. Through them the child comes to know that there are certain very special things *he* can do that the others cannot. These young children also like stories of familiar things—parents, pets, toys, animals; they enjoy hearing about children who feel angry, sad, disappointed, excited, or happy because they are trying to understand and cope with these feelings themselves. *My Book About Me* by Dr. Seuss and *Pat the Bunny* by Dorothy Kunhardt are good selections for the very young. Maurice Sendak's *Where the Wild Things Are* is a terror story built around the common fears of childhood. It helps the child to understand that bad boys are not really so bad and that their parents will still love them.

Following this period, the child comes to appreciate the somewhat less conventional story about little people who break rules, challenge authority, and in some way or other experiment with the familiar. Books like *Winnie the Pooh*, *Pinocchio*, and *Peter Rabbit* are favorites at this stage. These books mix comic elements with serious moments and help to prepare the child for the naturalism that will characterize stories at a later age.

Between the ages of six and ten, children enjoy folk tales, myths, and legends. By then they can grasp and follow a narrative. They can move from the familiar simplicity of *Jack and the Beanstalk* to the more sophisticated literary works of Andersen's *Wonder Stories Told to Children* and Perrault's *Tales for Children from Many Lands*. Later in this period, heroic stories containing moral struggles, violent emotions, and sometimes tragic endings are excellent sources of story material. The stories of Robin Hood, King Arthur, and Hiawatha are full of episodes that will deepen the child's understanding of human conflict and passion. During the school years, children can recognize the difference between the unworldly and the real, and such stories will stimulate their own creative work at a level beyond concrete understanding.

Although myths, fables, and legends will continue to interest children on into the early adolescent period, real-life story themes become important again in the teens. Children are now interested in hearing about characters very much like themselves who are coping with life's problems with courage and independence. *Avalanche* by Rutgers van der Loeff and *The Journey of Johnny Rew* by Anne Barrett are examples of stories with much appeal at this age. Poetry is often appreciated too, since romance and sentiment run high during these years.

In addition to the expected interests of the child based on developmental level, it is important that you consider the individual child's personal experiences when selecting a story. For example, if your patient is lonely without his pet, a story that focuses on kinship with animals might help him to cope with his feelings through identification with the theme of the story. He may even wish to make up his own story drawing out some of his own experiences.

Finally, in selecting a story ask yourself whether the story line is clear with an easy-to-follow sequence of events in which the characters seem alive and real. If your answer is yes, you have probably made a wise choice.

Telling the Story. Once a story is selected attention is turned to the telling of it. While every storyteller has a unique style, there are some common rules which underlie an effectively presented tale whether one is reading to one child or to a group. In the first place, the reader should know the story well so that she does not have to rely on a word-by-word reading (except when exact duplication of original narrative is essential to the meaning of the story). Both the reader and listeners should be in comfortable positions so that excessive movement, headturning, and stretching will not distract from the story. Be sure that the child (or children) can see your face, since your facial animation will express much about the action in the story. Also, for the young child, eye-to-eye contact is an important source of security. If you do need to read directly from the book, avoid burying your voice in it. Remember to use inflections and appropriate pauses and give word explanations where needed; however, the explanations should not be so lengthy that you digress from the story's primary theme. If pictures enhance the story, be sure that the child sees the picture from the proper perspective.

When introducing the story, it is generally best to get right into its action. One often hears a storyteller begin with, "This is a story about a little dog." It is preferable to capture immediate attention with something like, "I know a little dog who learned how to blow a whistle."

Use gestures when telling the story to enhance meaning and give proper emphasis to the action. Whenever possible, encourage active involvement of the children in the story itself. If the owl in the story hoots, let the children make the hooting noise themselves—you may first have to teach them how. This technique is especially good for the young child whose attention span does not permit listening for long periods of time.

By following these simple suggestions, you will be able to provide a varied and personally enriching experience for the child under your care as well as for yourself. A story can give form and depth to life's experiences in a way not duplicated by other forms of communication.

Books About Hospitalization. Children's books specifically about hospitalization are often useful in clarifying the unfamiliar routines, procedures and personnel that a child will encounter in the hospital. Books of this type can encourage expression of feelings about anticipated or past experiences. The parents and the nurse can both participate in the reading of the story and in the discussion likely to follow. The proper selection of books is most critical to a growth-producing outcome for the child. In the first place, the story should match the child's needs as closely as possible. Some books refer to specific illnesses such as appendectomies, *Linda Goes to the Hospital* by Nancy Dudley, or broken bones, *Mom! I Broke My Arm!* by Angelika Wolff. Others describe particular hospital procedures such as x-ray, *The Hospital See-Through Machine* by Nancy Cline, or anesthesia, *The Hospital Sandman* by John Welzenbach.

Secondly, the book should be appropriate to the child's reading level. If the language is too advanced, the story can be read by an adult and adapted to the child's cognitive stage. A new series of books that includes *A Hospital Story* and *About Handicaps*, both by Sara Bonnett Stein, combines large print and simple narrative for the child along with more detailed explanatory information for parents.

Lastly, the story should present a realistic picture of the hospital experience. A good book will neither ignore the unpleasant aspects of the hospital experience nor will it overdramatize them to the point of arousing needless fear. Be aware of the use of false clichés—that shots feel like mosquito bites or that ice cream tastes wonderful after a tonsillectomy. Children should not be mislead because it weakens their natural defenses and fosters distrust of hospital staff.

An annotated bibliography—prepared by Anne Altshuler—of good, quality, appealing books related to hospitalization can be found in the June 1973 newsletter of the *Association for the Care of Children in Hospitals.*

Resources. Children's books are not uniform in quality of writing style, content, or artwork. In selecting books for the library in your particular facility or unit, you may wish to refer to some source materials where quality books are listed and reviewed. Books that have been awarded the John Newbery Medal and the Caldecott Medal are especially worthwhile. These awards are made by the Children's Service Division of the American Library Association and represent the finest standards in children's literature. A source book that will acquaint the adult reader with the recipients of these and other literary awards is *Literary and Library Prizes, 8th edition* (New York, Bowker, 1973). *The Horn Book Magazine* is another useful reference. This periodical is devoted entirely to books for children and young adults. Literature is not only listed, but is reviewed and only books of the highest quality are selected.

THE NURSE, THE PARENT, AND PLAY

It has been repeatedly emphasized throughout this chapter that children enjoy play. It is a time when they are truly themselves. That parents and other family members should participate in the enjoyment of play

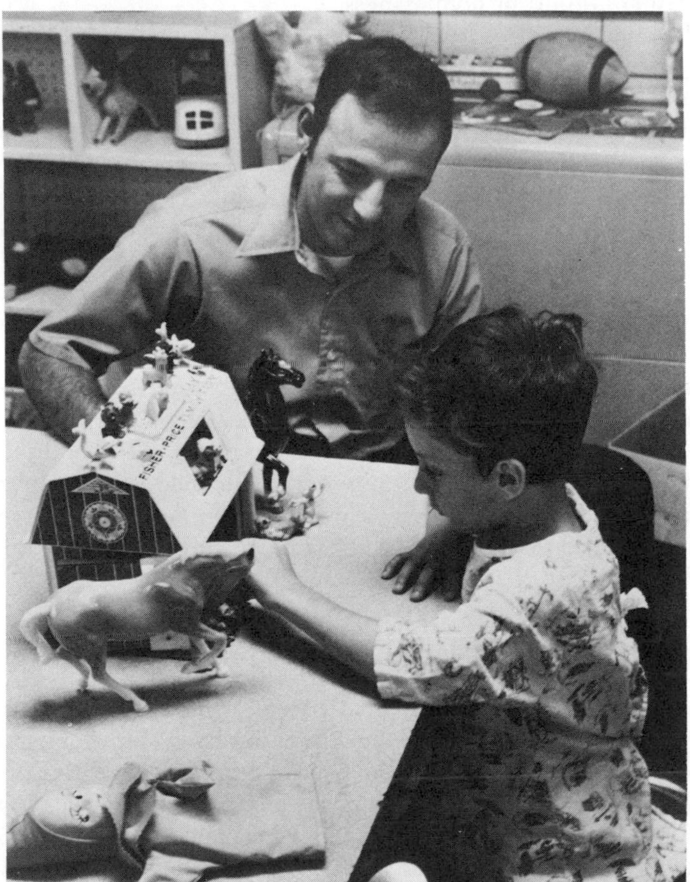

FIG. 30. Daddy is obviously enjoying this "little farmer's" play. A noninterfering, appreciative adult reinforces the child's "good feeling" about the arrangement of the animals.

should be a foregone conclusion. However, it is likewise well known that parental anxiety is increased when children are ill.

Many parental prerogatives are weakened or totally removed by the presence of an illness. Some of the components normally found in the parental role are taken on by specialized professional persons. Because so much depends on doing the "right thing," parents become increasing sensitive about the possible consequences of their actions.

For instance, they are uncertain about the limits of play. When asked about play during a clinic visit, I have heard them say, "I wasn't sure that he could do that without becoming sick again," or, "I didn't want to take any chances." This lack of confidence may indicate deeper feelings of anger, fear, disappointment, guilt, or helplessness.

If the illness is severe and has many observable signs, the parents' attention may be wholly directed towards the child's limitations. His assets, while certainly present, may be overlooked in the parents' grief and disillusionment. As a result, play deprivation may occur. The nurse can be instrumental in helping the parents evolve a positive viewpoint about play and, in so doing, revive interest in its beneficial outcomes (Fig. 30).

I wish to make pointed reference to the fact that nurses in all settings—hospital, out-patient service, and community—can provide the support that I will describe. Hopefully, the future will see more nurses moving freely among all of these settings to better coordinate the child's care. In the hospital, the nurse has the opportunity to observe play behavior over an extended period of time. The community nurse is in the position of seeing the child in his home setting where parental guidelines for play will have greatest practical significance. The clinic nurse, bridging the hospital and home, can evidence on-going interest in the child and note changes in play behavior occurring over time. Communication among these nurses is essential so that continuity in planning a meaningful play program can be achieved.

Evaluation of Play Responses

What are some of the things that parents will find helpful? Realizing that play should be fun, many ask how they can know with some assurance that the child is really enjoying his play. There are some reliable clues. Watch for facial expression and body posture. Expression reveals absorption in the activity and the child who is enjoying his play is generally relaxed and moves his body freely. Listen for verbalization during play. Children will use all avenues of expression to convey excitement and pleasure. Parents who are good listeners encourage play simply by giving a sympathetic, interested ear to the descriptions of the "great things" their children do or imagine themselves doing. Look for indications of pride in accomplishments and be alert to assure that there are more successes in play than failures. Note how much adult assistance is required. If parental presence is needed a great deal of the time, look to see whether the complexity of the activity exceeds the child's capabilities or whether it simply reflects the child's need for the personal presence of a supportive adult. If the latter explanation seems accurate, perhaps the play should be interrupted so that the parent can stay with the child for a while. This will reduce the energy expended to call someone every few minutes. A short period of undivided concentration on the child's primary concerns can provide the child just enough support and encouragement to enable him to proceed on his own to independent play. Time and effort is saved in the long-run for both child and parent. Also, note whether play is restless or aimless. This may indicate that the child is not ready to play, has too much to play with, or, possibly, too little stimulation.

Parents can expect this age-old rainy-day question from their children, "What can I do now?" The question certainly poses a challenge to parents, especially since play options will be somewhat hampered by the child's illness. Helping the parent to select play experiences that are balanced in scope is important. A bit of preplanning does not really limit the spontaneity of play. Look ahead for a month or so to see if there are any special events. Perhaps a holiday, a birthday, a visit of a relative, or a family excursion is forthcoming. The child who is ill must have his activity properly paced so that he is not stretched beyond the limits of his endurance. If one month contains a birthday and a holiday, perhaps the family excursion could be planned for a less busy time. Preplanning helps in another way, too. It provides a wellspring of ideas for play activities. If a holiday is coming, some activity to prepare for it might appeal to the child; if daddy's birthday is on the horizon, the child can make plans for the celebration or even make his "present." The parents should know that periods of quiet play should alternate with physically active play so that release of tension can be accommodated. The aspect of finding an aggressive outlet for the child often presents a major problem for parents. They do not always realize that anger, hostility, and fear are normal responses to the frustrations of illness. Materials such as clay, paint, pounding boards, and punching bags are good for draining off excess energies.

Selection of Play Materials

Criteria for selection of play materials can be useful information for the parents. Qualities of safety, durability, washability, color, and appropriate size and weight should be emphasized. Consideration of family resources must take high priority in this matter. Reasonable suggestions are fine, but unrealistic expectations are likely to meet with understandable resistance, since they make the parents feel inadequate to satisfy the child's needs. If guilt is already a problem, this merely magnifies it. Stress the idea of constructing toys from available household materials. Many parents feel that a toy is not a good one unless it comes from a toy store. Actually, simple household materials can bring many hours of delight to the child. Pots and pans, plastic bottles, spools, pieces of linoleum and rugs, sewing remnants, and discarded clothing provide endless opportunities for imaginative play. Making play materials also gives the parents something constructive to do for their child when other avenues of caring may be thwarted because of illness.

Family Participation in Play

Parents of a child with a long-term illness often need to be reminded that the child will be returning to a family. Therefore, he should have a visible role to play in family life and should share in family responsibilities. Participation in family-centered activities may require a rearrangement of space and furnishings to permit accessibility to the conduct of family affairs both indoors and out. A child who is confined to an upstairs bedroom misses a good deal of the interaction.

A child whose activity is grossly and permanently limited will place many strenuous demands on all members of the family. This child will consume an extraordinary amount of time and space and will tax the emotional reserves of the family. If serious social and economic constraints are also present, the stress is proportionately greater. However, although some of the problems will exist in the best of circumstances, satisfying outcomes can result.

Sibling acceptance of a child's disability will affect how the ill child views himself. Unless the brothers and sisters are given assistance in coping, siblings may be uncomfortable in the presence of a sick child either because of the way he looks or acts or because they are afraid of the illness itself. It is not always easy to find common interests for them to share. Yet a mutually satisfying experience is absolutely necessary for the child's integration into the family unit. The shared activity does not have to be elaborate, but all members must have significant input. For example, each of the children could select a dinner menu each week or, on occasion, the whole family could participate in preparing a meal. The bedbound child might make the placemats, shell peas, or peel the potatoes. The well child's responsibility might be the arrangement and serving of the dinner for the sick brother or sister. It can be an exciting and festive occasion with lots of opportunity for creativity for all involved. Another idea might be to have a continuing art exhibit. All the children can use graphic materials in their own way and then display them in some visible area. Paintings can be exchanged so that brothers and sisters can exhibit each other's work. This encourages appreciation of their individuality.

A child whose mental ability is grossly below that of his siblings or whose physical movements are bizarre presents an added challenge. One such child, who had cerebral palsy with multiple handicaps, was learning elements of balance and equilibrium. It was suggested that he roll around the yard in the center of a large cylinder. His brother and sister really enjoyed their participation in this activity of tumbling him round and round. The child with the disability obviously enjoyed the fun and the siblings felt satisfied that they were a part of his laughter. Family members themselves may come up with many more ideas if they are encouraged to do so. Persistence in the face of discouragement pays off in this significant area of family play.

The nurse can also be instrumental in encouraging play experiences outside of the family. Peer relationships are important to children, and when close friendships have formed during a hospital stay, it might be beneficial to sustain them. Make sure that the parents are aware of the new chum and know how he can be contacted. Also, parents are not always aware that organized groups such as the Scouts and 4H clubs can adapt activities for chronically ill children. The child's participation in such groups, even though limited, is ego-supporting and socially beneficial.

Parents can be encouraged to use the assessment tool previously described. Using the listed categories as guidelines, the parents can periodically observe their child at play and when the nurse makes her visit they can describe the positive outcomes and point more clearly to the problems that still seem to exist. The use of the profile is an aid to memory and reinforces the important role that play should be assuming in the child's way of life.

Overall, it is important to realize that not all parents have an intuitive feel about children's play. They will appreciate some concrete suggestions. To be most helpful, the nurse must convey to the parents that he/she has confidence in their ability to meet the child's needs. He/she must respect their own personal resources and the sincerity of their efforts. The nurse must also be convinced about his/her own ability to offer worthwhile guidelines, but must be flexible enough not to cling tenaciously to the plan. Perhaps the most valuable contribution that he/she can make is to help the parents feel a genuine respect for the creative urge that exists in every child and for the freedom of expression that the creative urge demands. This represents the child's most important "play right."

SUMMARY

Children learn about themselves and the world in which they live through intense involvement in play. They discharge physical energy while enjoying pleasantly satisfying sensory experiences; they expand and intensify social relationships; they explore the environment while actively manipulating materials in creative ways. Play is a freely chosen activity that, above all, is fun.

Each child has a style of play that is uniquely his own. Factors such as age, past experience, degree of physical limitation, and suitability of environment influences the way in which a child plays.

When a child faces a stressful experience, such as illness or hospitalization, he can work out many of his concerns and frustrations through the medium of play. He can re-create situations that aroused anxiety under circumstances in which he has control. Play can be used in preparing a child for a new experience. And, of course, play can simply be fun-filled activities that occupy the many hours of confinement that illness implies.

The nurse who hopes to meet the physical and psychologic needs of young patients must understand the child's view of play. Play behavior becomes an important part of the nursing assessment of the young patient.

In order to satisfy the child's play needs, the nurse must know what materials the child likes to use, who his play companions are, where and when he prefers to play, and the kinds of interactions that typify his play. By learning about the child's style of play, the nurse will be able to provide a rich play environment that will be a pleasurable experience for the child and will also serve to relieve the stress of illness and hospitalization. The nurse's role extends beyond the child to include the parents since play is an ongoing activity that is useful and necessary during every stage of illness—including convalescence.

Play is a major resource for resolution of the psychologic conflicts that accompany illness. Provision of appropriate opportunities for play encourages intellectual and creative abilities that will help the child to cope with his illness in a constructive way.

If the nurse is impressed with the importance of play and sees that his/her convictions are expressed in operational terms, he/she can be instrumental in adding a dimension of enjoyment and learning to the lives of children under his/her care.

BIBLIOGRAPHY

Alper T, Blane H, Abrams B: Reactions to finger painting as a function of social class. J Soc Abnorm Psychol 51:439, 1955

Alschuler RH, Hattwick LW: Painting and Personality: A Study of Young Children. Chicago, University of Chicago Press, 1947

Altshuler A: Children's books about hospitalization. ACCH Newsletter 1:7, 1973

Ames LB, Learned J: Imaginary companions and related phenomena. J Gen Psychol 69:147, 1946

Barton PH: Play as a Tool of Nursing. Nurs Outlook 10:162, March 1962

Blake F: The Child, His Parents and the Nurse. Philadelphia, Lippincott, 1954

———: Immobilized youth—a rationale for supportive nursing intervention. Am J Nurs 69:2364, November 1969
Burns SF: Children's art: a vehicle for learning. Young Children 30:193, 1975
Caillois R: Man, Play and Games, Barash M (trans). New York, Free Press of Glencoe, 1961
Call JD: Games babies play. Psychology Today 3:34, 1970
———, Marschak M: Styles and games in infancy. J Am Acad Child Psychiatry 5:193, 1966
Caplan F, Caplan T: The Power of Play. Garden City, NY, Anchor Books, 1973
De Nevi D: Fantasy and creativity. Child and Family 6:23, 1967
Dennis W: Group Values Through Children's Drawings. New York, Wiley, 1966
———: Infant reactions to restraint, (Abridged from Trans. N.Y. Acad Sci, 2:202, 1940), in Dennis W (ed) Reading in Child Psychology, 2nd ed. Englewood Cliffs, Prentice Hall, 1963
Di Leo JH: Young Children and Their Drawings. New York, Brunner/Mazel Publishers, 1970
Erickson FH: Play interviews for four-year-old hospitalized children. Monogr Soc Res Child Dev 23(3):77, 1958
Erikson EH: Childhood and Society, 2nd ed. New York, Norton, 1963
Fink PJ, Goldman MJ, Levich MF: Art therapy—a new discipline. Pennsylvania Med 70:61, 1967
FitzGerald C, Gunter D: Creative Storytelling. Dallas, Leslie Press, 1971
Frailberg S: The Magic Years. New York, Scribner's, 1959
Friedenberg EZ: The Vanishing Adolescent. New York, Dell, 1959
Gallagher JR: Medical Care of the Adolescent, 2nd ed. New York, Appleton, 1966
Gilmore JB: Role of anxiety and cognitive factors in children's play behavior. Child Dev 37:397, 1966
Goldberg S, Lewis M: Play behavior in the year-old infant: early sex differences. Child Dev 40:21, 1969
Green C: Larry thought puppet-play "childish." But it helped him face his fears. Nurs '75 5:30, 1975
Groos K: The Play of Man. New York, D Appleton and Company, 1901
Hartley RE, Frank LK, Goldenson RM: New Play Experiences for Children. New York, Columbia University Press, 1952
———: Understanding Children's Play. New York, Columbia University Press, 1952
Hartley RE, Goldenson RM: The Complete Book of Children's Play. New York, Crowell, 1963
Havighurst RJ: Developmental Tasks and Education. New York, McKay, 1952
Herron RE, Sutton-Smith B: Child's Play. New York, Wiley, 1971
Huizinga J: Homo Ludens: A Study of the Play-Element in Culture. New York, Roy Publishers, 1950
Jersild AT: The Psychology of Adolescence, 2nd ed. New York, Macmillan, 1963
Jolly H: Play is work: the role of play for sick and healthy children. Lancet 2:487, 1969
Jones A, Buttrey J: Children and Stories. Oxford, Basil Blackwell, 1970
Josselyn IM: The Adolescent and His World. New York, Family Services Assoc of America, 1952
Kellog R: The Psychology of Children's Art. New York, Random House, 1967
Kramer E: Art Therapy in a Children's Community. Springfield, Ill, Charles C Thomas, 1958
Lewis H (ed): Child Art: The Beginnings of Self-Affirmation. Berkeley, Calif, Diablo Press, 1966
Lonie D: Playing. Med J Aust 2:745, 1974

Lowenfeld M: Play in Childhood. New York, Wiley, 1967
Marcus IM: Costume play therapy—the exploration of a method for stimulating imaginative play in older children. J Am Acad Child Psychiatry 5:441, 1966
Matterson EM: Play and Playthings for the Pre-school Child. Baltimore, Penguin Books, 1967
Maurer A: The game of peek-a-boo. Dis Nerv Syst 28:118, 1967
Morgenstern FS: Facilities for children's play in hospitals. Dev Med Child Neurol 10:111, 1968
———: Psychological handicaps in the play of handicapped children. Dev Med Child Neurol 10:115, 1968
Noble E: Play and the Sick Child. London, Faber and Faber, 1967
Opie I, Opie P: The Lore and Language of School Children. London, Oxford University Press, 1959
Piaget J: Play, Dreams and Imitation in Childhood, (Cattegno C, Hodgson FM, trans). New York, Norton, 1962
———, Inhelder B: The Psychology of the Child. New York, Basic Books, 1969
Pickard PM: The Activity of Children. London, Longmans & Green, 1965
Pickett LK: The hospital environment for the pediatric surgical patient. Pediatr Clin North Am 16:531, 1969
Plank E: Working with Children in Hospitals, 2nd ed. Cleveland, Case Western Reserve University Press, 1971
Rahner H: Man at Play. New York, Herder and Herder, 1967
Ross R: Storyteller. Columbus, Ohio, Charles E. Merrill, 1972
Sapora AV, Mitchell ED: The Theory of Play and Recreation, 3rd ed. New York, Ronald Press, 1961
Schiller F: Essays, Aesthetical and Philosophical. London, George Bell, 1875
Shedlock M: The Art of the Storyteller. New York, Dover, 1951
Slovenko R, Knight JA (eds): Motivations in Play, Games and Sports. Springfield, Ill, Charles C Thomas, 1967
Spencer H: Principles of Psychology. New York, D Appleton and Company, 1873
Stone LJ, Church J: Childhood and Adolescence, 2nd ed. New York, Random House, 1968
Sutton-Smith B, Sutton-Smith S: How to Play with Your Children. New York, Hawthorn Books, 1974
Takata N: The play history. Am J Occup Ther 23:314, 1969
Taylor L: Storytelling and Dramatization. Minneapolis, Minn, Burgess Publishers, 1965
Torrance EP: Constructive Behavior: Stress, Personality and Mental Health. Belmont, Calif, Wadsworth, 1965
———: Problems of Highly Creative Children. Gifted Child Q 5:31, 1961
Winnicott DW: Playing: Its theoretical status in the clinical situation. Int J Psychoanal 49:591, 1968
———: Playing and Reality. New York, Basic Books, 1971
Zivin G: How to make a boring thing more boring. Child Dev 45:232, 1974

SUGGESTED CHILDREN'S BOOKS

Andersen HC: Wonder Stories Told to Children; Hans Christian Andersen's Favorite Fairy Tales. New York, Western Publ Co, 1974
Collodi C: Pinocchio. Chicago, Rand-McNally & Co, 1972

Kottmeyer WA et al: Robin Hood Stories. New York, McGraw-Hill, 1962
Kunhardt D: Pat the Bunny. New York, Western Publ Co, 1962
Lang A (ed): King Arthur: Tales of the Round Table. New York, Schocken Books, 1967
van der Loeff R: Avalanche. New York, Wm Morrow & Co, 1958
de la Mare W: Jack and the Beanstalk. New York Alfred A. Knopf, 1959
Milne AA: Winnie the Pooh. New York, Dell, 1974
Perrault C: Perrault's Fairy Tales. New York, Dover, 1969
Potter B: Peter Rabbit (revised ed.) New York, G & D Publ, 1962
Scribbins J: Hiwatha Story. Milwaukee, Kalmback, 1970
Sendak M: Where the Wild Things Are. New York, Harper & Row, 1963
Dr. Seuss: My Book About Me. Westminister, Maryland, Beginner Books, 1969

HOSPITAL STORIES FOR CHILDREN

Bonnett-Stein B: A Hospital Story. New York, Walker & Co., 1974
Bonnett-Stein B: About Handicaps. New York, Walker & Co., 1974
Wolff A: Mom! I Broke My Arm. New York, Lion Press, 1969

SHIRLEY STEELE

3 General Ideas in Relation to Long-Term Illness in Childhood

The increasing incidence of long-term illness (chronic illness) in the child population is partially due to life-saving medical advances, which have offered new opportunities for children who are born with or develop life-threatening conditions. The increasing incidence of long-term illness makes it imperative for health professionals to focus special attention on the health needs of these children.

Many of the problems associated with children with long-term illness originate from the fragmentation of health services which they receive. Bogg (1975) reported on one state:

> In 1963, the staff of the Division of Services to Crippled Children of the Michigan Department of Public Health began a study to determine the expenditures necessary for the long-term treatment of children with specific handicaps. Expenditure records of the 15 years studied showed that only a few children actually received long-term services. The typical handicapped child received services in only 3 or 4 different years, and many eligible children had never received more than $5 or $10 worth of care. (p 2)

The findings in Michigan in 1963 were not inconsistent with services offered in other states; they merely helped to document the fallacy that children with long-term illness receive consistent, adequate health care services.

The reasons that children with long-term illness do not receive adequate health care supervision are many and complex. The Michigan research conducted in 1965, attempted to determine why there was a discontinuity in the care delivered to these children (Bogg, 1975). One of the factors associated with dropping out of the program of care was a high alienation score on the Seeman and Middleton tests. Mothers who scored high on the alienation scale withdrew their children from the program earlier. Alienation scales correlated inversely with health knowledge, favorable attitudes toward preventive and curative health care, and specific planning for the future. The alienation described in these scales was related to feelings of powerlessness and meaninglessness and a sense that customary norm-abiding practices are insufficient for reaching goals. The alienated person is lonely and socially estranged. This finding can help to predict the health behavior that some parents might exhibit. Identifying a mother who scores high on the alienation scale should help health professionals to alter the services they render in an effort to meet the needs of the mother so that she is able to seek and continue receiving services for her disabled child. Mothers who did not score high on the alienation scale and had adequate socioeconomic status tended to continue receiving services for a longer time and were less likely to miss appointments. Mothers who fall into this category would need less professional assistance to help them continue with health supervision.

The financial burden of a long-term illness has often been cited as a cause for discontinuity in services. Certainly this is a more significant factor for families with limited income than for families with higher incomes and third-party health insurance. The health insurance industry is expanding and it is beyond the scope of this discussion to try to document which services are covered by which insurance programs. Likewise, the state aid programs are continually changing and it is imperative to keep up to date with current area coverage in order to help families assess their eligibility for financial assistance.

A third possibility for the lack of consistency in health care services to children with long-term illness may be related to geographic distance. Services are still clustered near large medical centers and tend to be less accessible for persons who have the most difficulty providing their own transportation. The decline in availability of public transportation has added further to this problem. In assessing your community, you may find circumstances such as the following: families are not eligible for particular services because they do not live in a prescribed geographic area, they are not in a particular economic category, or their child is mentally retarded as well as physically handicapped. Each community has unique requirements for eligibility for services which may exclude certain children who could potentially benefit from the services that are available.

A fourth reason that these children do not receive comprehensive services may relate to "professional territoriality." Although this subject has received less emphasis in the literature, in practice it is probably more common than professionals care to admit. Pluckhan (1972) describes the behavior of professionals that illustrate the concept of professional territoriality. She suggests that man's possessive needs probably extend beyond physical territory and include a need to defend his institutions, his role, his profession, and his area of operation. In my personal experiences, there have been instances where children with a particular disease would benefit from other local services offered specifically for his condition, but the child was not referred because the professional providers did not wish to relinquish their care to others. Another example occurs when one professional discipline will not share the care of a child with another; as when a nurse does not recommend a child for intensive physical therapy, even though the child would benefit from this referral.

Pluckhan suggests that the nurse is prohibited from using her judgment by specific policies and rules that delimit her ability to deliver expert services. She suggests that other professionals as well as employing agencies tend to establish practices that underutilize the nurse in the general health care delivery. This is also seen in the delivery of services to children with long-term illness. Some agencies that provide services to these children do not employ a nurse, and tend to underestimate the services that a nurse could provide to enhance the child's ability to reach his maximum potential. When a nurse is employed, she is frequently utilized to keep records, check on follow-up appointments, and so forth rather than in a professional nursing capacity. This underutilization of qualified nursing personnel may partially explain why some children and their families do not get adequate help with learning skills for daily living, or sufficient assistance to make use of community agencies and get proper placement and services in school. In addition, the whole nursing area related to health teaching and counseling is frequently not available to these children and their families on a consistent basis.

The territorial concept also partially explains why some outpatient services have been slow to materialize. The hospital, which formerly held the most prestigious position in health care delivery, houses professionals who strongly support the acute-care setting and tend to impede the progress of outpatient and home-care delivery that are more conducive to the care of children with long-term illness.

Closely related to the concept of territoriality is the idea of health professionals as a work-force group as described by Longest (1976). He suggests that health professionals have a high need for achievement and self-actualization, and a keen interest in their work and in developing new knowledge. He further states that health professionals generally have low loyalty to employing organizations, but high commitment to specialized role skills. This description would favor inpatient services as the professional is able to maintain a greater control over the client population and their families. Outpatient care would give greater control to the parents.

The emerging role of the nurse as a primary giver of care is beginning to gain acceptance. The territorial issue must be considered and professional roles reevaluated to guarantee that the consumer receives the best care possible. Epstein (1974) states, "with self-awareness, a lessening of fear, and a repertory of skills, we (health team) may together—the old and the new, the different professions, the sexes, the races, the diverse personalities —develop a continuing process of communication and self-evaluation with the primary objective of improved patient care" (p 67).

Hannam (1975) states that the parents of handicapped children whom he interviewed were relatively self-reliant and competent people. He states that they frequently expressed the opinion that they felt they had to fight for anything they got for their children. This "fight-minded" approach led to some parents becoming isolated, and if such a situation prevails, it is easy to see why some children did not receive adequate services. They become the victims of the resentment built up toward their parents by the health establishment. If services are lacking and the professionals do not institute new ones, it appears that only parents who have enough initiative and insight will eventually stimulate the right people to get the services that they feel they need for their children.

Another salient reason for inadequate health services is that it takes time for parents to absorb the information they are given. If too much responsibility is given to them when they are anxious, they may forget or become confused by the suggestions. Written, as well as verbal, directions are helpful in clarifying what is expected of the parent. Opportunities to check back with the parents about progress will also help to facilitate follow-through on plans.

Six potential reasons why children with long-term illness do not receive adequate health care services have been presented. They include the accessibility of services, the lack of services, professional territoriality, financial considerations, and areas which relate to the parents. The latter are, specifically, high scores on tests related to alienation, as well as lack of understanding, and isolation due to their insistance on better services. These reasons are not meant to be all-inclusive, but they do represent a variety of reasons that might explain why children have received limited health services even when they are offered.

The child with a long-term illness can be a real challenge to nurses, as well as to other medical personnel and to his family. The child develops some unique qualities which are formulated as a result of living with an illness. The way the child learns to live with his disability will be influenced by the way others respond to him.

IN THE HOSPITAL

The hospitalization of the child is covered in several sections in this book. This chapter focuses on a general discussion of the hospitalization experience and how it facilitates or impedes the care given to a child with a long-term illness. Hospitalization is also discussed in Chapter 4; focusing on the child's perception of his illness. Hospitalization is also addressed under the management of specific long-term conditions.

Profile of the Child. The child with a long-term illness is more likely to want to know the nurse's name. He very often prefers to call the nurses by their first names. However, he will abide by the customs of the institutions.

He also expects everyone to know his name and he delights in showing the other children how popular he is.

He is well aware of his rights on the hospital unit. He is often very authoritative when demanding or asking for things. He frequently finds a very prominent place, such as the nurses' station, to spend a great deal of his day. Another favorite spot is by the elevator, where he can watch everyone get off and on. If there is an acutely ill child on the unit, he frequently guards that door to learn all he can about what is going on.

Hospital Vocabulary. The child who is hospitalized a great deal develops a hospital vocabulary, although he does not always know exactly what he is verbalizing. The terms may sound very convincing, but if you explore further with him he frequently does not really know what he is talking about. The child uses his hospital vocabulary to impress people. He especially likes to use it when new personnel arrive. He uses terms like NPO, OR, and OT as though every child knows them. These terms are less impressive, however, than his very scientific-sounding description of his medical condition and its treatment.

Despite his apparent satisfaction gained from using hospital jargon when it meets his needs, he will pretend he does not understand you when you use it. An example is when you tell the school-age child he is NPO for blood work. The blood work is late and he gets hungry. He decides to eat a piece of candy from his bedside stand. When you ask him about it, he says you did not tell him he could not eat. You point out the NPO sign on his bed and he explains he does not understand what it means.

Breaking the Rules. The child will also know the rules of the institution and frequently learns how to break them. He delights in "outsmarting" the authority figures, such as the nursing supervisors. He learns their schedules and plans his wayward activities around them. He soon learns that he can be mischievous without much chance of being caught. In his planning he usually uses children with less knowledge about hospital routines. He seems to feel that children who are less well known are less likely to get reprimanded. His need to be independent and explore are usually met during these escapades.

An illustration follows. Ed was a teenager who was hospitalized for physical therapy and fitting of braces. During the early part of this hospitalization he was in a wheelchair. He was allowed up most of the day, with the exception of an enforced afternoon rest period and an early retiring time —much too early to meet the needs of the adolescent. Ed knew the time the evening supervisor made rounds. He knew the rounds were started at his end of the hall. He also knew it was rare to see the regular staff nurses for a few minutes following the supervisor's rounds. He mapped out a plan for the two school-age children in the next room to get out of bed immediately after the rounds and go across the hall and push the elevator button. (The elevator was frequently still there as the supervisor got off.) Ed quickly got himself into the wheelchair and scooted out to the open elevator. All three children went to the main lobby and wheeled around innocently exploring the area. Approximately 10 minutes later they entered the elevator and returned. Not much was accomplished by adult standards, but for these children it was fun and exciting to "outsmart" the nurses. It was also fun to tell "understanding" adults about the excursion.

Hospital Routines. The child also may become very involved with hospital routines and he may get quite upset when the routines are not carried out on schedule. He is used to having his wishes granted immediately because of the large number of helping adults surrounding him; when these wishes are not granted he may become quite intolerant.

The child is quite aware of the treatments he should receive and he likes to direct the nurse with these procedures. As a means of manipulating his environment, he may refuse to have them done by certain individuals. Any deviation from the usual way of performing his treatment may result in great anxiety to the child. If he has had a tracheostomy for a long time he may prefer to suction and clean it himself. If the nurse attempts to do this, it may result in any number of unfortunate circumstances. The child may also wish to have his parent perform his treatments to simulate his home routines as much as possible. The child with a long-term illness frequently is much more dependent on his parents than is the normal child.

Tattling. The child also has a tendency to "tattle" on professionals. When you are doing his dressing he tells you: "Miss Jones did not use the forceps when handling the 4 × 4 dressings." He watches you eagerly to see if you react to this piece of information. If he gets a response, he is likely to continue to tell you "items" whenever he has the opportunity.

He also spends a great deal of time tattling on other children. This should be discouraged so that the child does not begin to act as the unit "security officer." A certain amount of tattling is normal for children, but it is easier to handle when the child is not hospitalized with so many people as the recipients of "information."

The use of "tattling" is probably an attention-seeking phenomenon. It is essential to provide the child with recognition so he does not have to resort to this activity for prolonged periods of time.

Seeking Information. The child with a long-term illness also feels free to question how much you know about his particular problem. He has had a great deal of experience with people with varying degrees of competency and has learned to fear those who are least expert in the field. This is especially true in relation to blood work, injections, and other painful procedures. He likes and demands the most skillful person. This may present problems to the nursing student who is just learning child health nursing techniques and may show a degree of hesitancy. The child may have a need to ask many questions that do not seem realistic to the professionals administering his care. He may show an unusually keen interest in minute details that frustrate busy people. Simple explanations specifically related to his questions will help to meet his needs. His persistence in seeking information is probably a reflection of his insecurity in the situation. If he is not answered abruptly or sarcastically, he will probably be satisfied and reassured by the answers.

Placement in the Hospital. The child with a long-term illness may also develop a desire to be on a specific unit or in a specific room. He may be far less comfortable when put in an area which is not his choice. As he gets older it may be increasingly difficult to make him happy in his hospital placement. He may resent being in with toddlers or hearing them cry. As an adolescent, he frequently does not fit in with adult patients as he is often less mature than would be normal for his age. An adolescent unit would be ideal for meeting his needs. Conversely, sometimes a change in hospital placement results in an improvement in the child's behavior.

I am reminded of a child, Lenny, who had hemophilia. He was frequently hospitalized on a general pediatric unit. He was a "behavior problem" during much of his hospitalization. He knew all the personnel on the unit and the contribution each one made to his care, directly or indirectly. His hospitalizations were often "planned" to coincide with certain predictable changes in the staff. He would try to be admitted on or near the first of July when the medical house staff changed. He took great delight in "scaring" the new physicians. He knew the rotation schedule of the student nurses through the unit. He often had "an accident" so as to see a favorite student nurse before she rotated to a new unit. This type of abnormal and manipulative behavior was a definite pattern of this child's lifestyle. (Unfortunately, there were many complicating factors, which I will not discuss here, that precluded psychiatric help for this child.)

The child continued this pattern during his school-age and early adolescent years. Despite several serious illnesses, he reached adolescence. He had an injury and needed hospitalization when the pediatric unit was filled to capacity. The decision was made to admit him to an adult unit. As he was cared for as a service patient, he was admitted to an adult area which frequently had the "sickest" patients. It was a busy time on this unit, and there was little opportunity to select the "best placement" for the adolescent. He was admitted to a four-bed room. As was his usual pattern, he screamed loudly as he was moved from the wheelchair to the bed. He started screaming about his incurable disease and how much better everyone else was in the hospital. At first, the other men frowned and felt sympathy as well as dismay at their new roommate. However, these patients were also quite ill and their impatience quickly overtook their immediate emotions. First one and then another complained quietly to the nursing personnel about their noisy roommate. The nurses tried, in vain, to control him. Then the doctors tried to quiet him, first by "friendly persuasion" and then by medication. All this failed. They called the nurses from the pediatric area to come to their aide. Lenny seemed to be happy to see them, but he was acting much as he did on the pediatric area; so their presence did not improve the situation. It may have even worsened it! Lenny continued his plan to disrupt the unit and get attention. The other patients were becoming increasingly impatient. They began to yell back when Lenny yelled. They shouted "Shut up" or "Quiet-down," and their booming voices startled Lenny. He was more used to a nurse suggesting he be quiet so as not to disturb the babies or other sick children. The shouts of the men were very similar to the commands he received from his alcoholic father. Lenny began to "settle in" and the men took increasing interest in him. His change to an adult area actually improved his mental status. His admissions to the hospital decreased and it would seem that Lenny had actually "grown up" as a result of his change in the long-term care he received.

In the foregoing illustration, the child seemed to have benefited from his change in medical environment. This is not always the case, however, and the child may have to undergo several different placements before he is able to adjust.

Changing Hospitals. The child who has received medical supervision from a children's hospital may find it disturbing to be ineligible, by virtue of age, to continue with his familiar health care. On the other hand, some children with long-term illnesses are eager to change their care so they do not have to tell their friends they are going to a "children's hospital." The reputation of the facility in the community also has a bearing on how the child perceives it. This is especially significant to the adolescent. If the hospital has a positive program for adolescents, the child may be more content to continue going to it. If the adolescent is treated as a second-rate citizen, he may be eager to change.

As a Family Member. A child who is hospitalized for long periods may have a very superficial idea of what it actually is to be a member of a family. He has frequent or long periods away from the family, which loosens his ties. The family may consider the child as a burden, financially or socially. They may use the periods of separation caused by hospitalization to recuperate from the strain caused by the long-term illness. This separation is often interpreted by the nursing personnel as lack of interest or even neglect. The staff, which has become very attached to the child, may become resentful of the family. This can result in a very poor nurse-parent relationship. The child gets in the middle of this and begins to try to get the staff to side more and more with him and create a bigger gap between the staff and his parents. The child then decides to ignore the parents when they do visit. The child's attitude makes the family further deny their importance to the child and their visits are made even less frequently.

The separation from his siblings can be lessened if visiting restrictions are made more flexible. It is beneficial to have the other siblings visit the hospital and vicariously learn what hospitalization means to their brother or sister. Visiting provides them with an opportunity to witness, first hand, some of the situations that their kin must face. They are better able to appreciate that hospitalization can be stressful as well as beneficial. Visiting also allows for a continuity in the peer relationships of the children.

(See the section "The Family of the Child with Long-Term Illness" in this chapter for a more in-depth assessment of the family constellation and the responses of individual members.)

Privacy. The child needs an area that he can identify as his own. The child with long-term illness does not feel so comfortable if he is moved frequently to "make room" for new admissions. There should be an area where he can have his private belongings and not worry that they will be moved when he is not present. He should be encouraged to clean his own area, and if the nurse needs to assist he/she should only do so with the child present.

Possessions. The child's possessions can be very important to him and their true significance is rarely fully appreciated by the nurse. The child's possessions may take on an additional significance if the child is separated by long distances from significant others. The possessions tend to help to decrease the distance between home and hospital. Possessions used in this way are frequently referred to as transitional items. They help in the transition from a home to a hospital environment. They help in the transition from a free person in the outside world to a less free person in an institutional setting. They provide visual evidence that the child is still connected with the outside environment.

If any of the child's possessions are taken home by the family, it should be with the child's full knowledge. This will save a great deal of searching for missing objects.

Simple Chores. The child will also benefit by having simple chores that help him feel a part of the hospital. He may be expected to put the tablecloth on the table, or distribute the mail, or help compile new charts. If he has a chore it is important to insist that it is done. Also, the chores should be changed periodically so he does not become bored. He may request certain tasks to do but he easily tires of them. Competition with other children with long-term illness may be healthy. Children are used to competition and it can be beneficial if one child is not consistently the loser. All children need to have some positive experiences in order to be willing to become involved in competition.

Handling Money. The child will also need help in learning to manage money. He has fewer chances than the "normal" child to spend money. If he is hospitalized for long periods, he should have an allowance like his peers. This is especially important for the late school-age child and the adolescent. They can use their money to buy newspapers, magazines, or small purchases in the gift shop. If they are interested they may buy supplies and make small articles to sell or give as gifts. The child will not always buy wisely, but this is also part of the learning experience. The child should not be allowed to "solicit" money from visitors. This will establish a pattern that is difficult to break. The child needs to know how to make his money "safe" and precautions should be taken to insure the money is not stolen.

The availability of coins to use in the pay telephone is a frequent problem. Many facilities are not equipped with change makers and the child may become bothersome because he needs change at an inopportune time. Helping him to make early plans about his day's expenses enable him to seek change early in the day so that it is ready when he wants to place his calls. This attention to financial matters will give the child responsibility for planning activities; it will also foster better adult-child relationships.

School. School is an especially essential experience for the child with long-term illness. If there is no school provided in the setting, the nurse is responsible for setting aside a time for the child to do schoolwork. If it is not possible to get books from the child's teacher, books with very explicit directions are readily available in stores. The child should be encouraged to do an assignment a day. In addition there may be school activities such as drawing which will increase his interest. To study, the child needs an area comparatively free from distractions. It is usually more interesting if more than one child is studying together. This more closely assimilates an ordinary class situation.

The key criterion in relation to school is to provide consistency. In order for school work to meet this criterion it should be planned and implemented in a systematic fashion. The child should know exactly when school times are scheduled and he should be ready to participate in his school activities. If the school times are not consistent the child will tend to underestimate its importance and tend to forget to attend to this very vital part of his life.

Church or Chapel. Depending on the institution, chapel or church services may or may not be easily accessible. Most institutions have an area provided for quiet meditation. However, many do not actually have church services conducted. If the child is used to attending Sunday school classes he will usually miss them. Inexpensive, illustrated books of children's prayer and hymns can provide a substitute. An area supplied with children's hymnals and an altar can also be made available for the children to hold their own church services. If the nurse feels comfortable participating with the children, she/he should feel free to do so. The children enjoy learning simple hymns and prayers. These can also be said at bedtime, either as a group or individually. In addition, representatives of major faiths are usually available to most institutions. Many church-affiliated hospitals have very active programs in the children's area. The parents will usually be helpful in contacting the religious advisor of their choice.

The adolescent may be able to leave the hospital and attend a local house of worship. This, of course, requires a physician's approval.

Many television and radio stations provide services for shut-ins. If these are chosen, every opportunity should be made to have the child actively participate in the program. Passively watching the television or listening to the radio will not be as beneficial as incorporating the child into the process.

Admissions of other Children. Admissions of other children to the unit may pose a threat to the child. He may view them as infringing on his territory or his adopted family. The new child may require extensive care, and this cuts down on the time given the child with less acute problems. The newly admitted child may also receive a great deal of parental attention as well as gifts, and this may make the child with a long-term illness resent him. The child who has been there a long time may greet the new parents and he often will request gifts and favors from them. He learns that parents easily feel sorry for children who are hospitalized for long periods or children who do not have visitors. Frequently the child is able to manipulate the parents so much that they have difficulty visiting with their own child. The parents may feel obligated to bring gifts of toys and food to the child. This often complicates the nurse's role as she/he tries to discipline the child or maintain a therapeutic diet. The parent who becomes involved with long-term children on a unit may need to be consulted and informed about the needs of the child with the long-term illness. This consulting need not be considered as a violation of the child's privacy. It is rather a necessary part of the medical and nursing supervision needed to guarantee the best possible care to the child who is hospitalized for long periods.

It is important to introduce the children to each other. Sometimes children have difficulty introducing themselves. It is wise to add an additional statement such as, "John has been in the hospital a long time, probably much longer than you will need to be, he can help you find your way around." This statement will help allay any anxiety the new child might have about an extended hospitalization and also help to acknowledge the fact that John has something special he can offer to the new child. An illustration follows.

John was 12 years old when he was diagnosed as having a malignant tumor. The medical plan was to have John receive radiation therapy. He lived in a shack in a rural area. The shack did not have running water or toilet facilities. It was not adequately heated and John shared a floor (as a bed) with several adults.

Because of poor transportation and the above conditions, John was hospitalized many months. The family did not visit him, and he was very lonely. He became friends with children of all ages. He helped the younger children accept bed rest by spending time playing with them or getting them needed supplies. The children eagerly introduced their new friend to their parents. John was most appreciative of the attention he received. The parents began asking him about his family and they were amazed at the conditions John described. They often checked with the nursing staff to see if all John described was true. Then their next move was to buy things for John. This generosity confused John. He did not know how to respond. It was felt that the parents' gifts could be better spaced. When a parent asked about John, the nurse took the opportunity to explain that he was not used to receiving gifts; and he actually did not use many that he received. The nurse suggested that if a parent wished to donate toys that they be used in the play area and John would benefit, mutually, with the other children. In this way, John did not have to wonder why he was being singled out to receive numerous unsolicited gifts from people he had just met.

If the parents were still interested in giving directly to John, a suggestion such as contributions to his holiday celebration or to his wardrobe may have helped to cut down on the daily contributions he received—thereby providing him with special surprises when the other children also received them. This would make the gifts seem more natural. Another practical suggestion would have been to have the parents send cards to John rather than gifts. Then he would receive mail, like the other children.

Discharge of Other Children. Discharges can also be a stress situation for the child. He sees children admitted after him return to home, and he wishes he could be discharged. He also makes friends from within the hospital and his group relationships are broken each time a child is discharged. While he may long to go home, he may fear losing the security he feels in the hospital. The hospital may protect him against many of the inflictions he receives on the outside. This is especially so in relation to children with physical disabilities who are subject to being stared at or made fun of in the outside world. They like the security of medical personnel who are not so likely to be "shocked" by their appearance. At the time of discharge, the remaining child may wish to exchange addresses or telephone numbers in order to keep up his associations with his temporary friends.

Activities of Daily Living. The child who is hospitalized for long periods may lack many of the outside experiences of daily living. The child who is physically handicapped may be more deprived in this area, since even when he is sent home he may not receive enough stimulation and exposure to everyday experiences. Every attempt should be made to take these children out for walks or to give them weekend passes so they do not become completely deprived of normal experiences. Utilization of volunteers would be especially helpful in this area.

Volunteers. The volunteers utilized in the care of children with long-term illness should include persons in a variety of age categories. The grandmother or grandfather is as important as the young high-school student. The college student serves another function. The role of the sexes cannot be underestimated. The boy with a long-term illness needs male figures who do not constantly hurt or examine him. He needs the attention of healthy males with male roles after whom he can model himself. He needs to see ordinary street wear of the male. He benefits by the male slang. Diversity is extremely important for both the girl and boy with long-term illness. They are exposed to more than the average amount of medical personnel, and it will take many nonmedical persons to balance this exposure.

Street Clothes. The child with a long-term illness may benefit from wearing his everyday street clothes as opposed to hospital garb or pajamas and robe. The more natural attire may make it easier for him to retain his contacts with the outside. It also helps the nursing staff and visitors relate to him in a more ordinary fashion. Somehow, the child seems "less sick" if he is up and dressed (Fig. 1).

Wearing his own clothes will also give him a reason to look after his belongings, which more closely resembles his responsibilities at home. The child can be responsible for washing out his socks or small items. This may serve as his chore that I discussed earlier in the chapter.

Hobbies. The child can also be encouraged to continue with hobbies he had at home. Tropical or gold fish can easily be accommodated in his hospital unit. Children frequently respond quickly to new pets that are easily maintained in the hospital, such as turtles or hamsters. These smaller animals can sometimes take the place of the bigger, more familiar pets the children have at home.

Another means of supplying pets to children with long-term illness is to have a program similar to a lending library. The animal is brought in for a few hours from a veterinarian or a zoo to visit in the playroom or hospital lobby. The animal is specifically chosen for his love for children. A responsible adult is present for the entire time the children are visiting the animal. Children who are used to having pets will gain a great deal from this exposure. The period can also be used to introduce children to animals they did not previously know or have close contact with.

Trips. The child with a long-term illness can also be taken to the local zoo to see animals. A museum visit may also be beneficial. This trip might stimulate an interest in a hobby of collecting pictures of animals such as butterflies. The trips to these areas can be less expensive of professional time

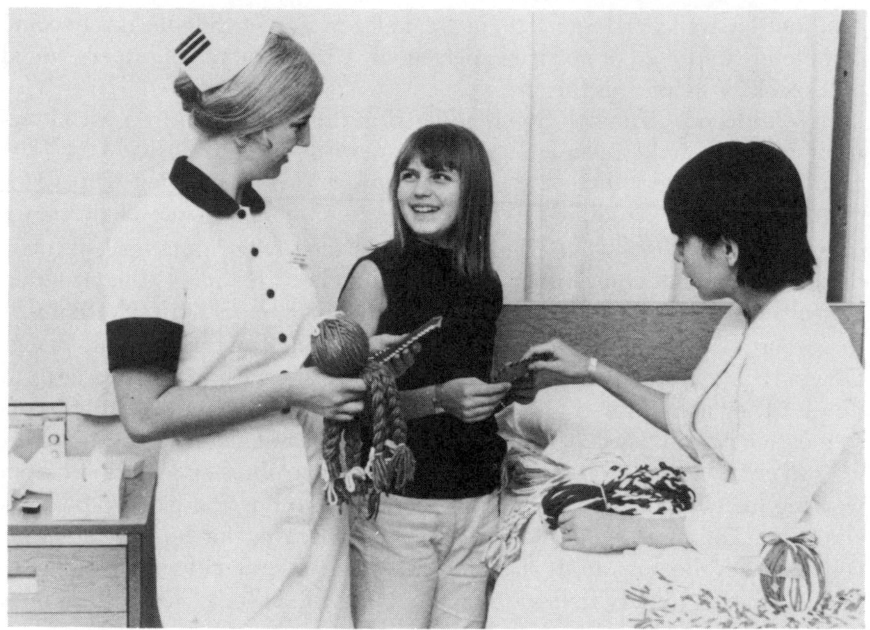

FIG. 1. Teens together help to pass the long hours of hospitalization. Note that the child who is ambulatory dresses in her own comfortable attire.

if volunteers are effectively solicited for the project. Volunteers are frequently very knowledgeable about these areas. Any activities planned outside the hospital will, of course, require permission of the physician and the child's parent or guardian.

Limit-Setting. The child should be exposed to reasonable and realistic limits while hospitalized. This should also be carried on even after discharge. Limits are very important to the child so that he knows his boundaries and feels free to function within them. He should not have free reign as this does not adequately prepare him to live in our society. (See Chapter 1 on normal growth and development for further guidelines.)

Bathing. The child's care should be planned to be as homelike as possible. The normal child is rarely bathed from a basin. He is more familiar with the bathtub or shower. If his condition warrants it, the home routine should be continued. This bath period can be a water-play period for the preschool child who delights in it. For the older child it is a close association with home.

The bath time should be scheduled with the assistance of the child. If he prefers to bathe at bedtime, this routine should be established. Special care should be taken to be certain that his bathing supplies are always replenished. He should be given responsibility for taking his own bath if he is old enough and capable of assuming responsibility for this aspect of his care.

Children with developmental lags will need definite programs established to help them achieve the goal of independent functioning in relation to activities of daily living. The plan should be simple. One task should be mastered at a time. Repetition and rewards are essential to the program. The child should be given adequate time to master the task before the adult providers give assistance.

Recreation and Play. Play activities are covered in Chapter 2. They are an important component of the nursing plan for the child. The nurse will utilize other available team members such as the play therapist, volunteers, and occupational therapists to provide this component. Recreation is an essential element and other interested citizens can provide movies, slides, or film strips for evening entertainment. The more adequately equipped facilities will have swings, slides, and monkey bars provided for the children. Hospital excursions can also be planned. A planned scavenger hunt —collecting inexpensive hospital items such as tongue blades, cotton balls, and soap—can be great fun. With a little preplanning these items can be satisfactorily hidden in the area chosen for conducting the hunt.

Settling-In. We sometimes underestimate the differences between home and hospital. The child admitted from a fairly segregated community may experience "culture shock" when first admitted to an integrated hospital setting. He may quickly be exposed to children of many cultural and ethnic backgrounds. This experience can be very valuable to the child. However, he needs help in adjusting to the situation. A child who has heard bigoted remarks about another race may begin to incorporate this into his own thinking. He may find it extremely difficult to find himself sharing a room with a child of a different race. Fortunately, children seem to accept others for what they really are and adjustment periods usually turn into keen friendships. The exposure the child has to other cultural and ethnic groups can prove to be one of the most positive factors derived from long periods of hospitalization. The sharing of experiences during periods of stress, with children from all backgrounds, may make him better able to function in the outside competitive world.

Maturation. An important factor to keep in mind is that this child will grow socially, mentally, emotionally, spiritually, and physically during his hospitalization and illness if we provide an adequate environment. This implies that we must adjust our plan of care to meet his changing needs. It also means that we must not always remember all the unpleasant things the child did when he was younger. Each time he is seen, a new evaluation of his progress should be made. It is also falsely assumed that if a child has a large comprehensive chart that everyone knows all about him. It has been my experience that large charts are often avoided as it takes too much time to read them. So, despite a good resource, people may know very little about his past medical or nursing history, and even little about his present reasons for hospitalization. An outsider who does not know the child may be a valuable asset to a team conference on the child. Some very significant things can easily be overlooked when the child is hospitalized a long time. An outsider, who has no vested interest in the child, may see other approaches or suggest further evaluation or treatment.

Goal Setting. The short-term and long-term goals of nursing care should be spelled out specifically. We are too prone to rely on day-to-day care rather than spelling out our plans and trying to meet them. These goals can be made independently by the nurse, in conjunction with the patient and his family, or in conjunction with other members of the professional team. The long-term goals should include, in addition to the plans for the hospitalization period, specific discharge planning.

An example of this goal setting follows. A child with a long-term illness is admitted to the unit. His parents live 60 miles away and have four younger children. Your goal is to maintain as close a child-parent relationship as possible. One approach is to have the parent plan to telephone at a certain time on a definite day of the week. Another approach is to provide the child with postcards and stamps to write to the parent. Still another approach is to have pictures of the entire family taped to the inside foot of the bed so he can easily see them. You have thus specified the long-term goal of maintaining the child as part of the family unit. You have also identified short-term goals which can easily be met. If this is done on admission, you are more likely to take care of this because it is fresh in your mind. If it is put off, a significant gap in the child-parent relationship may already take place, and neither the child nor the parent may have any interest in starting the program.

Charting. Modalities for charting information vary from one agency to another. The important point to remember is that the nurse has a responsibility to collect and record information. The way it is collected or recorded will be influenced by particular work situations. However, nurses have the responsibility to record observations and to systematically assess the child's progress. Otherwise we may fall victim to providing only custodial care for the child with a long-term illness. The progress notes in relation to the foregoing goals of nursing care would relate items such as the child's response to the parents' telephone call or the child's enthusiasm or lack of it for sending postcards. They could note also whether the child reacted positively or negatively to suggestions offered by the parent. They should also include information about whether the parent wanted to talk to the nurse about the child's progress or whether this information had to be given to the parent without a specific request. The progress notes should also include new ideas for maintaining a child-parent relationship. An example would be scheduling a visit from the parent and any request the parent has for this visit, such as an interview with the physician or a financial counselor. The progress notes should include nursing intervention taken in relation to these requests.

Parents of Children with Long-Term Illness. The parents of the child who is hospitalized frequently are not always well informed about hospital policies. It is often falsely assumed that repeated exposure to a situation makes one extremely knowledgeable. This is not always true and it is especially important to help the parents receive the information they need or desire. One very important area of concern to parents is the use or misuse of "specialists." Frequently, a specialist in a particular field of pediatrics is utilized. The parent may not be aware that a new physician is being utilized. They may not realize the need for the physician and, in their ignorance, they may be opposed to having her/him on consultation. The specialist may be known to the parents only by a bill they receive for services rendered. This type of incident rarely occurs with acute illnesses but is quite common with children with long-term illnesses. It is imperative that parents receive the same consideration and information when their child is in continual need of medical supervision.

THE FAMILY OF THE CHILD WITH LONG-TERM ILLNESS

To understand the implications of long-term illness to the family, one must draw upon the work of sociologists and social psychologists. They help to put into perspective the family as it exists in present-day society. We can then more easily understand some of the reasons that families react the way they do to illness. It is not my intention to try to break the various types of family structures in our country into minute categories. The student should consult the work of sociologists and anthropologists who are dedicating their talents to understanding particular groups for this information.

The individual roles of family members have been increasing in variety. Many authors are hesitating to categorize roles of family members because these roles are undergoing a period of transition. During this transition it is difficult to explain role expectations without being open to criticism. Generalizations about families are also difficult to make. Laing (1972) states, "We speak of families as though we all knew what families are. We identify, as families, networks of people who live together over periods of time, who have ties of marriage and kinship to one another. The more one studies family dynamics, the more unclear one becomes as to the ways family dynamics compare and contrast with the dynamics of other groups not called families, let alone the ways the families themselves differ" (p 3).

First, I should like to discuss the family as a unit. Knowing perfectly well that it is difficult, if not impossible, to describe the role expectations of families of children with long-term illness, the following broad guidelines are offered as an orientation in beginning to understand this complex social unit.

The unit may be comprised of many small systems depending on the numbers and types of participants. Within this unit there are a number of interrelationships which exist. Anything which affects one member of the family, directly or indirectly, affects all the other members. The degree to which people are affected varies from member to member. We must assume that the family is not an entity unto itself. It is also affected by and altered by the environment in which it exists.

These factors are especially important to professionals working with children with long-term illness. They are probably even more significant when the long-term illness is acquired rather than congenital. In an acquired illness the role of the child in the family has already been established and has to be adjusted to the new illness. The interrelationships the child has in the family may be drastically changed due to his illness, whereas the child who is born with a long-term illness derives his role in the family with the health condition being considered. This does not mean, however, that his condition makes the role of the other family members in relation to his illness any easier.

To understand this more thoroughly we will now look at roles within a family structure. Spiegel (1957) has stated that interrelationships of roles are crucial, as no role exists in isolation; it is always patterned to fit the complementary or reciprocal role of a role partner. He states that as long as the role each family member occupies is complementary with and conforms to the role expectations other members have for him, the family lives in dynamic equilibrium.

This explains why it is important to understand what the family feels about the child with a long-term illness. If they assume that he is going to live a long productive life and this is not the case, the family equilibrium may be shattered when the child does not succeed. If the family has cast the child in the role of a helpless individual and the child assumes an active role, this may shatter the family equilibrium. If another sibling reacts negatively to the role of the child with the long-term illness, this can interrupt the family equilibrium.

Why worry about family equilibrium? Spiegel (1957) states that the equilibrium which is brought about by complementary roles is a rewarding state of affairs. He further contends that the disequilibrium serves to motivate family members to attempt some form of resolution of existing role discrepancies. The rewarding nature of equilibrium stems from the fact that when roles are clearly defined and mutually agreed upon, the individual is spared the necessity of almost constant decision-making about the acts he performs.

This can be illustrated by the child with a cardiac condition. A mother casts the child in the role of a "cardiac cripple." The child feels well enough to go to school and participate in nonstrenuous sports. The child assumes a role not consistent with the one another vital family member has for him. The mother writes a note to the school forbidding her son to participate in any sports. The school acts as the environmental factor. The principal requests a note from the physician. The mother tries to influence the physician to take her side. The physician intervenes in favor of the son. The son participates in sports. The mother then is faced with a role which is not conducive to the one which she has established for her son. Disequilibrium results and role expectations must be modified if equilibrium is to be reestablished.

The role a parent ascribes for a particular child may also influence the way the other family members accept that child. A child with a cardiac condition is often "coddled" by his siblings because they take their cues from their parents. Consequently, the other siblings may wait on the child with the cardiac problem and lessen his chances of establishing independence. The child with the cardiac condition may then expect that his needs will be consistently met in this way. When he gets to school, he finds it difficult not to have his siblings able to continue their indulging role.

Spiegel (1957) states that there are four principal ways in which an individual acquires his social role. In each case the individual can accept the role assigned to him or he can refuse it, such as in the case presented above. Some roles are ascribed, that is, universally accepted—such as age and sex roles. Other roles, such as occupation, have to be achieved and others adopted. The fourth role he calls assumption, when the role has playful qualities. Such assumed roles are taken in make-believe and it is important that all members concerned realize the playful character of the assumed role. The adoptive roles are informal in character. They are adopted by one member and usually relate to another member. This can be illustrated by a 10-year-old sibling adopting the mother role to the child with a long-term illness, rather than the sibling role usually adopted by two children in the same family.

There are two other terms used by Spiegel (1957) which are useful in this discussion. One is the term allocative discrepancy and the other goal discrepancy. Allocative discrepancy is used when the individual refuses the role allocated to him or when others fail to complement his role. Goal discrepancy exists when the goal of one family member is to obtain some form of gratification from another, but the other fails to meet the demand because his goal is related to withholding or because he is unable to gratify the demand, for some reason. Goal discrepancy is especially significant, as long-term illness can cause a member not to be able to gratify the demands of other family members. A number of examples can be cited. The child born without limbs obviously cannot achieve his father's desire for him to be a football player. The child with advanced cystic fibrosis cannot take dancing lessons. The daughter with asthma will not be able to exist comfortably in the frilly bedroom signifying to the mother the height of femininity.

The severity of the discrepancies between what is expected and what is attained can greatly influence the family equilibrium. The severity of the discrepancy may vary from family member to family member. What may be a severe disappointment to the mother may be only a minor disappointment to a brother or sister. However, the degree to which it interrupts the relationships within the family is of major importance.

Current Roles of Family Members

In the foregoing discussion we have talked about roles in the family. It is useful to examine some of the present roles that influence the care given the child with a long-term illness.

Mother role. The role of the mother has always been concerned with the health of the children. Recently the role has changed from being not only one of concern with physical health but also the psychologic well-being of the child. This expanded role has put new and more demanding responsibility on the mother. She is forced to read about new developments in child care and to keep up with advances in medical practices. Formerly, it was sufficient for her to get to a doctor when the child was ill. She is now faced with understanding preventive health practices and the responsibility for meeting the emotional components of development.

The more educationally advantaged the mother, the greater are the demands for her to be informed.

In comparison are those mothers who have little or no education and derive their roles by modeling after a mother or grandmother, or by word of mouth from some other educationally disadvantaged mother.

When looking at the mother role in relation to illness, Bell (1966) states that the middle-class mother usually assumes the role of mediator between the impersonal, rational role decision of the medical expert and the application of those decisions within the highly emotional contexts of her relationships to her husband and children. This mediating role of the mother further extends the impersonal relationship between the medical personnel and the patients.

This is dynamically illustrated by the adolescent patient with a long-term illness. The medical person usually feels an obligation to talk to the parent before talking to the patient. The parent then makes some decisions which are not always the best for the patient. The medical person then proceeds, incorporating the parent's decision. The relationship between the medical personnel and the patient may suffer as a result. The decision that directly affects the adolescent has been mediated by an outside source, and the adolescent frequently has to live with this decision. It is fortunate that the adolescent has the capacity to rebel, as this rebellion may provide an opportunity for him to be consulted about his own care.

The mother from a disadvantaged family may be so strained by other responsibilities that she has little or no time for illness. According to Rainwater, as cited in Bell (1966), her attitude toward illness even when it becomes chronic is apt to be a tolerant one. People in lower socioeconomic families learn to live with illness rather than using their small stock of interpersonal and psychic resources to confront the problem.

These attitudes about illness are influenced by the degree to which the family members regard the crisis as a threat to the present or future life of the family. The parent responding to an ill child is responding to both the illness and the dependent status of the child in our society. In other societies, in which the child is less dependent, the parents' need to protect the child may be less.

The mother with a child with long-term nutritional anemia may bring the child to the hospital only when the child is dangerously close to death. The child is treated and responds. The mother is counseled on the dietary requirements of the child and seems to understand. However, the child is readmitted a few months later, in the same condition. The mother again is responding only when she considers herself incapable of handling the situation. She is not worrying about the sequela of the frequent brushes with death. Her aim is to keep the child alive but the overall well-being of the child may be an unknown concept to her. Even if it is known, she may have so many overwhelming crises to handle that she is not physically able to respond to them all and handles each one as she interprets its importance.

Father Role. The role of the father in relation to child-rearing practices is beginning to be presented as more significant. Young fathers are beginning to speak out on their right to influence the nurturing of their offspring. They are expressing a desire to change their image from one of a financial provider to one of an interacting essential member in the family process. This approach to child rearing will influence the way professional personnel deal with families. It will not be enough to talk only to the mother about child-rearing practices. Fathers who are integrally involved in the nurturing process will have to be included in the discussions and planning.

Implications of Long-Term Illness on Parental Roles. Bell (1966) has stated that some families have the tendency to resist the facts that a problem really exists. However, he has found that the parents of children with long-term illness tend to be less sociable and more withdrawn than the parents without such children. He found the mothers less likely to work outside the home than "normal" mothers. He also found that the community of "normal" families was not supportive of the revised norms of child care that must be established by families with severely handicapped children. Furthermore, the norms and values regulating participation in the community of normal families are hostile to the demands made upon the parents of severely handicapped children.

An illustration of this point is found in this picture given by a parent of a child with severe cerebral palsy.

> I was young and a newly married college graduate when I moved into the community my husband grew up in. I quickly settled into his friends and family and felt right at home. Our only child was born less than two years later. It was a difficult birth and Janie was 'brain-damaged.' The fight she put up for survival deserved everyone's praise and exultations. My period following delivery was filled with complications and necessitated an extended hospitalization. Everyone was very kind and extended themselves to include visiting me and my infant daughter as well as extending meals to include my husband.
>
> Since that early time many adjustments have been made in our lives to accommodate our severely handicapped daughter. Our opportunities to be with friends and family have decreased as baby-sitters are difficult to find or keep. When friends visit our home, we must alter our lives to make them comfortable. Few friends accept our dinner invitations, as they do not like to eat with our daughter whose awkward movements make eating seem primitive. Our friends are not sympathetic to her needs, when their own needs seem more important. Even our families do not understand why we eat at the same table with our own daughter, when she makes such a mess. Why don't we feed her? Why don't we put her in a nice home with other children with the same problem?

These questions and other similar questions serve to illustrate that other families do not have patience with the revised lifestyle of the family with a child with a disability.

The hostility is not always overt, but may be of a much subtler nature—such as when the friends merely refuse or find excuses not to accept another dinner invitation to the involved family's home. The hostility can further be manifested by the invited guests' telling other friends about their experience "to spare them from the same ordeal." This form of hostility tends to further isolate the family with the child with a disability and decreases their motivation to try to keep ties with their former close associates.

In discussing implications to family roles, it is necessary to keep in mind that people raise their children according to their own standards. These standards include those regarding what is health and what is illness. What is "normal" may be very different from one family to another. A minor handicap due to a long-term illness may not have any implications to roles in one family, but in another it is a major crisis.

The comparison of two families with children with phenylketonuria will illustrate the last statement. One mother learned her child had this condition. She did not see any reason to be alarmed. The girl was 12 years old and functioning at a moderately retarded level. The mother did not change her role. She always let the child get her own meals and eat what appealed to her. Meals were never a source of enjoyment and the family did not come together for them. The child was told of her health problem and for a short period she tried to comply with the medical management. Her role reverted back to the one she was comfortably occupying prior to the medical discovery, and the phenylketonuric diet was discarded.

The second mother learned the medical diagnosis and immediately set out to control the diet of her daughter. She became an amateur dietician, nurse, detective, and all around "commander-in-chief." She experimented with new ideas for preparing the limited diet and willingly shared them with other parents and medical personnel. Her role as mother was being camouflaged by her desire to be a crusader for her daughter's cause. Needless to say, the role of the child changed dramatically. She found her mother less capable of giving the love and support needed to her daily growth because she was too busy with her newly found chores. The change in the mother-child relationship influenced the entire family. The mother began quizzing her husband on his observations of increased intellectual functioning of the child. The other sibling resented the restricted dietary intake enforced upon her sister. The size of the family was also stabilized as a result of this long-term illness. It would be possible to go on and on about the implications of this illness to this family and its place in the community, but I believe what has been said adequately illustrates the point.

The parents often have difficulty finding baby sitters to accept the responsibility to care for a child with a disability. This may partially be due to their own fears or lack of knowledge about the special needs of the particular child. There is more emphasis being given to respite services through agencies which provide services for children with long-term illness. These respite services include short-term baby sitting and long-term accommodations to allow the family to vacation without the child. These respite services are a welcome addition to the services provided for children with long-term illness.

The need for parents to get away from the constant day-to-day responsibility of the child with long-term illness is dramatically illustrated in the quote from Hannam (1975), "I think the strain is that I am managing a large organization, by the end of a week sometimes Monday morning that the weekend has been a dead loss from my own selfish angle. That's because relationships in the house have been strained, perhaps because of a broken night's sleep, perhaps he has been naughty" (p 44).

Hannam still suggests the father is less affected than the mother by the child with a long-term illness. The situation is explained in that the father can at least get away to work and by immersing himself in his work, forget the problems which are at home.

The fathers are probably more affected when the child does not achieve anticipated developmental milestones such as going to school or being able to secure a vocation. At these times it becomes more obvious to the father that the child is not an average normal child succeeding in expected developmental tasks.

It is well to remember that all children can "get on their parents nerves at times." The child with a long-term illness is no exception. He is able to cause discomfort and put additional periodic stress on the parent's individual roles and their reciprocal roles. The stress can be increased if the parents do not agree upon and discipline the child consistently. Maddison and Raphael (1971) suggest that mothers caring for a child with a chronic illness should include an increased gratification of the child's dependency needs. They suggest the child needs this attention in order to feel loved and secure. Conversely, they caution that excessive gratification of the dependency needs may impede the child's development and deprive him of the maximum pleasure from passively receiving his mother's attention. Maddison and Raphael note that mothers, like their children, are inclined to view the child's condition as punishment for their own wrongdoings or mistakes. They emphasize that material conflict with a particular child may be based on a variety of factors. Included in their list of suggestions are the following: conception coinciding with a personally devaluing experience, attempted abortion, a crises situation during the pregnancy, or poor family planning. These attitudes may lead to aggressive feelings towards the child that may make the mother feel guilty, and she responds by overprotecting the child.

Implications for Sibling Roles. A fair amount of material has been written in relation to the changes in parents' roles in relation to illness. The effects on the other siblings has been less well defined. In the chapter on terminal illness I have included some thoughts in relation to the other children, but I would like to include a few more in this section.

As the emphasis in child rearing has focused on the individual rights of the members of a family, children have tended to become more egocentric. Their individual demands are frequently granted until a crisis arises. In time of crisis, the individual's rights are relegated to a lower level of priority and the crisis situation emerges with top priority. Let us take, for example, a family with two children. Henry and Mary have been treated with equal concern by their parents. Their needs were individual but easily met with a degree of give and take by the family. Henry has an accident and is severely injured. His developmental level regresses to that of a toddler. The family begins to expend all their energies on behalf of Henry. Mary's normal requests and demands are now considered unreasonable. The parents have no time to spend on the ordinary activities of daily living. They are burdened by going to the hospital, seeing that the best doctors are brought in, obtaining and maintaining private duty nurses, getting people to donate blood, checking on medical insurance coverage, and so forth. Mary is very much in the background of the medical crisis. She is painfully on the other end, where living conditions have deteriorated. Her meals are forgotten or thrown together, her clothing is neglected, no one is available to answer her questions or to ask her about her day. The phone rings frequently but the calls are always about Henry. In her childlike way she tries to adjust her sibling role to meet the crisis, but she becomes more and more painfully aware of her own desires and needs.

This traumatic beginning influences the way Mary will be able to handle her new role in relation to Henry with his long-term illness. Her role of equal competitor may change to one of hostility. Her position may be further in jeopardy when Henry returns home in a more dependent role. She may be asked to assume some of the responsibility for his care, casting her in a mother role or nursing role. She may adopt the role of mother willingly, and compete with her mother for this position with Henry. She may assume a role of cheerful happy young lady while in reality she very much resents her new responsibilities. Her exterior facade gives her parents confidence that she is delighted with her new responsibility. This creates a comfortable feeling in the parents and they do not look past it into Mary's true feelings.

This example illustrates why I believe that health care must be family-centered rather than patient-centered. The needs of Mary may well get to crisis proportions before anyone is aware that they even exist.

The changing role of siblings can be detrimental to the children's normal life pattern. With some degree of predictability, Mary might experience loss of normal activities of her age group. She might resent the premature role of mother and choose never to accept it again. She might become hostile toward her parents and not be able to establish a warm and loving relationship again.

A professional person, working with the family, might identify some of the clues to Mary's unhappiness and help her to handle her feelings.

In families that attend clinics for long-term health supervision, it is becoming evident that siblings have an increase in emotional problems. These emotional problems have been manifested in obesity, nail-biting, school failure, etc. The severity of the symptoms is not necessarily correlated with the degree of disturbance.

If it is unrealistic to have all the siblings included in the health supervision of the child with long-term illness, we might at least plan group sessions in which they can get together and ventilate their feelings about their roles and responsibilities. These sessions could be planned in the evening, so they do not interfere with school. Another possibility is for the school nurse to assume the leadership for these sessions. They can be successfully integrated into the health education program.

Just as respite care was suggested for the parents, it is also suggested for the siblings. Siblings need a chance to be free from the special considerations given to the child with a long-term illness. This is very important if the affected child has a mental impairment. The siblings may wish to entertain their friends without the potential embarrassment that may arise from the irrational acts of the child with a mental impairment. They may feel that their friends will not come to their homes if they are repelled by their sibling's behavior. Parents need to appreciate the need of siblings for periods of separation and to make sure these are provided. This does not mean that the child with long-term illness is neglected. He is merely excluded for certain times the same way he is included at other times.

Perhaps the best guide for assessing sibling situations is to try to provide respite for all the children. Each has special needs at particular periods and these needs should determine when a child's requests are reasonable and when they are unreasonable.

Maddison and Raphael (1971) report that the neglect of siblings results in hostile and aggressive responses to the affected child. They document that the siblings have an increased incidence of school problems and delinquency tendencies, which indicate that the siblings' needs are not being adequately met.

Implications for the Extended Family. The membership in the extended family has decreased in importance as today's families are separated by vocational and other interests. Mobility has ranked high on the list of reasons responsible for the decreasing importance and support available from the extended family. Frequently, there are only a few close relatives living nearby and they have families of their own to care for. Therefore, the relatives are able to maintain a psychologic distance which allows them to feel little or no pressure from the effects of the child with the disability.

Implications for Professional Roles. The role of the professional nurse in relation to the child with long-term illness is addressed in each chapter as it becomes appropriate. However, it seems appropriate to include the professional team during hospitalizations since they periodically become highly significant caretakers for the child. The hospital is geared toward cure of acute episodes of illness. This orientation frequently jeopardizes the care administered to children with long-term illness. In a teaching hospital, the child may not be considered "an appropriate learning experience" by the medical staff for their medical students or residents. Therefore, they may apply pressure to have the child discharged. The social worker or nurse, feeling that the family is not ready for the child to be returned home, may try to delay the discharge. This situation can result in friction between the members of the health team. It is during these periods of disagreement that it is extremely evident that the team is not really a team, but rather a group of professionals all working in the same institution.

Health professionals like to feel that they can cure illness. They feel frustration that they cannot cure the child's long-term illness. This realization is likely to make the professionals feel inadequate in their roles. In order to protect themselves against constant reinforcement of their imagined failure, professionals may tend to avoid the child with long-term illness.

Another point about working with these children is that we tend to focus only on the major problem areas and on how the child is responding in relation to them. If the child is making progress in these areas, the professionals tend to be optimistic, but if the child is not responding in the expected ways then we tend to be dissatisfied. The difficulties which may arise from too narrow a focus on a particular area are many:

1. The child receives impersonal treatment.
2. The professional may be unduly discouraged by lack of progress in his particular problem even though the child is making satisfactory progress in other areas.
3. The professional may be focusing on the one area where the child is least likely to show his best side. Therefore, the child also appears as uncooperative, moody, and so forth.
4. The child is not rewarded for progressing in the areas that may be most significant to him.
5. The child begins to anticipate rejection from professionals and dreads keeping his health-care appointments.
6. The child and professional tend to miss potential breakthroughs in the delivery of care because the focus is on a particular problem, rather than on how a particular patient responded to a particular situation in a given set of circumstances.

In order for professional personnel to achieve satisfaction from managing the care of children with long-term problems, the educational programs preparing health professionals need to focus less on the acute care situation and provide positive learning experiences with families over longer periods of time. This kind of association will provide a more realistic picture of the way the family is able to adapt to family stresses.

Implications for Members of the Community. The goal of care of the child with long-term illness is to make him a productive member of the community where he lives. This might be his private home or it might be an institution. The child needs to be able to cope with his illness and learn to live with it on a day-to-day basis.

Strauss (1975) emphasized that any given disease has the potentiality of causing many problems related in daily living. The day-to-day management of the illness is more complicated than the management during acute care episodes, since the conditions of the daily situation can be so diverse. Clients with long-term illness are beginning to realize the value of sharing their experiences of living with a disability with other individuals with similar problems. Strauss (1975) suggests that the key issues in the management of patients with long-term illness center around the prevention of medical crises, control of symptoms, carrying out prescribed treatments, adjusting to changes in progress, avoiding social isolation, normalizing social interactions, and financial assistance. In order to manage these key issues a great deal of planning must take place with significant others who will be intimately involved with the child. The special needs of the child will change as the child grows and the significant others change. In order to make the child's adjustments as easy as possible, it is best to anticipate these needs created by maturational crises and to plan for them. A network needs to be established to monitor the child's progress and to establish realistic goals to enhance his progress. The child should not miss out on going to school, for instance, because no one anticipated his special needs far enough in advance to plan for his entry. A child's discharge from the hospital should not have to be delayed because the equipment needs in the home have not been taken care of. Numerous examples of management schemes can be cited to give insight to the special planning that has to be done to facilitate the successful integration of long-term illness with the life-style of the child and his family or significant others. The special implications of the long-term nature of these conditions makes it difficult to have all the roads paved with a smooth surface. There will always be rocky spots as the child grows in awareness and as he periodically becomes disenchanted with his special routines.

A special mention needs to be made regarding the noncompliance with prescribed regimens. Noncompliance indicates that the child or significant other has not consistently followed through on the routines suggested by health professionals. Noncompliance can imply that there is a lack of cooperation on the part of these people. In long-term care it is necessary to explore the reasons for and the times when noncompliance takes place. Even the slightest request by health professionals may require a significant amount of rearranging of family lifestyles to accommodate the request. For instance, a clinic visit scheduled on a monthly basis during the day may necessitate a parent taking off from work, or arranging for a baby-sitter or for the car to be at a different place, or changing meal times or nap times, and so forth. In addition, the ongoing attention to regimes sometimes blows them out of proportion. After all, even brushing one's teeth or shaving can get to be boring.

Long-term management of many of the childhood conditions require relatively simple routines that can be learned by the family. Adjusting the routines so that they fit best into their busy lifestyles will help to delimit noncompliance. The more complicated, threatening routines will demand a great deal of assistance from health professionals. The community health nurse needs to be attuned to the regime and be available to assist in a variety of ways. Frequently, health professionals limit their services to specific times and days. Unfortunately, patient needs cannot be limited in this way.

Health care delivery must be available around the clock each day if families are to receive the help they need; otherwise, noncompliance might be a term associated with health professionals as well as the clients they serve.

Evaluation of Child's Assets: Nursing History

The nursing history may be used to collect data in hospital and outpatient settings. I have included a form (Fig. 2) that has been developed by using formats suggested by other nurses and by adopting this form to get the information needed in a particular setting.

The excuse that a form does not fit a particular institution or agency's needs and, therefore, is not used, is an outdated idea. The form is just a

UNIVERSITY HOSPITAL
U.S.A.
Nursing History (In-Patient Pediatrics)

Name: ____________________

Date: ____________________

Number of hospital or home care admissions

Duration of hospital admissions

Age(s) during hospital stay(s)

I. Appearance

II. Patient's understanding of illness—preparation for hospitalization

III. Events leading up to present hospital admission

IV. Place in family constellation—identification of family members

V. Significant information relative to:
   - a) feeding
   - b) toileting
   - c) sleep
   - d) play
   - e) language development
   - f) independent and dependent activities of daily living

VI. What is important to this child to make him feel secure in this situation?

VII. What are the policies of this agency which will interfere with or promote the well-being of this child?

VIII. What is the medical plan of care that will influence the nursing plan of care?

IX. What are the shot-term goals for this child?

X. What are the long-term goals for this child?

XI. What methods can be identified and tried to meet these goals?

XII. What are the significant principles of growth and development which will be incorporated into the plan of care?

XIII. What community or team resources will be utilized or approached to meet the nursing objectives?

XIV. What nursing intervention needs to be done with the family at this time?

FIG. 2. Suggested Form for Nursing History.

suggestion and should be tailored to meet your current needs. It is merely a guide for collecting data. If it is a deterrent to gathering data then it should be discarded in favor of another method.

Any child admitted to the hospital feels much more secure if he realizes that you know and understand him. One way to get to know the child and his parents is to do a nursing intake history. This history will help to identify significant factors to develop a realistic nursing care plan. The history will be taken on admission for most long-term patients. However, if the child is admitted in an acute crisis, the information may be more easily obtained a day or two after admission. Figure 2 is a guide for obtaining pertinent nursing information. If the information is stored easily, some of it can be saved from admission to admission and just be up-dated.

Pertinent information obtained from this interview should be immediately placed in the child's chart for utilization by the entire health team. Some of the aspects are gathered specifically for the Kardex. Other information, such as use of community resources, is utilized for instituting proper referrals.

Of the information gathered, some—such as feeding, toileting, and so forth—will need to be further evaluated by direct observation. An example would be: Mrs. Jones says that 2½-year-old Johnny feeds himself. When you make out his Kardex you include this fact. Johnny experiences regression due to hospitalization and refuses to eat. The Kardex should be revised to read: encourage self-feeding, needs assistance.

The question in relation to policies which interfere with meeting certain objectives may lend itself to changes in policy. For instance, you find that Johnny is very attached to his six-year-old brother. The hospital does not allow children under 14 years of age to visit. If you gather enough information indicating that the child's progress is hindered by being separated from his siblings, a change in policy may be considered.

Physicians have always identified, on admission, a plan of care and methods to be tried in relation to this plan. Nurses should also identify their care plan and ways they intend to facilitate this care. The physician then keeps progress notes in relation to things he has tried and their results. Then he adds more ideas and ways to meet the revised plan of care. Nurses seldom keep progress notes and rarely do we spell out why we changed our plan or what our future plans will be. Let us take as an example Mary, who is admitted with myelomeningocele with paralysis of her lower extremities. She is admitted with a decubitus ulcer on her ankle. Presently we begin a plan of care and chart on the nurses' notes in relation to size, location, discharge, and treatment given. A few days later we chart a different treatment given. Our only clue to what the treatment may be is the doctor's order sheet. However, nowhere is the independent nursing function charted. We may have tried to leave the area uncovered for three days without apparent improvement. We may have tried treatment by a heat lamp. We may have used a bedcradle or footboard to eliminate pressure from bedclothes. We may have positioned the child at night to keep her from rolling over and getting the decubitus on the sheet. We may have bathed the area in warm water three times a day. All of these independent measures should be charted with their results or lack of results; and when a new approach is started, the rationale should be clearly stated so that everyone reading the chart can easily see that the independent nursing functions as well as the dependent nursing functions are being met.

Needless to say, gathering of information is only one step in the process of improving care. Ways must be devised to disseminate this information to make it readily available and to eliminate some of the duplication that exists. We do not want to follow the medical profession's policy of several levels of medical personnel all gathering the same information. The use of computers to conveniently store and retrieve information will greatly improve our present methods of sharing information. It is imperative to establish how to identify pertinent nursing information, so we can identify what we can contribute to the computer input.

When one studies Figure 3, it becomes evident that the role of the nurse is greatly expanded and encompasses a longer time span than it did formerly. The nursing history just sets the stage for more dynamic types of nursing intervention. The information gathered helps the nurse to identify areas of care that uniquely belong to nursing or are shared by nursing. The

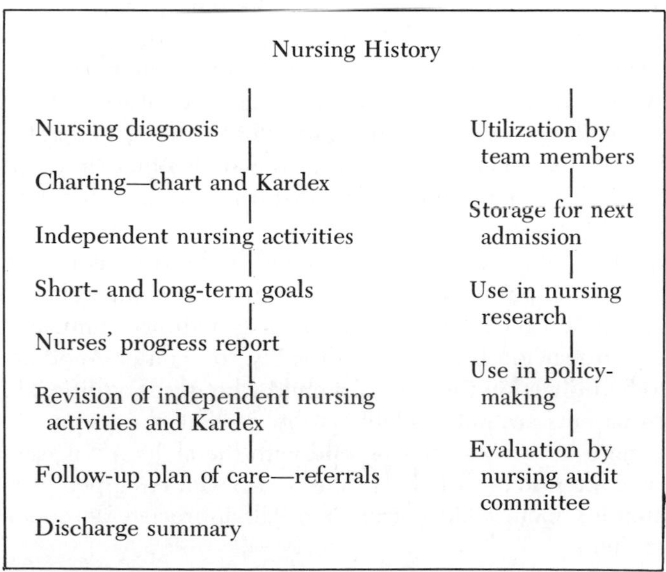

FIG. 3. The Expanding Role of the Nurse in History-Taking.

nurse makes a nursing diagnosis and then formulates the plan of care to meet the patient's needs. Patients with long-term illnesses may have so many medical diagnoses that we hesitate to add a nursing one to the list. However, this nursing diagnosis is somewhat different. The diagnosis is partially derived from factors relating to growth and development and normal developmental tasks (see Chapter 1). It is made by considering constraints made by the hospitalization process, and by considering the medical diagnosis and the scientific limitations imposed by this diagnosis. It is made by considering the child as an integral part of a family unit by considering the social forces that are present. It is made by the types of services available for aiding this child. It is made by the time element we have available to minister to the child.

An example might be that you make a nursing diagnosis of extreme environmental deprivation causing failure to thrive. You would like to have the same nurse care for this child each day on each shift. You would also like to provide the child with consistent visitation of the parents, and to have them participate in the care of the child—especially in regards to feeding and handling. After the diagnosis is made and plans tentatively formulated, you learn from the parents that they live far away and they will not be able to visit consistently. You also find the staffing of the unit is inadequate for the next few days and per diem nurses will be utilized to supplement the regular nursing staff.

It is now necessary for you to revise your thinking in relation to this child and to see what other resources you can draw on to supplement the care. You then decide that a volunteer may be used with this child, that she could provide the cuddling necessary for the child, that she would have more time to rock the child, and that she might even be in a position to feed the child. You will also want to be sure that the per diem nurses have the benefit of a very complete Kardex or verbal report to utilize when caring for the child so that they know the parents will not be there, so that they do not wait feedings if the volunteer is not there, and also that they will provide some of the stimulation the child will need during the time they are responsible for the child's care.

In addition you decide that toys should be used to assist you in your plan of care and you put up a mobile, or you use some musical wind-up toys that can be wound up periodically and used as auditory stimulation for the child. You also provide the child with a toy to cuddle. Another valuable resource to be utilized in the care of a child who needs additional attention because his parents are not available is the student of nursing. Frequently he/she has more time available to spend with the child and is eager to give the additional attention needed. He/she is also well equipped with some of the new theories about child rearing and will appreciate an opportunity to implement them.

In line with Figure 3, the next step—in addition to getting information in the Kardex in relation to this child—is to be sure that the charting states exactly how the child responded to the additional handling, to the toys, to sound, to feeding, etc. It is especially important that the chart shows when the child begins to eat better, what types of things contributed to his eating better, and if there were particular conditions under which he ate better. It is not unusual to have the child, even with additional handling, eat poorly at the beginning of his hospitalization. A child who at home has his bottle propped may not like the change of being held to be fed and may take quite some time before he begins to respond, and enjoys having somebody hold him and rock him while he is eating. The fact that the child seems to like having his bottle propped better than being hand fed does not mean that the nurse should use the propping procedure. It merely means that the child becomes programmed to propping; and because he knows no other way, he has learned to adjust to this. However, we know that because the child fails to thrive that he is not getting the full value out of feeding. The nurses' notes should clearly indicate when the child begins to improve or at what points the child might regress. We should be able to pinpoint very clearly on the notes some of the factors that contributed to progression or regression. We should also begin to accumulate a list of foods that the child likes or dislikes in his diet.

In designing goals for this child, it has already been indicated that we have established some short-term goals. The long-term goals may be to send referrals to the local community health nurse to visit the home and to help the mother with feeding the child, or in listening to the mother to see what types of things have contributed to the weak—or what seems to be weak—mother-child relationship.

The referral to the community health nurse should be made early so that he/she can provide the hospital team with information that may be very valuable while the child is hospitalized. He/she may have known the family for a long period of time prior to this hospitalization. The mother may need a great deal of reassurance while the child is hospitalized; and perhaps the mother might even have some guilt feelings about this child, especially if anyone has told her that it is the result of her behavior that the child has poor feeding habits and failure to thrive. This is not an unusual occurrence when a child with failure to thrive is admitted to the hospital.

The nurse's progress report should clearly state that he/she has contacted the community health nurse in the area and should also indicate any information that he/she has collected through this resource so that other members of the health team can also utilize this information. The independent nursing activities and the Kardex must be revised frequently in order to give the best possible care to the child. Having outdated information is no better than an empty Kardex.

We should also put in the Kardex some of our follow-up plans for the child. They may include such things as return to clinic so that we know that the child does have some after-care, or it may include the name of the physician to whom the child will be referred on the outside and, of course, the name of the community health nurse who can be contacted easily in the child's community. It is very important also to include in our charting a discharge summary of this child, indicating the progress the child has made during hospitalization, as well as some of the key nursing interventions that were made in order to meet the nursing needs of this child. This discharge summary should be sent to the community health nurse in the area and to the follow-up health care, wherever it will be given for this child.

Problem-Oriented Method

Since the first edition of this book, the problem-oriented record introduced by Weed has been gaining acceptance by all health disciplines for the collection of health data. Therefore, it is introduced into this volume as one alternative to the nursing history form, which is still retained in this edition for those geographic areas where the problem-oriented method is not and perhaps will not be adopted. The method used to collect the data must be accurate and complete.

The problem-oriented care process is based on the problem-oriented record. The written material in the chart should form the basis for the care plan. The plan begins with the compilation of an accurate, initial data base. The data base is obtained from a variety of sources: old records and charts, patient interviews, physical examinations including the review of systems, description of present illness, and family and social profiles. This initial data base should also include the patient profile and the information corresponding to items I through V (Fig. 2) of the nursing history—specifically, the age of the child, his school placement if any, his place in the family constellation, significant information about his feeding, toileting, sleeping, play, independent and dependent activities of daily living, and language development. The problem list derives from the data base. Each problem is numbered individually. Next, data are obtained in relation to each of the identified problems. The problems should not be confused with diagnoses. There does not need to be a diagnosis to support the identified problem. However, a patient may identify a particular disease as a problem. The list of problems should include social as well as medical concerns. There are columns for the date of onset and resolution to be recorded for each problem. After the problem list is completed, each problem is assessed and evaluated and appropriate plans are made for management. This step is generally referred to as SOAP, or soaping or soapie. The four initials stand for Subjective information, Objective information, Assessment, and Plan. Nurses have added two additional areas of Intervention and Evaluation. This information is the progress report for the patient.

The value of the problem-oriented record over the nursing history is that the problem-oriented method has all professionals participating in the same format and sharing of all information. In the past, much of the information gathered on the nursing history was not adequately shared with the rest of the health team. Indeed, the name "nursing history" made it seem a tool specific to the needs of one professional team member rather than data that offered challenges to a variety of health team members. The problem-oriented method will be of more value than the nursing history only if all health professionals are included in the formation of the problem list and encouraged to help resolve the problems that relate to their particular expertise.

The involvement of nurses in recording the initial data base will be dependent upon their educational preparation. Many nurses are learning the art of history-taking and physical examination. Nurses who are prepared in this way may take on added responsibility for the initial data base. In most cases, the physician will probably assume the responsibility for this aspect.

The problem-oriented method of data gathering is a systematic way to gather and analyze data pertinent to patient care. The easy accessibility of information related to each problem will facilitate the care and follow-through for the child. Having each problem numbered individually will help to focus attention on all the problem areas. The quick reference to past problems and their resolution will aid in the long-term management of these children. It should not be necessary to ask the parents many questions about past treatment, since the resolution data is clearly identified. For example, a child with recurrent sore throats may have this problem resolved by a T&A. If sore throats were to become a problem at a future date, they would receive a new number and be treated as a new problem.

CONCLUDING STATEMENT

The foregoing information is only of value to the student of nursing if it is utilized as a guide in delivering nursing services. Each child must be considered on an individual basis and treated within his own particular set of circumstances. The general ideas are given as guidelines for what the student might expect in learning the specific skills needed to deliver the best nursing services to the child with long-term illness.

CASE STUDY PRESENTATION AND STUDY QUESTIONS

Presenting Diagnosis: Blindness

Bobby was 12 years old when I first met him. He was blind from birth. Bobby was a premature infant tipping the scales at a mere 2 lbs. He was the fifth child in four years for his young Irish parents. He was born in a city hospital with a medium-sized obstetrical department.

The family physician delivered Bobby. The delivery was quick, uncomplicated, and performed without episiotomy or anesthesia. There is no Apgar score, but by the mother's recollection the child was "lifeless." A great deal of attention was already focused on the hazards of oxygen therapy to the eyesight of prematures. According to the records, the physician ordered higher concentrations anyway, as he expected the child to die soon.

The physician felt a great deal of guilt regarding Bobby's blindness and gave Bobby free medical supervision and care. The parents were very upset when the physician died (when Bobby was 2½ years old), and it was at this point that they began to feel the real burden of having a child who was blind.

The parents were contacted by someone from a preschool facility for blind children. They enrolled Bobby at three years of age in this school. Bobby was not ready for this socialization process and did not adjust to school. He was termed "retarded" by the professional personnel and the family was counseled to keep him home until he showed more signs of school-readiness.

The history is vague regarding Bobby as he came to be the middle child in a family of 10 children. Mrs. G. did not write down developmental achievements and therefore was not able to keep one child's record straight from another. Bobby received less and less of his parent's individual attention as they attempted to stretch their attention to reach ten active children. Mr. G. took a second job to help with the expenses of raising his large family. This made his personal contributions to his family decidedly fewer.

Bobby received individualized attention from an elderly aunt who was a retired elementary school teacher. It was her creativity that was responsible for Bobby's early educational endeavors. Miss W. taught Bobby the alphabet by designing boards with small, shell-macaroni letters. Bobby traced the letters with his fingers and after much persistence and dedication he could print his alphabet. Miss W. had no formal training with the blind, but she read everything she could get in regard to teaching. She played the piano and decided to teach Bobby how to play. After many hours of practice, he achieved several beginning piano pieces. At this time, Miss W. bought a piano for Bobby to have at home. Prior to this, he played only on Miss W.'s piano. Her home was within walking distance but approximately three-quarters of a mile away, making it seem inaccessible to the less ambitious members of the family.

It seemed like an excellent idea to have Bobby demonstrate his ability at the piano. None of the other siblings could play and this seemed like Bobby's opportunity to excel. However, it turned out to be a sad situation. Bobby was asked to demonstrate his talent for anyone that came to the home. His minimal talent was blown up out of proportion to his actual achievement. Bobby began to resent this and eventually he lost interest in playing the piano for anyone other than his aunt.

A routine check was made of all blind children in the community and Bobby was "rediscovered" by the school authorities. He had passed the most appropriate ages for achieving particular developmental tasks and he lacked many simple skills needed for entering school. The school officials suggested Bobby be thoroughly evaluated by an interdisciplinary team concerned with handicapped children.

When the evaluation was completed, it uncovered some interesting factors and raised several questions. After a conference with the parents, Bobby was enrolled in a special school and a tutor was hired by the school to work specifically to teach Braille to Bobby. Her individualized teaching was greatly responsible for the many educational advances made by Bobby. In addition, he needed to have his large muscles more thoroughly developed. This was partially achieved by swimming and gym classes. It was at swimming that Bobby's skills regarding dressing and undressing were perfected. Bobby was also taken on walks outside and was taught to cross the street by pushing the traffic control button and listening for the cars to stop. Bobby's walks were also used to introduce him to grass, flowers, curbs, people, and weather. Teaching Bobby was a challenge, a pleasure, and, occasionally, a frustration. It is difficult for a sighted person to describe things without including sight. It is too easy to take words for granted and assume they are self-explanatory. For instance, one day we were walking and a voting booth had been put on the sidewalk where we ordinarily passed freely. The booth was green, wooden, and rather plain. Before reaching the booth I explained to Bobby that the booth was there and to be careful as he approached it. Bobby got to it and started feeling it. He asked, "What did you say it was?" I replied, "A green house." "Oh, no," said Bobby, "a greenhouse is glass."

The same type of things can happen in the hospital setting. What seems to be a perfectly logical and simple explanation can be misinterpreted or rejected by the blind child because it is not consistent with his past experiences.

The needs and accomplishments of Bobby could fill many pages, but he is introduced here only to raise questions for nurses involved in the care of blind children. I pose the following questions for consideration:

1. How much can a family be expected to do on its own in seeking care for a child with a disability?
2. What can a community health nurse do to enhance the learning of a blind child excluded from formal schooling?
3. What clues would suggest the child is ready to be taught self-feeding?
4. How can nurses teach blind children to feed themselves?
5. How can a nurse provide needed stimulation for a hospitalized blind child?
6. How does a child "compensate" for being blind, or does he compensate?
7. What tasks could the other children in this family be delegated to help teach Bobby?
8. What types of information about Bobby's life-style could be obtained by interviewing one or two of the other children in the family?
9. If you were the one who uncovered Bobby's semi-isolation, what agencies would you contact for help and guidance?
10. What other types of activities could be suggested for developing Bobby's large and small muscles?

Presenting Diagnosis: Granulomatous Colitis

Harry is a 13-year-old white male and John is a 16-year-old white male. I introduce them as their long-term illness is the same: granulomatous colitis. Harry is presently hospitalized and receiving hyperalimentation therapy.* John is hospitalized on the same unit and is receiving medication therapy that presently consists of Imuran, ozulfadine, prednisone, multivitamins, and Librium. Harry has been through the medical route and has had a combination of medical and surgical therapy, but his disease has progressed to the serious condition which necessitated this admission.

Let us look at Harry's 13 years in more detail. Harry is the youngest of two children. His brother is 19 and has a spina bifida. His father has diabetes and his mother has anemia and a coagulation disorder. Harry's early years were without history of illness. His development is noted as normal, but little is known of the parent-child or sibling relationships. At age seven, his life-style was changed by serious illness which was diagnosed as colitis.

Hospitalizations occurred at ages seven, ten, twelve, and thirteen. Treatment during these confinements included medical regimens, surgery resulting in an ileal colectomy and closure of a ileal rectal fistula, and tracheostomy for respiratory distress resulting from laryngotracheobronchitis.

His present hospitalization followed a period of months of medical management that did not control rashes, fever, loss of weight, or diarrhea. For nearly a year, he was unable to attend school and a tutor came to Harry's home.

Harry is in a private room and one of this parents is allowed to room-in. The mother stays the majority of the time and assumes the majority of Harry's physical care. Mrs. J. is considered "overprotective" by most of the nursing staff. She has been accused of "interfering" with the occupational therapist's plan of care for Harry. When Mrs. J. leaves the room, several professionals have described an "improvement in Harry's attitude." He seems to open up and is willing to vent his feelings regarding his illness and hospitalization.

An example of Harry's interaction with a student nurse while his mother is present follows.

Nurse: "Do you have any friends visit?"
Harry: "No."
Nurse: "Are any of those cards from friends?"
Harry: "Yes, from James age 10, Mary, 13, and Joe, 14."
Nurse: "Would you like paper to write to them?"
Harry: "No, nothing to say."

Even open-ended questions resulted in short answers, and attempts to encourage interest in games were in vain. Mrs. J. left the room and the following conversation took place.

Harry: "I'm tired of this routine [hyperalimentation]. I know it's essential but I miss not eating."
Nurse: "I can appreciate that."

**Parenteral administration of glucose, amino acids, vitamins and electrolytes through a catheter into the child's right atrium (other hospitals report using the superior vena cava). Heparin is added to the IV solution to decrease the possibility of thrombosis formation.*

Harry: "I'm tired of being in the hospital. The worst part about being in the hospital is going home. All the kids laugh at me because I'm sick. They tease me because I can't keep up."

It is obvious from Harry's conversation that he needs more opportunities to be with a professional person without his mother being present.

There are several other factors that are significant in making Harry's hospitalization tolerable. He is retarded in growth due to the large amounts of steroids he has received over the years. The hospital school teacher knows his age and grade placement, but relates to him as a younger child. Harry resents this and finds the school work too easy. He needs to be challenged more on his intellectual level.

Harry's hyperalimentation therapy requires diligent and continual monitoring. The hourly check of the intravenous bottle does not guarantee Harry quality nursing care. The child frequently takes second place to the bottle. People frequently enter the room with their eye contact being made with the bottle high over Harry's head. Harry's morale is an important consideration in his therapy. During one hospitalization it was necessary to discharge him because of his "profound depression."

John's history includes several hospitalizations for medical management. He is currently having several bloody stools a day and requires transfusions for replacement. John is fully informed of his disease and knows about Harry's hyperalimentation routine. John does not feel he needs this therapy. He knows that Harry has had surgery without success and he doubts that surgery is the answer for control of his own disease.

John's parents doubt that he has colitis despite his long history and feel it is really "dysentery." John dropped out of school as a freshman in high school. He states he was an honor student and bored. He lives in an apratment with his brother. The brother is teaching him a trade.

John has visited Harry at Mrs. J.'s request. John feels Harry "lets his disease get to him." He feels Harry gives in too easily to cramps. John says, "I take my pills and stay up and go to work. That's why I do better than him."

Both boys show an adolescent understanding of their disease process. Both have a large hospital vocabulary. Both show effects of a long-term illness on peer relationships; neither seems to have many close friends. While John's parents continue to deny his disease, Harry's family is intimately involved in learning all they can about the disease and passing the information on to their local medical personnel. Both boys live a fair distance away and come to this hospital—"where the experts are," according to John.

The effects of the long-term illness on Harry are quite obvious. His ability to express himself is greatly impaired when his mother is present. He spends much time picking lightly at his arms and face. His eye contact with people is infrequent. He smiles very little and perhaps with good reason.

John seems much more self-sufficient despite his long-term illness. He knows he feels better when he takes sitz baths during periods of acute diarrhea. He swabs xylocaine viscus on his mouth ulcers when needed, and discontinues it when the ulcers are improved. He chooses his own diet, which is liberal but discourages large amounts of roughage. He has definite likes and dislikes in food and feels free to order meals. He refuses to let the hospital routine interfere with his ordinary personal hygiene habits. He is used to bathing in the evening and continues this practice in the hospital. He feels free to question his medical management. One example is in relation to giving blood for laboratory examination. He felt he needed a blood transfusion because the laboratory technician took so much blood. In an attempt to show him he was wrong, an empty intravenous bottle was filled with water collected in a blood tube. This demonstrated that even eight test tubes of blood would not necessitate a replacement transfusion.

John also showed some rebellious traits. He refused to save stool specimens needed for collection. He was allowed out of bed and used the toilet instead of the accessible bedpan. He did seem, however, willing to keep track of the number of stools he had a day. John also had difficulty relating to or empathizing with his 13-year-old roommate. This boy was newly diagnosed as having multiple sclerosis. He had sudden and profound loss of muscle tone on the left side and needed a great deal of assistance. John considered him "a baby" and told anyone that would listen. John and his family monopolized three-quarters of the two-bed room, leaving only one-quarter for the other boy and his family. In addition to space, John had the advantage of the window and close proximity to the bathroom.

John and Harry illustrate how two adolescents are reacting to an acute stage of their long-term illness. Their acceptance of some of the therapy is an example of a positive response of honest interpretations by health care personnel. Their difficulties in adjusting to school may be a result of how others view their illness or it may be the result of their own personalities. The emotional predisposition to their particular disease cannot be underestimated. How they interact with their peers and family may be a major link in their disease process. No less important during hospitalizations is how the nurse interacts with them.

Nursing intervention should focus on how best to meet their emotional needs during hospitalizations. I pose the following questions for consideration.

1. Is rooming-in a desirable practice for adolescent patients?
2. What can be done to compensate an adolescent on NPO for approximately 30 days?
3. Are selected diets a way to make the child feel he has some "control" of the situation? (Selected diet is one the child chooses.)
4. How much "support" does an adolescent with a milder form of a disease need when he is exposed to an adolescent with a more serious form of the same disease?
5. In what ways can the nurse be instrumental in channeling the child's educational pursuits? Or should the nurse get involved?
6. What types of recreational activities can be utilized during a child's bed rest to help him mature?
7. Is the room placement of either of these boys adequate? What would you consider a realistic placement on the unit?
8. Are there any other team members who seem essential for improving the quality care of these boys?

9. What role can a student nurse assume in her/his short experience in the clinical area? Should she/he assume any role, and why or why not?
10. Are the medical routines being used consistent with providing emotional support, or by their nature should we expect the child to be depressed? Why?

Nursing intervention is also concerned with the nursing tasks necessary for providing safe care. I pose the following questions for consideration in relation to these nursing tasks.

1. Who can safely assume responsibility for collecting, observing, and recording stools?
2. Is it possible to have the adolescent assume responsibility for recording his own intake and output? What factors would influence this decision?
3. Who is responsible for monitoring and recording the fluid administration? When the fluid is administered into the atrium, does this make the situation "too charged" for the usual consideration given an intravenous?
4. When the child is allowed out of bed only to be weighed, are there any special precautions necessary?
5. Who should be responsible for doing the urine specific gravity tests? Can the family be utilized for this task?
6. What special considerations are necessary when taking blood pressure readings? What significance do you think the taking of blood pressure has to these adolescents?
7. When the medication routine is changed, how much explanation should you give the child? Should adolescents with long-term illness be candidates for self-medication routines in the hospital or at home?

CHILDREN'S MISCONCEPTIONS AND INTERPRETATIONS

The jargon of the hospital easily becomes known to the child with long-term illness. However, the child is like every other child during his original orientation to the hospital. Children's misconceptions are casily made when a nurse fails to explain things in understandable language. Some illustrations follow.

Nurse: On admission, the child is seen by the intern.

Child's interpretation: I'll be seen in turn, but for what? I hope it doesn't hurt. Whose turn is first? We take turns in school, but the teacher tells us for what. I hope the bell rings before my turn comes up.

Nurse: John is to have blood work, a CBC, and x-ray pictures.

Child's interpretation: What is this blood work? I know a needle. I hope the doctor doesn't come. I need my blood. I hope I don't die. See Bea See, sounds like they think I'm a girl. Wonder what they want me to see. Hope it is nice. Pictures I like, but these x-ray pictures, I don't know. Wonder why they want my picture? Do they keep a family album of all the kids that come here?

Nurse: We need a urine specimen from John.
Child's interpretation: What is this your in? In what? Specimen, wonder what this means? Better ask mom.
Nurse: John should put on his Johnny shirt.
Child's interpretation: This isn't my shirt. Why did she call it Johnny's shirt? What a funny shirt all opened down the back. Why do I have to wear a shirt? Where are the pants? Look how short!
Nurse: Here is your call light.
Child's interpretation: Why call a light? Where is the bulb? Does the light talk? Must try to call the light, but what do I do with it?
Nurse: This is your bedside stand.
Child's interpretation: Why do I have to stand by the bedside? That looks like a cabinet to me. Wonder what's in there? Why does she call it mine? I never saw that before. I don't even like it.
Nurse: Visiting hours are from 11 a.m. to 8 p.m. for parents only.
Child's interpretation: Where are my parents going? Isn't daddy going to work? They didn't tell me they were going away. Imagine putting me in here and then leaving town. I think I'll put up a fuss. Maybe it isn't so bad—Alice will have that terrible old baby-sitter.

The next day John is introduced to several other confusing situations. He looks around the room and sees the following signs on the children's beds.

NPO
Child's interpretation: Must be some kind of sign language. Good, a secret language, these kids are really cool.
HOLD
Child's interpretation: Hold what? I'll just watch and see why they hold that kid. Maybe it's part of this secret game.
Late Breakfast
Child's interpretation: Oh no! Just when I'm starved they decide to serve breakfast late. Mom always has my breakfast ready when I come downstairs. Wonder how late it will be?
Force Fluids
Child's interpretation: Wow! Wonder what they do for force. Hope it doesn't hurt. Feel sorry for that poor kid. Fluids, that sounds familiar, but really don't know why they'd force lighter fluid. Mom says it's dangerous.
Save Urine
Child's interpretation: That urine is really going to the bathroom. I learned that yesterday. But, why save the urine? Wonder what they do with it. Supposing someone flushes the toilet when you're not looking? Do you get punished? Or maybe you use that urinal thing. Hope it doesn't overflow, that would be awful!
Daily Urine
Child's interpretation: Guess they like those urine specimens. I better get ready if you have to do it daily. Hope that nurse doesn't look, it's hard to go with her standing here.
Note Bleeding
Child's interpretation: Gosh that poor kid's in rough shape. I wonder

when he bleeds? I don't like to see blood. Wonder why they want us to watch. I'll just cover over my head with the sheet.

OR

Child's interpretation: That's a funny sign. Or what? This place has to be nuts. Nothing makes sense.

The nurse enters the room and talks to John.

Nurse: John, I will take you to the treatment room for a finger prick.

Child's interpretation: Treatment room, what's that like? I like my room. I'm scared to go there. And a finger prick—I don't want to get stuck. That's all they do here everytime a guy turns around they give him a shot. Wish mom were here to go to this awful place with me. Wonder how I get there, on an elevator, by wheelchair?

Nurse: The doctor's orders state that you must have blood work done by the house officer.

Child's interpretation: Orders. I guess they give out a lot of those around here. The doctor seemed like a nice guy in his office. Why did he have to give orders to hurt me? I'll get even with him. I won't talk to him. Big bully! House officer sounds like the cops are around. Anyone can see this isn't a house, it's a hospital. A big, mean old hospital and I hate it. I want to go home; wish mom would come. I'm real mad at her; she left me here, left me and went on vacation. Forgot to ask her about that, wonder when she'll be back. Anyway, she wasn't going until 11 A.M. Maybe she'll come here just in time to save me from this blood-sucking monster. But, what good will it do? She'll never know where this treatment room is. Bet it's down in the basement, down in a dark dungeon! Wish I was home, I miss Alice. Alice is my very best friend. Maybe she'll run away and come find me.

As the nurse and John walk down the hall, the nurse begins to identify things for John.

Nurse: That is the linen chute.

Child's interpretation: Linen shoot, linen shoot. Shoot is something you do with a gun. Why would they want to shoot linen? Maybe they shoot people, too. Or maybe it's a shoot like a slide. Yes, that's it—a slide. Wonder if the kids can slide down it? But, linen that makes it a special slide. I haven't seen a tablecloth anywhere, wonder where the linen is. Perhaps there's a dining room with these linen tablecloths. Maybe that's where they serve the late breakfast. I hope she shows it to me soon.

Nurse: That is the dumbwaiter that goes to Central Supply.

Child's interpretation: I knew that waiter was dumb before she told me. Late breakfast when a guy is starving! Central supply must be the place where they keep the food, wonder why they don't call it a kitchen or pantry like mom does. That door seems awfully high for that dumb waiter to pass through. Maybe he has a stool or they wheel away the stairs like on an airplane. Or maybe he's like Superman, magic. Gee, I hope I get to meet him. Maybe he's not such a dumb guy after all.

Nurse: There are two people you will see a lot while you're here, John. The cleaning lady and the security guard.

Child's interpretation: Cleaning lady—she doesn't look like Minny. Wonder what she cleans, maybe it's the other kids. Not me though, mom will clean me. Minny irons the clothes, but anyone can see they don't iron these terrible Johnny shirts. Glad I have my bathrobe to cover it up. I don't want anyone to see me running around in this thing. It must have shrunk in the wash. Maybe if she irons it, it will be longer. I'll ask her next time I see her. And that security guard. What a spooky place, your very own policeman walking around looking in the rooms. I see him smiling at the kids but I won't smile back when he gets to me.

Nurse: That boy is in the oxygen tent.

Child's interpretation: Fine tent that is, you can see right through it. How does the poor guy sleep? I don't like the tent—it's so small the bed doesn't fit all the way in. Wonder what that pipe is doing shooting fog into the tent? Maybe they're trying to kill the kid. He doesn't look so good. Hope his mom comes to save him. That tent makes an awful lot of noise, wonder how the other kids sleep? Maybe they get soundproof tents at night.

Nurse: This is the treatment room, John. That is an intercom to use in an emergency.

Child's interpretation: Emergency, boy I knew things were getting rough. Maybe I better use it now to call mom. I'd rather go home, this emergency stuff is not for me. This whole room is filled with terrible things. Just look at that—hard table, wonder what they're for. Surely not breakfast. Who could eat in here anyway. I feel sick to my stomach just looking at all those tubes and needles and machines. Even that scale is big enough to weigh a giant! There's a refrigerator, I guess it must be the dining room after all or maybe that central supply place—wonder where the dumb waiter is? Here he comes now with the white jacket. He doesn't look too dumb.

Nurse: Hello, Dr. Jones, this is John.

Child's interpretation: Foiled again, it's not that house officer guy or the dumb waiter. It's not my doctor, either. They must have me mixed up with some other kid. I'll set them straight and beat it out of here.

The doctor prepares to take the blood and John complains he feels faint.

Nurse: I'll have oj ready for you as soon as it's over.

Child's interpretation: Imagine, a real live football player waiting to see me after he sucks out the blood. Maybe this place isn't so bad after all.

Nurse: Doctor, would you like to talk to John about going to the OR, recovery room, and possibly the intensive care unit?

Child's interpretation: Intensive care, wonder why you get that. No one cares here. They just stare at you and take urine and put up signs on beds. OR—that must be one of those words they don't want me to know. Just like all the other big people, they spell when they don't want you to know what they're talking about. But, what's this recovery bit? How can I recover when I haven't seen a ball being thrown. Imagine a whole room for ball games. Maybe they'll take me there after breakfast. Gee, but I'm hungry. I should have read that sign on

> the bottom of my bed. Maybe it said, no food, ever. If I could only get some of that intensive care or just someone who cared even a little when a guy is hungry.

The foregoing examples are given to emphasize to the nurse that teaching the child about the hospital is more than relating facts. The child will interpret information by utilizing experiences in his life experience. It is difficult for him to understand new concepts without help. Time must be spent to help the child interpret facts in a new way. The child enjoys learning new things and will be more comfortable when he gets the intended meanings, rather than his garbled interpretation. There are numerous examples which can be cited. The nurse must be certain to communicate with the child on his own level, and then spend time being sure the child really understands what is being said.

BIBLIOGRAPHY

Bell RA: Discontinuity of care in a crippled children program. Studies in Handicapping Conditions. Rockville, Maryland, HEW, 1975
Bell RR: The Impact of Illness on Family Roles: A Sociological Framework for Patient Care. New York, Wiley, 1966, pp 177–89
Bright F: The pediatric nurse and parental anxiety. Nurs Forum 4:30, 1965
Bowlby J: Grief and mourning in infancy and early childhood. Psychoanal Stud Child 15:9, 1960
Debusky M (ed): The Chronically Ill Child and His Family. Springfield, Ill, Thomas, 1970
Diller L: Psychology of disabled children. In Rudick E (ed): Pediatric Nursing, Dubuque, Iowa, Brown, 1966
Epstein C: Breaking the barriers to communications on the health team. Nurs '74 4:65, September 1974
Farber B: Family: Organization and Interaction. San Francisco, Chandler, 1964
Fields G: Social implications of long-term illness in children. In Downey JA and Low NL: The Child with Disabling Illness. Philadelphia, Saunders, 1974
Green M: Care of the child with long-term threatening illness: some principles of management. Pediatrics 39:441, 1967
Green M, Durocher MA: Improving parent care of handicapped children. Children, 12:185, 1965
Hannam C: Parents and Mentally Handicapped Children. England, Penguin, 1975
Illingworth RS: The increasing challenge of handicapped children. In Rudick E (ed): Pediatric Nursing. Dubuque, Iowa, Brown, 1966
Kline J, Schowalter JE: How to care for the "between-ager." Nurs '74 4:43–51, Nov, 1974
Laing RD: The Politics of the Family. New York, Vintage, 1972
Longest BB: Management Practices for the Health Professional. Reston, Va, Reston, 1976
Maddison D, Raphael B: Social and psychological consequences of chronic disease in childhood. Med J Aust 2:1265, 1971

Mattsson A: Long-term physical illness in childhood: a challenge to psychosocial adaptation. Pediatrics 50:801, 1972

Petrillo M, Sanger S: Emotional Care of Hospitalized Children: An Environmental Approach. Philadelphia, Lippincott, 1972

Pluckham, ML: Professional territoriality: a problem affecting the delivery of health care. Nurs Forum 11:300, 1972

Ramos S: Teaching your Child to Cope with Crisis. New York, McKay, 1975

Rapoport L: Working with families in crisis: an exploration in preventive intervention. In Parad HJ (ed): Crisis Intervention. New York, Family Service Assoc of America, 1965

Ross AO: The Exceptional Child in the Family. New York, Grune & Stratton, 1964

Rubin M: Caring for children with illness requiring long-term hospitalization: In Anderson E (ed): Current Concepts in Clinical Nursing. St Louis, Mosby, 1967

Shore MF, Geiser RL, Wolman HM: Constructive uses of a hospital experience. Children 12:3-8, 1965

Smith DM: A clinical nursing tool. Am J Nurs, 68:2384-88, Nov, 1968

Smith M: Ego support for the child patient. In Rudick E (ed): Pediatric Nursing. Dubuque, Iowa, Brown, 1966

Spiegel JP: The resolution of role conflict within the family. Psychiatry 20:1-16, 1957

Strauss AL: Chronic Illness and the Quality of Life. St. Louis, Mosby, 1975

Weed LL: Medical Records, Medical Education and Patient Care, 5th ed. Chicago, The Press of Case Western Reserve, 1971

Wooley FR, Warnick MW, Kane RL et al: Problem-oriented Nursing. New York, Springer, 1974

DONNA JUENKER

4
Child's Perception of His Illness

The life span of a child consists of a multitude of experiences that he assimilates into his reality. His "reality" depends to a large extent on how he perceives those experiences. This attachment of meaning to stimuli is a complex process for the child. When one compares the relative insensitivity of the newborn infant with the sophisticated modes of perception that characterize the adolescent, one is immediately aware of the magnitude of change in perceptual development.

The infant first perceives emotional significances (Stone and Church, 1957). The meaning that an object has is perceived well in advance of the characteristics of the object itself. Later on, an awareness of "action" relationships is added to "feeling" associations. Objects are perceived in relation to what they do to the child. As the objects in the child's world assume more stability and permanence, the child learns to perceive objective properties. Once able to attach labels to objects, he can more easily note differences between them. For instance, he learns that "dogs" have properties that are different from "cats" or that "yellow" and "orange" are different colors.

When confronted by an unfamiliar stimulus, such as a picture of an unusual object, the young child tends to react to the entire stimulus as a whole rather than to its parts. The older child, on the other hand, can see distinct aspects of the same new stimulus. His initial perception will include a more complete description of the details in the picture.

In spite of perceptual constancy in areas such as shape, color, and depth, perception is a very individual matter since it is constantly being altered by past experience. Throughout the evolution of perceptual development, experience broadens the child's repertory of cues so that he can be increasingly adept at recognizing similarities and differences among the objects in the environment. As the child grows older, a stimuli perceived earlier can have increasingly complex meanings because of the child's ability to see new properties in a particular object or to see new alternatives in a particular problem situation. By repeated experiences involving seeing, hearing, tasting, smelling, and touching, the child improves his powers of discrimination, and gradually his perceptions become more objective. This process is an important part of cognitive development.

Perception is affected by the intensity of the stimulus—that is, the degree to which it absorbs the child's attention. A very strong stimulus blocks out distracting influences. Such intense involvement or absorption in an experience can open one's sensory receptivity to a point at which maximum learning can take place. However, if the stimulus is very stressful, the perceptual field can become extremely narrow so that attention is directed solely on the alleviation of the stress.

The child's perception is also affected by the scope of the stimulus—that is, the number of parts in the whole. If his senses are simultaneously affected by many stimuli such as sights, sounds, and internal stirrings, he is likely to select from the total those parts that have special meaning or are in some way connected to a familiar past experience. While this selectivity is an understandable way of coping with a new situation, the child's perception of the experience may not conform with consensus reality. He may have missed many significant aspects that were quite evident to onlookers.

Many children face the experience of being ill. Illness brings with it an endless combination of disquieting symptoms, variation in intensity of objective stress, and marked changes in the social and physical aspects of the external environment. Each of these components constitutes a unique experiential phenomenon, which the child assimilates into his reality as best he can. Each new experience is somehow linked to previous ones. A child who is confronted by a situation that is unlike any previous experience is left without a ready response. He has to call on what may be a limited number of mental configurations or images and immature psychologic defenses to accommodate the new experience.

This chapter seeks to identify and describe the factors that influence the child's perception of illness. Emphasis will be placed on those that are most essential in planning nursing care. For example, it is well known that illness alters body image to some degree. To understand the impact of change in body image, it is important that the nurse knows how the body-image concept evolves in childhood and how important such a concept is to a child.

Another section of the chapter examines the child's view of the structure and function of the body. It is obvious that the child's reality is different from that of the adult. When a health professional with sophisticated knowledge about the body attempts to communicate with a child about his illness, many false assumptions can be made. If the nurse understands what the child thinks about the healthy body, her communication can be guided by the level of knowledge which the child possesses. If she is aware of common misconceptions that children have, she is not likely to presume that they have a realistic grasp of their problems.

Every child attaches a wide range of meanings to his illness. The variety of factors that determine his interpretation will be discussed, as will be the influences of age and past experience.

Still another section of the chapter will explore the impact of hospitalization. Viewed as one aspect of illness, the hospitalization experience will be examined primarily in relation to the environmental changes it produces.

Since the attitudes and actions of parents are among the most important of the factors affecting the child's perception of his illness, this chapter will conclude with an analysis of parental influences.

This collection of information will hopefully increase the nurse's awareness of the perceptual process as it relates to a child's view of illness. An important by-product of this awareness is an increased empathy for young patients and their families. With empathy, the nurse will be better able to interact meaningfully about a very significant experience for any child —illness.

CONCEPT OF BODY IMAGE

Gorman (1969) defines body image as the concept of one's own body, based on present and past perceptions. Body image is a dynamic concept —constantly undergoing changes in keeping with one's perceptions. The ability to give one's body the characteristics of unity and distinctness from others requires an integration of external stimuli and internal sensations. Such a concept evolves over a lifetime, with its beginnings traceable to infancy.

The young infant, of course, cannot grasp the notion of his separateness. He perceives himself and the world to be identical. One of his important tasks, then, is to learn about his distinctiveness. Because of his concentration on oral activities, it seems likely that the infant begins to note the differences between things coming into the mouth from the outside and the internal feelings that ingestion of food brings with it. The constancy of the mouth and tongue as opposed to the changing nature of the solids and liquids entering the oral cavity serves to identify the mouth as a body boundary. The infant's increasing observation and use of his arms and legs and fingers and toes along with the assumption of an upright posture further extends feelings of "you-ness" and "me-ness." The "out-of-sight, out-of-mind" cognitive stage gradually gives way to the realization that the extended arm or leg can be maneuvered into the range of vision, that its function remains constant, and that it is "me." Thus maturational changes affect body image.

There are several other factors that contribute to the infant's "body feeling." One mechanism is pain (Schilder, 1935; Bender, 1963). Although the young child may not be able to verbalize the location of pain, pain is felt as a localized phenomenon and consequently it is associated with the organization of the body image. When there is pain on the surface of the body, that body part becomes overemphasized. Attention is drawn to it. Through repetition of painful experiences, the infant not only learns about his own body boundaries, but he also comes to realize that only he can feel "his" pain.

Another sensation that contributes to the body-image concept is touch (Anthony, 1968). Touching one's own body arouses a different feeling from that experienced when touching the body of another. Being touched by another is yet a different experience. The infant who chews on his own fingers evokes a feeling-state that is quite different from that achieved by chewing on his mother's fingers.

Anthony also describes a fourth mechanism in the process of self-differentiation—the mirror image. By looking into a mirror the infant sees himself in the way that others see him. As social awareness increases the child recognizes the reflection as his own image.

Psychosexual stages of development have considerable bearing on concepts of body image in the young child. For instance, the child develops erotic interests in particular parts of his body—especially the oral, anal, umbilical, and genital zones. The satisfaction derived from exploring these areas draws attention to body configuration and helps to consolidate an understanding of body boundaries.

In "toddlerhood," language becomes an important contributor to body image. Body parts are named and classified. The frequency with which certain body parts become a part of the approved vocabulary makes the child attach a certain level of significance to them. If a part of the body and its accompanying terminology are purposefully avoided or are spoken about in hushed or emotional tones, the child may learn to repress this knowledge or consider it taboo.

Learning control of body functions occupies much of the toddler's energies. This preoccupation and "fussing" with the body may resemble a hypochondriac reaction. The power over elimination symbolizes power over all body processes and is another mark of differentiation between the self and others.

During the preschool period, one of the most significant discoveries about the body is that of sex differences. This discovery gives rise to the Freudian concept of the castration complex. The little boy's "pride" in his penis coincides with his extreme fear of losing the organ (as he thinks happened to girls). Girls, on the other hand, feel cheated and deprived and may wish to grow a penis. Recognition of and response to these concerns, when they occur, may have a bearing on how these children perceive the male-female aspects of their body image.

Children continue to expand their awareness of body dimensions as they progress from the early stages of development when initial discoveries about the body are of great magnitude. They still perceive the body in terms of what it can do for them. However, as they move into the school years (and perhaps even before), these concrete body concepts are modified by more subtle interpretations of the meaning of body type. For example, Staffieri (1967) studied 90 boys between the ages of six and ten to determine the extent to which they associated body build with social-personal behaviors. Responses differed depending upon whether the children were viewing silhouettes of mesomorphic (muscular), endomorphic (fat), or ectomorphic (thin) body types. All of the adjectives that the children assigned to the mesomorph figure were favorable. They were rated as strong, healthy, good looking, brave, smart, and as having lots of friends. Characteristics assigned to the endomorph and ectomorph figures were generally either socially or personally unfavorable. The fat child was often viewed as naughty, mean, ugly, dirty, and stupid. On the other hand, the thin silhouette evoked descriptions that included words like quiet, afraid, sad, and weak. Although the boys in the study had a reasonably accurate perception of their own body type, they showed a clear preference for looking like the mesomorph image. This preference began to be evident between six and seven years of age.

Accuracy of the perception of one's body appears to increase with age. Nash (1969) studied a group of seventh- and ninth-grade boys to determine the extent to which they could recognize photographs of parts of their own bodies and those of their acquaintances. The facial regions (forehead, eyes, mouth) were better recognized than other parts of the body. In this sample, because of the age (puberty), recognition of some of the features seemed to be related to developmental factors such as acne and changes in body proportions.

The study group was racially heterogeneous. The greatest accuracy in self-recognition was found among minority group children. Furthermore, majority race children tended to be more accurate in recognizing minority group children than they were in recognizing acquaintances of their own race. Recognition seemed to be related to stereotyped concepts associated with the anatomical features of minority races. While the results of the study are certainly not conclusive, they lead one to speculate that a child's personal interest or concern about his body is sustained during the school years and possibly heightened at times when normal physical changes in the body become evident, especially at the time of puberty. It seems possible that a child's membership in a stigmatized group may also heighten body interest. One might wonder whether alteration in body image is more disturbing to these children whose bodies are apparently well scrutinized by themselves and others.

A group often thought to be stigmatized in our culture is that composed of obese individuals. Children who are significantly overweight are thought to have more difficulty in forming a differentiated and mature body image than nonobese youngsters. Nathan (1973) studied 36 children with obesity and compared them to 36 nonobese control subjects in relation to their ability to draw the human figure. (An obese subject was one whose weight was at least 30 percent in excess of stated weight for height.) In the three age groups studied (7, 10, and 13 years), drawings made by the children with obesity lacked more differentiation and detail than did those of the control group. It is generally known that obesity in our culture is often ridiculed.

The attitudes held by others toward one's appearance certainly contribute to the development of a concept of self. Also, the bodily activities that contribute to the kinesthetic sense are a necessary element in structuring the body image.

Illness also seems to affect the formation of body image. Fleming (1972) studied 136 healthy and ill children between the ages of five through twelve in relation to differences in human figure drawings. Drawings by groups of chronically ill, physically disabled, and acutely ill children were compared with those of a matched control group of healthy children. Each child was asked to draw a person and then to draw his family. After each drawing was completed, the child was asked to tell about the person or people he had drawn. Figures that psychologists judged as representing a disturbed self-image were found more frequently among physically disabled children than among the healthy controls. Interestingly, the drawings of the chronically ill children were more complete than those of the physically disabled, indicating less conflict with body image.

Drawings from each group of ill children showed more overall abnormalities (differences were noted in detailing, shading, pencil pressure, placement of figures on the paper, and omissions and distortions of body parts) than did those of the healthy controls, indicating that these children may have a greater tendency to develop disturbed self-images. Fleming feels that ill children, especially the physically disabled, have a smaller margin of adaptability, and because of hospitalizations have greater limitations in experience. Both of these factors affect self-image. Recognition, through the use of drawings, of those things that are troublesome for the child may be the first step in helping a child cope with his lowered self-image. It is not the only tool the nurse can use, but in collaboration with a psychologist it can be a most meaningful one.

It seems reasonable to conclude from the foregoing statements that one's body image evolves from multiple factors—biologic configuration, physiologic function, developmental maturation, and social reinforcement. The intensity of the child's interest in his body varies, but it seems obvious from the literature that body perceptions are quite keen fairly early in life. This should lead us to examine more closely what a young child thinks about his body when it undergoes unanticipated changes during illness.

PERCEPTIONS ABOUT THE INSIDE OF THE BODY

While children appear to have some sophistication about the external dimensions of the body, the internal organs and tissues are shrouded in considerable mystery. The fact that there is substantial ignorance about the inside of the body is really not too surprising when one realizes that most bodily sensation is concentrated on the body surface. When the body systems are functioning normally, children are not acutely aware of organic activity. The lungs, heart, and intestines are not in the mainstream of consciousness as they carry out their daily activities. Nevertheless, in spite of a vague awareness of body organs and little theoretical background, children do construct frameworks of body functioning—sometimes very elaborate ones, indeed.

Schilder and Weschler (1935), among the earliest to describe children's concepts about their bodies, asked children what was inside of the body. Most of them (especially between the ages of five and ten) replied that the inside of the body contained food. Some used more concrete terms and pictured themselves filled with bread, milk, or meat. One boy of 8½ expressed a combination of ideas when asked what was in his belly. In response to the query, he replied, "Food, my stomach, sweets, and ice." The children expressed interesting ideas about the self. When one child was asked to describe what was under his skin he answered "me." For some it seemed to be an envelope of the self. In other words, if the skin were peeled off, the whole self would be revealed.

This five-year-old boy's discussion with his teacher reveals his thoughts about his skin. (Words in parenthesis are comments of the teacher.)

> (Inspecting his abdomen as he dresses after nap.) You know a thing? There is something funny about my skin. It fits all smooth mostly, but when I do this, there are extra skin crumples. What is that for? (It's loose so you can move and stretch, etc.) No it is not loose or it would show. It would hang down. It would be too big. (Like a rubber band.) Would it break if you pulled it too much? (Can stretch a lot.) I had this same skin when I was a baby. It fits very nice. It is me. (Stone and Church, 1957, p 160.)

Concepts about body processes were studied by Nagy (1953). She focused on brain function, breathing, and digestion. The children in the sample ranged in age from about four to twelve years. Nearly all of the children associated the brain with intellectual activities. It was not until the age of eight that other functions began to appear in the children's descriptions. Predominance of mental function over emotional and physical factors is not surprising because children are often reminded to use their brain when mental effort is required. Nerves—with functions such as feeling, working, and moving—were mentioned by some of the older children, but such sophisticated answers occurred rarely. Children did not refer consistently to the process of breathing (ie, taking in and expelling of air) until around nine years of age. The nose, mouth, and throat were frequently mentioned in relation to breathing. This seemed to indicate that children believed that air circulated in the head region, primarily between the nose and mouth. A high percentage of children believed that breathing was necessary for life but generally did not know why. The digestive tract was thought by most to consist of the mouth and stomach. The stomach was the place for "keeping our food" or for "eating;" the purpose of eating was very vague—"to live," "to grow," and "to keep healthy."

Gellert (1962) also conducted an extensive study aimed at examining children's perception of the content and functioning of the human body. The children ranged in age from 4 years and 9 months to 16 years and 11 months. All of the children were hospitalized, so it is likely that their ideas about their bodies were affected by their illnesses. As in the Schilder and Weschler study, Gellert found that younger children listed food, blood, and excreta as being inside of the body. As age increased, digestive, urinary, nervous, and respiratory systems were mentioned with greater frequency. The numbers of body parts that children could name dramatically increased at about age nine. For example, children between 5 and 7 years could name an average of three parts; those between 9 and 11 listed an average of nine parts.

When children were asked about the most important part of the body, the heart was given this distinction by most of the children in all age categories. Organs associated with nervous, sensory, and intellectual activity were next in order. The importance of an organ was generally rated on the basis of its capacity to "run and/or control vital functions." It was interesting to note that some of the very young children associated importance with the amount of care and attention given to a particular body part. One youngster claimed that his toes were the most important part of the body "because you have to scrub between [them] which is real hard" (Gellert, 1962, p 320).

The children were asked to describe the parts of the body that they consider dispensable. Doing without a part of the body was inconceivable for some; 20 percent of the children quizzed firmly believed that they needed all their parts and could dispense with none. (All of these children were under the age of 11.) Of the dispensable parts recorded by the children it was surprising to note that arms and legs were mentioned with greatest frequency in spite of their importance in the daily life of the children.

There is some evidence in the study to support the influence of the mass media on concepts that children have about the body. For instance, Gellert discovered that several children were aware of the existence of organ transplants. The impact of illness was also evident since many children attached special significance to the diseased parts of their bodies.

The methods used to gather the data in these studies included interviews, graphic representations, written essays, and paper-and-pencil tests.

A variety of methods had to be used in order to accommodate the cognitive abilities of the children. The investigators are careful to point out the findings reveal only what the children are willing to talk about or write down. Very likely the information given does not reflect all that they know. As mentioned before, certain parts of the body may be considered as "forbidden" areas and the child may not express his knowledge because he thinks it is unacceptable to do so.

Children's human figure drawings reveal a great deal about how children view their bodies. The head predominates in the child's first recognizable drawings, and arms and legs appear as projections from the head (Di Leo, 1970). The head, arms, and legs are significant in the child's life since they are the primary foci for sensory input. They serve locomotion needs and permit exploration and experimentation with people and objects in the environment. Generally speaking, the trunk is ignored. Eyes are the dominant facial features, appearing as large circles in the head. The frequency of their presence in early drawings suggests the importance to the child of expressive eyes. Other facial features will be added before the body is consistently included in the drawing. It is not until about age five that the trunk is added.

As the child grows older, he perceives more of the fine details of the body and has the manipulative ability to depict his perceptions. Yet, his figure drawings do not truly reflect actual body dimensions. Rather, they seem to coincide with body image—not as we see the child, only as he conceives himself (Gorman, 1969).

CHILD'S INTERPRETATION OF HIS ILLNESS

Illness has meanings for every child. Interpretation depends upon a wide range of factors: age, the nature of the illness and its treatment, family relationships, and past experiences. Illness is stressful at all ages—even when illness is mild, family relationships are satisfying, and past experiences are basically untraumatic. However, each child experiences his own set of concerns to a degree of intensity that is uniquely his.

Perceptions About Cause of Illness

A primary concern of the ill child is resolution of responsibility for the illness. It is commonly assumed by children that illness is a punishment. Sometimes the child can recall a specific deed that he perpetrated that is of sufficient magnitude to cause illness. Recollection of mother's warning, "If you don't wear your rubbers, you'll get sick," suddenly becomes very meaningful. That blame and illness or injury go hand-in-hand in the child's mind was readily noted when a young boy of eight reacted to a picture of a child with a bandaged head by saying, "It was his fault; he probably didn't watch the cars when he crossed the street."

The idea of punishment is not just related to bad deeds. Illness can also serve as a retribution for bad thoughts. During the preschool years, for instance, children are known to wish their parents dead because of competition for affection. There is much ambivalence about this notion, so they also experience guilt. When illness or injury strikes, they can associate the discomfort with "evil" thoughts. Feelings of anger often accompany the guilt, but sometimes the opportunity to "suffer" relieves some of the child's anxiety.

The school-age child associates the cause of illness with "germs" (Nagy, 1953). Many children believe that germs are animals, identified especially with insects such as flies and spiders. They are commonly thought to enter the body through the mouth and once inside the body children say that they invariably cause illness. Germs are believed to have properties such as walking around inside the body, eating and breeding. Although the child connects disease with an external causative factor, he may continue to hold himself responsible for the entry of the germ into the body. Sometimes, children will extend the blame to parents and peers.

Consequences of Illness

The sick child can be visibly concerned about the tangible consequences of his illness apart from the physical aspects of his disease. For instance, the child may worry about a loss of position in the family. This might be an especially critical issue if his status is already a bit shaky because of the arrival of a new sibling or if an older brother or sister has just returned from college. In the case of the new sibling, however, the illness may provide the child with the added attention that he craves.

School absenteeism, accompanied by interruption in the social and competitive aspects of peer activities, is also a major worry for the sick child. If the duration of the illness is prolonged, the child may be fearful about his ability to resume normal activities. Not "measuring up" to his own expectations and the expectations of others is an age-old concern of all children in the middle years of childhood. However, if residual effects of illness complicate the situation, the problem can be enormous.

The restrictions of movement that often accompany illness can exert hardship on the child. There is no uniform reaction to restraint. Many factors will influence how a particular child will respond. An important one is the child's usual temperament. If he is characteristically a very active child who satisfies many of his needs through body movement, his resistance to restraint may be more aggressive than a child whose behavior is more passive. Also, the stage and type of illness is an important determinant. For example, in preparing a child preoperatively to tolerate necessary postoperative restraint, the parent or nurse may encounter much resistance—tossing, turning, pulling against restraints, attempting to stand or sit—suggesting that the postoperative period will be a battle of wills. Postoperatively, however, the same child may be quietly tolerant of limited movement, not because he has accepted it but rather because the physiologic stress does not allow him to be an active resister. Instead children in this situation often resort to regressive activities, such as sucking, withdrawal, and visual vigilance. However, once he begins to feel better, these restrictions are increasingly difficult to bear. Of course, the reaction to these limitations is affected by the meaning that they have for a particular child and family: an active, sports-minded, outdoor enthusiast will experience more stress than a child whose interests are more sedentary.

Restriction of food often poses another problem. In a family in which enjoyment of food plays a dominant role, limited food intake is stressful not only for the child who is ill, but also for the mother who must enforce the restrictions. Many mothers judge the effectiveness of their mothering role by how well they feed their children.

All illness brings with it a certain degree of dependency. In moderation this is good because it permits the individual to focus attention on himself and conserve energy that he might otherwise expend in trying to sustain independent function. However, if the degree of dependency is great, it becomes threatening. Dependent independent conflicts are frequent occurrences in childhood. The autonomy for which the toddler strives hinges on the achievement of a variety of important developmental tasks such as walking, bowel control, self-feeding, and talking. When illness disrupts the normal progression of these developmental landmarks and robs the child of new-found independence, the effects are clearly visible and the child takes backward steps in all of these areas. This regression wounds the ego, and it requires sensitive handling to reestablish self-satisfying independence.

The dependency problems experienced by the older child are not quite so obvious. Dependency on others, after a period when the child has mastered complete control over his body, arouses feelings of shame and embarrassment. Strong feelings of modesty conflict with the invasion of privacy that attends bodily illness. The adolescent resents dependency in a special way. In some ways the intensity of his feelings and his self-interest parallel that of the toddler—but there is a difference. The adolescent, in his search for identity, is concerned with how he appears in the eyes of others as compared to his view of himself. Dependence, in this instance, can be devastating because it puts the adolescent out of touch with his peers and places the reins of control in the hands of authoritarian adults from which he is trying to loosen ties.

The older child who is sick can be very conscious of the hardships that his illness exerts on the members of the family. He may struggle with the realization that his own needs are in conflict with family needs. In his sincere attempt to reduce his demands on family resources, he may inadvertently appear to reject his family's attention. Youngsters also worry about the financial burden that the treatment may impose. The father who has to work a double job to make ends meet is a reminder to the child that he has strained family resources. The concern is especially acute during the school years when contributions to and responsibility for family affairs is an important aspect of social development. A child who thinks that he is not doing his share thinks less of himself.

Family vacations and other activities may be postponed in deference to the needs of the sick child, whether he is treated at home or in the hospital. The child's needs may require someone in attendance at all times. Parents can well understand the need (although they realistically experience disappointment when anticipated plans are changed), but siblings have greater difficulty in handling the conflict of interests. The sick child is often quite aware of the turmoil he thinks that he has caused and this may intensify already present guilt feelings.

Physical Aspects of Illness

I have just pointed out that the behavior of a sick child has many psychosocial determinants. It is also important to discuss the relationship between behavior and physical aspects of the illness itself. This concept is not quite so clear, although the existence of some type of relationship seems likely.

Infants and toddlers do not perceive the significance of altered body function in its real sense; râther, they view it as an interruption in the usual sequence of the meaningful events to which they have become accustomed. To them, illness amounts to a collection of deprivations and overstimulations. No doubt these children experience internal stirrings that beg for satisfaction along the tension-relaxation continuum. Frustration of oral drives and restriction of movement are major sources of tension.

The toddler, of course, perceives more of his body than does the infant, but as yet he has not incorporated the concept of self and therefore does not see himself clearly as a separately functioning unit. While it is true that toddlers can identify visible parts of the body, especially facial characteristics, they do not have the cognitive faculty of associating illness with threat to body function.

The preschool period brings with it increased awareness of body structure and function. Control of excretory function draws attention to the body and its products. The child attaches great significance to physical sex differences and, generally, is taken up with the notion of physical identity. Fear of injury to the self is common. All parts of the body are essential to its wholeness. Thus a break in the skin or a removal of a body part, such as the tonsils, fragments the child's concept of his unity.

Stone and Church (1957) record the following comments made by a five-year-old boy, which well illustrate feelings about being complete:

> Once there was Stuart with a tooth and in it there was a hole. So it was fixed. The man had many little streams there, very nice. There was a pain, a bright pain. It was bright when he pushed with a noise and a bar. But there was no blood. No blood. . . . Can I get a hole in my hand like the hole in my tooth? Will it have to be filled with a loud noise? . . . The queen was in the garden hanging up her clothes, there came along a big thing to snap off her nose. . . . Her nose was not. It bled and bled and she died. Humpty Dumpty did die, too. He fell off and couldn't put together again. . . . When I have my tonsils out—what will happen when I have my tonsils out? Will it bleed? Will I be dead? Being blood is being dead. Why do I have my tonsils out?
>
> *I do not like myself not to be myself, and that is what will happen if even my littlest tonsils is taken away from me.*
>
> . . . Sad it was to have a nose taken off. So it will be sad to have a tonsil out. Blood, blood, blood. When the nose—the tonsil is out (p 161).

Older children have more realistic conceptions of their bodies. However, because they can connect illness with impaired body function and then relate impaired function with a threat to their well-being, bodily changes can arouse marked anxiety. This is especially true if misconceptions go undetected. Death fantasies are quite common during later childhood. The consequences of illness such as physical limitation or dietary restriction are more impressive to children in this age group. This may contribute to the increased incidence of withdrawal and depression.

At all ages, certain parts of the body have symbolic significance. Diseases of the heart, brain, and eyes seem to cause a high degree of anxiety (Blom, 1958; Langford, 1961). This coincides with the importance attached to these organs by children themselves. Anna Freud (1952) postulates that genital operations arouse castration fears at virtually all levels of development. Of course, any part of the body can be charged with libidinal significance if, for some reason, it is made the focus of an unusual amount of attention.

The visibility of the illness may also be a factor in determining the child's reaction. Bergmann (1965) describes differences between children with orthopedic illnesses and those who had cardiac conditions. The orthopedic patients, as a group, seemed to adjust to their illnesses in a more positive manner than did the cardiac children. Part of this reaction seemed to be due to the fact that the malady was so evident. The child and his roommates could see the disorder and the apparatus that was used to treat it. The illness, in effect, could be touched and manipulated. In fact, it could not be hidden even if there was a desire to do so. Explanations about the illness could be given matter-of-factly with a predictable timetable of progress. The undeniable reality of the illness seemed to discourage excessive use of fantasy. The realization that other children were in the same circumstances also seemed supportive.

Bergmann proposes an interesting basis for acceptance of the illness. She suggests that children might view their period of immobilization as a time of "suspense" in a way similar to atonement in fairy tales, in which "a happy ending is reached only after great hardship has been endured, such hardship not only being accepted but sought after and endowed with pleasurable anticipation" (p 61). She goes on to point out, however, that although these children appeared to adjust well to the period of immobilization, they behaved in quite a different way when ambulation was begun. The slow progress of ambulation undermined their magical expectations. Once the element of freedom was reintroduced, they were unwilling to be patient with any further restriction no matter how slight it was.

Cardiac patients, on the other hand, were generally depressed and discouraged and tended to be hypochondriac. In the absence of clear-cut evidence of illness, these children had to find something on which to focus their attention. Often, they became preoccupied with their heartbeat and identified even normal variations in it with a deterioration of their condition. Part of the children's problem in dealing with this type of illness seemed to be related to their inability to comprehend the nature of heart action. The progress of their recovery was not predictable and they constantly compared themselves with others and viewed relapses as premonitions of their own fate. Their mental construct of the importance of the heart often had ominous overtones.

It seems likely to me that the staff's own attitude toward a particular illness could have an important bearing on the attitude of the child. The staff could probably be more open about orthopedic illnesses than they were about cardiac conditions. When the outcome of an illness is obscure or when treatment is unpleasant or introduces a threat to life, the medical and nursing personnel can experience much ambivalence in interacting with the child. It is always easier to tell a child that he is getting better than to explain why he is not.

The extent to which ill children look alike or different from other youngsters may also affect how they view their own illness. In Gellert's study, it was noted that children verbalized that arms and legs were dispensable parts of the body. However, when other children were confronted by a child with an amputation, they had difficulty identifying with the disability (Bergmann, 1965). The impact of the reality of the situation overshadowed the intellectual awareness that, indeed, one can live without an arm or leg.

The existence of scars is a significant factor to consider when one is trying to assess the child's reaction to illness. The adult's perception frequently centers on the scar's appearance. The older child, especially the adolescent, is concerned about appearance, too. However, the scar may cause great upset because of such a seemingly inconsequential matter as the strange numbness that may occur around the scarred area.

I remember caring for an 11-year-old girl who was badly burned on the upper trunk and legs. She was a black child and the extensive skin grafts left unsightly changes in the pigmentation of her skin. Her primary concern, however, was not the scar itself but rather that the scars would restrict development of what little breast tissue remained after the burn. She was likewise very anxious about the fact that she would not have any breast nipples.

The kinds of symptoms associated with an illness may also affect the type and intensity of the child's reaction. When illness is accompanied by diarrhea or vomiting, children may experience a psychologic as well as a physical insult. Especially to the preschool child, it represents loss of control over a function of the body that had previously been managed at his discretion. Signs such as pronounced edema and severe postural defects are of special concern to adolescents whose self-identity hinges on the body's appearance. Dizziness, nausea, and dyspnea are frightening sensations for which the child is unprepared. He feels strangely different but has no way to judge the degree of threat posed to his well-being. Treatments such as intubation, enemas, rectal temperatures, spinal taps, and forcible administration of medicine can be viewed by the children as purposely intrusive acts.

Significance of Pain

One of the physical consequences of illness and treatment is pain. It is generally assumed that very young infants lack a sophisticated mechanism to perceive and respond to painful stimuli. Evidence to support this assumption from a physiologic point of view is scanty. Although it is generally agreed that the fetus and the newborn (at least for a few hours) have a high degree of tolerance for pain (Pratt, 1954), it has also been noted that there is a developmental decrease in electrotactual thresholds of infants as early as one day of age (Kaye and Lipsitt, 1964). Therefore, it seems that sensitivity to pain increases quite rapidly. It does not take long before the infant withdraws the part of his body that has encountered a noxious stimuli.

The physiologic basis for pain involves the functioning of a complex interwoven network of fine, beaded, subcutaneous nerve terminals, chemical substances that activate nerve impulses, and an intact central nervous system (Crowley, 1962). However common this physiologic make-up might be to all individuals, children do react in various ways to what might be considered the same intensity of objective stress. Many reasons for these variations have been proposed.

Engel (1962) states that early in childhood, pain and punishment become linked. This is understandable if one remembers that a considerable amount of childhood pain results from such stimuli as spankings when one is bad. Guilt is associated with the pain of punishment. If the experience of reconciliation after punishment constitutes the only love and support that a child receives, it is probable that some children may actually enjoy the pain of punishment because they anticipate love and forgiveness. If an insecure child notices that his complaints of pain call forth expressions of concern and sympathy from usually undemonstrative parents, the child may use pain as a means of getting love from them (Hardy et al, 1952).

Children can also associate pain with aggression and power. Threatening or inflicting pain can give the child control over persons or objects in the environment.

Child-rearing practices and sex roles can determine the limits of acceptable responses to pain. Boys generally are discouraged from crying in the interest of avoiding "sissy-like" behavior; girls, on the other hand, are expected to be more emotional, so that a show of tears is seldom punished. Apart from this cultural determinant, the parent's own attitude toward pain affects how the child will behave. If the parent attaches great significance to the slightest bodily hurt, the child will likely respond with a heightened sensitivity to pain. Lack of protection from pain will be just as detrimental and will also result in a low pain threshold. Total avoidance of painful experiences is certainly improbable and actually unwise. However, when a child experiences pain he obviously needs support from significant persons. Given such support, it is probable that repeated exposure to moderately noxious stimuli helps the child to cope with the stress of pain.

Any one or any combination of these factors may be operating when a child's illness has the element of pain associated with it. They must be considered in evaluating the significance of the pain. The child who screams from pain following a finger prick deserves attention as does the child with severe incisional pain following surgery. In both cases, the child's pain is real to him and it must be dealt with in terms of his experience.

Recognition of the existence of pain has always been a nursing dilemma. The very young child has difficulty expressing feelings of pain and localizing it, partly because of maturational factors and partly because of fear. The nurse must rely on nonverbal cues to spot evidence of pain. Tense body position, inability to be comforted by ordinary means, rolling of the head, rubbing or pulling on a part of the body, and restlessness and overreaction to the environment are indications of the child's discomfort. The older child can be more explicit in his description of pain, but is also more sophisticated in covering up real pain when he feels that it might be to his advantage to do so. A child anticipating discharge from the hospital, for instance, might withhold a complaint of pain since it might be an obstacle to leaving.

In the same sense, the older child can also willfully exaggerate pain to serve his own needs. The presence or absence of strained facial expression, unusual quietness, and disinclination to move a part of the body are subtle indications that even the older child finds difficult to hide especially if "no one is looking." Pain causes tension of skeletal muscle and if it occurs for prolonged periods of time it produces fatigue, lethargy, and additional aches and pains elsewhere in the body. Consequently prompt relief based on early recognition is important.

Perception of Types of Treatment

If the treatment involves motor restraint, the nurse can expect heightened aggression in some children; in others, there may be increased docility. Restraint of one part of the body may inhibit nonaffected parts (Freud, 1952). A deficient or malfunctioning part of the body, wherever it might be, will capture the child's attention. For the period of illness, that part stands isolated and will distort the body image to some extent.

Illness, especially if it requires surgical treatment, arouses the child's fantasies. As previously mentioned it might bring to the foreground ideas about being attacked or castrated. These notions appear most frequently in the conversations of young children. Anna Freud suggests that an operation might be experienced as mutilation in punishment for penis envy or masturbation. Other fantasies may center around episodes of abandonment and uncontrollable animated properties associated with diseased parts of the body. The construction of an elaborate body model can be illustrated by the case of a five-year-old boy described by Anthony (1968). He was referred for treatment of severe constipation, headaches, sinus trouble, and a dry cough. The little child explained these symptoms in the context of this coherent framework: "The 'plops' that didn't come out were turned back and wandered instead into his chest (to give bronchitis), into his face (to produce sinus trouble), and into his head (to produce headaches)" (p 111).

The child's age and past experiences will play a part in his fantasies. As children grow older and enter middle childhood, they are concerned with how the world really is. They are preoccupied with how things work and the concrete outcomes that result from their endeavors. Fantasy, while still present, is modified by added experience. There is an increased awareness of the difference between fact and fantasy so that, when fantasy occurs, the child tends to repress it. To the casual onlooker, it is sometimes difficult to sort out the fantasy in the child's expression because he has so well incorporated it into a quasi-realistic framework. A child's preoccupation with a function of his body or his constant testing of the limits of bed rest may be deeply rooted in fantasy. For instance, he may imagine, as did a child in Gellert's study that "if you didn't have ribs, somebody could hit you and you'd collapse like a feather." A child with this impression may be overwhelmed with fear if he was about to experience chest surgery. Fantasy, of course, is a well-recognized coping strategy. It can be a very acceptable way of tolerating a stressful experience (Murphy, 1962). It is a rather common way of adjusting to losses of body parts and injuries such as severe burns. However, when it becomes a dominant mechanism of defense, fantasy leads to isolation (Lidz, 1968).

Langford (1961) describes a type of anxiety experienced by sick children that he calls "organismic." It is an unconscious phenomenon in which the child perceives a threat to the life or integrity of the organism. Evidence to support this idea comes from Langford's observations of children who developed neurotic symptoms prior to the onset of physical illness. Acute overwhelming anxiety that is out of proportion to the stress is sometimes reported by parents before signs and symptoms appear. Anna Freud explains this as resulting from the heightened demand of the ill body for libidinal cathexis.

Coping Mechanisms

Each child responds to these stressful feelings with a unique pattern of behavior. In essence he learns a series of coping strategies to fit a variety of environmental demands. Murphy (1962) defines coping strategies as "the child's individual patternings and timings of his resources for dealing with specific problems or needs or challenges" (p 274). Some of the common mechanisms can be summarized as follows:

The child can sort out those aspects of a stressful situation that he can reasonably handle. Some children are hesitant in facing a new situation and proceed one step at a time; others are eager to explore many aspects of an unfamiliar situation simultaneously. The little child who fights to "put on his own Bandaid" may not only be concerned about keeping himself intact, but may also be saying that his involvement in a familiar activity relieves some of his stress. Older children may show exorbitant concern about a minor defect such as an old scar or birth mark, rather than focus on the uncomfortable symptoms of their illness.

Children can avoid a stressful situation by denying reality. By resorting to fantasy, they can make their illness temporarily less real. This gives them time to absorb the effects of the stress more gradually. Sometimes children will insist that they are completely well. Langford (1961) reports the case of one boy who had gangrene of the foot. He insisted that his mother not be told of the impending amputation until after his foot had grown back on. Forced gaiety is another manifestation of denial used as a temporary defense mechanism.

Another method of reacting to unwelcome pressures is simply to escape from them. "You never told me, so how was I to know?" Excuses give the child some tentative control over a situation when he feels that he is losing ground. The teenager who turns off potentially stressful conversation by burying himself in a book or television is using this mechanism. Other children, when faced with the stress of an unpleasant procedure literally run away from it. Children have fled the hospital on more than one occasion in obvious rebellion against what they considered a hostile environment. Stalling and other delay tactics are also common devices used for escape.

The tension in some anxiety-producing situations can be contained by exercise of insight or through conscious evaluation of the nature of the threat. If the stress is not overwhelming and the child is assured of appropriate support, he can tolerate an uncomfortable experience. A young child may lay quietly in bed as directed by the doctor but may be sullen and noncommunicative about it; on the other hand, another child faced with the same restriction might creatively look for new ways to pass his time. An older child may tolerate—but certainly not enjoy—his injections. Some are convinced only that "shots" constitute an inevitable evil, but others do see their connection to a greater good, eventual recovery, and consequently endure the pain with good-natured resignation.

Stress can be managed through compulsive repetitions or continued practice of elements in the situation. The child expends extra effort in mastering the particular task. Moderate practice generally consolidates a skill. However, if a child feels compelled to repeat an activity over and over again, his attention may be so fully absorbed with the task that he loses his ability to cope with even minor additional stresses. Ritualistic behavior, such as repetition of body movements (foot-tapping, scratching, etc.) can facilitate release of tension. In observing children at play, one can often overlook repetitive motor movements involved in the interest of focusing on the objects of play or the symbolism expressed through play.

Looking past these aspects to the movements themselves is often quite revealing. Dzik (1974) describes the behavior of a five-year-old boy undergoing a repair of a cleft lip in terms of his motor expression. On one occasion, for example, the child repeatedly ran around an aquarium tapping the glass to make the fish move away. One could interpret this to mean nothing more than interest in the fish and aquarium. However, the most important outcome might have been the tension release that the activity itself afforded. For some periods during his early postoperative period this boy's movements were partially restricted by elbow restraints limiting motor expression. The impulse to discharge energy once restraints are removed is natural and opportunities to do so should be provided in an effort to reduce stress.

Children may balance a threat with security measures that include reassurance. In effect, they protect themselves with available gratifications. "Can I go to the playroom after I take my medicine?" is a query that children often make. An affirmative reply cushions the discomfort and helps the child to cope with an unpleasant situation. Children visiting a clinic in which I work are given a candy sucker to take home with them. On repeat visits, many youngsters head straight for the sucker box. A tight hold on the sucker stick while they wait to be examined seems to give them a tighter hold on themselves.

Children frequently regress under tension. Resorting to earlier patterns of behavior reduces the level of anxiety to a more manageable proportion. A lower level of operation is less demanding intellectually, socially, and emotionally. By allowing others to assume responsibility for care, the child feels more secure. Regression in the face of illness is a common manifestation, especially in young children, and can be almost invariably predicted in situations involving hospitalization. The young child's classic regression in areas such as toileting, eating, and sleeping is well known. However, the older child, too, can manifest behavior such as whimpering, baby-talk, and demands for show of affection.

Some children are able to change or transform elements in a situation in order to deal with it constructively. This is often evident in the child's play experience. In coping with the stress of being a patient and consequently the recipient of the intrusive actions of doctors and nurses, the young child will reverse roles so that he can have the experience of being the doctor or nurse himself. This manipulation helps him to better tolerate the patient role.

Many children look to the "things" in the environment as potential measures of comfort. Sometimes lacking continuity in close interpersonal ties, the ill child may counterbalance this need by a temporary but constructive interest in things rather than people. Fleming (1974) showed a group of ill and healthy school-age children pictures that portrayed hospitalized children in situations where there were people present with and without a variety of hospital equipment and toys. Physically disabled children focused on the pictures that had more "things" in them. The control group focused more on the "people" pictures. This finding suggests that children can become very attached to objects in the environment and possibly can derive comfort from their presence and use. Too casual a disregard for this relationship can be a source of unnecessary upset for the child who is trying to find alternative methods to cope with the stress of his illness.

The older child may react to anxiety by a show of depression. Often this is related to the fact that the child blames himself for the illness. He tends to feel hostile toward himself and unconsciously wishes to be punished. Nothing is worthwhile and the well-meaning attempts to help are met with further withdrawal. The juvenile period itself contains its share of "normal" anxieties and depression; illness simply exaggerates the situation.

Hypochondriac reactions are sometimes evident in older children. This overconcern with bodily functions directs feelings to the self. Many times the parents of these children are themselves hypochondriac and symptoms of illness are frequently discussed in the home. Often it results from a convalescence that is unnecessarily prolonged or from an overemphasis either by parents or physician of a particular type of symptom. Children who are labeled "potential cardiacs" because of a murmur are examples of a particularly susceptible group. Anxiety and unconscious fears and fantasies may also lead to hypochondriac behavior.

Sublimation is a more sophisticated way of coping with stress. With appropriate support, the ill child can be helped to employ this mechanism. It is a device whereby a socially unacceptable activity is redirected into a more approved channel. The child with rheumatic heart disease who desires to be the running back on the football team will have to make a goal-substitution in order to cope with his illness.

THE IMPACT OF HOSPITALIZATION

The reactions to illness described thus far may occur in response to any illness and may happen whether the child is treated at home or in the hospital. If the illness does require hospitalization, stress is likely to be intensified in all the dimensions already discussed. Added to these factors is another set of unique variables which hospitalization, by its very nature, imposes.

Impact of Separation

Hospitalization implies separation—separation from loved persons and familiar environment. For the young child (especially under three years of age) separation from the mother is the most frequently mentioned source of psychologic upset. The effects of this kind of stress are well documented (Robertson, 1958; Bowlby, 1960; Spitz, 1965; Fagin, 1966; Branstetter, 1969). Since the child is too young to interpret the reason for hospitalization properly, he can see it only in terms of the loss of his mother or at least of mothering care. He feels abandoned and lonely. Loss of the mother's care interferes with the fulfillment of basic needs for affection, food, elimination, and sleep. The young child thinks that his parents are all-powerful and expects their protection when he is threatened with harm. Their absence, at what is for him a critical time, arouses hostile feelings which the child cannot deal with comfortably. The child's conception of comfort and protection as synonymous with love seems contradicted in his mind and his confusion is psychologically disrupting.

Bowlby (1960) and Robertson (1958) describe the behavioral results of such stress. Three phases of disturbed behavior are noted during periods of separation—protest, despair, and detachment (denial).

> The initial phase, that of Protest, may last from a few hours to a week or more. During it the young child appears acutely distressed at having lost his mother and seeks to recapture her by the full exercise of his limited resources. He will often cry loudly, shake his cot, throw himself about, and look eagerly towards any sight or sound which might prove to be his missing mother. All his behaviour suggests strong expectation that she will return. Meantime, he is apt to reject all alternative figures who offer to do things for him, though some children will cling desperately to a nurse.
>
> During the phase of Despair, which succeeds protest, his preoccupation with his missing mother is still evident, though his behavior suggests increasing hopelessness. The active physical movements diminish or come to an end, and he may cry monotonously or intermittently. He is withdrawn and inactive, makes no demands on the environment, and appears to be in a state of deep mourning. This is a quiet stage, and sometimes, clearly erroneously, is presumed to indicate a diminution of distress.
>
> Because the child shows more interest in his surroundings, the phase of Detachment which sooner or later succeeds protest and despair is often welcomed as a sign of recovery. He no longer rejects the nurses, accepts their care and the food and toys they bring, and may even smile and be sociable. This seems satisfactory. When his mother visits, however, it can be seen that all is not well, for there is a striking absence of the behaviour characteristic of the strong attachment normal at this age. So far from greeting his mother he may seem hardly to know her; so far from clinging to her he may remain remote and apathetic; instead of tears there is a listless turning away. He seems to have lost all interest in her. (Bowlby, 1960)

Disruptive behavior often extends into the posthospitalization period. It is important that parents be apprised of this fact so that they can better respond to the child's needs.

Fagin (1966) found that young children who were separated from their mothers during hospitalization continued to show regressive behavior one month after discharge from the hospital. The children demonstrated behavior such as emotional dependence, food finickiness, resistance to going to bed, and regression in urine training. Some children may show an emotional coldness at first and then follow this by intense and demanding dependence on the mother. Jealousy and outbursts of anger are also common posthospitalization behaviors.

Prugh et al (1953) also noted that infantile behavior persisted for several months in many children under the age of five. Nightmares, bed-wetting, and undue fear of needles were found in older children, but these behaviors disappeared more quickly than in younger age groups.

So much concern has been expressed about the effects of prolonged separation from loved ones, as well as other forms of psychologic and social deprivation, that a new diagnostic category has been suggested. Clancy and McBride (1975) have identified elements in what they call the *isolation syndrome*. Four behaviors are associated with the syndrome: (1) the child lacks the normal attending responses to the mother, such as eye contact and social smiling; (2) the child fails to respond appropriately to sensory stimulation, such as not showing any reaction to his mother's verbal communication; (3) the child engages in self-stimulation activities, such as rocking, head banging, or masturbation; and (4) the child shows developmental deficits especially in the area of language.

There are many situations in which this syndrome can occur. Separation occasioned by prolonged illness is one of them. If the illness occurs very early in infancy, it interferes with the initial establishment of bonding between mother and child. If it occurs at a later stage in development, the effects of separation, though they may be less severe, result in a disruption of the existing bond that will ultimately have to be reestablished. Another factor affecting the ill child extends beyond the problem of physical separation. The nature of the illness itself can be very significant in the sense that parents perceive certain illnesses differently from others and adjust their responses accordingly. Under these circumstances abnormal relationships can develop that perpetuate the existence of the isolation syndrome, even in cases where the child is cared for in the home. For example, if the child's illness (eg, blindness, retardation, etc.) results in a limited capacity to respond positively to the mother's care, the mother, often without realizing it, may diminish the quantity and quality of the care she gives in return. Because there are so many variables in these situations, it is sometimes difficult to identify the primary problem as related to some form of isolation. Unfortunately, therefore, treatment is often misdirected.

Although there are many behavior changes in young children in response to hospitalization, the responses of adolescents are even more numerous. Some adolescents are passive and cooperative, others are openly rebellious, and still others respond maturely and use the hospitalization as a constructive experience. Problems and developmental considerations of special importance during adolescence affect the teenager's response to this event. Narcissistic attitudes toward the body coupled with a reality-oriented concept of illness and death create a heightened awareness of their physical selves. Confinement, relative isolation, and dependence upon the care of others are in direct conflict with the need for independence. Although their thinking is generally reality based, it is occasionally marked by contradictions and the desire to do impossible things, which is sometimes translated into bizarre and unpredictable actions. Naturally these circumstances create a challenge for both parents and nurse.

It is well then to understand some of the specific concerns of adolescents who are hospitalized. Schowalter and Lord (1970) reported on the content of informal, weekly discussions between patients and staff of the adolescent unit of Yale-New Haven Hospital. Although the focus of any particular meeting was related to the recent experiences of the patient group, some common subjects were discussed by many. Interestingly, hospital food uniformly elicited much animated comment. It was always poorly cooked or poorly served. Even the timid members of the group joined in with these complaints. Since food represents nurturing, care, and longing for home, it becomes a safe-to-discuss symbol of these treasured but now unavailable comforts. Ward routine frequently enters the conversation, but most often is presented in a fairly favorable light. Staff who wish to obtain a critique of their service from the otherwise vocal teenager may be disappointed, since even the teenager surmises that it is seldom worth the risk of "biting the hand that feeds you." Complaints about care that are brought before the group are usually in reference to care *other* patients have received. Speaking as an advocate for another is apparently a less risky disclosure.

Concerns about their lack of control over situations affecting them surface frequently in adolescent discussions. The feeling of helplessness even extends to fears of contracting others' illnesses or succumbing to death. It appears that surgery marks the ultimate "helpless" experience and consequently is frequently discussed in the adolescent group. It is of much interest even to those who have never experienced it. There is general consensus that even though such discussions can be worrisome, it is better to be forewarned about what to expect.

Group meetings such as those held at Yale-New Haven Hospital serve several important purposes which may apply to other settings as well. They provide an opportunity, in a nonthreatening way, for patients to become acquainted with each other and, through group support, mobilize their efforts to cope with a stressful situation. There is also advantage in having an ongoing patient-staff communication system which can be readily used when especially disrupting events occur on the unit. Perhaps most important, the meetings help to keep the staff in touch with the needs of patients.

While there is considerable agreement that sustained behavioral changes can result from hospitalization, it is likewise generally agreed that the emotional and physical environment of the hospital can be constructively modified to minimize such ill effects. Permitting maternal attendance during hospitalization reduces the number and intensity of adverse reactions for the young child (Fagin, 1966). When the mother cannot be present in the hospital, substitute mothering will reduce trauma since it is possible that some of the emotional distress experienced by the young child results from need deprivation rather than from separation anxiety per se (Branstetter, 1969).

Relaxed admission procedures, liberal visiting hours, early ambulation (to minimize effects of immobilization and sensory deprivation), play programs, and purposeful preparation for traumatic procedures are additional ways in which the environment can be modified to reduce the child's anxiety level (Prugh et al, 1953).

For the older child, more sophisticated techniques can be used since anxiety can be dealt with in a different way. Group discussions seem to be a profitable method of managing anxiety. Psychotherapy sessions in which children are encouraged to explore their concerns and fantasies seem to have more long-range benefit than mere information-giving tutorial meetings (Rie et al, 1968). Although the latter group "learned," communication in this type of setting tends to be unilateral and demands a singular response from the children. When anxieties are confronted directly and actively explored by the children themselves, there may be no actual reduction in anxiety; however, through the open method of interaction, older youngsters can reduce their need to cope with anxiety in a defensive manner. In effect, this method tends to encourage a child to search for a solution to his problems in an independent way.

Preparation for Hospitalization

There is scarcely anyone writing on the subject of effects of hospitalization who does not emphasize the importance of preparation for the new experience. Preparation for illness and hospitalization is an ongoing process and is a part of every new experience. Often it is presumed that because a child has been in the hospital before or has had a doctor's examination on many occasions, he does not need much preparation. Two factors make this an unfair assumption. In the first place, each time a child returns to the hospital he is literally a different person. He is at a wholly new stage of development with correspondingly different fears and expectations that must be dealt with at his present level of comprehension. Secondly, the past experiences with illness may have been upsetting ones which he imagines will be repeated. It is therefore essential before any preparation is attempted, that the nurse find out how the child views the circumstances of his illness. Once this information is obtained, the nurse has a sound basis on which to begin.

Age is an important factor in determining the method and style of preparation. The preschool child thinks primarily about himself—how he feels, what will happen to him. He is in the animistic or magical stage of thinking in which reality and fantasy are indistinguishable to him. He also thinks in very concrete terms. However, his capacity to understand far exceeds his verbal ability. Therefore, when preparing him for hospitalization or treatment, one should keep a few simple rules in mind. The preschool child requires only about two days' advance notice of an upcoming hospitalization or operation. A longer period of preparation awakens fantasies and arouses unnecessary fears. Yet he does need some time to absorb the idea of a new venture and to ask questions. Keep the actual preparation simple. Direct attention to what will happen to him and how he will feel when things happen. Playing out anticipated events gives the child something tangible to cling to as he faces new and strange situations. Do not hesitate to explain things, even though the child has not verbalized his curiosity and concern. Because the preschool child considers adults to be all-knowing, he expects that those caring for him understand what he is thinking.

The thinking of the school-age child begins to be based on logic. He is able to classify and label objects. He has more realistic concepts about his body and its functions. Consequently, he requires and seeks a more detailed explanation of the illness and its treatment. He can benefit from more time to prepare so that he can make some decisions about controlling his environment. He can decide, for example, what to bring to the hospital, and how to tell his friends about the hospitalization. Bringing his own clothes and other familiar items helps to preserve his own identity. Proper timing will also permit him to voice his inevitable concerns which are often quite realistic. Questions about possible death and residual disability are not infrequent. While these youngsters appreciate a fairly comprehensive preparation in keeping with their increasing knowledge about the body, care must be taken not to overemphasize self-control. The discomforts and anxieties that illness will arouse may cause a temporary breakdown in the child's emotional control, which is very understandable. Children must not be made to feel that they are failures because of this.

The adolescent is capable of abstract thought and conceptualization and can assume initiative in solving his problems. He should have considerable say in making decisions that affect his own welfare. If the hospitalization is elective, he should be involved in the decision about timing. Social and academic affairs might reasonably have priorities over hospitalization in certain situations such as graduation, a swimming meet, or a senior prom. Again, avoid falling into the trap of omitting important information because the teenager gives the impression of knowing all about everything. Do not be discouraged when the adolescent greets your efforts by a blasé, disinterested "ho-hum"! It is not a valid indication of the real impact that the teaching had.

Repetition may be necessary at all age levels, depending upon the reason for hospitalization and the extent of personal threat involved. When preparation has to be hurried, it is generally advisable to give less detailed information and supplement the gaps by being present during the experience so that ongoing explanation and physical and emotional support can be given.

The use of props or teaching tools is recommended for all age groups. Puppets, coloring books, storybooks, and doctor and nurse kits are appropriate for preschool children. Older children appreciate simple diagrams of the body or diseased organ. Instructional films, videotapes on closed-circuit television, or self-instruction materials are all effective media. Self-instruction tools are especially beneficial because the child can learn at his own pace. There are few child-oriented materials available for this purpose. More attention could well be directed to their development.

Hospital Environment

Hospitalization introduces the child to a wholly new environment. Hall (1959) has expounded on the idea that when persons move from one country to another, they experience a condition known as culture shock. He defines this phenomenon as "a removal or distortion of the many familiar cues one encounters at home and the substitution for them of other cues which are strange" (p 156). Gellert (1958) comments that in the child's eyes the hospital is like a foreign country. It is a place with its own customs, language, and schedules to which the child must adapt. Certainly, the familiar cues that help a child feel secure are either absent or distorted—sometimes beyond recognition. Established routines for daily care that provide continuity from day to day are altered to suit hospital protocol. Equipment is often noisy and overpowering. This is especially true if the child is hospitalized in an institution primarily geared to the care of adult patients. Consequently, the child can view hospitalization as a type of culture shock.

The child tries to attach meanings to unfamiliar vocabulary and often misinterprets what is said. "Diagnosis" can be mentally construed to be "dying noses"; children can give a literal interpretation to the doctor's statement that he will "sit on" the case until morning; "resolution" of pneumonia easily turns into "revolution"; "blood work," for a child unfamiliar with the jargon and still in the stage of animistic thinking, can mean that his blood is "working" inside of him.

There is a considerable amount of sensory distortion in the hospital environment. Normal cycles of day and night are not always clearly discernable, particularly in special-care units in which windows are high-set and often at a premium and bright lighting is maintained around the clock. Auditory stimuli may consist of the continuous sound of the respirator, isolette, or mist tent, or the unintelligible garble of distant voices. A very disquieting sound is that of the cries of another child. Visual stimuli take on an unnatural perspective, too. Sometimes, because of confinement to bed or to a particular room, range of vision is limited. If the child is immobilized the restrictions are even more severe. What the child does see leaves much to be desired—the same four walls, the same arrangement of furniture. As the child peers into the hospital corridors, sometimes through several glass partitions, the people he sees are often distorted and literally unrecognizable.

Interpersonal spatial distance is also distorted in the hospital. It is well known that the spatial distance between interacting persons is a cue to the type of social relationship existing between them (Hall, 1959). As the degree of acquaintance increases the distance between members of a dyad decreases. This connection between physical closeness and closeness of interpersonal relationship is understood by children as young as the age of eight (Blood and Livant, 1957). Such ideas are quite clearly utilized by age 11 or 12 (Guardo, 1969). Since children do use these cues of physical proximity to interpret relationships, I wonder what difficulty is posed for the child when perfect strangers assume positions of considerable intimacy. Often, the child has no time to develop an acquaintance with the many people who take care of his body. A real friendship with them is a rarity. Since children do value personal space, it would seem likely that close physical contact with the school-age child ought to be used with discretion. Of course, it must be remembered that these children were not studied under conditions of stress.

The same set of circumstances does not seem to operate for the young child. Rosenthal (1967) introduced preschool children to an anxiety-provoking situation and studied their dependency behavior in relation to their mothers and to strangers. Under nonstressful circumstances, dependent behavior was observed with mothers more frequently than with strangers. However, anxiety increased dependency behavior toward both mother and stranger. This appears to conflict with the common notion that when under high anxiety, a child will withdraw from strangers. Therefore, the diminished ability of young children to cope with stress such as that of hospitalization demands behavior from the nurse that is physically comforting and responsive to the child's dependency needs.

One of the most unsettling aspects of hospitalization is the inconsistency of care. The number of interpersonal contacts in the course of a single day is phenomenal. Many persons who enter the child's world come for a very specific purpose and once it is accomplished they are gone. This kind of disturbance is relatively self-limited in its effect. However, inconsistency among the nurses who have prolonged contact with the child is less well tolerated. After a certain number of unsettling, confusing experiences, the child realizes that he really cannot prepare himself for the next day's plan of care because each nurse approaches him differently. In an environment in which interruptions and surprises are frequent occurrences at best, the child is robbed of one element of consistency that he could come to depend upon: his nurse. In the interests of scheduling limitations, one nurse cannot work around the clock nor take care of a child with a long-term illness without interruption. However, the child can feel more secure if he knows one nurse in a special way. He can adjust to the inevitable changes on her days off because he knows where she is and that she will return. Gradually, the space barrier between them can be broken down so that meaningful matters will come up for discussion.

Hospitalization is often necessary because surgery is planned as a part of the treatment. An operation brings with it many anxieties. One obviously relieved child told me that, "I had my operation today. That means I won't have to have it tomorrow." The anticipated loss of or entry into a part of the body is very threatening especially for the preschool child. If the surgery will result in disfigurement, anxiety is heightened and self-image is significantly altered. The operating suite itself is the object of many fantasies for children of all ages. Because it is largely unknown to them and even to those who must prepare the children, it takes on ominous and mysterious characteristics; and when they are actually confronted with the environment, it is admittedly austere and impersonal—with masked faces and gloved hands. Children fear anesthesia not only because of the traditional mask and "smelly gas" (which incidentally are seldom used for induction), but also because they fear losing self-control and consciousness. The postoperative presence of such things as oxygen, drainage tubes, and intravenous tubing is quick to arouse anxiety. The taking of medicines, both oral and parenteral, are compounded by fears of being attacked or of having the body penetrated. The preschool child frequently is convinced that "his insides will run out through the hole" made by the needle. The insistence on Bandaids following intramuscular injections is often based on this conviction.

All of the environmental variables mentioned thus far have been stressful. While the subject has not been extensively studied, there is some indication that, for some children, psychologic benefit may result from hospitalization (Jessner, 1952; Solnit, 1960; Shore, 1965; Rie, 1968; Oremland and Oremland, 1973). Shore cites several areas in which benefit has been noted; encouragement of normal growth patterns; support in parent-child relationships; provision of refuge in emotional storms; and provision of identification models for parents and child. Langford (1961) comments that children who come from unstable family circumstances may find that the hospital provides them with more consistent care and acceptance than they receive at home. He recalled one child's appreciative exclamation, "Gee, sheets and a pillow!"

In a symposium on effects of hospitalization (published in a volume edited by Oremland and Oremland, 1973), Spielman suggests that, since hospitalization often speeds recovery from physical illness, it may interrupt the cycle of suffering experienced by the sick child and reduce the escalating effects of mood and behavioral changes manifested by both child and parents. At the end of an uncomplicated hospital experience, parents may feel more competent, having successfully intervened in a supportive way in a crisis situation. The inevitable need to rely on professionals during hospitalization may encourage parents (and child) to see them as helpful resources in resolving future problems.

Feelings of competence may emerge for the child too. Hospitalization is a stressful event which must be faced, coped with, and mastered. Having done this, the child may feel proud of himself in much the same way as the young athlete proudly shows off his broken arm as evidence that, though the battle was rugged, he survived. The fearful fantasies that surround hospitalization can often be dispelled through real-life experience in the hospital. Reality wins out in most circumstances and this in itself can be growth producing. For those children who have few social experiences or who come from a socially disruptive situation, hospitalization can provide a sympathetic, protected environment in which the child can find models for more constructive behavior and in which the friendly atmosphere is conducive to the development of social ties that extend well beyond the actual hospital confinement. Another circumstance that may yield positive outcomes for the child is that the entire family is often mobilized around his needs during hospitalization. Everyone can understand the fantasy of attention that comes through physical illness. We all like to feel indulged and forgiven and there is no more deserved time than during illness.

Hospitalized children, particularly those who have a long-term illness, have occasion to see more illness than do healthy children. They see children in all stages of illness and, undoubtedly, during repeated hospitalizations, have witnessed some catastrophies. The sight of many people and strange equipment coupled with an atmosphere of tense urgency arouses all sorts of fearful fantasies concerning the child's own safety. A sudden upsetting event may leave the child no time to support himself through anticipation of it.

Care ought to be taken in planning room assignments so that children are not introduced to more stress than they can tolerate. A child with an amputation should not be indiscriminately placed with a preschool child whose normal fantasies concern mutilation. It will only confirm his worst fears. An older child can be expected to have difficulty adjusting to such a disabled child, but he can be better supported because of his appreciation of reality. The situation obviously needs to be discussed so that misconceptions do not brew under the surface. Placement of a child severely scarred with burns requires the same considerations.

Careful judgment has to be exercised when children with the same illness are placed together. Sometimes it can be mutually beneficial, but inevitable comparisons will be made. If the condition of one child is precarious, comparisons between the two children could undermine the progress of each. The sick child can become jealous of the other's progress and the other can fear that a setback is bound to happen to him.

Young children suppose that other children harbor the same fears that they do (Lazar, 1969). If they are highly anxious and therefore believe others to experience the same kinds of fears, the child may see no avenue of help for himself in the stressful situation. The child can become fearful through close contact with anxious people. The child who hears another patient cry plaintively for his mother may be as frightened as the crying child. This factor of fear transmission and fear interpretation must also be considered when one is assigning patients to rooms.

Because of the emotional aspects involved in meeting the needs of sick children, ongoing staff education is essential. Staff members may often experience high levels of anxiety as they attempt to support parents and children through very traumatic experiences. All staff members have certain biases about children stemming from their own attitudes toward child rearing. Consequently, some behavior in children and in parents can arouse strongly charged reactions in the nurses who care for them. Recognition that this situation is natural and not something to be ashamed of is part of realistic nursing intervention. When such attitudes go beyond the nurse's control and directly interfere with effective function, outside assistance should be requested without shame. Group conferences where feelings can be "aired" openly and without fear of reprisal do improve the level of care. Inappropriate attitudes and inappropriate skill in working with children accentuates the child's adverse reaction to the stress of illness.

PARENTAL INFLUENCE ON THE CHILD'S PERCEPTION OF ILLNESS

"Like father, like son; he's a chip off the old block; as the tree is bent." These phrases are common clichés pointing to parental influence on the child's behavior. Through the experience of early mother-infant and father-infant relationships, the child learns to recognize cues that express parental approval and disapproval and adjusts his behavior accordingly.

Child's Incorporation of Parental Emotions

The theory of symbiosis helps to explain how the child incorporates the emotional reactions of his mother. The symbiotic relationship existing during pregnancy enhances feelings of motherliness. The hormonal changes occurring with pregnancy arouse libidinous feelings of well-being that are intimately related to motherliness. During this time, the mother's fantasies not only incorporate her desires for a child but also include wishes and ambitions that she hopes to fulfill through the child (Benedek, 1949). Thus, the child is viewed in terms of the mother's predetermined goals before he is born.

After birth, the need for symbiosis continues in the mother. The woman's desire to care for the infant and to experience the close bodily contact that symbiosis implies, really represents the original symbiotic relationship for both the infant and the mother. The motherliness that develops when needs are gratified expands the mother's personality and, in a cyclic manner, enhances her capacity to meet the infant's demands. The resulting closeness affords the infant the opportunity to experience a transfer of the physiologic effects of a warm, relaxed body, and the psychosocial effects of a smiling face and soothing voice.

As experiences accumulate, the infant becomes able to distinguish between tension and relaxation; between anxiety and contentment; between fear and confidence. His cues may take the form of voice change, muscle tightness, facial expression, or spatial distance. Whatever form they take, the child's early and sustained scrutiny of his mother makes him uniquely sensitive to her moods.

As he develops, the child's interpersonal relationships envelop the father and the siblings. When the process of imitation and identification becomes dominant, sensitivity to the behavior of others increases correspondingly. The child begins to see himself as a "contributor" to their reactions and experiences "good" feelings or "bad" feelings depending on his perception of the outcome of the interaction.

When a child becomes ill, he has a great need for parental support. His search for assurance heightens his sensitivity to parental behavior. If the parents appear very anxious or seem to lack control over the situation, the child's fears about his well-being will be accentuated. For example, if an infant is ill and cannot accept, or even appears to reject (by crying, vomiting, diarrhea, etc.), the mother's ministrations, the symbiotic relationship referred to earlier is weakened. The infant lacks confidence in the mother's ability to meet his needs and the mother also loses confidence in her ability to assume her idealized mothering role.

A similar phenomenon occurs when the child is older. The preschool child believes that his parents are all-powerful and that they will protect him from harm. When they appear to condone painful experiences, the child may express anger and resentment toward his parents. Parents often react by becoming overindulgent. The child, consequently, is unsure of their expectations. He may become quite unsettled when previously unacceptable behavior is suddenly rewarded or at least overlooked.

What is happening in this "feedback" mechanism is that changes in both parent and child behavior affect responses in each other and complicate ability to interpret the behavior with objectivity. If the behavior of one could be guided toward some degree of consistency, the behavior of the other might be more comfortably stabilized.

Parents have the capability of mature thought and hence can respond to rational interaction. Therefore, nursing intervention directed toward reducing parental anxiety would be a very productive means of allaying the fears of sick children. If the child had not learned to be so "in tune" with parental feelings, parents could have more latitude in the expression of their worries.

As it is, parents are called upon to exert great self-control under difficult conditions. To carry out this responsibility, they will appreciate opportunities for expression which the nurse can provide.

Parental Behavior During Periods of Illness

Before the nurse can respond to the parent's need for help, it is important to know what factors are likely to contribute to parental behavior.

The presence of a prolonged and possibly debilitating condition constitutes a potential threat to the child's life. This alone is stressful enough for the parents, but if there are already other psychologic or social problems in the home, the stress is greatly magnified. Since illness never comes at a convenient time, it must always be viewed in the context of the total family experience along with other crises the family members may be facing.

Other factors affecting parental reaction, of course, include the type of illness and the availability of effective treatment. If the physician can assure the family that there is every hope of a good recovery, the family is buoyed up by the favorable prognosis. If, on the other hand, the outcome is doubtful even after a period of lengthy treatment, the anxiety will be heightened and depression and a certain amount of hopelessness may become a dominant mood. Adjustment to inherited and congenital disorders is particularly difficult for parents because of their tendency to feel responsible for the illness.

Another consideration that should not be overlooked is the stress due to the high cost of the illness and its treatment. Families with limited incomes are often hard pressed to provide adequate resources for all the members of the family. Frequently, simple pleasures have to be sacrificed so that the needs of the ill child can be met. This can be a source of jealousy and hostility among the family members. At times, parents may feel resentful and bitter about their plight. These feelings may be directed toward family, friends, or the physician but are sometimes focused on the ill child himself.

Parents are not always fully aware of the so-called normal behavioral changes that are concurrent with childhood illness and hospitalization. Consequently, it is easy for parents to misinterpret their child's behavior.

For example, many mothers view the child's demanding behavior as "being spoiled." Consequently, they may react by vigorous attempts to correct this, which the child in turn can interpret as rejection. Parents sometimes have a difficult time seeing things from the child's point of view. From their adult perspective, many of the events that provoke aggressive or "naughty" behavior are not of sufficient consequence to cause such violent outbursts. They expect the child to demonstrate more control over his feelings than is possible for his age or condition.

The rejecting child is another source of parental concern. Children can withdraw from their parents just when the parents wish to be most consoling. This may happen for a variety of reasons. Sometimes the child is simply disappointed or angry with his parents because they do not "rescue" him from the strange, unpleasant environment. Other children may fear losing self-control if they give free expression to their feelings; and so they withdraw into themselves. This frightens parents and accentuates feelings of guilt and helplessness.

The child's misbehavior threatens the parent in another way. Parents are well aware of their dependency on the members of the health team and they do not want to risk losing their good favor. If the child misbehaves, parents may feel that the disruptive behavior will alienate the staff who will then retaliate by withdrawing attention. This is, perhaps, one reason why parents tend to worry more when their children are troublesome and aggressive than when they are quiet and fearful.

Children in the hospital sometimes manifest behavior characteristics that are completely different from their "at-home" personalities. Parents are genuinely at a loss to explain the change; and, if it is a change for the worse, they are embarrassed and concerned that the staff will consider them unsuitable parents. We all know the frustration of trying to defend a situation when the evident circumstances do not reflect "the way it really is."

Occasionally, parents must bear some of the responsibility for their child's maladaptive behavior. Parents may inadvertently contribute to the stress of hospitalization because of unfortunate associations they have created in the child's mind. Often parents assign punitive meanings to going to bed, confinement to a room, or food restrictions. Thus, when the child faces these circumstances during the course of his illness, it is not unreasonable for him to attribute his confinement to punishment for "bad" acts or thoughts. And, of course, any child can find something in his real or fantasied past that deserves retribution. This may confirm the child's fear that even his most secret thoughts will somehow be punished. Another common threat voiced frequently by parents is "to stop crying or I'll have the nurse give you another shot." This does little to cement friendly nurse-patient relationships; but however much the nurse cringes at this unfair description of her role, she must understand that the parent is generally motivated more by a strong desire to stop the child's crying than by any conscious attempt to undermine a therapeutic relationship.

Hospital Rules and Regulations

Hospital rules and regulations also contribute to parental anxiety. They can readily upset parents by seeming to interfere with their style of child care. Food restrictions and limited visiting hours are perhaps the most obvious recipients of criticism, but they may serve merely as available scapegoats for more subtle concerns. There is a code of conduct or hospital protocol to which parents feel obliged to adapt. Unfortunately, the code of expected behavior is not always explicit. Whom to ask for what thing can become a real problem. How to get needed information without becoming a bother is often an important parent concern. Another question parents ask themselves is, "How far do I go in ministering to my child's needs before I assume the nurses' prerogatives?" How frequently are parents unsure about whether to stay with their child during treatments? Placing the burden of such decision-making solely on the parents predisposes them to the development of a lack of self-confidence. Failure to find reassurance from others further heightens the anxiety that can be so readily transmitted to the supersensitive child.

Inflexibility in the management of some units occasionally presents the parents with grave hardships, which are not always evident to the staff. I can remember one father whose desire to be with his sick child caused him to lose his job because work and visiting hours conflicted. A call from the physician explaining his absence reinstated him, but this would have gone undiscovered had the nurse not been interested enough in the total family to make the significant inquiry about employment.

Socioeconomic and Cultural Factors

Socioeconomic and cultural factors may intensify parental anxiety. A significant experience gap may occur between parent and nurse. It is important to bear in mind that persons in the low-income strata may have different ideas about health and illness than those in the middle-income group. The fact that parents may bring a child for treatment when it seems to be too late may not be due to neglect but rather may be a function of their definition of illness. For the poor, symptoms of physical discomfort do not always constitute sickness; actual incapacitation is viewed as a more realistic criteria (Koos, 1954; Rosenblatt, 1964).

Persons who live in poverty may have goals and values that differ from those who live in a more affluent environment. The effects of economic deprivation may be expressed in four life themes: fatalism, orientation to the present, authoritarianism, and concreteness (Irelan, 1967). It becomes difficult for persons with this orientation to make plans for the future since they are more concerned about immediate happenings and sensations. If they consider their destiny to be controlled by fate, it is unlikely that they will look seriously at the consequences of their actions. Authoritarianism is based on belief in the validity of strength; decisions are made on the basis of authority rather than reason. This attitude can pervade health and child-rearing practices. Awareness of some of these factors becomes especially important in providing anticipatory guidance to parents which is such an important part of the nursing role.

I can recall a situation in which the clinic nurse was having a conference with a Puerto Rican mother about her daughter's nutrition. The seven-year-old child was convalescing at home following a bout of rheumatic fever. The mother reported that her appetite was poor. Among other things, the nurse encouraged social interaction at mealtime, and more variety in choice of foods, implying that the predominance of rice, beans, and starchy vegetables typical of this family's diet was nutritionally inadequate. The mother seemed uninterested in the well-intentioned information. Had the nurse first explored cultural preferences, her advice could have been more meaningful.

The benefits of making mealtime a social exchange was not appreciated in this family. As a rule, meals were not eaten by all the family together. Usually the father was served alone out of respect for his position in the family. There was little conversation at the meal. Disruptions of any kind were looked at unfavorably. Some parents consider eating, "like praying, a time for seriousness, quiet and devotion" (Landy, 1959, p 104).

Instead of trying to change the cultural dietary pattern, some slight modifications can improve nutritional quality without drastically changing preferences. For example, white polished rice is highly valued by the Puerto Rican. Consequently, attempts to persuade the purchase of unpolished rice are not likely to be successful. Rather, the nurse can encourage fortified rice enriched with vitamins. The red kidney bean is a valuable source of protein, but the nurse can suggest the addition of other beans such as soybeans and chick-peas that are far more nutritious. Cafe con leché is a common drink for all ages from childhood up. Rather than discourage young children from the drinking of any coffee, encourage minimal coffee and more milk in view of the child's need for protein. These examples illustrate the concrete value of cultural awareness.

The examples just described should not in any sense encourage the stereotyping of particular socioeconomic and ethnic groups. There is great danger in ignoring the diversity of individual lifestyles within groups. Certainly not all poor people are fatalists and many Puerto Rican families are so "Americanized" that any resemblance to island culture is remote. Unless one's ordinary biases are balanced by a genuine openness to individual differences, meaningful communication is blocked.

If the nurse is aware of the existence of such anxiety-provoking factors as inevitable changes in child's behavior, environmental insecurity, and experiential gap between parent and health worker, she/he can then plan how to intervene constructively.

Parental Preparation and Support

Preparation for any new experience enriches the learning that can come from it. The occasions of illness and hospitalization are no exceptions. Parents play an important part in the child's preparation. Nursing intervention ought then to assist parents with this task. Perhaps the most meaningful part of the intervention takes place long before the actual illness. I am referring to the anticipatory guidance that is part of the supervision of well children. While preparation at the time of crisis is important, studies have indicated that the number and severity of adverse reactions to hospitalization depend to a great extent on the quality of the parent-child relationship prior to the illness. For instance, children who are poorly adjusted emotionally before surgery have more severe postoperative reactions, even though they have been thoroughly prepared (Jessner, 1952). Emotional trauma prior to illness seems to predispose the child to a stronger reaction. Therefore, through anticipatory guidance designed to assist parents in developing sound, mutually satisfying relationships with their children, the nurse is actually "preparing" the child to weather the crisis of illness with less upset.

When actual hospitalization is anticipated, specific preparatory intervention is important. The parents, physician, office nurse, and clinic nurse should participate in the process. Before the parents can be helpful, they must have a reasonably accurate idea of what will happen. The physician should explain in detail the reason for the hospitalization and what the treatment regimen will entail. The nurse can reinforce the doctor's statements and add her/his own unique knowledge about illness and hospitalization to the parents' background information. She/he can explain the hospital environment. Booklets that describe hospital policy and procedure should be given in advance of the time of admission so parents can become familiar with them. Very often such brochures are handed to parents when they arrive at the hospital. This can be wasted effort because the parent's natural focus at this time is on the child—not on hospital policy. The nurse can also be helpful in suggesting teaching methods that parents might use. Books designed for children with colorful pictures about the admission procedure or the trip to the operating room are good tools, but only if they depict the situation realistically and appropriately to the particular hospital environment to which the child will be exposed. Suggestions about role-playing episodes and timing of preparation are also appreciated by parents. Office and clinic nurses ought to have a collection of props available for parents. Caps, masks, tongue blades, and bandages can be given out when appropriate; nurse-doctor hand-and-finger puppets can be loaned out for use in the home (Fig. 1). Arranging for an actual visit to the hospital and/or group teaching of parents commonly involved in a particular situation such as open heart surgery are well within the range of nursing intervention.

A telephone call to the family shortly before admission to the hospital would give the nurse an opportunity to allay some of the last-minute apprehensions and to answer questions which inevitably arise as plans are made for a stay in the hospital. The nurse may not be able to do this for all patients, but she/he can set priorities. Families about to experience treatment

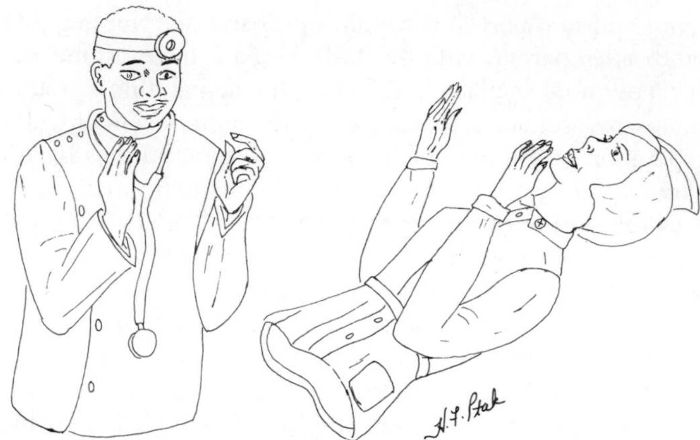

FIG. 1. Puppets commonly used with children. They can be used by parents, the child or nurse.

that has a high degree of risk or families that are already known to be highly reactive to stress would be selected for such contacts. All families, however, should be encouraged to make telephone contacts with the nurse whenever they feel the need to do so.

Once the child is in the hospital, ongoing support is essential. Roy (1967) describes three very practical ways in which the nurse can intervene. The nurse's actions are aimed at supporting the mother's adequacy in relating to her hospitalized child. I believe that these actions could be employed in interacting with any significant person in the sick child's environment. The supportive interaction techniques are congruent orientation, involvement, and role reference. Congruent orientation means that the nurse aligns the focus of her/his attention with that of the mother. For example, if the mother is concerned about her own fatigue, the nurse would focus her/his comments on this area, too. Involvement refers to specific communication with the mother about the child's condition. The nurse, in this case, might tell the mother that the child slept well or that he ate a good breakfast. Role reference is used when the nurse defines for the mother what she can do for the child. Teaching the mother how to apply a dressing is an example of this. When mothers are supported in these direct ways early in the course of hospitalization, they demonstrate a greater degree of adequacy in meeting their child's needs. By introducing to the mother these cues for care, the nurse indicates her/his understanding and acceptance of parent needs. By taking the initiative in these traditional areas of parent concern, she/he removes the burden of inquiry from the parents.

Skipper and Leonard (1968) also describe the value of purposeful social interaction between the mother and the nurse in reducing the anxiety level of the hospitalized child. They measured the effectiveness of the interaction in terms of somatic measures of children's stress such as temperature, blood pressure, pulse, postoperative vomiting, and oral intake of fluids. Communication of information and emotional support to mothers, especially when begun at the crucial time of admission, significantly reduced the child's manifestations of stress. This study reinforces the need to give more than mere lip service to the social process between parent and nurse as a means of reducing stress in the child.

The way in which these cues are offered is important. Avoid cutting off communication by the thoughtless use of professional jargon. Parents are sometimes hesitant to admit their ignorance of medical terminology, and consequently valuable information can be clouded with distortion and half-truth. Also, do not judge parents solely on the basis of first impressions. As has been pointed out, parents are not themselves when their children are ill. Their usual calm objectivity often melts into emotional subjectivity when they are faced with a personal crisis.

Parents can also benefit from informal group discussions designed to help them explore their concerns about their sick child or hospital policies or any of a number of issues that may arise in the course of hospitalization (Glaser, 1960). Such conferences, if properly guided, offer direct benefit to parents not only because of the information they receive from the hospital staff, but also from the support that they receive by sharing experiences with each other. It can be a valuable teaching tool for continuing education of the staff since it reveals how parents view the hospital environment. Suggestions by the parents as consumers of health services can also stimulate constructive administrative changes in unit management. In order to achieve these benefits, however, it seems important that an open, nonpunitive atmosphere be maintained by selecting a group leader who is not directly involved in the management of the unit or the care of the children.

Adjustment At Home

Adjustment to living at home after a period of hospitalization may be a difficult experience for the child, his parents and his siblings. For one thing, it may require a change in roles among the family members. One should not forget that once home, the ill child actively resumes his many identities as son, brother, grandson, or boy next door. Internal role-consistency and congruence between role expectation and actual performance have been cited as important elements in adequate family functioning (Glasser and Glasser, 1966). The long-term illness may leave residual effects, both mental and physical, that will alter the degree to which social obligations and self-responsibility can be resumed; and making it necessary for other family members to add additional behaviors to their customary role-taking.

When the patient holds one view of how he should behave in the context of his chronic illness and the parents or siblings hold a contrary view, conflict is inevitable. For example, if the child with heart disease believes himself to be completely normal without any restrictions and the parents, on the other hand, limit his activity, stress will be produced. Parents, however, may have more unrealistic conceptions than their ill child. They can completely deny a disability and thus hold unattainable goals. Neither of these extremes is conducive to normalizing behavior within the family.

The family's concept of the origin and treatment of the illness can be critical to home adjustment and the patient's well-being. Often gaps in understanding are not fully appreciated in the hospital setting where sophisticated resources seem to promote a false sense of security. Family members, including parents, may have nonscientific concepts of disease. This is especially true in cases of chronic illness where the effects of the disease may not be outwardly apparent. Once symptoms seem to disappear, the patient may be considered as cured and maintenance therapy felt to be no longer necessary. Realization that the child must *always* take the medicine, must *always* have follow-up visits to the clinic, or must *always* limit the intake of certain foods may be clear enough to the health professional, but the immediacy of the need may become clouded in the minds of the most well-meaning parents when at home, and under the influence of neighbors and other family members. This is even more true if strong economic, cultural, or social constraints would argue against preventive maintenance. In these instances, although they may be rare, alternative ways of managing the child's care should be sought.

Another consideration in facilitating home adjustment of the child with long-term illness is the extent to which the family's physical environment has to be altered to accommodate the ill child's special needs. For example, in order for the child to be included in family activities, it might be necessary for him to have a downstairs bedroom that had been occupied by a sibling. Depending upon the age and understanding of the sibling and the amount of preparation he receives for this invasion of his territory, this could be a very disruptive experience for the entire family.

In helping a family cope with homecoming, the nurse should also determine whether the family can assume the nursing role required by the child's illness. Parents and older siblings may be reluctant to admit that they feel unable to master the stress of cleansing draining wounds or changing feeding tubes. If a daily procedure of this type is the occasion of much tension and uneasiness, its effects can spill over in a negative way to every person in the family.

In summary, the major factors that influence a child's adjustment after he has returned home are the state of his health and the nature of his home environment, both in terms of its psychologic and material resources. The nature of the nursing intervention that is required will depend upon whether or not the disease is benign or has a prolonged, perhaps fatal, course or whether the home has adequate resources. However, regardless of circumstances, careful discharge preparation in which family members participate in decision making is an absolutely essential point.

SUMMARY

The way in which a child interprets illness depends upon his body image, his view of body function, and also on such variables as age, nature of the illness and its treatment, family relationships, and past experience. Consequently, a child's view of his illness is a very individual matter. The child may view his illness in the light of psychosocial consequences. Absence from school, loss of position in the family, threat of dependency, and financial strain on the family are examples of common concerns. Physical aspects of illness determine, in part, how the illness is perceived. The symbolic significance attached to the diseased part of the body, the visibility of the illness, and the symptoms associated with it all contribute to the child's mental construct of his illness. Through experience every child develops his own strategies of coping with stress. These mechanisms range from complete escape or denial to temporary regression to a positive restructuring of the stressful situation into manageable dimensions.

Hospitalization during the illness crisis introduces a new set of variables. It causes separation from loved ones. This induces behavioral reactions that include tearful protest, hopeless withdrawal, remote disinterest, and regression in normal age-appropriate activities. The hospital setting introduces the child to a new environment with which he is often ill prepared to deal. The familiar cues that help a child to feel secure are missing. Sensory distortion is a common occurrence, as is inconsistency in care.

Much of the stress of hospitalization, especially for the young child, can be minimized by maintaining a close parent-child relationship during the confinement. Provision of appropriate support is important in order to assure adequacy of the parents' role. Also, the nurse can ease the child's stress by carefully planned and implemented preparation for new experiences.

Parental feelings and actions also influence the child's perception of his illness. A child is extremely sensitive to the changes in his parents' behavior that inevitably accompany his illness. Parental anxiety can stem from unexplained changes in the child's behavior, hospital rules and regulations, socioeconomic and cultural gaps between parent and health worker, and lack of confidence in ability to assume the parental role. Involvement of parents in the care of the child along with provision of cues to help them participate effectively is an important way of relieving some of their anxiety. Encouragement of self-expression through group discussion is another productive way of improving the hospital environment and thus indirectly lessening the stress of hospitalization for the child.

The nurse who understands the many possible ways that illness can be perceived is in a position to deal with the stress in a manner that is appropriate for the family and also satisfying to herself/himself.

BIBLIOGRAPHY

Anthony EJ: The child's discovery of his body. Physical Therapy 48:1103–14, 1968

Bakwin H, Bakwin R: Clinical Management of Behavior Disorders in Children, 3rd ed. Philadelphia, Saunders, 1966

Bartoleschi B, Novelletto A: Child Analysis and Paediatrics. The influence of severe bodily illness in early childhood on mental development. Int J Psychoanal 49:294–97, 1968

Bender L, Faretra G: Body image problems of children. In Lief H et al (eds): The Psychological Basis of Medical Practice. New York, Harper and Row, 1963

Benedek T: The psychosomatic implications of the primary unit: mother-child. Am J Ortho-Psychiatry 19:642–54, 1949

Bergmann T: Children in the Hospital. New York, International Universities Press, 1965

Berman DC: Pediatric nurses as mothers see them. Am J Nurs 66:2429–31, 1966

Blau A et al: The collaboration of nursing and child psychiatry in a general hospital. Am J Ortho-Psychiatry 29:77–93, 1959

Blom GE: The reactions of hospitalized children to illness. Pediatrics 22:590–600, 1968

Blood RO, Livant WP: The use of space within the cabin group. J Social Issues 13:47–53, 1957

Bowlby J: Maternal Care and Mental Health. Geneva, World Health Organization, 1952

———: Separation anxiety. Int J Psychoanal 41:89–113, 1960

Branstetter E: The young child's response to hospitalization: separation anxiety or lack of mothering care? Am J Public Health 59:92–97, 1969

Breckenridge M, Murphy M: Growth and Development of the Young Child, 7th ed. Philadelphia, Saunders, 1963

Clancy H, McBride G: The isolation syndrome in childhood. Dev Med Child Neurol 17:198–219, 1975

Coffin M: Nursing Observations of the Young Patient. Dubuque, Iowa, Brown, 1970

Crowley D: Pain and Its Alleviation. Sacramento, Regents of the University of California, 1962

Davidson A, Fay J: Phantasy in Childhood. New York, Philosophical Library, 1953

Di Leo J: Young Children and Their Drawings. New York, Brunner/Mazel, 1970

Dzik H: The use of motility by a pre-school boy during hospitalization. Mat Child Nurs J 3:169, 1974

Engel G: Psychological Development in Health and Disease. Philadelphia, Saunders, 1962

Fagin C: The Effects of Maternal Attendance During Hospitalization on the Post Hospital Behavior of Young Children: A Comparative Survey. Philadelphia, Davis, 1966

Fleming J: Hospitalized physically disabled children focus on things not people. Percept Mot Skills 39:1002, 1974

———: Understanding children through drawings. In Eighth Nursing Research Conference, Albuquerque, New Mexico, March 15–17, 1972. New York, American Nurse's Assoc. 1972, pp 133–47

Freud A: The role of bodily illness in the mental life of children. Psychoanal Study Child 7:69–81, 1952

Friedman DB: The parent in the parent-child relationship. California Med 86:25, 1957

Garrard S, Richmond J: Psychological aspects of the management of chronic diseases and handicapping conditions in childhood. In Lief H et al (eds): The Psychological Basis of Medical Practice. New York, Harper and Row, 1963

Gellert E: Children's conceptions of the content and functions of the human body. Genet Psychol Monogr 65:293, 1962

———: Reducing the emotional stresses of hospitalization for children. Am J Occup Ther 12:125, 1958

Glaser K: Group discussions with mothers of hospitalized children. Pediatrics 26:132, 1960

Glasser P, Glasser L: Adequate family functioning. In Glasser P, Glasser L (eds): Families in Crisis. New York, Harper & Row, 1970, pp 290–301

Gorman W: Body Image and the Image of the Brain. St. Louis, Green, 1969

Guardo C: Personal space in children. Child Dev 40:143–51, 1969

Gutelius M: Child-rearing attitudes of teen-age Negro girls. Am J Public Health 60:93, 1970

Hall E: The Silent Language. Greenwich, Conn, Faucett, 1959

Hall J, Weaver B (eds): Nursing of Families in Crisis. Philadelphia, Lippincott, 1974

Haller J (ed): The Hospitalized Child and His Family. Baltimore, Md, Johns Hopkins Press, 1967

Hardy JD et al: Pain Sensations and Reactions. Baltimore, Williams & Wilkins, 1952

Hirt M, Kurtz R: A reexamination of the relationship between body boundary and site of disease. J Abnorm Psychol 74:67, 1969

Howe J: Children's ideas about injury. In ANA Regional Clinical Conferences. New York, Appleton, 1968

Irelan L (ed): Low-Income Life Styles (No. 14). Washington, D.C., HEW, 1968

Jessner L, Blom G, Waldfogel S: Emotional implications of tonsillectomy and adenoidectomy on children. Psychoanal Study Child 7:126–29, 1952

Kangery R: Children's answers. Am J Nurs 60:1748, December 1960

Kaye H, Lipsitt LP: Relation of electrotactual threshold to basal skin conductance. Child Dev 35:1307, 1964

Kessler JW: Impact of disability on the child. Physical Therapy 46:153, 1966

Kliman G: Psychological Emergencies of Childhood. New York, Grune & Stratton, 1968

Koos E: The Health of Regionville. New York, Columbia University Press, 1954

Landy D: Tropical Childhood. Chapel Hill, N.C., University of North Carolina Press, 1959

Langer J: Theories of Development. New York, Holt, Rinehart and Winston, 1969

Langford W: The child in the pediatric hospital: adaptation to illness and hospitalization. Am J Ortho-Psychol 31:667, 1961

Lazar E: Children's perceptions of other children's fears. J Genet Psychol 114:3, 1969

Lidz T: The Person. New York, Basic Books, 1969

Linkheim R, Glaser H, Coffin C: Changing Hospital Environments for Children. Cambridge, Mass, Harvard University Press, 1972

Mabrey J: Medicine and the family. In Glasser P, Glasser L (eds): Families in Crisis. New York, Harper & Row, 1970, pp 241–50
MacGregor F: Social Science in Nursing. New York, Russell Sage Foundation, 1960
McCandless BR: Children: Behavior and Development, 2nd ed. New York, Holt, Rinehart and Winston, 1967
McNeil E: Human Socialization. Belmont, Calif, Brooks/Cole, 1969
Mechanic D: The influence of mothers on their children's health attitudes and behavior. Pediatrics 33:444, 1969
Mellish RWP: Preparation of a child for hospitalization and surgery. Pediatr Clin North Am 16:543, 1969
Murphy LB: The Widening World of Childhood. New York, Basic Books, 1962
Nagy M: Children's conceptions of some bodily functions. J Genet Psychol 83:199, 1953
———: The representation of "germs" by children. J Genet Psychol 83:227, 1953
Nash H: Recognition of body surface regions. Genet Psychol Monogr 79:297, 1969
Nash J: Developmental Psychology. Englewood Cliffs, NJ, Prentice-Hall, 1970
Nathan S: Body image in chronically obese children as reflected in figure drawings. Eng J Personal Assessment 37:456, 1973
Olshansky S: Chronic sorrow: a response to having a mentally defective child. Social Casework 43:190, 1962
Opler M: Cultural values and attitudes on child care. Children 2:45, 1955
Oremland E, Oremland J (eds): The Effects of Hospitalization on Children. Springfield, Ill, Thomas, 1973
Orsten P, Mattsson A: Hospitalization symptoms in children. Acta Paediatr 44:79, 1955
Padilla E: Up from Puerto Rico. New York, Columbia University Press, 1958
Piaget J, Inhelder B: The Psychology of the Child. New York, Basic Books, 1969
Pickett L: The hospital environment for the pediatric surgical patient. Pediatr Clin North Am 16:531, 1969
Pratt KC: The neonate. In Carmichael L (ed): Manual of Child Psychology, 2nd ed. New York, Wiley, 1954
Provence S, Lipton R: Infants in Institutions. New York, International Universities Press, 1962
Prugh D et al: A study of the emotional reactions of children and families to hospitalization and illness. Am J Ortho-Psychol 23:70, 1953
Rie H et al: Immediate and long-term effects of interventions early in prolonged hospitalization. Pediatrics 41:755, 1968
Robertson J: Young Children in Hospitals. New York, Basic Books, 1958
Rodrigue E: Severe bodily illness in childhood. Int J Psychoanal 49:290, 1968
Rosenblatt D, Suchman E: Blue collar attitudes and information toward health and illness. In Shostak A, Gomberg W (eds): Blue Collar World. Englewood Cliffs, NJ, Prentice-Hall, 1964, pp 324–33
Rosenthal M: The generalization of dependency behaviour from mother to stranger. J Child Psychol 8:117, 1967
Roy, Sister M: Role cues and mothers of hospitalized children. Nurs Res 16:178, Spring 1967
Scahill MP: Preparing children for procedures and operations. Nurs Outlook 17:36, 1969
Schilder P: The image and appearance of the human body. Psyche Monographs (No. 4). London, Kegan Paul, 1935
———, Wechsler D: What do children know about the interior of the body? Int J Psychoanal 16:355, 1935

Schowalter J, Lord R: Utilization of patient meetings on an adolescent ward. Psychiatr Med 1:197, 1970
Shontz FC: Perceptual and Cognitive Aspects of Body Experience. New York, Academic, 1969
Shore MF, Geiser RL, Wolman HW: Constructive uses of a hospital experience. Children 12:3, 1965
Shrand H: Behavior changes in sick children nursed at home. Pediatrics 36:604, 1965
Skipper J, Leonard R: Children, stress, and hospitalization: a field experiment. J Health Soc Behav 9:275, 1968
Simmel M: Developmental aspects of the body scheme. Child Dev 37:83, 1966
Smith M: Ego support for the child patient. Am J Nurs 63:90, October 1963
Solnit AJ: Hospitalization. An aid to physical and psychological health in childhood. Am J Dis Child 99:155, 1960
Spitz R: The First Year of Life. New York, International Universities Press, 1965
Staffieri JR: A study of social stereotype of body image in children. J Pers Soc Psychol 7:101, 1967
Steinhauer P, Muskin D, Rae-Grant L: Psychological aspects of chronic illness. Pediatr Clin North Am 21:825, 1974
Stone LJ, Church J: Childhood and Adolescence. New York, Random, 1957
Thomas E: The problems of disability from the perspective of role theory. In Glasser P, Glasser L (eds): Families in Crisis. New York, Harper & Row, 1970, pp 250–72
Torrance EP: Constructive Behavior: Stress, Personality, and Mental Health. Belmont, Calif, Wadsworth, 1965
Vernon D et al: The Psychological Responses of Children to Hospitalization and Illness. Springfield, Ill, Thomas, 1965
Walters CE: Interaction of the body and its segments. Am J Phys Med 46:280, 1967
Williams T: Responses of a twelve-month-old girl to physical restraint during hospitalization. Mat Child Nurs J 4:109, 1975
Wolff S: Children Under Stress. London, Penguin, 1969
Wu R: Explaining treatments to young children. Am J Nurs 65:71, July 1965

JACQUELINE THOMPSON

5 Current Nutritional Considerations: Manipulation of the Internal Environment and the Role of the Nurse

The primary focus of this chapter will be an attempt to take a look at current nutritional information, particularly as it affects children through their growing years (through adolescence). Also considered will be the role of the nurse in relation to the nutritional aspects of care as seen in a variety of nursing settings.

The following general topics will be discussed throughout this chapter. First, a short discussion of the nurse's commitment to the manipulation of the patient's internal environment. Second, the normal nutritional needs of well children from infancy through 18 years of age—with a short discussion of the various nutriants, their function, and interrelatedness. Third, an exploration of various kinds of stress experienced by ill children and its effect upon their normal nutritional needs. Fourth, a look at several current nutritional problems and their influence upon the growth and development of the child. Finally, nutrition, nursing, and how we can find this aspect of nursing more reinforcing to ourselves and our patients.

MANIPULATION OF THE INTERNAL ENVIRONMENT

When one first considers the title of this chapter, one might at first suspect that manipulating and stimulating the internal environment of an individual is less complicated than manipulating and stimulating the external environment of an individual. To my mind, the many variables that interact, all in their own unique way, to achieve "normal" internal functioning are neither less diverse nor more stable than the variables which interact with the child to achieve "normal" external functioning.

The human body with its multitude of functioning cells may be best visualized as a free-form mass. Its constructs and very existence are bombarded with internal and external stimuli. These stimuli may be so destructive or negative that they change or threaten the very existence of any or all of the constructual parts. Or the stimuli may be so constructive or positive that they strengthen and enhance any or all of the constructual parts. We can consider this barrier of functioning cells as life. Our task is then to define the nurse's role as she/he interacts with and mediates the stimuli on either side of this "barrier."

The professional nurse seems to have little difficulty understanding her/his role as an interactor with respect to the external stimuli. The nurse is able to interact and mediate even external stimuli that are only mildly negative. Thus she/he is able to manipulate relatively small changes in the external environment. Unfortunately, some nurses feel great reluctance when interacting with and mediating stimuli which are internal. These stimuli must largely be manipulated by changing various ingested materials, usually food nutrients. The internal environment is generally adjusted either by drugs that bring the internal environment back to or within the normal viable range or by manipulation of ingested nutrients. I realize that the administration of a yellow pill can be less trying than persuading a child to eat his lunch. In fact, one of the most unrewarding times of the day for many nurses is when they are attempting to manipulate the internal environment through food intake. In a real sense this is one of the nurse's dilemmas. It is not that nurses do not understand the importance and purpose of food in the recovery of their patients, but many nurses will not or cannot define their own role in this area in positive terms. More often than not, the whole role centers around who is going to "pass the trays." This is hardly the most paramount issue.

Why is there such an obvious rejection of this manipulation of the internal environment? It is certainly just as important as any found in the area of external environment. What is there about the feeding situation that makes many of us reject any positive thoughts about our involvement?

Let us reflect for a moment on the subject of food in our world —particularly, the concrete experience of being fed. Both "love" and "food" will have some impact upon our attempts to "set a scene" for the ingestion of food during that stress-provoking lunch time. Fortunately or unfortunately, since an interaction is a reciprocal relationship, the impact of our own previous experiences related to feeding must not be overlooked. I sometimes wonder how aware we are of the impact of our own early feeding experiences on our current day's action! To reiterate my point, how significantly do our feelings about food interfere or enhance our ability to set the scene for the manipulation of the internal environment through the ingestion of nutrients?

Another area of concern, along with our own feelings about food and the kinds of foods that we considered good to eat, is the difficulty of separating the role of the nurse from the role of the dietician. Many believe that our role should be very limited when a dietician is a member of the team. Justification for our limited role is based on the assumption that the dietician has greater expertise in the area of nutrition. This assumption is certainly granted; she/he may also have greater or as great technical knowledge in the area of feeding and the two roles augment and interact daily. However, despite this expertise, success or failure to change the internal environment most often lies in creating a positive atmosphere at meal time, which is entirely dependent upon the nurse's overall relationship with the child.

As adults we know that the same menu served by candlelight with people we enjoy is more palatable than an identical meal eaten hurriedly with less congenial people. We must recognize this is also true for the child. If the child is not feeling well, if he does not like the person he is with, and if the environment is new, strange, or hostile, the likelihood of his eating is lessened.

NORMAL NUTRITIONAL NEEDS OF WELL CHILDREN

The field of nutrition has undergone rapid advancement within the last one and a half decades. As White (1969) pointed out, we now have enough knowledge concerning human physiology that we can determine the food intake each individual in our society needs for optimum health. White believes that nearly every aspect of human development can now be controlled to some extent by nutritional manipulation during the first months of life and thereafter.

This startling statement certainly encompasses the world, but the logistic possibilities of delivering this kind of service to each individual is minute. While it seems, academically, to be a very interesting point of view, it actually is not very useful at this time. However, it does point out the knowledge explosion in the area of normal nutrition and the rapidity with which it is changing. Nutritional books are sometimes outdated by the time they are published. White therefore recommends that the subject of normal nutrition be taught through the readings of current published articles. If this suggestion is not practiced, the chosen text should be heavily supplemented by current published articles.

The rapid unfolding of new information in the area of nutrition is exemplified by new recommended daily allowances that are released every few years. The food and nutrition board of the National Academy of Science, National Research Council, publishes a recommended daily allowance which is designed for the maintenance of good nutrition of practically all healthy people in the United States. The last revision was in 1968 (see Table 1 for pertinent excerpts from these recommendations). When one reviews the recommended daily allowances it is imperative to keep the goals of the Council in mind. These recommendations were devised for planning food supplies and as a guide for the interpretation of food consumption by a large group of people. Therefore, you may see individual diets that you believe are inadequate when viewed in context with the recommended allowances. This does not necessarily mean that for a particular individual it is an inadequate diet since the recommended allowances are standards established to meet the needs of the majority of the people. Because individuals have their own internal and external environmental needs, we find that for some people the food recommendations are too small and for others they are too large. The recommendations include enough nutritional value so that daily allowances are aimed at what the Board considers optimal health for persons needing the maximum. All biochemical functions can be maintained with desirable storage levels. It is not merely providing enough nutrition to avoid deficiencies.

With the above in mind, let us consider some of the nutrients that we find included in the recommendation for infancy through 18 years of age. Let us also consider a brief review of the various functions and in some cases the important interrelatedness of one nutrient to another.

Calories and Energy Expenditure

Let us first discuss the recent information relating to the area of caloric and energy expenditure in the child. As you look at the recommended daily allowances you will note that the period of infancy has now been broken up into three age levels. The recommended allowances for the various ages are based largely on the general composition of breast milk and on the general intake of thriving infants because there is a real lack of information of normal infant needs. Unfortunately, from 1 year of age to 18 years the recommendations are based on rather scant available experimental information when compared to adult nutritional requirements.

When we consider energy metabolism, we should recall that the daily need for energy fluctuates within the individual from one day to the next as the body attempts to maintain its equilibrium with the external environment. Watson (1967) discusses the clinical signs of an increased pulse rate as reflected in an increased heat reduction and muscle action resulting in an increased energy need. Climate also makes a difference in the day-to-day fluctuations of energy needs. Hot weather will decrease the body heat production, while cold weather increases it. Food intake itself will influence energy expenditure by raising and lowering the basal metabolism rate. An insufficient diet will tend to lower the basal metabolism rate, while a regular diet will raise it approximately 6 percent, and overfeeding may raise it as much as 40 percent. Growth, of course, tends to increase heat production. The individual child's ability or inability to adequately maintain normal body temperature will affect metabolism and thus energy expenditure. Temperature decreases during infancy will increase metabolism rate. This process is called thermogenesis. Thermogenesis in infants is similar to shivering in adults. Examples of factors which interfere with thermogenesis are respiratory distress syndrome, immaturity, the ingestion of some drugs, and so forth (Watson, 1967).

There are a number of rules of thumb which can be used when calculating caloric needs. Caloric needs can be predicted best on the basis of body height. Caloric intake closely correlates with the various stages of growth. Peak energy intakes coincide with the highest growth rates. Unfortunately, current studies tend to lump children together by age groups and do not take into account growth patterns—thus discounting, for example, the changes that occur during the preadolescent growth spurt. The studies particularly miss the high energy needs of the adolescent girls at menarche. Another significant factor is that of energy expenditure resulting from physical activity. Energy expenditure through physical activity in the child from four to six years of age is 35 percent of his total energy intake, while energy expenditure of the child from 10 to 12 years of age is 32 percent of his total energy intake in physical activity (Heald et al, 1963). Sex-based caloric need variances must also be considered. For example, in late childhood the boy exceeds the girl by a very small caloric margin—up to 13 years of age when the boy begins to increase his caloric intake and girls begin to decrease their caloric intake.

While grouping by chronologic age is not a very reliable indicator of caloric requirements, we do see some similarities in the various phases of growth and development. The caloric requirements of the infant are high when compared with his body weight. By body weight, infants are more active metabolically than adults but less active than the toddlers one through three years of age. The infant uses energy for his activities and stores large amounts of calories for growth and loss of heat. Heat loss is great because of his large skin surface in comparison to his body weight. His growth process is marked by increased cell number and sizes, cell mass, and to some extent cell function (*Dairy Council Digest*, Mar–Apr, 1969). One group of experimenters found that the caloric intake of the four- to six-month-old infant was more closely related to the degree of activity than to the size of the infant. Energy is also lost through the specific dynamic action of foods (approximately 5 to 7 calories per kilogram) and loss through excretion of body

TABLE 1

Food and Nutrition Board, National Academy of Sciences-National Research Council Recommended Daily Dietary Allowances,* Revised 1974 (Designed for the maintenance of good nutrition of practically all healthy people in the U.S.A.)

								FAT-SOLUBLE VITAMINS				
	Age (years)	Weight (kg)	(lbs)	Height (cm)	(in)	Energy (kcal)†	Protein (g)	Vitamin A Activity (RE)‡	(IU)	Vitamin D (IU)	Vitamin E Activity‖ (IU)	Ascorbic Acid (mg)
Infants	0.0–0.5	6	14	60	24	kg × 117	kg × 2.2	420§	1,400	400	4	35
	0.5–1.0	9	20	71	28	kg × 108	kg × 2.0	400	2,000	400	5	35
Children	1–3	13	28	86	34	1300	23	400	2,000	400	7	40
	4–6	20	44	110	44	1800	30	500	2,500	400	9	40
	7–10	30	66	135	54	2400	36	700	3,300	400	10	40
Males	11–14	44	97	158	63	2800	44	1,000	5,000	400	12	45
	15–18	61	134	172	69	3000	54	1,000	5,000	400	15	45
	19–22	67	147	172	69	3000	54	1,000	5,000	400	15	45
	23–50	70	154	172	69	2700	56	1,000	5,000		15	45
	51+	70	154	172	69	2400	56	1,000	5,000		15	45
Females	11–14	44	97	155	62	2400	44	800	4,000	400	12	45
	15–18	54	119	162	65	2100	48	800	4,000	400	12	45
	19–22	58	128	162	65	2100	46	800	4,000	400	12	45
	23–50	58	128	162	65	2000	46	800	4,000		12	45
	51+	58	128	162	65	1800	46	800	4,000		12	45
Pregnant						+300	+30	1,000	5,000	400	15	60
Lactating						+500	+20	1,200	6,000	400	15	80

*The allowances are intended to provide for individual variations among most normal persons as they live in the United States under usual environmental stresses. Diets should be based on a variety of common foods in order to provide other nutrients for which human requirements have been less well defined. See text for more detailed discussion of allowances and of nutrients not tabulated; †Kilojoules (kj) = 4.2 × kcal

	WATER-SOLUBLE VITAMINS						MINERALS					
	Folacin# (μg)	Niacin** (mg)	Riboflavin (B_2)(mg)	Thiamin (B_1)(mg)	Vitamin B_6 (mg)	Vitamin B_{12} (μg)	Calcium (mg)	Phosphorus (mg)	Iodine (μg)	Iron (mg)	Magnesium (mg)	Zinc (mg)
Infants	50	5	0.4	0.3	0.3	0.3	360	240	35	10	60	3
	50	8	0.6	0.5	0.4	0.3	540	400	45	15	70	5
Children	100	9	0.8	0.7	0.6	1.0	800	800	60	15	150	10
	200	12	1.1	0.9	0.9	1.5	800	800	80	10	200	10
	300	16	1.2	1.2	1.2	2.0	800	800	110	10	250	10
Males	400	18	1.5	1.4	1.6	3.0	1200	1200	130	18	350	15
	400	20	1.8	1.5	2.0	3.0	1200	1200	150	18	400	15
	400	20	1.8	1.5	2.0	3.0	800	800	140	10	350	15
	400	18	1.6	1.4	2.0	3.0	800	800	130	10	350	15
	400	16	1.5	1.2	2.0	3.0	800	800	110	10	350	15
Females	400	16	1.3	1.2	1.6	3.0	1200	1200	115	18	300	15
	400	14	1.4	1.1	2.0	3.0	1200	1200	115	18	300	15
	400	14	1.4	1.1	2.0	3.0	800	800	100	18	300	15
	400	13	1.2	1.0	2.0	3.0	800	800	100	18	300	15
	400	12	1.1	1.0	2.0	3.0	800	800	80	10	300	15
Pregnant	800	+2	+0.3	+0.3	2.5	4.0	1200	1200	125	18††	450	20
Lactating	600	+4	+0.5	+0.3	2.5	4.0	1200	1200	150	18	450	25

‡Retinol equivalents

§Assumed to be all as retinol in milk during the first six months of life. All subsequent intakes are assumed to be half as retinol and half as β-carotene when calculated from international units. As retinol equivalents, three fourths are as retinol and one fourth as β-carotene.

‖Total vitamin E activity, estimated to be 80 percent as α-tocopherol and 20 percent other tocopherols. See text for variation in allowances.

#The folacin allowances refer to dietary sources as determined by *Lactobacillus casei* assay. Pure forms of folacin may be effective in doses less than one fourth of the recommended dietary allowance.

**Although allowances are expressed as niacin, it is recognized that on the average 1 mg of niacin is derived from each 60 mg of dietary tryptophan.

††This increased requirement cannot be met by ordinary diets; therefore, the use of supplemental iron is recommended.

wastes (8 to 10 percent in breast-fed infants). We can extrapolate from this information that individual infants vary greatly from one another in their actual daily use of calories because of their varying energy expenditures.

Individual caloric needs and daily allowances will not be appropriate for every individual, but the recommendations can be used as a general guideline just as those connected with the basic four food groups. As the child grows from toddler age through adolescence, his energy needs are determined by his genetically programmed body size and growth pattern, as well as by his sex and his activity level. The child's basal metabolic rate reflects his high cellular activity and high body surface. The basal metabolic rate decreases slowly year by year with a temporary increase during adolescence with a final decrease to the adult maintenance level. The basal metabolic rate is higher for boys than girls because of the higher muscle mass. Males increase their rate of muscle cell growth over females, actually having a greater number of muscle cells at maturity.

Calories during the growing years are needed to compensate for expended body energy. Because of their critical role, deficiencies as small as 10 calories per kilogram body weight can result in failure to grow and decrease nitrogen retention. Excessive calorie intake will be discussed later in this chapter, as will lack of calories in undernutrition. Unfortunately, our ability correctly to estimate specific caloric requirements is not very reliable and becomes impossible when energy disturbances come into play; a well-known example is obesity (Heald et al, 1963; Proudfit and Robinson, 1967).

Protein

As you will recall from your earlier study of normal nutrition, protein functions as an essential ingredient for proper growth and development. It forms the basic building-block material needed for tissue growth. Protein is also used by the body in connection with various enzyme systems. An example of this function is seen in the infant's use of trytophan or phenylalanine in the production of antibody responses.

It must be remembered that the recommended daily allowances for infants are calculated on normal breast milk. While cow's milk has more protein by weight than human milk, it is not so well utilized because human infants do not have the proper enzymes for efficient digestion. Obviously, cow's milk was made for calves and not for human infants. However, some increase in utilization of cow's milk does result from the milk being pasteurized and homogenized. For example, one-half the protein in breast milk is lactalbumin, which is quickly digested by the infant. Only one-fifth of the cow's milk is lactalbumin. In the child, approximately 12 to 14 percent of the total caloric need is supplied by proteins. Some investigators believe that the current protein intake of children and adolescents provides more than the recommended daily allowances and that there may be some evidence that an overabundance of protein is being provided in the child's diet.

The need for protein tends to parallel such maturational events as growth spurts and sexual maturation during adolescence. Recommendations regarding protein must take into account sex differences, as they did for calorie intake. For boys the peak protein intake is reached at about 15 years of age, and gradually falls off until about 18—when the adult maintenance level is reached. Girls' protein intake rises gradually at about 12 years of age, and then begins to decline. Here again, information concerning protein and nitrogen metabolism in the normal adolescent is scarce. However, researchers have found that nitrogen retention is related to menarche in adolescent girls and that there is a greater retention of protein during the period of accelerated growth preceding menarche. Following this growth spurt in girls, nitrogen retention diminishes. Unfortunately, we have no acceptable data for boys during the period of the preadolescent growth spurt (Heald et al, 1963).

Vitamins

Vitamins function in a myriad of biochemical systems. The vitamin interrelates in a weblike fashion with the functioning body tissues and with all other nutrients. For example, vitamins function within the brain itself. They facilitate the transportation of amino acids across brain cell membranes. They serve as a co-enzyme in the enzyme system which is involved in the formation of catecholaminines. They participate in the formation of single carbon fragments that are incorporated into the chemical structure of nucleic acids, affecting their synthesis and limiting protein biosynthesis (Coursin, 1967).

Vitamin A. One important aspect of vitamin A and the next vitamin to be discussed (vitamin D) is that large amounts will produce toxicity and in small infants this is a most acute and dangerous side-effect. Deficiencies in vitamin A result in faulty bone and tooth development,night blindness, and keratinization of the epithelium and mucus membranes, as well as skin and xerophthalmia.

Vitamin D. Vitamin D is most often synthetically fortified in modern-day foods. Vitamin D functions in the regulation of calcium absorption. Deficiencies of vitamin D have been quite common in children in the past. The most widely known result is, of course, rickets. Classical ricket symptoms are rarely seen today in industrialized countries, although subclinical states may be more common than supposed. These subclinical states may be revealed by serum calcium, phosphorus, and alkaline phosphatase tests. Of course, patients suffering from renal insufficiency must be immediately suspect. Individual needs of vitamin D vary markedly because of differences in absorption and utilization, exposure to ultraviolet radiation, skin pigment, and so forth (*Current Aspects of Infant Nutrition*, 1962). Vitamin D deficiency can also cause convulsions in children.

Vitamin E. Vitamin E was included for the first time in the recommended daily allowances of vitamins in 1968. Its inclusion in the recommendations occurs primarily because of an increase in dietary polyunsaturated fats. As the intake of polyunsaturated fats increases, so does the need for vitamin E. Also, part of the problem is that vitamin E is not stored in the body to any extent and must be taken in each day. There are some questions as to whether the body can synthesize vitamin E in the intestine, but more research will have to be done in this area. The main sources of vitamin E are the plant tissues, rice germ, wheat germ, green leafy vegetables, and so forth. It functions in the body by reducing oxidation of vitamin A, carotenes, and polyunsaturated fatty acids. It also functions in hematopoiesis. Research has established that in experimental animals vitamin E also functions in the normal reproduction cycle and in the development of cholesterol. It also assists in the utilization of sex hormones.

There is a diversity of opinion concerning the amount of deficiency of vitamin E in the population at the present time. Some studies indicate that there is no deficiency so long as there is not a large amount of polyunsaturated fats in the diet. Other studies have found that there are indications of vitamin E inadequacy in infant diets, particularly in premature infants. This, again, depends on the amount of polyunsaturates in the diet. For example, some workers found a vitamin E deficiency syndrome which is characterized by edema, hemolytic anemia, and thrombocytosis. This deficiency was found in premature infants given commercial formulas high in polyunsaturated fatty acids. As vitamin E now is included in the recommended daily allowances, it is likely that more studies of its activity will eventually be published.

Vitamin K. Vitamin K, another fat-soluble vitamin, is not mentioned in the current recommended daily allowances. Vitamin K is found in a diversified array of food. There is also some question as to whether vitamin K is not synthesized in the gastrointestinal system. The Committee on Nutrition of the American Medical Associaton did show some concern about vitamin K levels in the newborn infant. They believed that infants diagnosed as having hemorrhagic disease of the newborn definitely exhibited a deficiency of vitamin K. They also found vitamin K deficiencies in older children due to such diseases as obstructive jaundice, and biliary and pancreatic insufficiences. Vitamin K is required, of course, for the synthesis of prothrombin or for blood clotting.

Vitamin C. Vitamin C is found in its greatest concentrations in the most active tissues. It forms and maintains intercellular substance. Vitamin C is used in the metabolism of some amino acids and it facilitates absorption of iron in the conversion of folic acid to folinic acid. Deficiencies of vitamin C result in cutaneous hemorrhages, improper bone development, weakened cartilages, muscle degeneration, anemia, stunted growth, susceptibility to infection and, scurvy. Vitamin C is found in most fruit and vegetables.

Folacin is used in the synthesis of protein and as such is necessary in the regeneration of blood cells. Folacin also regulates the metabolism of a number of amino acids. Folacin interrelates with ascorbic acid since ascorbic acid is used by the body to transfer folic acid (which is the dietary form of folacin) into the biologically active folinic acid. Deficiency of folacin is not likely to be found in normal man, but it may occur secondary to disease. Examples of diseases in which folacin deficiencies are found are macrocytic anemia, diarrhea and malabsorption, and so forth. It can also be present in infancy and during pregnancy. Sources of folacin are widespread.

Niacin, Riboflavin, and Thiamin. Niacin functions as the active constituent of enzyme systems primarily used to transform hydrogen. Its deficiency disease is the well-known pellagra, which causes changes in the gastrointestinal, skin, and neurologic systems. Niacin is found in all of the basic four food groups. Riboflavin, another water-soluble vitamin is primarily used as the constituent of enzyme systems. It assists in the transfer of hydrogen from one metabolite to another. Symptoms of deficiency of riboflavin include cracks at the corner of the lips, inflammation of the lips and tongue, burning and itching of the eyes, photophobia, and blurred vision. Riboflavin is primarily found in green leafy vegetables and in rich foods such as liver, kidney, and milk. Thiamine functions primarily as part of the enzyme system, carboxylase. Deficiencies of thiamine result in lack of appetite, nervous instability, depression, fatigue, gastrointestinal atony, constipation, and the well-known deficiency disease beriberi, which elicits symptoms of polyneuritis, cardiac failure, and edema. The committee on nutrition of the American Academy of Pediatrics discussed several experiments with children in connection with the vitamin thiamine. One author described symptoms of thiamine deficiency in breast-fed infants. He found that the infants failed to gain weight, were constipated, and vomited frequently. By and large the committee did agree that thiamine deficiency in infants was less frequent than thiamine deficiency in preschool and school-age children. Lean pork, beef, liver, whole or enriched grains, and legumes are foods with good sources of thiamine.

Vitamin B_6 and B_{12}. Vitamin B_6 functions in the carboxylation from amino acids, transamination from one substance to another, and transulfuration from tryptophan to niacin. It also participates in the conversion of linoleic acid to arachidonic acid. Deficiencies in vitamin B_6 are usually not seen in adults. Investigators have observed in vitamin B_6 deficiencies in experiments in which infants received a formula deficient in the vitamin. Disorders observed during the experiment were impaired growth, hypochromatic anemia, and convulsions.

Vitamin B_{12} is involved in purine metabolism and the synthesis of linoleic acids and nucleoproteins. Vitamin B_{12} is essential for the maturation of red blood cells in the bone marrow, synthesis of methionine, and the metabolism of nervous tissue. The level of absorption of vitamin B_{12} into the body is dependent upon the intrinsic factor, a mucoprotein enzyme secreted by the stomach. For years it was believed that vitamin B_{12} was needed for growth in infants and children. Recently there have been a great number of studies concerning the effects of vitamin B_{12} on the growth of infants and children. Primarily, those workers studying the premature infant found that infants fed vitamin B_{12} supplements did not show additional growth gains. Experimenters studying normal infants generally found the same results. The same lack of positive results was found in experiments dealing with older children (ranging from age 7 to 14 years). A conclusion was drawn from these studies by the Committee of Nutrition of the American Academy of Pediatrics, which stated that these workers thought it was clear to them that vitamin B_{12} did not encourage appetite so as to cause growth increase in children. Pernicious anemia, macrocytic anemia, and degenerative changes of the nervous system result from vitamin B_{12} deficiency (Hill et al, 1958; Blumberg et al, 1961, 1963; McWilliams, 1967; Proudfit and Robinson, 1967; Witkep, 1967; *Dairy Council Digest*, Mar–Apr, 1969).

Minerals

General minerals function in the following ways: (1) minerals in ionic form are components of all body fluid; (2) minerals are components of essential compounds within the body; (3) minerals regulate the metabolism of many enzymes; (4) minerals maintain the acid-base balance; (5) minerals influence osmolarity; (6) minerals facilitate membrane transfer of essential compounds; and (7) minerals functioning as ash are found in bones and serve as structural support and as hemostatic mechanisms.

The major prerequisites for mineral functions are that they be in the right place at the right time and at the right concentration. An example of the interrelatedness of the inorganic compounds with other nutrients is their relationship with proteins and calories. We see in protein calorie malnutrition such conditions as reduced length of bones, decomposition of matrix and total ash, and increased reabsorption of other nutrients effecting bone growth. The interrelatedness of vitamins A, C, and D and the minerals magnesium, manganese, copper, zinc, and phosphorus is seen in mineralization and modeling of bones. It appears as though the bonds between the nutrients are more important than the absolute amount of each of the nutrients in the body. It is believed that an inbalance in minerals will not occur unless one of the elements is missing or is deficient in the diet.

New to the field of mineral research are studies of the relationship of the internal environment and its influence upon the inorganic elements. There is some evidence to indicate that the interrelationships of the various minerals, as well as their absorption and excretion and their internal functionings, will affect the dietary needs of other nutrients. For example, the enzymes needed for the breakdown of glucose are influenced by the body's calcium and sodium level. Deficiencies of most minerals or their absence is rarely seen in normal man. However, when the body is under stress of infection or disease clinical evidence of mineral deficiencies may emerge (Dairy Council Digest, Sept–Oct, 1968).

Calcium. Calcium functions in the building of bones and teeth, in muscle contraction, normal heart rhythm, nerve irritability, activation of some enzymes, and blood coagulation. The absorption of calcium into the body is regulated by body need and aided by vitamin D, ascorbic acid, and lactose. Oxalic acid, phytic acid, and certain highly saturated fatty acids interfere with the absorption of calcium. When we discuss the metabolism of calcium, consideration must be given to a wide variety of differing opinions on the subject. First, it has been found that high intakes of calcium correlate with increased bone density—which one might assume. It has also been found that during periods of inactive growth the amount of calcium needed to maintain the balance reflects the previous calcium intake. For example, if a child has a high calcium intake during infancy, this same child will need more calcium to maintain his balance during the next period of low growth than the child who has gone through the growth period in a deficient state. Second, calcium is absorbed more efficiently at lower rather than higher levels of intake. For example, the retention of calcium at a low dietary level is 90 percent while the retention of calcium at a high dietary level would be something around 27 percent. With this taken into consideration, it has been found that chemical and histologic examinations of the bone fail to reveal any difference between high and low intakes of calcium. An increase of absorption does not necessarily mean increased retention. It appears that the problem with current studies is that they may be reflecting only the availability of calcium within the subjects. In any case, results of calcium studies may certainly be seen to be in conflict with one other.

The need for calcium throughout the child's life varies depending upon growth. The infant's need for calcium has been studied by Beal (1968). His study found that the maximum need for calcium during infancy was four times as high as the minimum need. He also found that during the first six months of life the need for calcium is at its highest. The median need for calcium was about six to seven months for girls and seven to nine months for boys. Studies show that adolescent girls function within normal range on a lower serum calcium level than boys. Experimenters have found a relationship between estrogenic secretions and calcium. They administered gastronic substances to normal girls. This depressed both calcium and nitrogen retention. They found an abrupt depression of calcium retention following menarche, after which some girls recovered to values higher than before menarche whereas others did not.

Another problem in estimating the individual's need for calcium lies in the area of maturation timing. For example, we see rapid gains in skeletal mass in early maturing individuals. This is in contrast to continuing long-term growth in late-maturing individuals. Obviously, the calcium needs of these divergent groups of individuals would be in error if the values were calculated by age alone. When we are dealing with the problem of calculating calcium intake for individual children we run into large numbers of problem children. These are usually boys with high calcium requirements because of tremendously increased bone growth, and late-maturing girls who are concerned with their figures, ie, their fat stores, so that their calcium intake is often inadequate. Unfortunately, discovery of low calcium stores is difficult. Inadequate intakes of calcium in combination with a caloric intake adequate for growth may have no discernible effect on the outer bone growth, but it definitely will effect the tubular of the bones and the size of the skeletal mass. Good sources of calcium are found in the dairy products and vegetable group (Heald et al, 1963; Garn and Wagner, 1967; McWilliams, 1967; Proudfit and Robinson, 1967; Beal, 1968; Dairy Council Digest, Sept–Oct, 1968; Dairy Council Digest, Mar–Apr, 1969).

Phosphorus. Phosphorus functions in the building of bones and teeth and is used in buffer salts. Phosphorus is a compound needed by every cell. It is seen in biologic material such as DNA, RNA, and so forth. Phosphorus is also important in the pH regulation of the body. Phosphorus absorption is aided by Vitamin D, thus interrelating with Vitamin A. Deficiencies of phosphorus are not likely to occur, particularly if an adequate amount of protein and calcium is ingested. However, in individuals subjected to prolonged therapy with certain antacids we may find a deficiency in phosphorus. Such a deficiency can be manifested by poor mineralization of bones, poor bone growth, or rickets.

Iodine. Iodine, a constituent of theroxin, regulates the rate of energy exchange. There is, of course, iodinization of table salt in this country. This practice is particularly recommended in areas in which food is low in natural iodine. A symptom of iodine deficiency is, of course, a simple goiter or an enlargement of the thyroid gland. A deficiency occurring prenatally results in a condition called cretinism, but this is very rare in the United States.

Iron. Iron is a mineral found in hemoglobin and myoglobin. Iron is also present in serum transferrin and certain enzymes. It can be found in all of the body's cells. Information regarding iron tends to suggest that the substance is deficient in most of our population. For example, investigators recommend double iron for infants of low birth weight or of low iron endowment. A number of studies have found that iron in infants and in preschool children is lower than the recommended intake. Andelman and Sered (1966) believe that iron deficiency anemia is a common and prevalent disorder throughout our environment, and that it contributes to infant mortality despite our advanced knowledge in the area. They also held that hospitalized infants had a higher rate of anemia. In their study of hospitalized infants only 25–44 percent were from the lower socioeconomic level but 76 percent were found to be anemic. This finding was stable even when their diets were recommended by a pediatrician and they were receiving adequate health supervision. The true incidence of iron deficiency is unknown, but the Committee on Nutrition of the American Medical Association maintains that the incidence of iron deficiency is relatively high in pregnant women and infants under one year of age. One study of children under six years of age in rural Tenessee found that 10 percent of the children were anemic. Children under one year old were even more anemic.

Since iron is not easily excreted by the body, iron level regulation comes from absorption capacity. As the child grows older the ability of his body to absorb iron increases. This increase usually happens between 7 to 10 years of age. In the older child, iron losses come from menstruation in the female and from fecal loss. Unfortunately, there are very few studies of iron requirement during adolescence, although we do know that the need for iron increases at this time. Boys' needs are increased because of the rapid growth of body mass. This is accompanied by increased blood volume, muscle mass, and respiratory enzymes. There is a real question as to whether girls above 10 years of age are able to ingest, through dietary means, an adequate amount of iron. Recent studies have disclosed that iron stores are reduced or absent in about two-thirds of menstruating women. A number of investigators recommend eating fortified foods as a desirable means of combating iron deficiency.

The average full-term infant has enough iron stores at birth for about the first six months of life. If the infant then has an optimal food intake, he will derive enough iron from his dietary sources alone. The term infant with deficient body iron at birth may require iron as early as three months and the immature infant as early as two months. The immature infant requires more iron than the term infant because of two factors: (1) lower total iron and (2) a proportional and greater growth rate postnatally. The absorption of iron by infants has been studied by a number of investigators. Some found that such absorption by infants under three months of age was faster than at any other age during life (Schulman, 1961; Heald et al, 1963; Andelman and Sered, 1966; Proudfit and Robinson, 1967; Committee on Iron Deficiency, Feb 5,

1968; Dairy Council Digest, Sept–Oct, Nov–Dec, 1968; and Mar–Apr, 1969).

Magnesium. Magnesium influences almost all of the bodily processes. Deficiencies are largely unknown in man, with the exception of secondary deficiencies caused by alcoholism, cirrhosis, severe renal disease, absorption syndromes, loss of body fluids, and some surgical procedures. Because magnesium is interrelated with numerous other minerals, its deficiency has a profound effect on the body. Magnesium is largely found in whole grain cereal and in dark green vegetables.

Sodium. Sodium functions in the regulation of osmolarity. It is used in buffer salts and as an enzyme activator by the body. It assists in the maintenance of water balance and regulates muscle and nerve irritability and is a constituent of hydrochloric acid. It is found mostly in the extracellular fluid, but a small amount is also found inside of cells. Deficiencies of sodium rarely occur. If they do, the symptoms are nausea, diarrhea, and muscle cramps. There are some investigators who believe that there is an increased need of sodium by the body during pregnancy. Sodium is primarily found in the meat group, milk, eggs, and also table salt.

Chloride, Potassium, Sulfur, Zinc. Chloride is found mostly in the extracellular fluid, along with sodium. Deficiencies are rarely found except in patients who have experienced prolonged vomiting. Chloride is found in the same food group as sodium, and is also found in table salt.

Potassium is found in the intracellular fluid with only small amounts in the extracellular spaces. It functions in the regulation of pH, osmolarity, cell membrane transfer, and carbohydrate and protein metabolism. Deficiency in potassium is rather unlikely, but conditions of secondary deficiencies may be found in patients with kidney diseases and diabetic acidosis.

Sulfur is present in sulfur-containing amino acids, in oxidation reduction reactions, and in the synthesis of a number of essential metabolizers. It also functions with thiamine, biotin, and other inorganic sulfurs. Sulfur is a constituent of hair and nails. It is found in eggs, cheese, milk, and meat.

Zinc functions as a constituent of carbonic anhydrase, for the transfer of carbon dioxide, and is a constituent of the digestive enzyme for the hydrolysis of protein. Zinc may also be important in the metabolism of nucleic acid. Zinc deficiency has been demonstrated in the population of some underdeveloped countries, particularly in persons whose diets are also deficient in proteins and iron.

Copper. Copper functions in the absorption of iron and in the metabolism of ascorbic acid; it also acts in normal hemoglobin synthesis, in the oxidation of fatty acids, and in the oxidation of tyrosine to melanin pigments. Some experimenters believe that copper may also be an integral part of the DNA or RNA molecules. The deficiency of copper will lead to retarded hemoglobin production, but it rarely occurs within our society. Copper is found in liver, shell fish, the meat group, and whole grain cereals.

Manganese, Fluorine, Cobalt, Molybdenum. Manganese functions in the body in the formation of urea and in thoroxin formation. Manganese is related to lipotropic active enzymes in the Krebs cycle. Deficiencies in manganese are not known in man. Manganese is found in whole grain cereals, in meat groups, and in green leafy vegetables.

Fluorine is used to increase the resistance of teeth to decay. It appears to affect teeth due to its combination with bone crystal in the forming of more stable compounds.

Cobalt, a constituent of Vitamin B_{12}, is essential in the normal function of all cells, particularly cells of bone marrow, of the nevous system, and of the gastrointestinal system. Primary deficiency disease is rare, except in persons in whom no animal products are consumed. Secondary deficiencies may be found in conditions such as lack of the gastric intrinsic factor, gastrectomy, and malabsorption syndromes. The source of cobalt is found in Vitamin B_{12}.

Molybdenum is a constituent of essential enzymes. There is little information about this micromineral (Proudfit and Robinson, 1967; Dairy Council Digest, Sept–Oct, 1968).

RECOMMENDED DAILY ALLOWANCES

When I considered writing this chapter on nutrition, I first thought that I would not even mention recommended daily allowances. I felt this way because I have found too many nurses who have had poor educational experiences concerning nutrition, and who promptly suppressed the information after it was "learned." But after reconsidering the total chapter I wanted to make an attempt to put the daily recommended allowances in their proper place—that of a base or starting point from which we can consider the individual's needs. It can serve as part of our concrete conceptualization of human nutritional needs along with the basic four food groups. Both of these suggested aids can be used as a core content to assess the current literature on nutrition.

I was asked to recommend a book on nutrition for distribution to several health aid service agencies for children. Rather than recommend a book, I recommended a notebook that would contain current copies of pertinent articles. Nutrition is indeed a dynamic discipline, but unfortunately many professionals still remember all the outdated information they memorized many years ago. My hope is that this chapter will give the reader current information so that she/he can begin to translate her/his new information into nursing practices.

Studies and Their Results

Now that we have at some length examined the recommended daily allowances for the average child, let us consider reality for a moment. Since the mid-1960s numerous experimenters have attempted to evaluate the nutritional status of the American child. Large numbers of children have been studied ranging in age from two years through adolescence. Several methods of study have been used—including interviews; food records; height, weight, skinfold thickness records; attitude scales; chemical analysis; and circulating levels of thiamine, hemoglobin, ascorbic acid, and so forth.

One study of children two to six years of age found the children's intake of iron sufficiently below the recommended daily requirement and in sporadic instances low amounts of the other nutrients, particularly ascorbic acid. These results are even more startling if one considers that 71 percent of the children were receiving vitamin supplements and had parents of a high educational level.

Another study of 150 children of six to twelve years of age from Burlington, Vermont, recorded height,weight, skinfold thickness, plus other clinical and biochemical measures in order to determine nutritional status. Besides these measurements, social adjustment, parental attitude, and dietary intake were determined. The investigations found that there were low-average intakes of calcium, vitamin A, and ascorbic acid. Other pertinent factors were that children of average weight rated higher on various tests of social adjustment and nutrient intakes than children who were either overweight or underweight. A study conducted in two suburbs in a Minnesota community examined 136 children. The children studied were nine through eleven years of age. Methods used in this study were dietary data collected from the children, and socioeconomic and attitudinal data collected by children, teacher, and parent questionnaires. The results showed that, on the average, the children were fairly well fed, but large segments had very low or very high intakes of vitamin A and ascorbic acid.

A multiracial study in New York City studied 642 10- to 13-year-old children. These workers investigated the levels of thiamine, biotin, riboflavin, pantothenate, nicotinic, carotin, ascorbic acid, total cholesterol, triglycerides, and vitamins B_6, B_{12}, A, and E. This study found that 12 percent of the children received protein below the amount accepted as adequate. It also found an association between diets low in protein and lower-than-average blood values of thiamine, biotin, and ascorbate. Another multiracial study was conducted in Onondaga County, New York, with 400 12- to 15-year-old children. The methods used in this study were biochemical analysis of blood and urine samples, interview data on race, age, father's occupation, and breakfast, as well as food supplements. The results of this study were as follows: the data on height and weight, skinfold thickness, and certain biochemical criteria indicated poorer nutrition in Negroes than in white children; also, girls were less well nourished than boys and were more likely to be overweight.

In a study done in 1965 in Burlington, Vermont, 401 school children of varying socioeconomic levels and from ages 12 to 15 were subjected to biochemical measures of nutritional status: hemoglobin, hematocrit, and thiamine, riboflavin, and ascorbic acid levels. It was found that overall nutritional status of these children was good, although hemoglobin and thiamine were found to be rather low or deficient in the highest number of children, with girls rating poorer than boys. Most of the children came from moderate to more affluent residential areas; 22 percent of the boys and 29 percent of the girls came from low-income areas.

In the late 1960s there were two studies of high-school students—one in Berkeley and one in a town in Iowa. The Berkeley researchers studied seven-day food diaries. Children were classified by degree of body fat, and it was noted that: (1) the calcium and iron intakes were low, especially for girls; (2) highest intakes of calories and nutrients were found in average-weight boys and in lean girls; and (3) Blacks and lower-socioeconomic-level whites tended to have lower intakes of nutrients than others. The Iowa study of 2045 high-school students conducted physical examinations of all the students, made biochemical analyses, and collected clinical and dietary data from 252 of the students. They found the average adolescent was healthy and well-fed, but a substantial minority omitted breakfast and ate diets that were not well-balanced. They also found that some individual diets were poor —not because of socioeconomic status, but rather because of diet fads and food preferences.

From these studies we can get some indication that even children from average families—children who are considered healthy and well—may indeed have nutritional deficiencies or may have a nutritional index that is borderline. From this we must assume that today we can no longer automatically state that if a child lives in America he must have an adequate nutritional status. If we believe this assumption to be true, how will it change the nursing role when caring for children? How can we begin to evaluate, in terms of our nursing role, the adequate nutritional status of our patient?

First let us consider what we would look for in a cursory visual evaluation of the child in our care. Proudfit and Robinson (1967) elaborated on several of the observations we can make when we are grossly evaluating nutritional status. One thing that stands out in most peoples' minds when they consider the usual behavior of well-nourished children is energy and vitality. Most children exhibit a high activity level throughout the day. They exhibit their ability to recover quickly from fatigue and fall asleep quickly at night after a long, rushed day. Well-nourished children are usually happy, interested in activities, and generally have a sense of well-being. Their posture is appropriate for their age, and teeth are usually straight and free of cavities. Their gums are firm and pink, without any signs of bleeding; they are slightly moist and have a healthy glow. The eyes, one of the major areas to observe, should be clear and bright—with no circles of fatigue around them. The well-nourished child's hair should be lustrous and shiny, with a healthy scalp. The well-nourished child will have a good appetite and eliminate regularly. His attention span will be appropriate for his age and he will tend to get along easily with others. The child's weight should be normal for his height, age, and body build. For ill children, weight-height information can be obtained from the chart. Signs of crying, irritability, and restlessness are significant signs of a disturbed or ill child. With the above in mind one should consciously make attempts to evaluate the children seen in the hospital (Dairy Council Digest, Nov–Dec, 1967; Proudfit and Robinson, 1968).

Nutritional Aspects of the Child Under Stress

We have discussed the recommended daily allowances and the general nutritional status of normal healthy American children. Now we must look at the changes in nutrition that occur when the child comes under "stress." What is stress? The Dairy Council Digest (May–June, 1966), defines stress as "the wear and tear on the human machinery that accompanies any vital activity and, in a sense, parallels the intensity of life." This body wear-and-tear includes such things as increased physical activity or decreased physical activity, immobilization of the body for any length of time, obesity or underweight, extreme hot and cold environments, infections and malnutrition, trauma or stress of psychologic origin, surgery, various gastrointestinal disorders, and drugs.

Some stress is not necessarily harmful to the individual, particularly if the individual is physically and mentally prepared to adapt to the stress. We all know that the body has a number of adapting mechanisms; the major one is the endocrine system. The nervous and endocrine systems help to keep the body structure functioning in equilibrium during times of stress. For example, the body's reaction to moderate to severe trauma is a net loss of protein. There is an increased secretion of glucocorticoid hormone which increases catabolism of tissue but is useful to increase the body's defenses in times of stress. On the other hand, there may be disturbances within the endocrine system itself that will affect the nutritional process and may consequently alter the needs of the tissue for the various nutrients. "An increase or decrease in the release of hormones is reflected in cellular metabolism and affects the cellular requirement for certain vitamins and other essential nutrients" (*Dairy Council Digest*, May–June, 1966, p 13). For example, in hypothyroidism there is an increase in metabolic rate that increases the caloric needs of the body as well as the requirements for almost all of the water soluble vitamins.

Physical Events and Changes in Nutritional Needs

Increased physical activity affects the body's requirements for energy-yielding nutrients. The amount of change in the need of energy-yielding nutrients is proportionate to the intensity of the physical activity. Along with this, an increase in thiamine, riboflavin, and niacin are recommended with increased calorie expenditure. Vitamins are particularly susceptible to changes in physical activity and the ability to perform work is impaired by vitamin deficiency. Of particular note in the studies was the decreased work capacity suffered with severe Vitamin C deficiency.

Immobilization. Immobilization is one stress that has a higher prevalence in children who are hospitalized. Immobilization produces alterations in the metabolic balance leading to a net loss of certain nutrients. Protein breakdown and excretion of nitrogen are drastically increased above normal during immobilization. Take for example a person immobilized for seven weeks; he has an average daily loss of 2.3 g of nitrogen and requires another seven weeks to recover from this stress. Nitrogen losses in persons immobilized with fractures are found to be even greater than this. One study found that 8.13 g/day of nitrogen was lost on an average with fracture patients.

Calcium is another nutrient that is lost in large amounts during immobilization. It seems as though the body needs a certain degree of stress on a skeletal system to maintain its calcium balance. For example, a patient immobilized for seven weeks might have a total loss of 13.1 g of calcium. Following bed-rest he would continue to lose calcium or to be in negative calcium balance for the next three weeks—even though he was actively losing approximately 4.4 g of calcium per day. Unlike protein, the calcium loss may take years (one to four years) to restore. Apparently bone that does not receive stress from the weight of the body or the pull of the muscle loses calcium. There are other negative balances in the area of electrolytes that also occur during immobilization. The whole area of nutrient loss during immobilization suggests the real need to look into passive exercises or isometric body position which increase gravitation pull on the skeletal structure of immobilized patients. How much good reinstituting the passive range of motion exercises during a bed-bath of the immobilized patient is something that might make an interesting and useful study for the nurse.

Obesity. Obesity must be considered as one of the body stresses. The problem lies in the oxygenation of so much adipose tissue. There is a high prevalence of impaired glucose tolerance or hyperglycemia in obesity. Now we find that diseases of bones and joints are complicated by excessive weight. (Obesity will be discussed at length in a later section.)

Hot and Cold Environments. We rarely think of an increase or decrease in environmental heat as stress, but it it certainly does change the need for certain nutrients. This must be considered one of the normal stresses of life. We can all recall that large amounts of sodium are lost during a heat wave, particularly if in addition to the heat the person is also doing physical work. But I believe that many of us fail to recognize that nitrogen is also lost in large amounts in high temperatures (anything above 70 to 80°F). Studies of moderate physical activity have found that the large amounts of iron are lost in tropical kinds of climate as well as calcium, copper, manganese, phosphorus, and potassium. It has been stated that nitrogen loss in sweat may be one of the several contributing factors to the high prevalence of protein malnutrition or kwashiorkor in tropical areas.

Infection and Malnutrition. The combination of infection and malnutrition often leads to more severe diseases than when either one is found alone. Some groups of Americans suffer more from this combination than others. Such persons are food faddists, elderly persons, or those on desired reducing diet, adolescents with erratic food habits, and individuals with depressed appetites or who are debilitated from chronic diseases. It must be remembered that all infection, no matter how minor, brings changes in the nutritional requirements in the individual body. The malnutrition connected with infections is brought about by three major faults: (1) faulty intake; (2) faulty digestion, absorption, or excretion; and (3) faulty metabolism.

Sebrell and Goldsmith (1967) found that malnutrition in the United States was usually secondary malnutrition—that is, secondary to physical, mental, or psychologic stress of the variety we have been discussing. The recommended daily allowances we discussed earlier were not devised for the ill, although they may form a buffer against increased needs during severe trauma. Health workers of the future must consider the metabolic status of every patient and correct the nutritional and metabolic imbalances produced as a result of some other disease. Unfortunately, not much information has been produced concerning the prevention and treatment of this kind of nutritional deficiency. One disease that we have seen frequently is acute diarrhea. Severe acute diarrhea and other disorders that grossly interfere with gastrointestinal functioning are often fatal, particularly in malnourished preschool children. Experimenters have also found that kwashiorkor usually follows from four to six weeks of acute diarrhea or acute infections in those undernourished individuals living in underdeveloped countries. Diarrhea occurring concurrently with the weaning of children in underdeveloped countries is an outstanding example of the synergistic interaction of malnutrition and infection.

One nutrient that is involved in the areas of infection and malnutrition is protein (nitrogen retention). There is usually a decrease of 10–15 percent nitrogen retention in severe cases of diarrhea. If the child is fed nothing but gruels and starchy solutions, this also results in protein malnutrition. This high carbohydrate diet can also perpetuate the diarrhea even after the infection has passed. It is far better to feed a child with diarrhea adequately since the absorption of nitrogen and fat increases quantitatively with intake even though it is less efficient because of the diarrhea. Vitamin A during an infection is greatly reduced in the blood. Childhood diseases frequently precipitate keratinization of the epithelium, particularly in underdeveloped countries. The same phenomenon may also occur in our own depressed areas, although the subject has not been studied.

Bordeline thiamine deficiencies can be seen in people who come under stress. Vitamin C in combination with infection will decrease blood levels and increase the urinary excretion of thiamine. It may also produce clinical scurvy. Infections also influence iron metabolism. Chronic infection may decrease iron's infection-fighting capacities, reduce iron retention, and shorten the life-span of the erythrocytes. One could call this phenomena the anemia of infection. The relationship between infection, malnutrition, and nutrition is very complex and more information concerning the relationship is being published almost monthly.

Trauma and Stress of Psychologic Origin. It has been found that stress of psychologic origin increases the urinary excretion of nitrogen. This is probably due to the fact that amino acids are released from the muscle and other dispensible tissues as a result of the increased secretion of glucocorticoid hormone. Severe trauma is expressed as an operation, injury, fracture, or burn. Nitrogen loss is caused partly by the increase of adrenal-stimulating hormones of the pituitary glands and increased steroid hormones of the adrenal gland. Severe trauma causes urinary losses of nitrogen, sulfur, phosphorus, potassium, and cretisin. It also increases the basal oxygen consumption and the losses of nitrogen and sulfur within the muscles. There is a decreased tolerance of glucose, and generally disturbed electrolyte balance. In moderate traumas the loss is less and can occur primarily because of food limitation, immobilization, and altered catabolism.

Surgery, Gastrointestinal Disorders, and Drugs. The nutritional need of the body when elective surgery is being contemplated will depend upon a number of factors: the extent of the surgery, previous nutritional status of the patient, the effect of the operation on the patient's ability to judge what he needs to eat, and the selection of specific operative procedures. Protein is the most important nutrient when we consider surgery; it must be used in tissue replacement. Other nutrients for nutritional consideration in wound healing include hydration of tissues and distribution of body electrolytes, vitamin C, vitamin K, and so forth. Postoperatively, the patient is temporarily immobilized and thus will lose nitrogen. Three to five days postoperatively there should be a great effort made to provide adequate calories to the patient to protect the dietary protein from being used up for energy. Usually supplementary thiamine is needed postoperatively because of inadequate dietary intake.

Experimenters found that the average weight loss was 6 percent within 10 days of a postoperative period, although these investigators believed that a significant portion of this weight loss was associated with preoperative procedures which included catharsis and restricted calorie intake. They found that there was a lessening of the protein loss postoperatively when protein was administered. There was a decreased destruction of muscle tissue and connective tissue with patients fed calories plus plasma or protein hydrolyse. This kind of feeding was compared with starving patients, who were supplied only with fluid electrolytes and not more than 3000 calories daily postoperatively. The aim of postoperative nutrition should be to replace the tissue loss and to enhance wound healing. Vitamin C given postoperatively will be used for collagen formation, and postoperative administration of zinc will hasten wound healing in zinc-depleted patients.

Gastrointestinal handicaps such as abnormalities occurring in the gastrointestinal tract and the organs leading to it (eg, pancreas and liver) lead to faulty digestion and absorption of nutrients. This usually leads to malnutrition. You may recall that iron is absorbed in the upper jejunum; glucose, electrolytes, and water-soluble vitamins are also absorbed in the upper jejunum; calcium, protein, fat, and fat-soluble vitamins are absorbed in the small intestine; and vitamin B_{12} is synthesized in the terminal ileum.

These facts should also be kept in mind after bowel surgery. The nurse should definitely watch for clinical secondary deficiencies of the abovementioned nutrients in patients who have had bowel surgery and gastrointestinal abnormalities or diseases. We should not minimize any disorders of the gastrointestinal tract. This is the primary system through which our life-giving nutrients are absorbed from the dietary nutrition ingested. Once malnutrition takes over it can also cause gastrointestinal disorders. For example, protein deficiency can damage the intestinal mucosa, causing malabsorption. Iron deficiency can cause achlorhydria. Niacin deficiency may cause diarrhea, riboflavin deficiency, and cheilosis. There are a number of other agents that can cause malnutrition because of their effect on the digestion and absorption system. Some diet therapy itself can cause digestive and absorption changes. For example, a gluten-free diet can effect the gluten enterpathy causing idiopathic steatorrhea. Organ diseases, such as those affecting the liver and pancreas, can affect digestion and absorption. Enzymes may cause metabolism errors. For example, biosalts may result in malabsorption. Diarrhea caused by an intestinal parasite will affect nutrition.

Let us for a moment discuss the interrelatonship drugs have to the digestion and absorption systems. Drug intolerance may be explained by differences in the metabolic system from one patient to another. These differences may be either hereditary or be caused by diet. Unfortunately, there is a limited amount of information in the whole area of nutrition, infection, and drug therapy. There are a number of animal studies which are likely to be significant when interrelationships are studied. Some factors to be considered in the area follow:

A deficiency of substrate or enzymes for drug conjugation may be due to malnutrition. Protein malnutrition may cause infiltration of the liver. This may make the liver more vulnerable to the biochemical affects of drugs because of diminished conjugation. Unfortunately, the very patients who receive the full amount of any given drug are the ones who are nutritionally impaired by primary disease, which interferes with their ability to conjugate, eliminate, or use drugs normally. Drugs and disease may affect the metabolic process both independently and jointly. While drugs may act synergistically in modifying the course of a disease, the disease, drugs, and food in combination may cause a toxic reaction. Protein depletion with an inadequate intake of sulfur-containing amino acids may inhibit conjugation and elimination of certain drugs. Starvation or caloric depletion may increase the affect of drug toxification. Drug intolerance may be caused by an enzyme defect (Dairy Council Digest, May–June, 1966; Roe, 1967; Watson and Lawrey, 1967; Christakes and Miridjanian, 1968; Gershoff et al, 1968; Dairy Council Digest, Sept–Oct, 1969; Weisberger et al, 1969).

Summary

To highlight the area: There are three factors which effect the nutritional status of the ill child. First, there are nutritional effects due to the use of therapeutic diets. For example, low-sodium diets decrease palatability of food along with the decrease in edema; high-polyunsaturated diets decrease serum cholesterol and increase depot linoleate, but may increase vitamin E requirements in infants. Although fat diets will decrease the absorption of creatine, a high-fat diet will increase the serum cholesterol and triglycerides. High-protein diets will increase the requirement for vitamin B_6. High-carbohydrate diets will increase serum triglycerides and thiamine requirements. Second, some diseases affect the nutritional status. For example, acute gastrointestinal disorders affect nutrition by causing anorexia, electrolyte, and protein losses from the symptoms of vomiting and diarrhea. These in turn cause hypermotility and malabsorption. Third, various types of drugs affect the nutritional status of the individual. For example, antacids tend to destruct thiamine; mineral oil decreases the absorption of creatine and vitamin A. Chelating agents decrease the absorption of metals. Cation exchange resins decrease sodium, potassium, and calcium absorption. The antimetabolytes affect folic acid by reacting as antivitamin agents; barbituates and anticonvulsive drugs are also antivitamin agents and affect folic acid. Corticosteroids decrease glucose tolerance, decrease muscle protein, and increase liver fat. Drugs may also increase or decrease the appetite; they may increase nausea, vomiting, and diarrhea; they may change the intestinal flora; and they may have a pharmacologic effect on the gastrointestinal tract. I think we must also watch for what current investigators call secondary deficiencies—those deficiencies that have come about because of disease trauma or stress. It seems to me most urgent that we begin to notice these nutrient deficiencies, whether primary or secondary, if we are adequately to manipulate the internal environment of the child (Christakis and Miridjanian, 1968).

SOME MAJOR NUTRITIONAL CONCERNS OF CHILDHOOD

Today's American exhibits an almost overwhelming concern with food. Nearly everyone has considered his diet for one reason or another. We have people on special diets because they are underweight or overweight, have a family history of heart attacks or diabetes, have in-born metabolic errors, and so forth. Vitamin supplements have become part of our daily nutrient intake. There are some people in America who are concerned just with getting enough to eat.

All this is to point out our great concern with food. Because of this concern I should like to discuss four of the numerous areas of concern to us as modern-day Americans and as modern-day workers in the area of child health. There are many other areas which could be covered; I chose these because they included a large segment of the population or were new and had a large potential for being seen in the child population we serve. The first three problems are of major concern: obesity, anemia, and malnutrition. While the last, malnutrition, is not usually seen in America it is of major concern in our world and we have recently been recognizing more malnutrition in this country. I will also include some current information on atherosclerosis in childhood, an area of great potential concern to us as nurses.

Obesity

When we consider the problem of obesity the first question which arises is cause. Barnes (1968) maintains that the delivery of nutritional services in the United States and the nutritional education of the population could not be blamed for obesity; the cause may stem from our need to modify the individual's total behavior. For example, obesity may be caused by excess calorie intake, but the solution, according to Barnes, does not lie only in the area of decreased calories but in how we influence food choices in order to improve health—or what kind of food choices are suitable for the individual's own body chemistry as well as with the child's activity levels.

Let us remember that the role of food includes its social function in our society. It is closely interwoven with ethnic, religious, and family customs. Food provides satisfaction and relief from stress—which, for some people, can be obtained no other way. Statistically obesity is largely found in persons of lower socioeconomic status. For example, 30 percent of lower-economic-group females were found to be obese. Stunkard (1968) found that obese persons who were given a free food access in privacy ate considerably more than obese persons who had a free food access not in a private setting. This suggests that part of the problem with obesity is general lack of bodily control. In other words: How well disciplined is the individual? There is some reason to believe from the literature that a great deal of the problems of obese people is their inability to control themselves, not only in the area of food but also in other areas of activity. It is thought that because obesity sets up a physiologic chain of events it tends to be self-perpetuating. In addition to this, there are some irreversible physiologic changes that make weight gain more efficient than weight loss after the person has once become obese; the abundance of fat cells being the most significnt factor. Obese people have an obsessive concern with weight that often leads to passivity, expectation of rejection, and greater inactivity. Unfortunately, the basic habits of childhood arc hard to change in the adult, and if the child has been overweight there will be a greater tendency to remain overweight in adulthood.

A very interesting side-effect of obesity is the potential for the distortion of body image. Obese people exhibit many forms of behavior, although there are only two that seem to be related to their obesity. The first is overeating and the second is distortion of body image. The distortion of body image often takes the form of overwhelming negative preoccupation with obesity, so that weight and sometimes weight control becomes a paramount concern of the person. Such a person often sees his own body in grotesque form and believes that others view his body with contempt. Stunkard (1968) believes that there are three developments which predispose obese people to distort body image. First, the age of onset of the obesity; second, the presence of neurosis of one kind or another; and third, perpetual evaluation of the obesity. He found that if obesity occurred during adolescence or during childhood there was a greater tendency to have distortion of body image than obesity which occurred during adulthood. How the family felt about the child himself and about his obesity was important. For example, some families might view being large in a positive way and connect it with strength, healthiness, and manliness especially in boys. Other families might feel that even being a little overweight was very negative and the child who exhibited these features might become a focal point of the family's hostility and contempt. So it seems that the adolescent, preadolescent, and childhood periods are critical points at which children should attempt to control their weight.

Unfortunately, one of the growth characteristics of the adolescent is change in body fat content. We see girls getting heavy, fatty deposits developing in the hips. These changes probably reflect alterations in the hormonal, biochemical, and other systems rather than any overeating or decreased activity. There are sex differences in fat deposits all the way from infancy. For example, infant girls have more subcutaneous fat than infant boys, and this persists all the way through childhood and adolescence. Around 8 to 12 years, the preadolescent period, children of both sexes increase their accumulation of fat tissue. Then, around 13, boys begin to decrease fat deposits as part of their growth spurt. At 13 girls have a tendency to increase their fattiness. What happens to the biochemistry of the adolescent that increases the incidence of obesity? Heald (1969) found that there are clear-cut changes in two areas: (1) glucose metabolism and (2) energy metabolism. Glucose metabolism is definitely different in obesity. Obese individuals respond to glucose tolerance tests with hyperglycemic reaction very much like diabetics, although they are not diabetic. Investigators have also found that there is hypertrophy of the pancreatic islet cells in the obese adolescent. There seems to be an inverse relationship between the amount of fat in the body and the increased resistance of the transfer of glucose into the muscles. In other words, obese people have a tendency to turn their glucose into fat rather than muscle. About 20 percent of all adolescents and adult obese persons show changes or differences in glucose tolerance. There is some question as to whether this is an inborn kind of deviation or whether it represents the body's adapting itself to a changed internal environment originally caused by overeating.

Diets

Thus we come to the dilemma of the diet. The amount of literature in this area is fantastic. Obviously I am not going to cover it in this chapter, but there are a couple of things I found interesting and which might interest you in delving more deeply into the problem of obesity. There are a great many diets that make use of rather serious fasting. We find these fad diets being used in large numbers by adolescents, particularly adolescent girls. There are serious risks involved, particularly with people who have any kind of infection, diabetes, liver disease, ulcers, or who are pregnant. There are many complications to serious fasting, which we certainly can call starvation. For example, there can be severe orthostatic hypotension, nonochromic anemia, and so forth. People who use diets that include fasting should be made aware of the fact that this amounts to starvation as far as the body is concerned. Of the weight lost during fasting, 60 percent will probably be in muscle tissue and only 35 percent in adipose tissue. Thus the weight loss becomes the result of catabolism of tissue. There is also considerable water loss. It appears as though the last kind of tissue to be decreased is adipose tissue. We do not destroy the number of adipose tissue cells. There is an interesting phenomenon in that once the body has laid down the amount of fat cells that the individual is going to have (this takes place during infancy), the body will have a tendency to fill these fat cells up whenever it can. The fat cells will not be destroyed by losing weight; they will only be emptied. Once the infant sets down the number of fat cells he is going to have, this number will be with him throughout his life. An infant who is very fat may have an abnormally large amount of adipose tissue cells. If this is the case it follows that this infant will either have to be in a semi-starved state his entire life to be thin, or express his tendency to be overweight.

When we think of weight reduction diets we should think of diets that contain sufficient protein to maintain the body structures, particularly during adolescence when children are growing. Children also need carbohydrates so they do not have to use protein for energy. We must remember that using protein for energy is very hard on the kidneys. It also should be mentioned that following fasting, when the person goes back on a normal diet, they will begin to increase weight even if the caloric intake is at equilibrium for their height and weight. This continued weight gain occurs because the body is restoring the protein lost during the fasting. When protein and caloric intake is resumed after fasting, the body will begin to start to gain weight again. As a matter of fact, for every pound of protein replenished the body will gain four pounds in body weight.

Exercise is another aspect of obesity. There is a great deal of literature on the subject of obesity and exercise. Obviously, this is one way to expend energy. Researchers have found that obese children do not exercise as much as normal children. The whole problem of weight control can be best summed up by something we could call preventive weight control. The populaton should be educated to the fact that the way to counteract obesity is never to overfeed the child, beginning with his infancy. There are a number of subcultures in the United States in which people really feel that if the child is of normal weight during infancy there must be something wrong with him—ie, that it is really the fat, chunky little babies that are the healthiest. Unfortunately, many things point to the fact that if the infant is overweight he probably is going to be an overweight adolescent and adult. It is important that health workers begin to advertise the fact that moderate eating habits from birth is the road to optimum health. It appears as though the numerous diets that are floating around our society are not working. In some way special diets appear not to be the problem. The solution appears not to be a quickie diet here and there. It is the problem of changing food intake, changing exercise habits, and, to some extent, changing how we feel about particular foods and about ourselves. It appears that most obese people need a total change of life-style, and we know that this does not take place very readily in adults or even in late adolescence (Stunkard, 1968; Heald, 1967; Barnes, 1968).

Anemia

Anemia is prevalent not only in the United States but also throughout the world. (Anemia caused by iron deficiency has been discussed earlier in this chapter.) Anemia is most often seen during growth spurts and as a secondary deficiency during illness. Thus we often see children in hospitals or children who are chronically ill suffering from anemia due to increased malabsorption. The child is able to maintain adequate iron until a tissue overload occurs during illness.

There is a high incidence of anemia during all the growth spurts, so that iron deficiencies should be watched for in infancy and during the preadolescent growth spurt. How can we prevent anemia? It has been suggested that there should be increased food fortification and mothers should be educated to use these fortified foods, particularly during the child's infancy and preschool stage. There should be careful observation in the hospital for children who have shown any amount of blood loss. Infants of low birth weight should be checked frequently since they may need two times the amount of iron than the normal infant needs. Infants with reduced iron endowment should also be watched closely.

In summary, it is known that anemia is caused by a deficiency in iron or folic acid or vitamin B_{12} or protein. It may also be caused by poor absorption, excessive demands upon the iron, or through blood loss or any of the disturbances in the red blood cell cycle (Brown, 1963; Patwardhan, 1966; Kimber and Weintraub, 1968; McNeil, 1968; Dairy Council Digest, July–Aug, 1969; Flock, 1969). It is imperative to monitor the child through hemoglobins or hematverit to detect deficiencies and correct them.

Malnutrition

Within the recent past malnutrition has been brought to the foreground through the medium of television. We have become aware, within our country, that malnutrition in a sense encircles our affluent society. It varies from severe malnutrition in infants to undernutrition in large percentages of population. In fact, undernutrition may not express the situation accurately enough.

In a country as wealthy and as theoretically able to feed its population as the United States, it seems hard to believe that we are so poorly nourished.

We have discussed poor nutrition throughout this chapter when we talked about poor nutrition in obese people and we discussed the different nutrient deficiencies. Woodruff (1966) defines nutrition as "the sum of all factors in metabolism necessary for growth as well as the maintenance of all body tissues." He holds that malnutrition is a disturbance of (1) neural processes, (2) the body's inability to maintain normal nutrient composition, and (3) the body's inability to respond to disease and stress. All of these biologic factors cause malnutrition. I think we can safely say that malnutrition is commonly found throughout the world; sometimes it is found in normal children in the United States, and it is commonly found in American children who are ill.

The causes of malnutrition within the United States and the world run all the way from congenital abnormalities and metabolic derangement to the secondary malnutrition of acquired disease. According to Girdwood (1969), twelve million American citizens living in poverty are subjected to primary and/or secondary malnutrition. The White House Conference in 1968 exposed some startling findings about malnutrition in this country. The Conference stated that malnutrition resulted in learning deficiencies, productivity loss, and in increased cost of care for diet-related illnesses.

Malnutrition has its most severe effects upon the very young. During infant growth spurts, it interferes with both physical and mental growth. For example, at birth the infant's length is 30 percent of his adult height; at one year of age it is 44.5 percent of his adult height. At birth the infant's head circumference is 63 percent of the adult circumference. Unfortunately after the age of 6 months, when breast milk is no longer sufficient and weaning is beginning, many children do not have their nutritional requirements. Protein deficiency becomes particularly common at this time. It results in slower head growth after one year of age, which becomes progressive throughout the preschool period. Children who have suffered decreased head growth will not recover the growth loss when the child is again well fed. Thus there is a permanent decrease in head circumference, which equals a permanent defect. If the malnourishment is of short duration, regardless of the severity, permanent-damage defects may be prevented. If the child is older or out of infancy when the malnourishment begins, he may make up his deficits later and probably will not have permanent stunting. Thus, decreased dietary intake will cause malnutrition and decreased physical growth. The opposite does not bring about physical growth increases above what is genetically programmed. Graham (1967) stated that "when a diet with an adequate calorie intake, a generous supply of high quality protein and a sufficient amount of micronutrients is consumed with good healthy care the prognosis for growth and body length is seemingly better but not strikingly so than when the very adequate usual diet is provided over long periods so that there is chronic malnutrition this deficit will probably not be made up by further increasing the amount of food." Thus overeating or overnutrition will not produce the same kind off bodily changes that undernutrition will. There are striking differences between average nutrition and undernutrition in resulting height, weight, and head circumference that are not seen between average nutrition and overabundant nutrition. Graham did maintain that following a malnourished period in the child's life, unless it has been for a long period of time, optimal care has definite advantages over average care in making up deficiencies particularly in head size.

Scrimshaw (1967) wrote that the nutritional disease characterized by food restriction—marasmus—was common during the first year of life when postnatal brain growth was at its peak. Food restrictions were frequently found in the populations of cities and stemmed largely from early weaning practices of low-income groups, which are patterned after middle- and upper-class behavior but are done without providing proper dietary substitutes. When protein was inadequate the disease that may follow after drastic protein inadequacy is kwashiorkor. It is generally a fatal disease and produces pronounced central nervous system damage. Scrimshaw, in reviewing animal studies, concluded that marasmus produced some behavior changes in the child; for example, they could still solve some problems. With kwashiorkor the behavior changes impair the capacity to perform tests that require learning from trials. Also growth characteristics are retarded. Retardation begins after the first four to six months of life and becomes progressively worse until the child passes the critical weaning period and succumbs to the disease or to another infectious disease. Scrimshaw also found a difference in children of industrialized countries and nonindustrialized countries in the average height and weight of the children. As far as the United States or other industrialized countries go, it is very difficult to separate nutritional aspects from psychologic and social aspects of deprivation. For example, in industrialized countries children exhibit intellectual deficiencies that are also similar to children who are malnourished. Scrimshaw hypothesized that in industrialized countries it may be something other than malnourishment that causes intellectual deficiencies. He also held that current programs such as the Head Start preschool programs for underprivileged children come a little late for children who are already suffering from malnutrition—that is, by this age there is already permanent physical and psychologic damage. But how much could be attributed to malnutrition and how much could be attributed to cultural deprivation, Scrimshaw was not willing to say. We know, for example, that adaptive capacity depends on the development of interrelations among separate senses, and there have been some current studies in this area of intersensory relationship. Cravioto et al (1966) studied the relationship of intersensory development in Guatemala, in both middle- and upper-class urban children and rural children. They found that the physical structure of rural children who were less well-nourished fell behind those of the middle and upper-class children. They also found that intersensory relationships of rural children, although they improved with age, lagged behind. Another finding was that when the children more nearly realize their genetic potential for growth differences in height, then nutritional and social aspects of development tend to lose significance (see also Woodruff, 1966; Calahan, 1967; Graham, 1967; Sebrell, 1967; Scrimshaw, 1968; Girdwood, 1969).

How does most deficiency come about? Usually very slowly. Heald (1969), in his article on biochemical nutritional status, lists three stages of deficiency. The first stage is characterized by depleted body storage, decreased nutrient concentration in the blood and other tissues, and depressed urinary excretion of nutrients and other metabolites; the second by manifestations of functional impairment; and the third by anatomical reflections of clinical disorders that are caused by (1) deficient diet, which is primary deficiency, and (2) poor absorption because of transportation decrease and utilization (secondary deficiency). Heald concluded that undernourishment in early life retarded growth rate more than it retarded the expression of availability of nutrients, protein in particular, thus giving the body a false impression of nourishment.

Heald also believes that the hemoglobin level is the best available single biochemical index of general health. He found that iron deficiency anemia was very common within the United States. For example, 42 percent of females from 13 to 20 years of age had intakes two-thirds of the recommended daily allowances in 1958. (The recommended allowance is even higher now.) Heald found that Vitamin A deficiency in the United States was usually found in persons with fat absorption defects such as infectious hepatitis, wasting disease, scarlet fever, pneumonia, and rheumatic fever. He found scurvy to be prevalent in the United States in the very young and very old patients, with clinical signs appearing as early as four to six months after deprivation started (Heald, 1968).

Cravioto et al (1966) reported on a number of experiments and also studied the ecology of malnutrition. They coined a phrase for the phenomenon, which they called the spiral effect: "a low level of adaptive capacity, ignorance, social custom, infection or environmental paucity of foodstuffs appeared to result in malnutrition which may produce a large pool of individuals who come to function in sub-optimal ways." The investigators saw this spiral effect as starting with parents who were themselves victims of ignorance, using less efficient ways to adapt socially. These parents in turn reared their children under the same conditions and produced a new generation of malnourished people. Cravioto et al maintained that serious degrees of malnourishment are caused from an inadequate source of foodstuffs and secondly from infection and the like.

Not too many years ago, professional child health workers believed that malnourished children would make up for their lost growth and development as soon as their nutrition again became adequate. Cravioto et al found that there is an initial growth recovery spurt when the child resumes adequate nutrition but that this recovery rate is the same rate as would be seen in a child of a younger age who is the same size as the malnourished child. Because of this, children who have been malnourished for a long time will end up with lower overall growth, particularly lower head circumference and shorter heights than their peers. For example, infants who are malnourished grow up to be adolescents who are shorter than their peers. Length and skeletal development remain reduced and retarded after this infantile malnutrition. They do not recover at an accelerated rate so they will not catch up with their peers. Therefore, we should not satisfy ourselves with the idea that a child will make up such losses. There is much to indicate that he will not make up the losses and he will continue to be behind his peer group, although growing at the same rate as a child who is much younger in age but similar in size.

Cravioto et al pointed out that not only was size affected, but that there was also some indication of arrested biochemical maturation producing "retrogressions to earlier age specific patterns of functioning." The malnourished child may function immunologically at a younger age level. For example, protein metabolism is modified following malnutrition—showing high ratios of phenylalanine to tyrosine. This suggests that deprivation results in a defective enzyme system that causes an inadequate conversion of phenylalanine to tyrosine. This is what we see in newborn infants with PKU, which reinforces the idea that the malnourished child is functioning at an age level much younger than his own age (ie, more in keeping with his metabolic or physiologic age).

Cravioto et al also cited some Russian studies in the area of essential nutrients. These workers found changes in the conditioned reflex in children even before clinical signs of malnutrition occur. Malnutrition modifies the acquisition of rate, maintenance, and extinction of conditioned reflex. The Russian investigators also found that there are marked disturbances in cortical functions, decreased capacity to elaborate new conditioned reflexes, and, if a malnourished state continued, previously well-established responses may be depressed or abolished. As the children recovered, through adequate nutrition, there was also a very slow reflex recovery.

This analysis (Cravioto et al, 1966) of exhibited psychologic disturbances seems to be most important for those professionals working with children with long-term diseases. For example, a prominent feature of clinical findings of a protein-calorie malnutrition syndrome is apathy. There was a decrease in normal curiosity and desire to explore on the part of the child. Of course, apathy may have multiple causes—such as emotional deprivation or separation, which usually accompanies hospitalization. Interestingly enough, recovery among those infants whose mothers showed the greatest interest in them during hospitalization exhibited a more rapid recovery than those infants whose mothers showed no interest or little interest during hospitalization. Cravioto et al maintained that the behavior of malnourished infants resembled infants who were abruptly separated from their mothers by hospitalization. They also noted that children who remained at home and were in the affectionate care of devoted but nutritionally misguided mothers also have psychologic disturbances that resemble children who have been hospitalized. In conclusion, the investigators noted that children with mild to moderate and severe malnutrition failed to respond and showed signs of progressive withdrawal or progressive behavior regression.

Heretofore in the chapter, I have discussed the physical signs of malnutrition. There are also psychologic changes during malnutrition that can be determined by observation. Psychologic changes that will affect the course of the child's cognitive development. It does make one wonder how much the apathy we see in the hospital among children is a sign not so much of psychologic changes caused by social external environment but of pure undernutrition or malnutrition.

Cravioto et al also studied the effects of malnutrition on the results of psychologic testing. He found that the average IQ was more stable in well-nourished children than in malnourished children. In fact, one group of malnourished children's IQs rose 18 percent following an improvement of their nutrition. A number of studies have been done in this area. A well-known one is the study done in Africa (Cravioto et al, 1966). Children from the same background were studied. One group was undernourished and the other one well nourished. The malnourished children showed lower values for height, weight, and head circumference, and their mean IQ was well below that of the children who were well nourished. In this study it was found that children developed well during the first month of life. Even those children who later developed kwashiorkor or severe protein calorie malnutrition developed well during the first month. But the children who later developed kwashiorkor showed signs of slowed motor development and particularly severe retardation of language development following the first month.

Another study conducted in Latin America (Cravioto et al, 1966), brought some interesting results. It was found that infants who were undernourished from four to six months of age had weight gains similar to the normal full-term infant in a highly industrialized society. But from 6 to 18 months the weight gain was progressively smaller than that of their peer group. At about 24 months there was a slow but steady gain. Following this there was a return to incremental values normal for the chronologic age, but the children never regained the weight loss that transpired during the earlier period of malnutrition. The investigators also found that psychologic deficits were most profound if distress took place during the first period (four to six months). These infants showed no signs of catching up, and increased developmental age only equaled the number of months the children remained hospitalized.

Garn and Rohmann (1966) found that protein-calorie malnutrition caused children to be progressively retarded in behavior following weaning. They evaluated this retardation by measuring gross manipulative motor skills and perceptual and linguistic development. They reported that, "the more the child falls behind in somatic growth, the more retarded he appears to become in such motor activities as block piling, in linguistic activities such as namings, in visual-perceptual activities such as form-board behavior, and the like." They also found that children with secondary malnutrition were behind in motor coordination. What is happening to the ill child is explained rather clearly by the statement, "A child who had dumped protein and lost bone is in no physical condition to improve his block piling activities nor in a mood to point out and name parts of his body" (Garn and Rohmann, 1966). We must include in our role of child health nursing the child's play. It is obvious that we can use the area of play to increase the children's development. But we must not forget that the child may not feel like participating in the activities we have planned. We must realize that this does not necessarily mean the child is being negative or is rejecting our planned activities. It may mean that the child is not absorbing or getting the amount of nutrients that will give him the energy or the physical stamina to participate in the play activity. I think we should look to inadequate nutrition for solutions to some of the problems in the child-nurse interrelationship.

As we have suggested, malnutrition not only affects the physical growth, height, weight, and head circumference, but it also affects the development of the nervous system. Central nervous system development and performance basically come from the chemistry of the nerve cells, their metabolism, their cell structure, their energy kinetics, and their integrity of function. Nutrition is fundamentally related to nerve development over the time continuum.

Ninety percent of the brain growth takes place by the fourth year. The period from infancy to preschool is highly critical. It is extremely important that the preschool child is well nourished. There is some indication from Waterlow (1968) that the body does not just "sit still" during protein deprivation. The protein-depleted body makes some attempt to adapt to the low protein intakes. Waterlow found that the body responded to low protein intake by lowering the rate of growth with protein synthesis used to maintain some organs while sacrificing other organs. For example, there might be a decrease excretion of nitrogen due to a reduced proportion of nitrogen being excreted as urea, rather than reduced protein synthesis. Waterlow found that the general protein synthesis may decline, particularly muscle protein synthesis, suggesting an adaption to low protein intake and accompanied by changes in patterns of endocrine and enzyme activity. With low protein intake, we see changing patterns of protein metabolism which are vital to body function (Barnes et al, 1967; Caldwell and Churchwell, 1967; Frankova and Barnes, 1968; Waterlow, 1968).

In summary, it may be said that poor nutrition in early life adversely affects mental development. Unfortunately, not much is known of the effects of undernutrition over a long duration, partly because of the inability of current experimenters to ferret out environmental factors such as social stimulation from their studies. Much has been surmised from animal experiments in the area, but there is still a great deal of speculation about the interrelatedness of malnutrition and learning behavior. This lack of information is unfortunate as it is critical to the lives of the next generation, whose members are being molded now with a lack of protein and nutrients. Thus it seems better to err in the side of assuming that malnutrition is causing some of the symptoms we see and proceed to decrease the malnutrition in young children, whether it be primary malnutrition which must be dealt with through public health, or secondary malnutrition that must be dealt with by the worker in child health in the hospital setting. We must also increase our ability to observe malnutrition and nutritional deficiencies in the children with whom we work. Otherwise, it seems that our efforts in the other areas of nursing care will be futile if the child loses his ability to develop into an interrelated, thinking human being (Dairy Council Digest, Mar–Apr, 1969).

ATHEROSCLEROSIS DURING GROWTH

Another interesting long-term disease that we are finding increased evidence of in younger persons is atherosclerosis. Heald (1969) discussed this at great length in his book Adolescent Nutrition and Growth. Apparently there are signs of early stages of atherosclerosis as early as infancy. Fatty tissue deposits are found in some of the arteries. There is also rupture, degeneration, and regeneration of elastic membranes in the coronary arteries. The laying-down of fatty deposit was found to be most prominent in infants of three and four months of age. Following this age it leveled off sharply and began to decrease. Whether the early fatty streaks that were found in the arteries of infants is the precursor to heart disease is not known at this time. There are definitely increases in lipids in the coronary arteries and the aorta during infancy. But we don't see mineral deposits in large amounts until the fifth decade of life. Almost all infants have these fatty deposits and it is not until 20 years of age that there became significant differences among peoples, individuals, and races.

Researchers also found that in adolescents the atherosclerotic patients showed signs of a prediabetic glucose tolerance level. In fact, there was some speculation that atherosclerosis may be an expression of a glucose metabolic defect. We see, of course, a full-fledged glucose metabolic defect in diabetes. Recent literature gives one the impression that perhaps diabetes and atherosclerosis both have an origin in glucose metabolism, but this has not been substantiated as yet. However, it is certainly something we should perhaps keep in mind. There is also some question as to whether these fatty lesions during growth are primarily related to nutrition or are merely a natural biochemistry defect of human beings. Heald (1969) concluded that nutritional factors may indeed play a more significant role in the complications which develop from these primary lesions of the arteries.

CONCLUDING STATEMENT

The foregoing only highlights the current concerns of modern-day nutrition of children. Researchers and professional workers in the area of child health have been concerned with the nutrition of children for decades. But only recently have we had enough technical knowledge really to see the true scope of the problem. The individual is indeed what he eats and to a great extent his body reflects the nutrition of his mother and her mother. This makes the analysis of normal individual nutritional needs highly complex. Illness further complicates the picture and long-term illness makes the constant evaluation of nutritional needs imperative. It is a critical area of health and one that warrants constant and detailed observation from the health workers who are constantly interrelating with the child.

BIBLIOGRAPHY

Adebonojo FO: Artificial vs. breast feeding: Relation to infant health in a middle class American community. Clin Pediatr 11(1):25–29, January 1972

Bender AE: Nutritional status of schoolchildren. Proc Nutr Soc 33(45):45–50, 1974

Bruch H: Psychological implications of obesity. Nutr News 35(3):9, 12, October 1972

Cook J, Altman DG, Jacody A, Holland WW: School meals and the nutrition of schoolchildren. Brit J Prev Soc Med 29:182–89, 1975

Crow RM: Why my babies are bottle fed. Am J Nurs 71(12):2367–68, December 1971

Dairy Council Digest: Malnutrition, learning and behavior. 44(6):31–34, November–December 1973

———: Recommended dietary allowances: revised 1974. 45(3):14–18, May–June 1974

———: Child nutrition programs. 45(1):2–5, January–February 1974

———: The biological effects of polyunsaturated fatty acids. 46(6):31–35, November–December 1975

———: Iron-deficiency anemia in infants and preschool children. 43(1):1–5, January–February 1972

———: Current concepts in infant nutrition. 47(2):7–12, March–April 1976

———: Functions and interrelationships of vitamins. 43(5):25–28, September–October 1972

———: Some aspects of protein nutrition. 43(6):31–36, November–December 1972

Dayton DH: Early malnutrition and human development. Children 16(6)210–17, November–December 1969

Freeland JH, Cousins RJ, Schwartz R: Relationship of mineral status and intake to peridontal disease. Am. J Clin Nutr 29:745–49, July 1976

Frisch RE: Fatness of girls from menarche to age 18 years, with a nomogram. Hum Biol 48(2):353–59, May 1976

Hambidge KM, Walravens PA, Brown RM, et al: Zinc nutrition of preshool children in the Denver Head Start program. Am J Clin Nutr 29:734–38, July 1976

Health FP: Adolescent nutrition. Med Clin North Am 59(6):1329–36, 1975

Horwitt MK: Vitamin E, a reexamination. Am J Clin Nutr 29:569–78, May 1976

Jacoby A, Altman DG, Cook J, Holland WW: Influence of some social and environmental factors on the nutrient intake and nutritional status of schoolchildren. Br J Prev Soc Med 29:116–20, 1975

Ladas AK: How to help mothers breastfeed. Clin Pediatr 9(12):702–5, December 1970

Latham MC, Cobos F: The effects of malnutrition on intellectual development and learning. Am J Public Health 61(7):1307–24, July 1971

Lauer RM, Filer LJ Jr, Reiter MA, Clarke WR: Blood pressure, salt preference, salt threshold and relative weight. Am J Dis Child 130:493–97, May 1976

Lutwak L: Dietary calcium and the reversal of bone demineralization. Nutr News 37(1):1, 4, February 1974

Mann GV: Obesity, the nutritional spook. Am J Public Health. 61(8):1491–98, August 1971

Moglissi KS, Churchill JA, Kurrie D: Relationship of maternal amino acids and proteins to fetal growth and mental development. Am J Obstet Gynecol 123(4):398–410, October 1975

Nurdaught Sister A, Miller AE: Helping the breast-feeding mother. Am J Nurs 72(8):1420–23, August 1972

O'Grady RS: Feeding behavior in infants. Am J Nurs 71(4):736–39, April 1971

Pediatrics, the ten-state nutrition survey: a pediatric perspective. Committee to review the ten-state nutrition survey. American Academy of Pediatrics 51:1095–99, 1973

Piccano MF, Guthrie HA: Copper, iron and zinc content of mature human milk Am J Clin Nutr 29:242–54, March 1976

Robinson HL: Learning to count the calories. Nurs Times 1062–64, July 3, 1975

Schmitt MH: Superiority of breast-feeding, fact or fancy? Am J Nurs 70(7):1488–93, July 1970

Sloan CL, Tobias DL, Stapeli CA, Ho MT, Beagle WS: A weight control program for students using diet and behavior therapy. J Am Diet Assoc 68(5):466–68, May 1976

Trawell H: Definition of dietary fiber and hypothesis that it is a protective factor in certain diseases. Am J Clin Nutr 29:417–27, April 1976

PART II

Specific Long-Term Illness and Nursing Care

SHIRLEY STEELE

6 Nursing Care of the Child with Kidney Problems

Renal function impairment is attributed to illnesses that are either etiologically obscure or identifiable. In addition, symptomatology can be minimal or variable to the degree that a diagnosis is not achieved or the distinguishing cause remains an unknown because of existent advanced involvement. Many of the childen seen today with complicated genitourinary problems are thought to have had early presenting signs that went unnoticed or were insufficiently treated. To prevent complications associated with urinary tract illnesses and to prevent their occurrence because of complicated preceding infections, in recent years emphasis has been placed upon early detection and aggressive treatment. Whether this approach will prevent long-term complications will only be determined by longitudinal studies.

Infections of the urinary tract are quite common in children. They are especially frequent in infants because of self-contamination directly associated with wet or soiled diapers. The occurrence of pyelonephritis, which is the most common renal disease of children, is six times as prevalent in females as it is in males. An exception exists during the neonatal period, when there is about equal incidence. The anatomic difference probably accounts for the higher incidence in females. The short urethra in girls permits easy access for bacteria to ascend to the ureters and travel to the kidneys. Vesicoureteral reflux and posture both at night and during micturition are probably important and closely interrelated (Smallpiece, 1969). Vesicoureteral reflux has been found responsible for a large percentage of the urinary tract infections in children. Girls with thin-walled bladders or congenitally deficient ureterovesical junction mechanisms are particularly prone to reflux.

Evidence exists which demonstrates a close relationship between urinary tract infections and structural or functional defects of the urinary tract. This factor may be responsible for the higher incidence of urinary tract infections in males during the neonatal period. According to Williams (1968), congenital abnormalities of the male urinary tract often cause more serious secondary effects than in females, and the secondary effects occur at an earlier age. Therefore, it is essential that congenital malformations are diagnosed and treated to decrease the possibility of serious early infection and subsequent renal damage.

Additional factors which predispose the neonate to urinary tract infections are the possibility of contamination through the cord, the poor resistance of neonates to gram-negative organisms, the risk of epidemic infections in the nursery, and the adverse influence of dehydration (Smallpiece, 1969).

The circulatory system is another route for transport of infection to the urinary tract. There is considerable disagreement as to the most common route, but some authorities suggest that the blood route is responsible when the causative organism is a streptococcus or staphylococcus. It is generally thought that there must be some interference with the urinary flow before infection can be caused by the blood route. In addition, direct spread from a localized inflammation in the pelvis of the kidney and infection of the kidney by way of the lymphatics have both been thought to be possible sources, but are considered less seriously in the recent literature.

URINALYSIS

General Considerations

The kidney function of the newborn infant is not completely developed, despite the fact that urinary excretion begins about the ninth week of fetal life. The infant's kidneys have a limited ability to concentrate urine and therefore they need a larger amount of liquid to excrete a particular amount of solute. The infant also has difficulty in conserving body water when it is needed and in excreting excess fluid. The child's urine is usually a paler yellow than the adult's and is odorless unless highly colored. Urine excretion is greater throughout childhood than it is in adulthood. It is influenced by the fluid intake of the child, the digestive and nervous systems, and the environmental temperature. After bladder control is established, the normal child will void six to eight times every 24 hours.

Urine Collection

Some general principles to keep in mind when collecting urine specimens are:

1. The specimen should be recently voided.
2. Use a clean container—specimen bottle with an appropriate top.

3. Be sure the container is dry; water will dilute the urine.
4. Avoid contamination; no feces or toilet paper should be in the bedpan.
5. If it is necessary to measure the urine, use a dry container and be sure to empty complete specimen into the graduate.
6. If urine sample must be retained, refrigerate to delay decomposition.

The time for collection of a single specimen is usually in the morning. A 24-hour quantitative specimen is obtained by discarding the first specimen and then collecting all urine for a 24-hour period.

A urine culture is obtained by collecting a clean-catch urine or a catheterized specimen. Each agency has its own procedure for cleansing the child with use of a variety of agents such as pHisoHex, Zephirin, and sterile distilled water. The procedure, if done correctly, frees the area of bacteria and the collected urine specimen is sent for analysis in a sterile container. If the child is not toilet-trained, after the cleansing, a sterile urine collector is applied to the perineal area to obtain the collection.

Plastic urine collectors have lessened the difficulties nurses previously had in collecting urine specimens from children. Single-specimen collectors are marked "sterile" if they are sterilized. Otherwise, the collectors are clean. There are also 24-hour collectors with tube attachments for continuous flow. The collectors have a sticky substance for easy application, but painting around the area with tincture of benzoin aids with adherence and serves to protect vulnerable skin. For best results, the collector should be applied before the benzoin dries. Adhesive tape is irritating to children's tender skin and should be used sparingly. If its use is required, the nonallergic type is best. With girls it is crucial to check carefully to see that the collector is appropriately placed on the perineum to prevent the loss of the specimen.

After the collector is applied, a loosely fitted diaper may help to prevent the younger child from pulling at the collector. If the child is on bed-rest, elevating the head of the bed may help to prevent seepage from around the collector. Some nurses have found it helpful to place a cotton ball inside the collector to "weight it down." This practice is not usually recommended as the cotton ball usually needs to be squeezed out to get enough urine for the specimen and, too, it interferes with laboratory results. If the child can be out of bed, it is usually easier to collect the specimen without spillage —providing the collector has been correctly applied.

Collection of the specimen is usually enhanced by giving the child fluid approximately 10 minutes before the collector is applied, and continuing to give fluids until the specimen is collected. Fluid intake, however, is determined by the fluids allowed for the child. (Fluid intake will be discussed in greater detail later in the chapter.)

Fortunately, the glass collectors previously used for collecting urine specimens from children are becoming obsolete. If they are used, adhesive should be put around the edges in case there are any small chips or slight irregularities in the glass. Much closer observations must be made to guarantee that the container does not get broken.

Regardless of the method utilized for obtaining the specimen, the nurse should check the child frequently so the specimen to be obtained is not lost. After removing the collector, the child should be washed and dried in case urine has come in contact with his skin.

In some agencies more elaborate methods may be available for collecting specimens from infants and toddlers. These methods usually involve specially designed beds and sheeting which provide for drainage of urine into a collecting receptacle. The advantages include freedom from contamination by feces, fewer restraints, freedom from skin irritation due to strapping or adhesive tape, and greater temperature control if the child is in an isolette.

With children who will be having numerous experiences with urine collections, it is especially important to give them good, simple explanations and preparations. It is imperative that a positive response is set for the initial collection as well as for future collections. Therefore, restraints should be used only as a last resort for getting the child's cooperation. If restraints are applied, it is necessary to help the child and parents to understand that their use is for the child's protection, not as a form of punishment. If restraints are used to obtain a continuous collection, such as a 12- or 24-hour specimen, the nurse must free the restraints and turn the child periodically. She must also observe the restrained areas frequently to be sure there is no circulatory constriction. In addition, the areas should be properly padded and the restraints loose enough to allow some motion without interfering with the urine collection. It is also possible to restrain children in the sitting position so that they can be taken to the play area while the collection is in progress.

Other methods for collecting urine specimens from children include catheterization and suprapubic aspiration. Catheterization is difficult to do in children, and also has been considered to produce a high incidence of urinary tract infection. If it is utilized, every measure should be taken to make the external area as clean as possible and to maintain sterility of the catheter. Bacteriostatic agents are sometimes instilled during the catheterization. Suprapubic aspiration has been suggested by Goldberg (1967) as a method rapidly becoming popular for obtaining urine specimens in children, especially under the age of two years. He suggests the method as safe and effective when there is urine in the child's bladder. It is a procedure usually reserved for the physician.

The presence of pus or bacteria in a voided urine specimen does not establish urinary infection. Therefore, clean-catch urine samples are a necessary aid to the establishment of a diagnosis. Organisms can enter the sterile urine from external areas such as the prepuce in boys or the vulva in girls. Proper cleansing techniques will decrease this possibility and give a more accurate picture of the urinary constituents. Urine is a good culture medium and any organisms which enter it during voiding multiply rapidly and increase in number with time. For this reason, specimens should be sent to the laboratory immediately and marked sufficiently so they receive proper attention. If the specimen has been obtained on nights and the laboratory is not open, the specimen should be refrigerated to delay the growth of bacteria. When the urine is examined, it is the number of organisms present which is significant, so it is important to guard against contaminants being counted in the process. A variety of bacteria infects the urinary tract, but the colon bacillus is responsible in approximately 80 percent of the cases (Rubin, 1964).

Laboratory examination frequently includes antibiotic sensitivity testing in addition to counting the organisms present. This information will be utilized in treating the child and combating the causative agent. In recent years, more virulent organisms are being found responsible for urinary tract infections (Burko and Rhamy, 1970) and organisms such as Klebsiella, Pseudomonas, and Proteus are being reported. These organisms are generally less responsive to antibiotic therapy than *E. coli* and demand more vigorous therapeutic regimes.

In addition to collecting urine specimens, it is important for the nurse to make observations and recordings about the color, odor, amount, and frequency or urgency of urination. Very often children with urinary problems are placed on routine intake and output recordings. If this is not the case, the nurse should take independent action and establish the child's pattern before assuming that the relationship ratio is unimportant. In addition, she must ascertain if the child is having any difficulty or pain on voiding. These symptoms may precede, coincide, or follow voiding, and they should be charted appropriately (see Table 1).

If the child has an ileal conduit, the following method is used to obtain a urine culture. The stoma area is prepared by using specific bacteriostatic agents such as those already mentioned. A sterile catheter (a rubber No. 14, 16, or 18 straight variety) is then inserted into the stoma under sterile conditions. The urine is aspirated by using a disposable 10-cc syringe and adapter. The urine is put directly into a sterile urine bottle to be sent to the laboratory.

The following example will illustrate what transpires after the specimen is requested.

Mary is four years old and has a history of frequent, burning urination for the past two days. She is seen in the out-patient department for evaluation. She is prepared for a urine culture collection and the nurse collects the specimen as previously described. The urine culture is sent to the laboratory for analysis. If the culture contains more organisms than 10,000/ml the child

TABLE 1
Nurses' Notes

John—age 3½ years.

TIME	OBSERVATION AND ACTION
1:00 P.M.	Requested urinal—tried unsuccessfully to void.
1:15 P.M.	Requested urinal—cringed with pain as he intermittently voided 15 cc's pink-tinged concentrated urine. Stream weak, time needed for voiding: 5 min. No pain after voiding. No abdominal distention noted.
3:30 P.M.	Requested urinal—voided 10 cc's pink-tinged urine—5 min voiding, weak stream—no pain—urine odorless—specific gravity 1.020. Specimen sent to lab for routine examination. No abdominal distention noted.

will be started on therapy. The agents commonly used will be Gantricin (sulfisoxazole) or Furadantin (nitrofurantoin). These medications will be continued unless the sensitivity testing indicates resistance or the child's clinical response is unfavorable. A repeat culture will be taken one to two weeks after treatment is completed, and then every four to six weeks until the patient has been abacteriuric and off therapy for six months. If any of these cultures return positive (10,000 or more organisms), the treatment is reinstituted and the cycle reestablished.

In children who are not toilet-trained, it is necessary to estimate the urinary output by examining the diaper. Urine spreads quickly in diapers and there is a tendency to overestimate the output. Consequently, it is sometimes necessary to weigh the diaper before and after voidings to get a more accurate estimate of the output.

It is also common for children to go long periods of times without voiding before they have obvious signs of bladder distention. When checking a child for distention, have him place his hands under his head or on top of your hands. Having him keep his hands occupied will help to decrease the "ticklish sensation" frequently illicited when palpating the child's abdomen over the bladder area. The child will also be more cooperative if your hands are warm and applied gently.

DIAGNOSTIC TESTS AND EXAMINATIONS

There are numerous diagnostic tests, in addition to urine examinations, done to determine the type and extent of urinary tract involvement (Table 2).

Preparation of the child and family for any of these procedures should include an explanation of the routine outlined in the particular agency.

TABLE 2
Diagnostic Tests and Rationale

EXAMPLES OF COMMON TESTS OR EXAMINATIONS	EXPLANATION
Intravenous pyelogram (IVP)	Dye is injected into the vein and excreted through the kidneys into the urine. Films are taken as dye passes through kidneys, ureters, bladder, and urethra.
Retrograde pyelogram	Dye is injected directly into the ureters by way of a catheter passed through the bladder. This test is done in conjunction with cystoscopy.
Excretory cystoure-throgram	A film visualization of the bladder after intravenous injection of contrast material such as sodium or meglumine diatrizoate.
Cystoscopy	Visualization of the interior of the bladder by cystoscope. Ureteral catheters and bougies can be passed through the cystoscope into the kidney pelvis for urine specimen. Stones can also be removed or biopsy taken.
Cinecystourethrogram	X-ray motion picture of voiding and bladder function.
Renal biopsy	Operation done if direct visualization preferred. Otherwise closed procedure using percutaneous needle. Used to identify an underlying renal parenchymal disorder.
Blood urea nitrogen (BUN)	Blood determination of amount of urea and waste product accumulation.
Phenolsulfonphthalcin (PSP)	Kidney function test. Dye injected intravenously. Urine specimens collected after ½ hr, 1 hr and 2 hr to determine amount of dyc excreted.
Addis count	Determines type of kidney disease; 6–8-hr urine collection to determine number of cells and casts in sediment.

Factors relating to the time the test is scheduled, the number of trips off the unit, and restriction of fluids or food should be included in the explanation.

An example of preparation of a 13-year-old for a PSP test follows:

"George, you are having a test today that will help your doctor know more about your kidneys and how they work under certain conditions. This test is called a PSP test, which is a simple way of saying phenosulfonphthalein. The doctor will inject PSP dye into one of the veins in your arm. Before he does this you will be asked to drink at least a quart of water. By doing this you will help to guarantee a successful completion of the test. Your other task will be to void at certain times into these urine bottles which are already labeled for your convenience. I will come in to remind you when a specimen is due. The doctor has requested three specimens. One is due 30 minutes after the dye is injected, one is due at an hour after the injection, and the other two hours after the injection. While the test is being done it is important that you drink a glass of water every half hour.

This will help you be able to void at the appropriate times. Sometimes it is difficult to void when you are asked, but please try to void each time a specimen is due. Also, the dye may change your urine to a pink color; don't be alarmed—this will disappear when all the dye is excreted. Do you have any questions?"

Mandleco (1976) expresses the opinion that children undergoing renal biopsy can be facilitated in a successful support system by assessing the child's feelings using the Hospital Picture Test. It is a projective test which allows the child to respond to a set of eight pictures which depict hospital scenes. The child responds to the pictures and so allows the nurse to assess his reactions. This modality is another way to gather data which will be valuable in providing support to the child. Mandleco administered the test during hospitalization and also during a three-month follow-up visit. She noted that the child's overt reactions were not always consistent with the child's inner feelings.

SPECIFIC CONDITIONS

Excretion Problems

A decrease in urinary output may result from a lack of fluid intake, a decrease in the formation of urine, or an inability to excrete urine from the bladder. Urinary output may decrease in amount or it may be temporarily nonexistent. The length of time the urinary excretion problem exists is of utmost importance. For instance, the child may be playing actively on a hot day and not yield to his physiologic request for fluids. He becomes moderately dehydrated and as a result his urinary output is decreased. This is a simple excretory problem which can easily be corrected by the child's taking oral fluids. In contrast is the case the child with impending uremia. He is temporarily not excreting urine and fluid intake will not result in a correction of the problem.

Another excretory problem common in children is frequency of urination. The exception to this fact is in the case of infants, as it is normal for them to experience frequency. This is one of the contributing factors in not trying to toilet-train infants at a very early age. However, after two years of age, frequency may be a sign of overhydration or a urinary problem such as cystitis. Frequency may be due to nervous excitement in young children, and therefore it is necessary to get a good intake history regarding the relationship of the frequency to the everyday activities of the child. Other causes of frequency are a highly concentrated acid urine, which has an irritating effect that results in frequent trips to the lavatory, and renal calculi, which cause a reflex action or polyuria. It is clear that these conditions will have differing signs that will help the physician to make a diagnosis. For example, with polyuria, the specific gravity will be lower, the urine will most likely be paler in color, and the amount will be larger than expected for a child of a particular age.

Urinary Incontinence

Urinary incontinence may result when the bladder becomes overdistended with urine, causing an overflow. The overflow may be constant dribbling or it may be an intermittent urinary flow resulting without the child's knowledge. Incontinence in children may be due to congenital malformations such as exstrophy of the bladder or myelomeningocele, which are obvious and serious conditions of childhood, or it may be due to less obvious conditions such as an abnormal opening of the ureters into the vagina. The psychologic—as well as the physical—implications of incontinence to children need considerable attention. A school-age child finds it extremely embarrassing to be unable to control his elimination.

Enuresis

A form of urinary incontinence which is fairly common in childhood is enuresis, more commonly referred to as "bed-wetting." Children differ widely in their age for completing toilet training. Frequently, a child is toilet-trained for urination during the day long before he achieves night-time urinary control. The wide range in establishing urinary control makes it difficult to state when a child should be free from enuresis. Each child's developmental achievements should be evaluated to decide if enuresis at a particular age is abnormal for him. A clue to abnormality can be gained by evaluating accompanying symptoms such as unexplained fevers, inability to establish a constant urinary stream when voiding, or pain during voiding which awakens the child from his sleep. The history should include details in relation to whether the child is completely wet or whether he seems to "leak" urine. The time of wetting should be established. Does he wet soon after retiring, closer to the morning hours, or on frequent occasions during the night? Does he wet every night or is the wetting sporadic? When he spends a night away from home, does he have enuresis there, too? The history should also include the fluid intake of the child for at least a day, including the times that fluids are taken. Many children develop a habit of requesting cold fluids at bedtime and it must be established if this late fluid intake is merely resulting in an expected physiologic response.

Pyelonephritis

In the introductory paragraphs reference was made to the relatively high incidence of pyelonephritis in childhood. The pathologic process is usually more extensive than the term implies. An infection rarely is limited to a single portion of the urinary tract. This explains the use of the encompassing term rather than the specific anatomic segments. In the milder cases, there is congestion and leukocytic infiltration into the renal pelvis. Throughout the interstitial spaces there are collections of bacteria and polymorphonuclear cells. It is possible to have hemorrhages throughout the interstitial tissue and the tubules. There may be extensive scarring with loss of functional renal parenchyma when the infection has been prolonged. The end result may be a small shrunken kidney (Rubin, 1964). Both congenital and acquired factors predispose the kidney to infection and should be considered in prevention. The growing kidney is more susceptible to infection than is the adult kidney.

The symptoms which frequently accompany pyelonephritis are chills, flank pain, frequency, malaise, and hematuria. The child may have any combination of these symptoms. The onset is usually abrupt and the child may spike an extremely high temperature. The temperature usually spikes intermittently over a period of a week to ten days. The urinary symptoms of frequency, urgency, and dysuria, if present, usually last for a period of about three weeks. Due to the debilitated condition, anemia, anorexia, or failure to thrive are other symptoms that may be present for weeks following the resolution of the urinary symptoms.

The diagnosis of pyelonephritis is substantiated by the identification of bacteria and pus in the urine along with an elevated white blood count. In addition, the urine may contain red blood cells, and in severe cases, granular and hyaline casts. The child who has persistent pus in the urine should have further evaluation to establish a definite kidney involvement as pus can be a contaminant.

To further complicate the process of correctly diagnosing pyelonephritis, some children do not have any of the specific symptoms ordinarily considered pathognomonic of urinary infection. This is especially true in children under two years of age. They may merely present with a change in personality. The mother describes the child as fussy or irritable and lacking a desire to eat. The child may also have periods of vomiting which makes the infection seem related to the gastrointestinal tract. If the child's urine is not examined, he may lose weight and develop a chronic infection before the correct diagnosis is made.

With repeated attacks of pyelonephritis, it becomes increasingly difficult to make the diagnosis. Symptoms are generally lacking and the child can have a recurrent infection without having any overt difficulty. The unfortunate part is that renal damage may result without any warning. For this reason, children who have a history of urinary tract infection should be followed with routine urine examinations on a regularly scheduled basis. If pus is discovered in the routine urine, it should be followed by a urine culture.

The treatment of an acute urinary infection usually consists of a combination of antibacterial drugs; such as Furadantin, Gantricin, thiosulfil, or penicillin, as well as bed rest (which may be enhanced by sedation), analgesics for the temperature elevation, and increased amounts of fluid intake. At times it is beneficial to manipulate the acidity of the urine through medication in order to control infection. An example of a medication used in this way is Mandelamine. This procedure is undertaken to reduce the possibility of survival of organisms by decreasing the conditions under which they survive and grow. It is used less frequently in today's therapy, as currently available agents have more favorable results than earlier antibacterial drugs.

Recurrence of infection may be due to the same organism or infection by a different organism. If it is the same organism, it is usually because the organism becomes resistant to the antibiotic or chemotherapeutic agent being administered. If it is a new organism, the relapse usually occurs after a significant time period (approximately six months) when the urine has been clear. The child is considered more vulnerable to urinary infections once he has had one. This vulnerability may be related to host resistance or it may be due to a condition caused by the original infection, whereby the defense mechanism of the urinary tract is weakened.

When there is a structural or functional defect that predisposes the child to pyelonephritis, surgical correction is indicated. An example would be exstrophy of the bladder or a bladder neck obstruction. Even after correction, it is imperative that the child be followed medically since predisposition to urinary infections has already been established.

The school nurse has an important role to play in follow-up for these children. She/he is also responsible for seeing that the child is receiving his medication. The usual length of time on medication is six months (Williams, 1968). The nurse is also aware of the current minor illnesses within the school setting, including rashes and respiratory conditions, which the child should avoid. If the child is inadvertently exposed, the nurse can call the parents so they can seek medical advice.

Preventive Intervention. The nurse in the child health conference can be instrumental in helping parents to realize that children tend to delay coming into the house to void because it interferes with their play. This delay may cause overdistention of the bladder and lead to changes which may predispose the child to urinary tract infections. The parent should be encouraged to call the preschool child into the house every three or four hours to encourage him to empty his bladder. Children should be encouraged to respond to the urge to void and thereby establish a normal voiding pattern. As children mature, they may have a tendency to be embarrassed by the need to void. To avoid embarrassment, they retain the urine and eventually the bladder may adapt itself to a position in which it can ignore the normal stimulus to empty (Smallpiece, 1969).

Preventive intervention should focus on establishing an atmosphere whereby micturition is considered a normal and necessary process unrelated to filth and free from disgrace. Even in today's modern society, there are still parents who teach their children that this normal physiologic response is dirty or shameful. They may not intentionally teach this, but their own reactions to wet garments speak louder than words. Another aspect of intervention should focus on teaching parents that children are curious and may tend to explore their own anatomy by handling the genitalia or by inserting foreign objects, which may predispose the child to urinary tract infections.

Parents should also be encouraged to periodically check the urine output of their children. This can easily be done by a quick check to see if the urine is cloudy or if the urine has an unusual smell. A "fishy" smell is sometimes associated with pus in the urine. Parents are quick to respond to blood-tinged urine, but this symptom is not readily present in pyelonephritis.

In infants and young children, emphasis should be placed on changing them soon after the child has urinated or defecated rather than basing changes on the mother's busy schedule. Despite high incidence of pyelonephritis in the diapered population, there is not strong evidence to support the fact that there is a direct cause and relationship to the disease process (Smallpiece, 1969). Evidence to the contrary is also lacking. Therefore, good hygienic practices should continue to be included in the nurse's teaching plan for the parent.

Acute Glomerulonephritis

Acute glomerulonephritis has its highest incidence in children three to twelve years of age. It affects males with twice the frequency of females. It is generally considered to be an "allergic response" or an antigen-antibody reaction to a particular organism. The response usually follows an acute infection by one to three weeks, with the most common causative agent being the streptococcus. By the time the renal involvement makes its appearance, the preceding infection may be completely forgotten.

A good reason to treat comparatively benign infections such as pharyngitis, tonsillitis, and sinusitis is to prevent secondary glomerulonephritis. In a small number of cases, however, there is no history of previous infection.

The literature gives some indication that acute nephritis may have a viral causation (Rusnac et al, 1967; Jensen, 1967). However, a viral etiology will be responsible for only a small number of the actual cases that will be seen in the hospital. The nursing care of children with viral etiology will be essentially the same, so the controversy over etiology is more significant, at this time, to the physician than to the nurse.

The onset of acute glomerulonephritis may be sudden or insidious. The child may complain of weakness, anorexia, or headache. There may be accompanying pallor and edema that is not readily recognized. The edema may merely be a slight puffiness of the eyes or feet. A good clue is the child's complaining of tight-fitting shoes. The child may appear more overtired than acutely ill. In other instances, the symptoms may be more obvious—with hematuria, nausea and vomiting, and elevated temperature. On closer inspection, the child may show an elevated blood pressure and have visual disturbances.

In this disease process there is usually bilateral renal inflammation and the kidneys are slightly enlarged. There is capillary damage, which permits blood cells and protein to pass into the glomerular filtrate. This property is responsible for the appearance of red blood cells, granular and hyaline cells, and albumin in the urine. In some children hematuria is not always obvious to the naked eye, but is usually present on microscopic examination. However, other children may have gross hematuria for the first few days. After the bright red appearance, the urine changes to a dark brown color before returning to amber and pale yellow.

Children who have gross hematuria are readily brought to the attention of medical personnel. The hematuria may turn the urine brown because hemoglobin is liberated by hemolysis in the urine and transformed into brown hematin by the acidity of the child's urine (Hamburger et al, 1969). However, despite their concern, the severity of the child's condition is seldom evident to the parent or child.

The child is usually hospitalized and placed on bed rest. The diagnosis is enhanced by a thorough history. If the parent has "played down" or ignored the previous infection, they may be reluctant to tell the doctor about it. The nurse can frequently elicit this information as the parent does not always feel so guilty when talking with the nurse. Infections are often ignored if they interfere with everyday routines. For instance, if both parents work, it is difficult to keep the child home from school. This might necessitate the mother's missing time from work or an additional financial burden of hiring a baby sitter. Most parents learn that mild infections run their course and have no untoward reactions. They may have had experience with similar infections which responded well to their trusted home remedy of fluids, aspirin, and early-to-bed. They are shocked to learn that on this occasion a mild infection has resulted in a serious disease process necessitating hospitalization of the child.

In addition to the urinary findings, the child may have an elevated antistreptolysin titer, an elevated sedimentation rate (refer to Chapter 12 for more detail on these tests), a decrease in the serum albumin, and a mild anemia. The serum albumin is decreased as a result of the losses of protein in the urine. The child may have a decrease in urinary output with an elevated specific gravity.

Occasionally there are changes on the electrocardiogram, which may be related to the changes in electrolytes. According to Rubin (1964), the heart may be enlarged and this is associated with pulmonary congestion, evidenced by x-ray and pulmonary rales. According to Paul (1967), abnormalities of the chest were found in 90 percent of the children with acute glomerulonephritis in Singapore, where the condition is common. He suggests that the pulmonary vessels are affected in the same way as the renal vessels in this disease, and recommends that more emphasis be placed on the pulmonary changes associated with the disease process.

Hypertension may also be present, usually subsiding after approximately a week of treatment. The child more than likely has had experience with having his blood pressure taken, but the superimposed trauma of hospitalization may make him leery of this procedure. (See Chapter 12 for suggestions regarding this procedure.) The elevated blood pressure usually responds well to the patient's bed rest, but one must be careful to check it closely as activity is initiated. Occasionally, the blood pressure does not decrease and this is associated with cerebral edema and cardiac involvement. Under these conditions, the child must be observed closely for convulsions and cardiac failure. Frequently, there is improvement of these symptoms when the child begins to diurese.

Weights. The child is weighed on admission to establish his base weight for this illness and to prescribe medication and fluid requirements. The child's weight prior to illness is also significant. The parent may be able to give you this weight during the nursing intake history. The child should be undressed for this procedure and guaranteed privacy during the weighing. Each day the child should be weighed on the same scale, at the same time, and in the exact dress. (Some agencies permit the child to wear his underpants while being weighed.) Accurate weights are especially important, as the edema may not be so easily detected in these children. With bed rest, even before medication is started, the child may begin to experience diuresis. Weight loss can also result from the child's elevated temperature and the resultant increase in body metabolism.

Daily weights are usually taken before breakfast and after the child has attempted to void, as it is fairly easy to keep a consistent pattern at this time. If weights are ordered every eight hours, as is sometimes the case when severe edema is present, a convenient pattern must be established and adhered to. The more frequent weighings will help to establish when the child is retaining most of his fluids and will help the physician regulate medication, fluid intake, and ambulation. It is also a second check if a urine specimen accidently gets discarded. The additional weights are not a substitute for output measurement, but rather a system of checks and balances.

If the child is unable to stand while being weighed, a bed scale, baby scale, or metabolic scale may be used. As with any balanced scale, it is necessary to check that the scale is accurately balanced before the child is placed on it. In addition, the scale should be balanced with the covering used for protecting the child's skin. Depending on the size of the child, covering which may be utilized are diapers, scale paper, draw sheets, or pillow cases. Some agencies may have pads or old sheets mended for this use.

General Considerations. The fluid intake of the child with pyelonephritis and acute glomerulonephritis is usually increased (restriction of fluids will be discussed with nephrosis). It is easier to get the child to accept increases in fluids if they are prescribed and distributed reasonably. The age and size of the child are essential to good planning. As a natural pattern, smaller children drink lesser amounts more frequently. This concept should be utilized in planning for their increased fluid intake. The fluids should be spaced throughout the 24-hour period in order to maintain normal body fluid levels and to make allowances for fluids lost during periods when the temperature is elevated. Insensible fluid loss (the invisible loss of water without solute) is also a consideration in children, as perspiration is not always so obvious in children. Fluids are also dispersed throughout the 24-hour period so they can act as a normal irrigating system for the urinary tract. So as to allow adequate rest, they should be given during the night at the same time the child is awakened for other therapy. The increased fluids will help to prevent waste materials from passing through the urinary system in a concentrated form. One additional consideration in fluid therapy is not to overhydrate the child at any one point in time. Careful spacing of fluids will guarantee this.

Children with urinary tract involvement may have considerable difficulty voiding. To enhance voiding, stimulating fluids such as cola, tea, or coffee can be given. In addition, after approximately 30 minutes the child can be placed on the bedpan or toilet and Credé's method be tried. The other time-honored adjuncts to voiding—such as running water within the hearing distance of the child, providing privacy, and having the child place his fingers in water—should also be used freely.

The amount of fluid needed to provide an excess of fluid intake must take into account the solid foods consumed, the weather conditions, any losses due to vomiting or diarrhea, as well as the items already mentioned.

Medication Therapy for Nephritis. The medication therapy in nephritis is based on the individual child's clinical profile. More acute symptoms will, of course, need more vigorous and complicated therapy.

Penicillin is usually prescribed to combat the streptococcal infection. When an elevated blood pressure persists, Reserpine and Apresoline may be added to the regimen. When there is cardiac involvement it is common for the physician to digitalize the child and place him on a maintenance dose of Digoxin. He frequently adds a sedative to the plan when Digoxin is necessary to assure rest. There may be a trial of diuretics when edema is present and pulmonary congestion ensues. The results of the diuretic regimen are not always successful. In very advanced cases, there may be acidosis and sodium lactate may be given to correct this situation before it advances to a serious state that requires a 10 percent glucose solution for correction.

With the addition, subtraction, or reduction of any of these drugs, close observation of the child is essential. For instance, a child placed on Apresoline may have a rapid decrease in blood pressure necessitating a decrease or omission of the next dose of the drug. A child receiving Digoxin may have a decrease in pulse rate, below 60, which again necessitates a decrease or omission of the next dosage of the drug.

With the addition of the pharmacist to the health team providing direct care to the patient, the administration of drugs may be deleted from the list of nursing functions. This health team member may assume the responsibility for the patient's drug profile, or divided doses of medications, and probably for direct administration. Therefore, the nursing responsibilities should strongly be in favor of recognizing and reporting findings in relation to the patient's clinical picture, which in turn will influence the pharmacist's and physician's drug plan. She/he will still need to be aware of the drugs and their expected actions and side effects, but she/he will probably be freed of the responsibility of delivering and carrying the keys to the medicine cabinet. In agencies where this change in health service can be instituted, the nurse will then have more time to make the essential observations which are her/his expertise and highly significant contributions to the health team.

Nephrosis

Nephrosis has its peak incidence in children under six years of age. Boys are more frequently affected than girls. The causative agent in primary nephrosis is unknown. Initially, edema is present in the child's face in the morning and in the lower extremities after a day at play. The edema is painless and does not cause functional disturbance; therefore, it may go unnoticed at first. Eventually, the edema increases and affects the entire body, being most noticeable around the eyes, abdomen, and feet. In boys, the scrotal area is also markedly edematous. If a tap is performed the fluid obtained is generally clear but occasionally milky.

A less common symptom is voice change due to laryngeal edema. During the period when edema is increasing, the child's urinary output is decreasing and the appearance is opalescent and frothy. During diuresis, the urine increases in amount and is clear in appearance.

The pathophysiology of nephrosis centers on the increased permeability of the glomerular capillary basement membrane to protein.* This increased permeability is responsible for the large amount of protein excreted in the urine. Under ordinary circumstances, the kidney is able to filter out waste products and retain the protein necessary for normal body functioning. The change in kidney function results in a lowering of the serum albumin with a resultant decrease in the oncotic pressure of the plasma. This leads to a loss of water and sodium into the interstitial space, causing edema of the tissues.

Because of this loss of protein in the urine, there is a decrease in the serum proteins and reversal of the albumin-globulin ration (A/G ratio). In addition, there is frequently a hyperlipemia and hypercholesterolemia present, which is also secondary to the depletion of albumin. Hypocalcemia is common but there is rarely tetany associated with it. In addition, nephrotic urine also contains increased amounts of copper and iron (Hamburger et al, 1969) with a corresponding decrease in the serum levels.

There is a substantial amount of literature in which authors have expressed their views concerning nephrotic classification and accompanying clinical findings. To avoid confusion, the minute categorizations associated with the varying types of nephrosis will be excluded. However, clinical considerations will be incorporated in broad categories.

Congenital Nephrotic Syndrome. The first variation in this disease entity is congenital nephrotic syndrome or infantile nephrosis. This disease is especially important to nurses in nurseries of the newborn and in well-baby screening clinics. It is known that children susceptible to this disease are born before term and are usually small in comparison to their actual length of gestation. In the case of such infants, the placenta is large and frequently weighs the same as the child. The real significance of the placenta is its apparent inability to nourish the infant adequately, despite its unusually large size. These infants, according to Hallman et al (1967) are likely to have polycythemia and advanced erythrocytosis secondary to the impaired function of the edematous placenta. Other stigmata seen in these infants include a distended abdomen, proteinuria, wide cranial sutures, low-set ears, and small snub noses and talipes. As in all diseases, not all of the signs are present in every child. It is possible that the condition is caused by an immune response between the fetus and the mother (Hamburger et al, 1969).

What is the significance of congenital nephrotic syndrome to nurses? First, nurses must be astute case finders in the delivery room and in newborn services. Accurate recordings must be made of all associated aspects of

**Management of the nephrotic syndrome due to primary renal disease. Can Med Assoc J, 96:52, 1967.*

the delivery and newborn period. It is no longer appropriate to chart "normal delivery" if both the mother and infant survived. The placenta must be weighed and the length of gestation clearly identified. It is unfair to jump to the conclusion that the mother calculated her expected date of delivery incorrectly. Much more emphasis needs to be placed on the child who is not up to expected standards at birth. Nursing has a major role to play in collecting data on this group of high-risk children.

After the newborn period, careful screening and developmental assessment will help to identify other clues to diagnosis. One frequently found symptom is the child's failure to thrive. These infants gain poorly despite the most conscientious feeding techniques. They are also frequently members of a family known to have kidney problems. It is believed (Hallman et al, 1967) that the condition is probably transmitted by an autosomal recessive gene. The nursing intake may help to identify other members of the family with little-known kidney problems. In addition, the nurse can observe the child in a lying position. The position which seems most comfortable to an infant with an edematous abdomen is frequently one described as opisthotonus (an arched-back appearance). The ankles of the infant are often in a flexed position (Hallman et al, 1967), and this can be a significant clue that the child has had interference with osseous growth in utero.

One of the most significant aspects of case finding is bringing the child to adequate medical supervision immediately. At this particular time, these children do not respond to the therapy given the child with acquired nephrosis and their life expectancy is very poor. Perhaps earlier diagnosis will result in more adequate control.

Acquired Nephrosis. After six months of age, the child is considered to have the acquired type rather than the congenital form. This group includes the children categorized as having lipid nephrosis or nephrotic syndrome. In these conditions, the therapeutic regimen has resulted in prolongation of life or even complete recovery.

In order to appreciate the extensive care plan needed to meet this child's needs, it is necessary to look at the many areas involved as a result of the disease process.

Eyes. The soft tissue of the eyelids and below the eyes are common sites for edema. The classical picture of a child with nephrosis is one with slits for eye openings and swelling which causes a transparent appearance of the eyelids. The child is seen with his head tilted back in an attempt to utilize his narrow visual contact with his environment. He may benefit from soothing eye irrigations and occasionally from the use of eye ointments. The edema is transient and elevating his head may help to reduce the edema in this area. The child who sleeps without a pillow may accumulate a large amount of fluid overnight and awaken in the morning to total darkness. This can be an extremely frightening experience for the child. It is especially frightening to the preschooler, who is most prone to the disease.

In addition to the edema, the child may develop xanthomatous lesions on the eyelids which are uncomfortable and may cause the child to rub his eyes and further irritate the area. The xanthomatous lesions are thought to be associated with the high lipid levels in the blood.

Skin. Nuring measures are intimately involved with preventing excoriation and breakdown of the overstretched skin. Careful cleansing and attention to skin areas that meet one another is paramount. Support of edematous areas by pillows may help to lessen tension on the skin and make the child more comfortable. Scrotal supports are used effectively. Creases of the groin may need to be padded with soft flannel or other cloth to prevent breakdown. During the hot weather, the child will perspire in these areas and need frequent washing, drying, and changing of the padding. The padding will also have to be checked for dribbling urine which will foster the growth of bacteria in this warm, dark area.

The child's fingernails should be kept short and clean to discourage scratching. The fingernails are frequently brittle and striated (Hamburger et al, 1969). The child's skin is dry and is prone to erysipeloid lesions which consist of red, blotching, tender patches and add an additional annoyance to the child. The skin is susceptible to bacterial and fungal infections. Bathing the child in the bathtub may be extremely soothing. The nurse should get help in transferring the child. It is essential to use good body mechanics to prevent strain to herself/himself in lifting the child whose weight will be greatly increased by edema and whose body does not have the usual contours.

It is difficult to keep the child comfortable during the acute stages of the disease. Frequent changes in position will decrease the amount of whining that signals discomfort. When the child is turned, the areas exposed should be gently rubbed to decrease the "wrinkle marks" that result from the contact of the edematous tissues with the bed clothing.

In hot weather, the child may get relief from using a bed cradle to support the bed linen and allow for better air circulation. The child should not be exposed to drafts or placed in direct exposure to an electric fan. He is very susceptible to infection and any predisposing factors should be avoided.

After the acute stages of the disorder, skin irritation is less common and the child can be allowed out of bed. The shifting in edema, due to the upright position, will focus concern on the child's feet. It will be necessary to check his footwear and remove constricting items. The skin areas between the toes will need to be cleansed individually and observed for excoriation. A soothing foot powder may be sparingly applied.

The child's teeth should be brushed frequently as there is an increased possibility of dental caries. Dental enamel is altered in the permanent teeth (Hamburger et al, 1969).

Hamburger et al also mention the diminished elasticity of the external ear and also the tip of the nose after the diuresis is completed.

Nutrition. Underneath the edema, there may be extreme wasting of tissue, malnutrition, and anemia. These factors are extremely relevant to nursing care. The nurse must utilize every possible method to get the child interested in eating. The anorexia which accompanies acute infection, an acute disease process, elevated temperatures, physical discomfort, and separation from home and family makes it essential for the nurse to be creative and patient in her/his approach to feeding the child.

Occasionally children are also placed on salt-poor diets or diets with elevated or decreased protein content. These modifications to the expected taste of food may further discourage the child from eating. There may also be the added stress provided by limitation or restriction of fluids that may be necessary when the child is excreting only scant amounts of urine or having diarrhea, which may result from an edematous bowel. During these periods, the child may be allowed hard candy to suck on to decrease his thirst.

In the course of limited fluid intake it is extremely important to space the fluids throughout the 24-hour period. A common plan for establishing fluid intake is to base it on the previous day's urinary output. Therefore, the doctor's order may read: Oral fluids 100 cc's plus the previous day's output (which provides only a minimal increase in the total fluid allotment). To make the child feel he is getting more fluid, a small glass should be utilized so the fluid can be easily seen in the glass. If a plastic medicine glass is used, be sure the child is aware that it is not medication.

Urinary Output. The urinary output of the child with nephrosis is usually scant or nonexistent during the acute stages. It is impossible to emphasize how important it is to keep an accurate account of every voiding. As previously indicated, the daily fluid allotment may depend on it, the child's response to corticosteroid therapy will be monitored by it, and the appearance will give clues to decreasing or persistent hematuria, which may indicate a nephrotic syndrome that is a combination of nephrosis and acute glomerulonephritis.

Collection of specimens, needed to follow the albumin excretion, may be difficult due to the extreme amount of edema and the decrease in urinary sensation due to the small amounts of urine reaching the bladder. The child should be tried on the bedpan or given the urinal rather than relying on his urge to void. Care should be taken not to unduly alarm the child by continually focusing on your desire to have the child void. Statements such as, "Haven't you voided today?" are taboo and should be replaced by a statement such as "It is time to try using the urinal now." The emphasis is thereby placed on the attempt to void, rather than on the success of voiding. It must be understood that the preschooler wants to please adults and he will be disappointed if he is unable to do so. He begins to get the impression that if he voids he will be rewarded and if he does not he will be punished. Continual failure to void results in increased frustration. This frustration added to his irritability and mood swings caused by corticosteroids can make the staff classify him as a "crabby" little patient.

Changes in Body Image. Boys need reassurance that their penis has not disappeared despite its less prominent position. A statement of reassurance that the penis is still there and that you can see it from your position should precede the voiding request. This statement should be followed by one that shows the child that you appreciate his concern for the changes in his body and that you know with time he will again return to his normal appearance.

The child should be provided with opportunities to express his fears regarding the changes in his body. In nephrosis, this is especially frightening because the child has to adapt rapidly to an increasing body size and then to adapt to a change in size, on almost a daily basis, when diuresis occurs. In addition, due to the intermittent nature of the disease, he may have to make this adjustment on numerous occasions.

The degree of stress caused by such changes should not be underestimated. Take, for example, the preschooler who delighted in removing his socks and shoes and now cannot reach his toes; or the preschooler who was toilet-trained in a potty chair and now cannot free himself if he sits on the potty. These changes make it extremely difficult for the child to identify his immediate environment and his position in relation to it. His increasing size takes up more of his immediate environment and may cause him to bump into doors or fall over the side of the bed. The real significance of this information relates not only to his preservation of a healthy mental outlook but also to provision of safety. Even the young school-age child may need siderails to prevent him from falling out of bed. The siderails will also help to guarantee that a nurse is available to assist the child getting out of bed until he is aware of the changes needed to remain upright when his center of gravity is changed due to his large abdomen.

Susceptibility to Infection. Prevention of infection is directly related to the child's care. Children with nephrosis have a lowered resistance to infection and frequently seem to develop acute infections superimposed on chronic ones. The child may seem to have a "stuffy" nose a great deal of the time. This is probably related to swelling of the mucous membranes of the sinuses and nasal passages. Care must be taken when cleansing the nose with cotton tip applicators not to irritate these edematous linings. A rolled piece of cotton may be safer to use than the cotton tip applicator. The same care must be taken when doing nose and throat cultures ordered to detect early signs of bacterial infection.

Antibiotics are usually administered during acute infections or exposure to known infections, but rarely prophylactically. During acute infections, antibiotics may be administered intravenously due to the decreased ability of the edematous intestine to absorb adequate amounts administered by oral or intramuscular routes. If intramuscular administration is utilized, it is especially important to insure that the medication reaches muscular tissue since the edematous tissue is prone to develop subcutaneous abscesses. Therefore, palpation for abscess formation and rotation of sites is paramount prior to giving injections.

There have been reported cases of complete remission resulting from a case of measles or chickenpox in a child with nephrosis. Prior to the good results now possible to obtain with use of corticosteroids, it was fairly common practice to try to find a child sick with one of these communicable diseases to provide exposure and cross-infection. This procedure is now less frequently used as it does not guarantee success and the child can suffer the ill effects of the communicable disease and be prone to complications without obtaining a remission. This risk was considered worthwhile when early treatment was not too successful and the disease more often proceeded to a fatal outcome.

The nurse should be aware that the child may not be immunized until he has been completely free of proteinuria and off steroids for at least a year (Soyka, 1967). This delay in immunizing is based on the assumption that there may be an association between an immune process in nephrosis and delayed hypersensitivity. These factors are thought to be responsible for exacerbations of nephrotic symptoms following routine immunizations. This factor is especially significant if the child receives his immunizations at a clinic or immunization center in which the staff is not familiar with the child's entire health and illness profile. It is a good idea to explain to the mother any proposed delay in immunizations so as to cut down on the possibility of error.

The placement of the child on the clinical unit should be based on decreasing the amount of contact with children with infections. Otherwise, the child should not be limited in his associations with other children and adults.

The same principle should guide the mother when the child is discharged. The child should be allowed freedom of activity, but should avoid other children and adults with infectious processes. Exacerbations of nephrosis can be directly related to infection.

Obtaining Blood Specimens. During the acute stages of illness it is necessary to obtain frequent blood specimens for analysis. This creates a problem which can be a real frustration to the nurse and person trying to get the specimen. The preschooler's veins are difficult to locate under normal conditions. With the addition of edema, they are even more difficult to locate.

The child should be brought to the treatment room for the procedure. He should be prepared simply and honestly. Even the application of the tourniquet to his edematous limbs can be extremely uncomfortable. It is often necessary to release it and reapply it several times before an adequate vein can be identified. This action increases the child's time to fear the procedure and provides him with additional frustration.

The child is usually in a supine position for this procedure. Care must be taken to watch the child's respirations, as he has decreased respiratory functions; ascites causes pressure on the diaphragm, which may be further aggravated by anxiety and crying. If there is a long delay in obtaining the specimen, the child may benefit by a rest period in the upright position.

At one time it was common practice to place the child's legs in a froglike position and draw blood samples from the femoral arteries which are easier to locate. There is now evidence that indicates that arterial thrombosis can result from using this site, resulting in circulatory failure and eventual amputation. This outcome may have been partly due to the steroid therapy, which is known to cause hypercoagulability, but the serious nature of the complication has significantly decreased the use of the area. If this route is necessary, the nurse must be sure to apply pressure after the sample is obtained to stop the bleeding. A small dressing is then applied with nonallergic tape. The site must be checked periodically to be sure bleeding does not reoccur after the child is moved back to his room.

Early signs of thrombosis include nausea, vomiting, or pain in the groin or leg. There can also be decreased femoral, dorsalis pedis, and posterior tibial pulses. As the condition progresses, the leg becomes cool to the touch and the pulse becomes weaker. If surgical intervention is necessary, the child is usually placed on anticoagulants postoperatively.

Medication Therapy. As already alluded to in the foregoing sections, a common therapy is to administer one of the forms of corticosteroid presently available. The dosage and schedule for this drug vary according to the child's age and weight, and the physician's choice. It is generally accepted that long-term therapy assures longer remission than short-term therapy.

The child may or may not be receiving diuretics. Diuretics seem to have limited value but are sometimes tried in an attempt to decrease the edema and make the child more comfortable.

During the period when rapid diuresis takes place, it may be necessary to place the child on potassium therapy, because the rapid loss of sodium causes the potassium to leave the cell; it enters the circulation and is lost by excretion. Replacement may be achieved by potassium medication or by providing more potassium in the diet. A common dietary supplement is orange juice or cranberry juice, which children usually accept readily. If the potassium remains in the circulatory system, the nurse should be alert for signs of hyperkalemia and refrain from offering high potassium fluids.

Newer additions to the drugs prescribed for children with nephrosis include the immunosuppressive agents. Presently the alkalizing agents and purine antimetabolites (referred to in the therapy of children with cancer) are being tried in some agencies. This more dramatic therapy is generally reserved for children who seem resistant to steroid therapy. The principles involved are similar to earlier attempts at using nitrogen mustard in treatment of children with nephrosis.

Other therapies, such as the administration of salt-poor albumin and the use of exchange resins, seem to be used with decreasing frequency due to the high costs of the therapy and the lack of long-lasting effects.

Antihypertensive drugs are included when the blood pressure is elevated. Antibiotic therapy has already been explained. Anemia may be treated by iron supplements or, if severe, a transfusion of packed cells.

Other medications will depend on the individual child's symptomatology. The nursing intervention again plays a big role in helping the child to accept and tolerate large and frequent doses of medication. The follow-up care is dependent on the mother and the child fully understanding and appreciating the value of the medication. One older child stated that the nurse only said to take the pills. He could not appreciate the value of the medication based on such a limited explanation. It was not until he refused to take the medication, resulting in an exacerbation, that he could appreciate the true value of the medicine. Children and parents should not need to go through this biologic and financial crisis to appreciate prescribed therapy. Prior to the discharge, the action and reasons for medication should be explained to the family. The use of a diagram of the kidney may help in this explanation. An explanation of medications will also provide them with an opportunity again to discuss and clarify their feelings and knowledge about the disease.

McCrorey et al (1975), studying mortality rates in New York City, found that there has been a decrease in mortality due to nephrosis-nephritis, in the last two decades. They note that the decrease may be due to a milder course of the disease, which they point out is not unlike other childhood diseases associated with the streptococcal organism. However, they also note that children were also considered candidates for dialysis and transplantation during the study period and that these procedures could also be responsible for the declining mortality rates.

Uremia or Renal Failure

Uremia or renal failure is a very serious sequelae of kidney conditions. It may result after a long series of infections or disease processes such as chronic pyelonephritis or intermittent nephrotic syndrome, or it may be the result of an acute condition such as a traumatic injury or toxic ingestion. The uremia may be poorly tolerated by the child if it is sudden and grave, or it may seem to be better tolerated if it develops over a slow gradual course.

Uremia results when the kidney is no longer able to excrete end products of metabolism, the most notable of which are urea and creatinine (by-products of protein). In addition, the kidney may not be able to free the bloodstream of other organic acids such as indoles, phenols, and similar toxic substances.

The symptoms exhibited by the child will not be solely attributed to nitrogen retention. They are most likely the result of a combination of nitrogen retention and fluid and electrolyte imbalances. For example, if a child has frequent bleeding gums or epistaxis it may not be merely the result of nitrogen retention. This hemorrhagic tendency is probably linked to a coagulation problem, a prolonged bleeding time, changes in capillary resistance, or it may be related to starvation. Proper attention to the child's dietary intake may lessen or correct the condition.

Other symptoms that are attributed to nitrogen retention and/or fluid and electrolyte changes include gastrointestinal symptoms: anorexia, vomiting, intermittent diarrhea, and abdominal pain. The mouth may have a "urinary odor," there may be increased salivation, and stomatitis or parotitis may develop. In advanced stages, the skin may have "uremic frost"—white crystal accumulation around the face, forehead, base of the hair, neck, and chest. Or the skin may just be "itchy." The child may be cold due to direct action of the nitrogenous wastes on his nervous system, which interferes with temperature control. The color of the skin is usually sallow, with the face and palms of the hands sometimes appearing darker. This sallowness is probably related to the anemia which is usually present in uremia.

Nursing measures will be directed at making the child as comfortable as possible during the time close medical supervision is being carried out. Depending on the medical regimen, the child may have to tolerate periods with very little fluid intake or diets restricted in protein. He may have numerous blood tests as it is imperative to monitor his electrolytes carefully, especially if exchange resins are being utilized, or there is a period of oliguria, or rapid diuresis. Intake and output, skin care, and mouth care have already been discussed in the chapter and are mentioned again because of their importance to this acutely ill child's comfort.

Two of the major electrolytes involved in kidney failure are sodium and potassium. As the kidney becomes unable to retain sodium, it is excreted in serious proportions causing a hyponatremia. The kidney develops an inability to excrete potassium and this results in an increase in potassium in the circulatory system (hyperkalemia). An increase of circulating potassium can cause irritability to the myocardium which is easily monitored by an electrocardiograph tracing (see Chapter 12 for more details on EKG).

In addition, acidosis can result as the renal tubules fail to excrete hydrogen ions ($H+$) and regenerate bicarbonate ions (HCO_3-). This is further hindered by impairment of nitrogen secretion, which reduces the buffer capacity of the urine and further limits the secretion of hydrogen ions. Phosphate filtration is also reduced further, minimizing the buffer capacity of the tubular fluid. The resulting acidosis is reflected in the lowering of the blood carbon dioxide (CO_2) and the blood pH (Creditor and Statland, 1963).

The phosphate elevation causes a reciprocal reduction in blood calcium by urinary excretion. This reduced blood calcium is responsible for the related symptoms of muscular twitching and weakness.

Treatment. Treatment of uremia or kidney failure must include consideration of the causation as well as the uremia itself. If the uremia was sudden, an attempt may first be made to establish urinary flow by administering a large amount of intravenous fluid in a comparatively short amount of time. The nurse must observe the child closely for signs of fluid overload during this procedure. If urinary flow is not established, then a more serious condition exists and fluids will be given with great caution. It is very important not to overload the child's circulatory system with fluids (hypervolemia). Consideration is given for insensible fluid loss via the skin and respiratory routes and modifications made when other fluid losses result from vomiting or diarrhea. However, the major way a child regulates his fluid is by way of the kidneys, and when there is impairment in kidney function the child can easily become seriously edematous. This edema can result in pulmonary edema and death if the necessary precautions are not taken.

An attempt might also be made to have some of the electrolyte changes altered by use of exchange resins. These agents can be administered orally or rectally. The resins work to exchange potassium ions for ammonium or sodium ions. If the resin therapy is successful there will be a decrease in the hyperkalemia. This decrease will be noted in a slowing of the pulse and a return to a regular beat.

The rectal instillation of resins is similar to any rectal instillation. The resins are mixed with a specific amount of water and instilled by gravity using a rectal tube and funnel or cannister attachment. The child is encouraged to breathe deeply through his mouth during the instillation and the fluid is administered slowly so that it does not stimulate a quick evacuation. To be most effective, the solution must be retained a sufficient amount of time for the potassium exchange to take place. If the solution is not expelled after two hours, a rectal tube may be inserted or a small enema administered to start the evacuation. The fluid returned should be subtracted from the original amount of the instillation to determine the amount of fluid retained, if any. This retained fluid will be used by the physician in adjusting the child's intake. This is the safest method of dialysis in present use.

Diet. The dietary regimen for children with renal failure is a controversial area. The opinions vary from little restriction in diet because it interferes with the child's growth (Edelmann and Bunstein, 1968) to ones that recommend very specific and stringent dietary restrictions by using a carbohydrate-fat diet (high caloric) with restriction of proteins and potassium

(Hamburger et al, 1969). The amount of restriction depends on the degree of renal insufficiency present. In addition to protein restrictions, water and sodium are also prescribed cautiously. Water is usually given in sufficient amounts to achieve adequate urinary output. Care must be taken not to cause excessive excretions which will force sodium excretion in large amounts. Salt may need to be added to the diet, but in cases with cardiac involvement salt should be restricted. The child on a restricted diet is usually given supplementary vitamins as a protein-free or restricted diet is poor in vitamins.

With these general ideas as to dietary treatment, the nurse can readily see that her/his role in the care of these children will be intertwined with the role of the dietician. Working effectively together, they may help to prevent refusal of food, dehydration, or the necessity for alternate routes of intake such as tube feedings or intravenous therapy.

Peritoneal Dialysis. Peritoneal dialysis is a procedure utilized in children with severe kidney damage or impending renal failure. In this procedure, dialysis is performed by using the peritoneum as the dialyzing membrane. In exchange resin therapy the intestine was used as the dialyzing membrane. The principle is the same: a sterile solution of electrolytes is introduced into the abdominal cavity and waste products are removed from the body by osmosis. The peritoneum acts as a semipermeable membrane similar to the nephrons in a normal kidney. Approximately a liter of fluid is introduced through a catheter inserted into the child's abdomen. The solution utilized is similar to extracellular fluid but it lacks potassium and it contains dextrose. Potassium and other waste products diffuse through the peritoneum in an attempt to equalize the solution on both sides of the membrane. The dextrose makes the solution of sufficient osmolarity to prevent absorption of the dialyzing fluid into the blood. After the solution is introduced it is allowed to remain in the abdomen for a period of approximately 30 minutes. The fluid is then allowed to drain out by gravity into a sterile bottle (Fig. 1A and B).

While the procedure seems very simple, it is not without dangers. It has certainly made dialysis available to more persons than was possible when only the artificial kidney (hemodialysis) was available.

According to Boen (1964, pp 69–71), the following are some of the major advantages of peritoneal dialysis compared with the artificial kidney:

1. Simpler equipment makes it available in nearly every hospital.
2. Abrupt changes in blood volume can be avoided.
3. There is ample opportunity to change the composition of the irrigating fluid. It is therefore possible to avoid an insufficient or excessive correction of disturbances in electrolyte or water balance.
4. It can be used after surgery or with patients with bleeding tendency.
5. When increased protein breakdown is evident, peritoneal dialysis can be used longer.

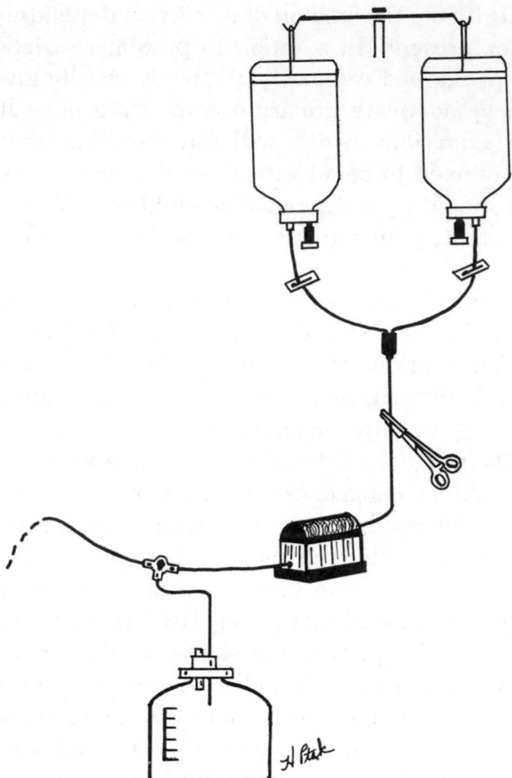

FIG. 1A. Equipment for peritoneal dialysis.

The major disadvantages to peritoneal dialysis cited by Boen (pp 69–71) include the following:

1. Water is removed more slowly by this procedure.
2. Infection is a possibility.
3. The intestine can be perforated during introduction of trocar.
4. A loss of about 40 gm of protein may occur.
5. Abdominal pain and discomfort may occur.
6. Not able to use where abdominal injury is present or with severe peritonitis.
7. Sterile irrigation fluids are necessary with peritoneal dialysis but not with the artificial kidney.

A closer look is now needed at some of the disadvantages and their implications for nursing. The first disadvantage relates to water excretion. The nurse must remember that the child can have respiratory distress due to the pressure of the solution on the diaphragm. She/he must also help the child to relax so that this increase in fluid does not cause undue abdominal discomfort. Preparation for the "full feeling" will help the child understand what is happening and lessen his fears.

The second disadvantage is danger of infection. This danger can be minimized by keeping the dressing and area around the catheter as clean and dry as possible. Periodic cleansing with antiseptic solution and application of sterile dressings under aseptic technique will lessen the possibility of infection. When new solutions are added, they must be accomplished under aseptic conditions and any medications, such as heparin or antibiotics, must be added with care.

The child should also be kept away from other children or adults with infections, as their resistance to infection is poor. If members of the health team or family are not feeling as well as usual, they should not visit the child until all doubt of illness is erased.

The disadvantage of loss of protein is especially significant as it further adds to the malnutrition and wasting prevalent in these children. It is especially important to have the child eat, as the child's anorexia improves due to

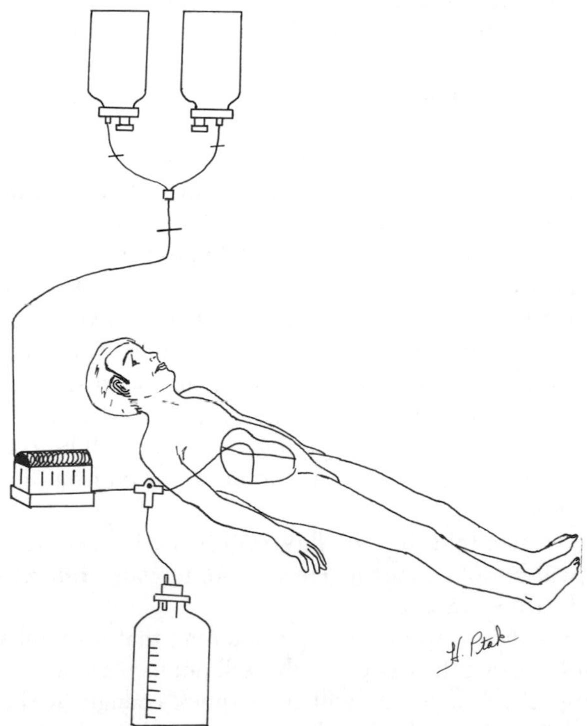

FIG. 1B. Schematic drawing illustrating intermittent peritoneal dialysis in use.

the removal of waste products. It is also common to have the child's disposition improve with dialysis and he may be more eager to choose foods and liquids that he has refused on other occasions.

Preparation of the Child for Dialysis. The child is prepared for peritoneal dialysis either before he is taken to the treatment or minor surgery area, or in the area before the procedure is started. He is asked to void the bladder. Sometimes the child is catheterized. A sketch of the dialysis set-up is useful in preparation as the child may get very confused by just an explanation (Fig. 1A). The child is asked to lie in a recumbent position with his pajama bottoms removed and his pajama top pulled up above the nipple line. The child is asked to lie with his arms up under his head or tucked under his buttocks on each side. This will help to keep his hands restrained without too much adult help. (The child is usually premedicated before coming to the area and this aids in limiting discomfort.)

The child is then told about the abdominal preparation, the cool antiseptic solution, and the sterile drape. He is told he will feel a prick of a needle which is special medicine for putting the skin to sleep so it will not feel any more pain. The nurse offers her/his hand for the child to squeeze and indicates it is OK to cry if he wants to. He is encouraged not to move as the covers will slip off and wiggling also interferes with the doctor's work. His cooperation is stressed as being a real asset to completing the procedure.

The physician then injects xylocaine (or similar substance) and prepares the area for the incision and introduction of the trocar. The child is then told he will feel pressure on his "tummy" or abdomen but it will not hurt. During the insertion the conversation can center on topics of interest to the child as he is prepared for the immediate procedure. If he cringes or wiggles, refocus on the procedure and make a supporting statement such as, "You are doing nicely, try to lie still, the doctor is almost through with this part."

After the catheter is inserted, a trial for proper functioning, considering patient comfort, is done by using 200–300 cc's of fluid. The child is prepared for the "full feeling" and observed for any overt or covert signs of discomfort. The catheter is either sutured or taped in place and a dressing applied. The child is told the procedure is just about over and he will be returned to his room as soon as the drape is taken off and he is moved from the table to his bed or a stretcher.

The child is then told that the fluid will be exchanged periodically and each time he will be told about it. He will not feel any different than when the doctor did it this time.

The nurse is then responsible for explaining that his vital signs will be taken frequently during the dialysis so he will not be alarmed. It is necessary to keep a close check as there will be a quick change in the electrolyte composition and too rapid fluid exchange can result in shock.

Nursing responsibilities will also include warming the solution before hanging a new bottle. A solution at body temperature is less likely to cause discomfort than a cold solution. She/he will also keep a very accurate intake and output (see Table 3). If the child retains the fluid, he may be turned carefully to aid the gravity drainage (the child is usually in a supine position with his head elevated approximately 45° during the dialysis). Care is also needed to prevent breakdown of debilitated skin (as was discussed earlier in this chapter). The tubing must also be kept free of kinks to provide adequate drainage and it must be observed for small clots or waste material which may interfere with flow. If flow cannot be reestablished by "milking the tube gently," the doctor should be notified. Heparin is sometimes ordered to decrease the clot formation or the physician may need to move the catheter to a better position. Coughing and deep breathing should be encouraged to decrease the possibility of pneumonia developing.

There are several signs which signal distress. Increased respirations may indicate that too much fluid is being administered for this particular child. Occasionally a child complains of shoulder pain, which is probably due to the same cause. Abdominal pain may be a sign of peritonitis or infection. Diarrhea is a common side effect of dialysis. A deterioration in the child's mental state may be related to the electrolyte exchange. All of these signs should be reported to the physician and recorded accurately.

After the dialysis is completed the catheter is removed and a small sterile dressing is applied over the incision. Intermittent dialysis is usually done by a new paracentesis puncture and new catheter. Using a new set-up each time seems to cut down the risk of infection. It does present a new stress situation to the child each time, however. Usually the child cries when he knows it must be done again, but that is the extent of his resistance. He seems quickly to equate the dialysis with an increase in well-being.

Medications. When a child is in renal failure it is necessary to monitor medication therapy much more cautiously. Many drugs are normally excreted by the kidneys and without normal renal function there may be toxic levels built up in the blood. A drug which is greatly affected is digitalis. Both digitalization and maintenance requirements are decreased when kidney failure is present. Several of the antibiotics also fall into this grouping; examples are streptomycin, kanamycin, and tetracycline (Schwartz and Dunea, 1967).

Some agencies do cultures on the first and last solution of the child's dialysis and order antibiotics if indicated. These antibiotics are sometimes added to the dialysis solution.

Medication given the child in renal failure is principally concerned with the underlying cause or with symptomatology. Therefore, if the child has tetany, calcium may be given; if there is cardiac involvement, digitalis de-

TABLE 3
Record of Peritoneal Dialysis Therapy

JOHN J.	AGE 12	AUG. 31, 1976		
Solution	**Medications**	**Solution In**		
		Start	End	Volume
Inpersol 1.5%	Added Heparin 0.5 cc	12:00	12:20	300

Solution Out			Differential
Start	End	Volume	
1:20	1:40	275	+25

rivatives and barbiturates; and if there is pneumonia, antibiotics. At present there is no drug which can satisfactorily treat nitrogen retention (Hamburger et al, 1969).

Hemodialysis. The use of the artificial kidney is to circulate the child's blood through a semipermeable membrane in order to draw metabolic waste materials and toxins from the blood. Raffensperger, Ferlit, and Fochtmen (1976), describe the procedure in this way: the child's arterial blood is fed into the artificial kidney machine and his dialyzed blood is returned to his body by use of a venous site. The child may have new incisions done for each treatment or he may have indwelling cannulas. The sites of the cannula insertions must be thoroughly prepared and kept clean and free of contamination. The dialysis is usually done three times a week.

The hemodialysis may be viewed by the parents as the "cure" for their child's disease. However, the child is frequently in the advanced stages of his disease before the treatment is chosen and a "cure" is highly unlikely.

The special attention surrounding the treatment, often on a special unit—with complicated-looking equipment, special nurses, medical experts, and a variety of persons in training—and the media reports of the need for additional kidney machines and the extreme financial burdens imposed on the family, certainly a reality, all combine to place a great deal of stress on the family that is chosen to receive this medical intervention for their child.

Raimbault and deRecherches (1973) suggest that the young child is unable to integrate the idea that the artificial kidney is essential to his life space. Due to this inability, he needs an adult at his side during treatments to lessen his fears of abandonment and alienation. They suggest that older children display their inability to assimilate the value of the treatments by outbursts of aggression, anger, and negativism. They also may act indifferently toward people with whom they must interact. The authors suggest that the child is searching for someone to help him integrate a "nonsymbolizable situation" through these covert responses (Raimbault and deRecherches, p 69).

This response situation is illustrated in the following case presentation.

Charles was six years old when his kidney condition demanded treatment with hemodialysis. It was necessary to transport him to another hospital for the treatment. At the hospital responsible for his primary care, he was responsive and friendly. He interacted effectively with the staff and he was able to maintain his composure when faced with treatments such as blood work and large doses of medication. He was able to cry when it was painful and verbally express his dissatisfaction at being interrupted to take medications. He readily returned to other activities and played with other children after his brief interruptions.

His behavior was much different at the second hospital. He refused to respond to the nurse or physicians when they greeted him, he turned his head towards the wall to avoid eye contact, and he screamed uncontrollably during initiation of the treatment, frequently requiring physical restraint to hold him in position.

The unfortunate part of this interaction was that the professional personnel reciprocated by becoming less responsive to him and their attitudes were easily reflected in their delivery of service.

To attempt to interrupt this mutually negative interaction, a nurse from the primary hospital took the responsibility for working with Charlie and his mother to make the hemodialysis treatments more tolerable. The nurse had Charlie draw pictures of the dialysis unit and helped him to express his anger in a more appropriate way, using puppets and toys. His pictures were filled with death symbols. He had airplanes crashing into walls and boats sinking. His mother was helped to tolerate his outbursts so she could feel comfortable sitting with him throughout the treatment without feeling embarrassed by his behavior. She was told that Charlie's response was not uncommon and that her presence would eventually help to decrease his fears of the treatment. She was encouraged to talk to him about the need for the treatments and to keep reinforcing the fact that the treatment could not be done at his primary hospital and so the transporting was necessary. It was important to have the child know the treatments were not punishment.

Charlie's outbursts became less intense, but he did not learn to respond to the personnel in the same way he had responded to health professionals previously.

If the child has indwelling cannulas the mother is encouraged to observe the dressing for oozing. Following strenous activity, it is common for a watery or pink-tinged drainage to appear. The dressing will be changed cautiously by a health professional to decrease the possibility of infection. If a site becomes infected, it cannot be reused for future cannula insertions. The infected part should be immobilized to try to localize the infection. Sometimes heat is applied to the infection site to help hasten the drainage and to provide comfort.

The cannula site must be protected during bathing. If the site (usually wrist or leg) cannot be protected from getting wet during the usual bathing procedure, then the mother will need to have assistance to help modify her bathing techniques. In addition, it may be helpful to put a plastic cover over the dressing to give added protection in case the child splashes unexpectedly.

A set of cannula clamps is kept in a readily accessible place. This is essential as a shunt can become separated, causing the child to bleed profusely. Each cannula tubing needs to be clamped immediately if this should happen. The connection should be reestablished as soon as possible.

Another aspect of the long-term management of these children is the dietary management. The mother will need the support of a dietician to help plan menus that will foster normal growth but limit protein, sodium, potassium, and fluid. The restrictions will be specifically ordered by the physician. Creativity will be needed to have a diet attractive enough to satisfy the child.

KIDNEY TRANSPLANTATION

The use of transplanted kidneys in the human is generally reserved for patients with irreversible renal damage. Successful transplants were first done between identical twins and are now successful between less closely related individuals because of tissue cross-catching and the use of immunosuppressive drugs. Early transplants used total body irradiation prior to surgery to decrease the possibility of rejection. This procedure is in less use now, since drugs such as imuron have proved effective. Total body irradiation is especially serious to children as it will interfere with future growth.

Obtaining satisfactory kidneys for transplantation is not a simple process. A living donor has to undergo major surgery without being promised any definite results for the recipient. A kidney from a cadaver must be selected very carefully to be sure it is healthy, and obtaining kidneys must be done after the person is officially pronounced dead. Obtaining kidneys raises many ethical issues and makes it more difficult to provide the organ necessary to try to prolong another's life.

While the child is waiting for a compatible kidney, he is maintained on intermittent peritoneal dialysis or hemodialysis. Between dialyses, the child is usually permitted to be discharged.

When a living donor is found, the child and donor are admitted to the hospital for more extensive blood work and kidney function tests, including arteriograms. If the donor is found compatible, both the donor and the child are scheduled for major surgery. The child is started on chemotherapy approximately a week before surgery. The donor may be discharged until the day before surgery. If the child is severely debilitated, transfusions may be indicated preoperatively. On the day of surgery, each patient will have his own surgical team responsible for his care. The donor kidney is removed and refrigerated (cooling to 4 C is achieved by immersing the kidney in cold saline solution for five minutes or direct perfusion of the kidney with a special solution cooled to 4 C). The cooling process prepares the kidney for prolonged ischemia without causing functional defects. The recipient is prepared to receive the donor kidney. The usual site for the kidney is the right iliac fossa (Fig. 2). The kidney is turned over so that its posterior side is anterior to make it easier to anastomose the renal vein to the external iliac vein and the renal artery to the hypogastric artery. The ureter is either anastomosed to the recipient's ureter at the kidney pelvis or directly into his bladder.

In some instances, the kidneys (bilateral nephrectomies) are removed approximately a month prior to surgery and the child is maintained on

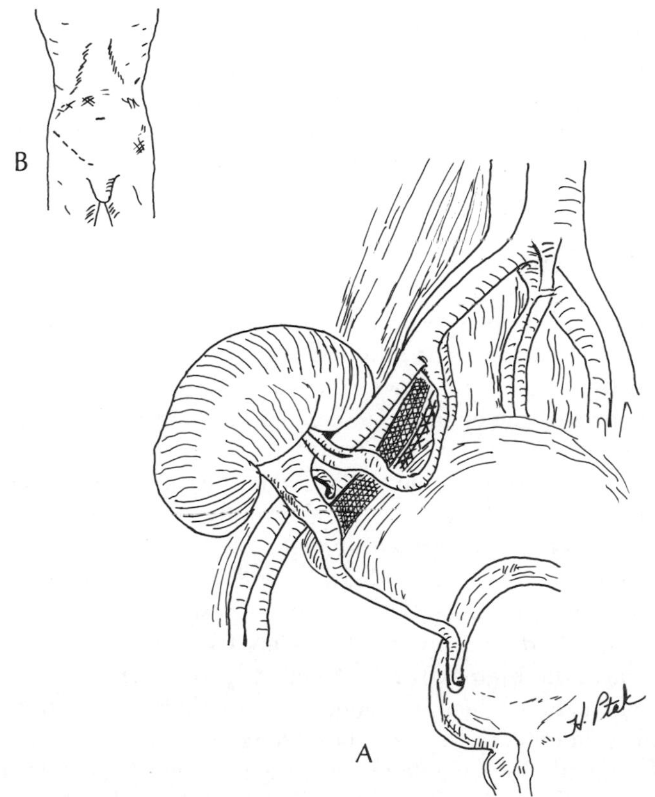

FIG. 2A. Kidney transplant. The new kidney is placed into the recipient's iliac fossa opposite the side from which it was taken. **B.** Incision site.

dialysis. This gives the child an opportunity to recover from major surgery before being subjected to the transplant.

In other instances, the surgeons prefer to remove the recipient's diseased kidney(s) and/or spleen at the time of transplantation. Mention is also being made of correction of urinary tract defects in combination with transplants. An example of such a repair would be a YV plasty. If these procedures are done, the child will probably have a more difficult postoperative course due to the more extensive surgery involved.

The spleen is considered to play a role in the rejection process, but many surgeons now believe its removal has not significantly reduced the possibilities of rejection and are not routinely removing the organ. The removal of the kidney(s) is based on the theory that the diseased kidneys can play a major role in postoperative infection. Each child will be considered individually for the best possible course of action.

It is also important to keep in mind that as the recipient surgical team is preparing the child to receive the kidney, they may decide that the child's possibilities of accepting the donor kidney are too slim and the surgery will not proceed. In this case, the donor surgical team is notified not to proceed with removal of the kidney. A reason for cancellation of the surgery would be severe cardiac failure in the child. Frequent communication takes place between the two surgical teams during the procedure to insure both patients the best possible care and consideration.

Postoperative Care

The child will be placed on reverse isolation because his resistance to infection is very low due to the immunosuppressive drug therapy. It is best if one nurse cares for the child during the early postoperative period. This will help to cut down on infection and also guarantee continual monitoring of the child's condition.

Immediately postoperatively, the kidney usually excretes adequate to large amounts of urine. This can make the family extremely optimistic, even if they have been told this is the expected outcome. The urine excretion has its darker side also; it is a hazard because with the excretion come resultant fluid and electrolyte changes. These changes pose a threat to the child's life and must be watched carefully. Vital signs are taken every 15 minutes during this early stage; the temperature is taken at least hourly. The child usually has a nasogastric tube which is connected to gentle intermittent suction. If a catheter or catheters are in place they are connected to drainage. Urine is checked frequently for specific gravity, sugar, acetone, protein, and color. The physician will usually leave specific directions for calling him/her regarding the results. For instance, if urine has +2 acetone, notify the physician. In addition, there will be specific orders regarding regulation of intravenous fluids. They will be given in accordance with the previous hour's urine output. In addition, intravenous flow is regulated to take into consideration nasogastric drainage, usually every four hours. Weights are also taken and may influence the intravenous intake.

After the period of diuresis the child's urine output will stabilize and a period of good renal function will exist. This quiescent period is usually followed by a period termed "rejection crisis." This attempt at rejection is signaled by scanty output, proteinuria, elevated temperature, weight gain, hypertension, or uremia. Immunosuppressive drugs are given to counteract the rejection; commonly used agents are imuran, prednisone, actinonycin C, and antilymphocytic globulin (ALG). In addition, local irradiation to the site may be tried. Peritoneal dialysis may be instituted if anuria persists or the electrolyte imbalance is severe. The large doses of steroids may cause gastric irritation (ulcers) and an antacid may be given to counteract this response. Stools may be tested for guiac as a precautionary measure.

During this postoperative period, the child may feel increasingly better than he has felt in a long time. This improvement in affect is very encouraging to the parents as they breathlessly await the outcome of the transplant.

As soon as the nasogastric tube is taken out, usually on the first postoperative day if bowel sounds are present, the child is started on oral fluids. If these are tolerated he is progressed to a soft diet. Any diet restrictions will be based on symptoms, but generally the diet will be fairly free to encourage the child to eat and begin to rehabilitate himself.

During the entire time the child is hospitalized, his decreased ability to counteract infection must be considered. If isolation is dicontinued, the child should be kept away from obvious sources of infection. The parents should be made aware that they will need to take the same precautions when the child is discharged. Some agencies keep the child on strict isolation prior to surgery and until discharge, but this practice is decreasing in frequency as bacterial studies have shown that most of the bacteria present are actually related to the patient rather than to the clinical areas. Bacteria are most often found in the patient's mouth, nose, feces, or on the skin and can be treated effectively by taking cultures and having them assessed.

The child will continue taking medications after discharge, so the parents must have explicit directions regarding them. Refer to Table 4 for side effects of particular drugs to include in the parent teaching. In addition, the parents must be aware of signs and symptoms that necessitate medical intervention (Table 5). Late rejection crisis usually occurs between the third and twenty-sixth month after surgery. This wide variation in time makes it difficult to prepare the family for the situation.

After discharge, the child will be followed very closely on an out-patient basis. The parents must understand the value and rationale for this continued close supervision. In addition, they must be helped to begin to let the

TABLE 4
Immunosuppressive Medications*

NAME	SIDE EFFECTS
Imuran (azathioprine)	Bone marrow depression (leukopenia)
Prednisone	Rapid withdrawal may cause severe rejection in addition to adrenal insufficiency. Transient retention of salt and water Increased blood pressure May raise BUN Euphoria or emotional instability Increased appetite Diabetes mellitus Cushnoid conditions: a. purplish or reddish striae of skin b. development of supraclavicular fat pads c. abnormal growth of hair d. rounded contour of face Delayed healing Masking effect on infections
Actinomysin C	Irritations of mucus membranes
ALG (Anti-lymphocytic globulin)	Severe pain, fever, edema, and swelling at injection site Chest pain Muscle cramping Shortness of breath Flushing or cyanosis Nausea and vomiting

*Adapted from Bois M.S., et al: Nursing care of patients having kidney transplants. Am J Nurs 68:1245, June 1968.

child develop independence so that his additional years will be well spent.

While many cases have successful outcomes, it must be kept in mind that death is a very real threat postoperatively. Transplantation of kidneys has resulted in improved techniques but success cannot be guaranteed.

Psychologic Implications

The chance that a child facing imminent death might survive almost seems to make any risk worth taking. However, kidney transplant is still a big risk, as already explained. In addition, another healthy person may be taking a risk by donating his healthy kidney based on his present excellent

TABLE 5
Signs and Symptoms Heralding Complications in Kidney Transplant Patients*

SIGNS AND SYMPTOMS	CAUSES
Skin infections ("herpes")	Lower resistance of the body
Dysuria, frequency or burning on urination	Urinary tract infection
Hematuria	Urinary tract infection or homograft rejection
Oliguria or anuria	Inadequate fluid intake or homograft rejection (urinary tract obstruction)
Pain in the kidney site, or any abdominal pain	Homograft rejection or gastrointestinal complications
Lethargy	Homograft medication side effects, rejection, or electrolyte imbalance
Elevated temperature	Homograft rejection or infection
Joint pain	Medication side effect (steroids)
Rapid increase in weight	Excessive fluid or food intake, or decreased renal function
Nausea or vomiting	Infections, gastrointestinal complications
Vertigo; postural hypotension	Antihypertensive medications or electrolyte imbalance
Headache	Hypertension, medication side effects, excessive sodium in diet, central nervous system infections
Chest pains and respiratory difficulty	Pulmonary embolism, pneumonia, atelectasis, or cardiac complications
Change in bowel habits and in color or consistency of stools	Hepatitis, ulcers, hemorrhoids, fecal impaction, or bowel obstruction
Visual disturbances (blurring, dizziness)	Medication side effects (anthihypertensives, steroids) glaucoma, cataract

*From Bois MS et al: Nursing care of patients having kidney transplants. Am J Nurs 68:1243, June 1968.

health. Today's good health does not guarantee tomorrow's good health, as is well known. If a parent donates a kidney to his child, is it unreasonable for him to feel he has made a real sacrifice and expect a return for this sacrifice? If a relative donates the kidney, is it unusual for the parents to feel they owe him something? These are the very questions that make the psychologic implications of kidney transplant almost as great as the surgical ones.

Let me illustrate by a clinical example.

Susan was five years old when first brought to the hospital with severe kidney damage. Her mother also had kidney damage and even with this history, she did not seek medical attention for Susan until the child's disease was too far advanced.

Susan was treated with intermittent peritoneal dialysis but her condition continued to deteriorate. The parents were informed that Susan's only chance for survival was a kidney transplant, and this held only a slim margin of hope. Mrs. G. convinced her husband he should donate a kidney, if he was compatible. Mr. G. was not enthusiastic about the surgery but agreed after many conferences with the physician and social worker.

Postoperatively, Mr. G. was a model patient. It was difficult to believe he had major surgery. His recovery period was uneventful and he was discharged after a week. But Susan's body did not accept the kidney and after a period of peritoneal dialysis and conscientious care, she died.

During Susan's hospitalization, Mrs. G. derived a great deal of satisfaction from the nursing staff. She did not seem close to Mr. G. or able to communicate readily with him. She spent very little time visiting him after his surgery. The relationship seemed strained and one wonders about the implications of the child's death to this marriage. If the child had survived would the mother be closer to the father for his role in the recovery? With the death will she blame her husband because it was his kidney the child's body rejected? Did the mother have such extensive guilt for not seeking medical attention that she had to offer the child everything possible before she could face the child's death?

This situation illustrates the magnitude of the psychologic aspects related to kidney transplants and especially in relation to decisions which must be made for the child by an adult. With adult patients, some agencies use psychologic testing to help in determining whether a patient should be considered for a transplant. It is not this simple with young children as they seldom understand what is truly involved. Perhaps with further advancements in the field, the problems will be eased and the decisions easier to make.

CASE PRESENTATION AND STUDY QUESTIONS

Kevin is a six-year-old white male with a history of nephrosis probably beginning at seven months of age when his mother noticed intermittent puffy eyes and rhinorrhea. He was treated for allergy until a routine urinalysis (at two years of age) disclosed proteinuria. The patient is now admitted with +4 protein and a sedimentation rate of 103.

1. The +4 protein and sedimentation rate of 103 are significant. Explain.
2. Is there any connection between the "allergy" and the disease process nephrosis?
3. What other laboratory determinations will be done?
4. How will you prepare Kevin for these tests?

After a more extensive work-up Kevin was given a trial of steroids and diuretics.

5. Why were these drugs chosen and what is the expected outcome?
6. What are the side effects of these medications?
7. As a nurse, what are your responsibilities in relation to medications both while the child is hospitalized and in relation to home care?

Kevin does not respond to therapy and a renal biopsy is done. It shows proliferate glomerulonephritis with sclerosis of the vessels. It is decided to start Kevin on intermittent peritoneal dialysis.

8. How will you prepare Kevin and his family for this procedure?
9. What are the expected outcomes from the dialysis?
10. After dialysis is started, what are essential nursing functions?

You are responsible for making a nursing referral to the community health nurse.

11. What information will you include?
12. What feedback can you expect from the community health nurse to be used by the health team in the hospital?

BIBLIOGRAPHY

Boen ST: Peritoneal Dialysis in Clinical Medicine. Springfield, Ill, Thomas, 1964

Bois MS et al: Nursing care of patients having kidney transplants. Am J Nurs 68:1238, June 1968

Butt K et al: Transplantation in children. Dialysis and Transplantation 5:59, 1976

Chisholm CD: Dialysis for renal failure in children. S Afr Med J 1169, 1967

Creditor MC, Statland H: Kidney diseases. In Statland H (ed): Fluid and Electrolytes in Practice, 3rd ed. Philadelphia, Lippincott, 1963, Chap 16

Daeschner CW Jr: Evaluations of the child with hematuria. Hosp Med 1967, p 59

Downing SR: Nursing support in early renal failure. Am J Nurs 69:1212, June 1969

Eckstein H: Enuresis. In Williams DI (ed): Pediatric Urology. New York, Appleton, 1968

Edelman CM, Bernstein J: The kidneys and urinary tracts. In Barnett H (ed): Pediatrics, 14th ed. New York, Appleton, 1968, Chap 24

Feldman W et al: Intermittent peritoneal dialysis in the management of chronic renal failure in children. Am J Dis Child 116:30, 1968

Girdany BR: Vesicoureteral reflux and renal scarring. J Pediatr 86:998, 1975

Goldberg I: The diagnosis of pyelonephritis in childhood. Manitoba Med Rev 1967

Gutch CF, Stoner MH: Review of Hemodialysis for Nurses and Dialysis Personnel. St. Louis, Mosby, 1971

Hallman N, Norio R, Kouvalainen K: Main features of the congenital nephrotic syndrome. Acta Paediatr Scand (Suppl) 172:75–78, 1967

Hamburger J et al: Nephrology. Philadelphia, Saunders, 1969, Chaps 6, 7, 18, 58

Hopkins J, Armstrong S: Psychotherapy for adolescent dialysis patients. Dialysis and Transplantation 5:54, 1976

Jensen MM: Viruses and kidney disease. Am J Med 43:897–911, 1967

Juzwiak M: Nursing the kidney-transplant patient. RN 31:34–41, 1968

Kanter A, Nadler N, Vertel RM, Pollak VE: Peritoneal dialysis: indications and technique in the surgical patient. Surg Clin North Am 48:47, 1968

Kaye M, Comty C: Nutritional repletion during dialysis. Am J Clin Nutr 21:583–89, 1968

Keuhnelian J, Sanders V: Urologic Nursing. London, Macmillan, 1970

Kreider N, Curtiss JW: A case study of a chronic, progressive physical disability. J Rehabil 34:35–36, 1968

Krupp MA: Diagnosis of medial renal diseases. In Smith D (ed): General Urology. California, Lange Medical, 1966

Lewy PR, Belman AB: Familial occurrence of nonobstructive, noninfectious, vesicoureteral reflux with renal scarring. J Pediatr 86:851–56, 1975

MacGregor M, Freeman P: Subclassification of childhood urinary tract infections as an aid to prognosis. In O'Grady F, Brumfitt W (eds): Urinary Tract Infection. New York, Oxford University Press, 1968

Mandleco BH: Monitoring children's reactions when they are hospitalized for percutaneous renal biopsy. MCN 1:288–92, 1976

Martin AJ Jr: Renal transplantation: surgical technique and complications. Am J Nurs 68:1240–41, June 1968

McCrory WW, Shibuya M, Yano K et al: Recent trends in the mortality rate from renal disease in children and young adults in New York City. J Pediatr 87:928–32, 1975

O'Doherty N: Urinary tract infection in the neonatal period and later infancy. In O'Grady F, Brumfitt W (eds): Urinary Tract Infection. New York, Oxford University Press, 1968

Pande SR, Mehrotra TN, Gupta SC: Electrophoretic studies of the serum and urinary proteins in nephrotic syndrome. Indian J Med Sci 21:800–3, 1967

Parrish RA, Scurry RB, Robertson AF III et al: Recurrent arterial thrombosis in nephrosis. Am J Dis Child 130:428–29, 1976

Paul FM: The roentgenographic changes of the lung in acute nephritis in Singapore children. J Singapore Paediatr Soc 9:82, 1967

Raimbault G, deRecherches M: Psychological problems in the chronic nephropathies of childhood. In Anthony EJ, Koupernik C: The Child in His Family. New York, Wiley, 1973, p 65

Raffensperger JG et al: Nursing care of the child with genitourinary abnormalities. In Raffensberger JG, Fochtman D: Principles of Nursing Care of the Pediatric Surgery Patient, 2nd ed. Boston, Little, Brown, 1976

Rubin M: Disturbances of the kidney. In Nelson W (ed): Textbook of Pediatrics, Philadelphia, Saunders, 1964

Rusnac C, Puskas G, Abraham A, Sabau M: Contributions to the problem of the viral aetiology of certain acute nephrites in children. Rom Med Rev 12:23, 1968

Samler LP: Clinical and immunological aspects of glomerular disease in children. Am Med Wom Assoc 22:743–50, 1967

Sato FF: New devices for continuous urine collection in pediatrics. Am J Nurs 69:804–5, April 1969

Scott JE: Urinary infection. In Williams DI (ed): Paediatric Urology. New York, Appleton, 1968

Smallpiece V: Urinary Tract Infection in Childhood and its Relevance to Disease in Adult Life. St Louis, Mosby, 1968

Soyka LF: The nephrotic syndrome: current concepts in diagnosis and therapy advantages of alternate day steroid regimen. Clin Pediatr 6:77–82, 1967

Schwartz FD, Dunea G: Acute renal failure. Med Times 95:1287–94, 1967

Watkins FL: The patient who has peritoneal dialysis. Am J Nurs 66:1572–77, July 1966
Williams DI: Paediatric Urology. New York, Appleton, 1968
Winter C, Roehm M: Sawyer's Nursing Care of Patients with Urologic Diseases. St. Louis, Mosby, 1968
———: Practical Urology. St. Louis, Mosby, 1969

MARY NORMA O'HARA

7

Nursing Care of the Child with Respiratory Problems

The respiratory problems described in this chapter were selected because of the long-term nature of the entity and the implications for nursing management. Allergy, with special emphasis on asthma, as well as bronchiolitis, tuberculosis, and cystic fibrosis are included.

The majority of these disorders will most likely require hospitalization at least once during the course of the disease. Some will require frequent visits to the clinic or physician's office. Regardless of the setting, all of these illnesses will require knowledge on the part of the nurse in relation to the disease process, significant observations for assessment and planning of care, instruction for the child and family, and evaluation of the plan for management.

In the mid-1960s, one of the major causes of early infant death was the respiratory distress syndrome. Respiratory disease was not a common cause of mortality in preschool and school-age children. Accurate statistics on morbidity are more difficult to find. The National Institutes of Health provides a picture of those illnesses which are more common in childhood and which tend to interfere with the child's normal activities. The majority of these conditions are a result of injuries or acute infectious diseases and respond to appropriate medical treatment. A significant number, on the other hand, are chronic in nature and require highly specialized care.

It is imperative from our knowledge of the effect of hospitalization on the child and family, as well as from an economic standpoint, that every effort be made to prevent complications when possible and to provide intensive care measures so that early discharge is possible.

The average number of days a child is hospitalized has declined rapidly in the past several years, but the number of children receiving care on an ambulatory basis has rapidly increased. It is vital that planning for discharge as well as patient-family teaching begin early in the hospitalization so that early discharge does not require readmission due to poor preparation.

In discussing long-term or chronic illness, the fact that they persist may be the only commonality. Some disorders are irreversible, while others may be transitory and respond to a therapeutic regimen. Some of these conditions may have their onset in infancy; others appear in early or late childhood. For example, cystic fibrosis, which causes severe respiratory problems in many instances, may be diagnosed in the newborn period through meconium ileus. Asthma may have its onset in infancy or in childhood.

Cultural and social factors must be considered. We should also examine attitudes of nursing personnel toward children with chronic disease. Caring for children with long-term problems can contribute to professional development not only in terms of learning nursing management but also in increasing one's depth of knowledge and clinical skills. The goals for treatment are different in a long-term respiratory problem from those in acute illness. Rewards are not attained so readily. The nurse must realize her/his limitation—as should other members of the health team. The combined efforts of the physician, nurse, physical therapist, occupational therapist, and social worker in complex cases will be necessary to attain the goals established.

BRONCHIOLITIS

One of the early respiratory problems affecting infants under 18 months is acute or capillary bronchiolitis. Usually occurring in winter or early spring, it is the main lower respiratory tract disease requiring hospitalization of infants and is considered to be primarily a viral illness. The symptoms are similar to asthmatic bronchitis, ie, wheezing, dyspnea, and cough. In addition, lethargy, cyanosis, and sternal retractions are present. There is no definitive evidence to date that the infant with bronchiolitis will or will not develop asthma in later years.

The concern in dealing with respiratory problems in infants is related to the size of various tubular structures of the respiratory passages. The small bronchioles are vulnerable to obstruction due to inflammation of mucosa, edema of the bronchiolar walls, and obstruction of the lumen with mucus and cellular debris. As a result of the widespread airway obstruction, hypoxemia occurs. Because the size of the airways is greater during inspiration than expiration, air is trapped in alveoli resulting in emphysema. The major problem is with the egress of air (Fig. 1).

The chest becomes overinflated and appears barrel-shaped and the chest wall retracts with each inspiration. Upon auscultation widespread fine rales are usually found occurring on both inspiration and expiration. If air entry is very poor no adventitious sounds may be heard. The liver and spleen may be palpable below the costal margins because of emphysema which depresses the diaphragm.

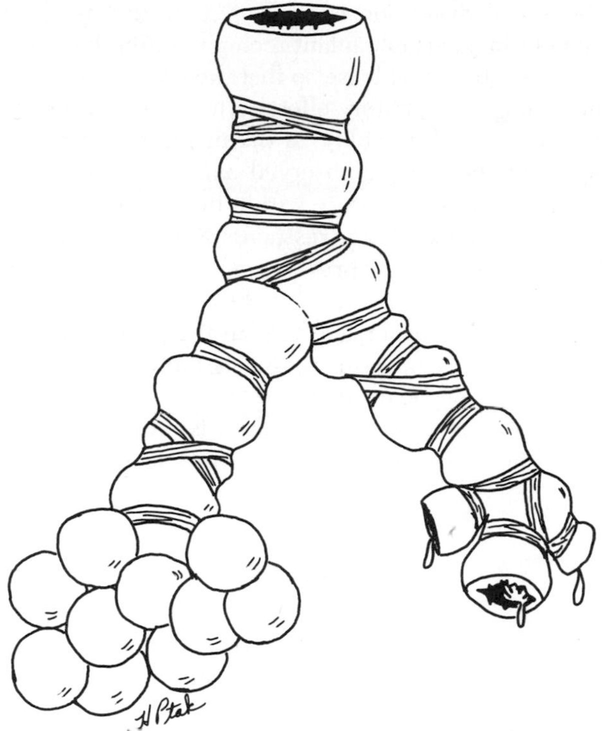

FIG. 1. Normal bronchiole and constriction of air passages during bronchospasm.

Clinical Example

John G., five months of age was admitted with rapid, shallow respirations and tachycardia. During inspiration the suprasternal notch and intercostal spaces and ribs retracted. A "hacky" cough could be heard frequently. Fever was absent. He was cyanotic, irritable and restless—appearing to devote all his energy to breathing. Only a feeble attempt was made to respond when a toy was presented to him. His mother reported that he had not slept and that she had experienced difficulty in feeding him during the past 24 hours. Dehydration and exhaustion were evident.

Therapeutic measures—which were intensive and life-saving-—included administration of oxygen and humidity in a mist tent and correction of dehydration with parenteral therapy. Blood gases were monitored. Since no evidence of secondary bacterial infection was noted, antibiotics were not prescribed during his hospitalization. Vital signs were monitored carefully. Oral feedings were instituted when respiratory distress subsided. Close observation and surveillance were most important. John's response to therapy was dramatic and he returned home to his family five days after admission.

When abdominal distention is present, elevation of the head of the infant or placement in a portable infant recliner within the mist tent may be beneficial. The shirt should be loose so that the chest can easily be exposed to observe and evaluate respiratory efforts. The nurse must assess the effectiveness of the oxygen and humidity. If the mist tent is functioning improperly, the increased restlessness observed may occur as a result of lack of oxygen and/or increased temperature within the tent rather than a progression of the disease process. When restraints are indicated for any reason, care should be taken to avoid any pressure on the chest or abdomen that will aggravate respiratory effort.

Personnel should be encouraged to plan the administration of medications, fluids, and comforting measures, during the acute stage, to guarantee that the child does not become exhausted.

The mortality rate is usually very low. It is, however, common to find that a child with chronic respiratory disease had severe bronchiolitis as an infant.

ASTHMA

Allergy is listed as one of the major chronic illnesses experienced by children today. It has been stated that over five million Americans suffer from asthma and approximately three-fifths of these people are children. Many children are often susceptible to infections. Absence from school may occur in the first or second week of the new term due to sudden exposure to nose and throat infections of classmates. In surveys which include chronic conditions causing days lost from school, asthma is often the single chronic condition causing the highest percentage of days lost. Since asthma is a long-term problem, the importance of early diagnosis and effective management is important in order to avoid complications of this chronic disease. Fontana (1969) believes that "the term asthma should only be applied to allergic reaction producing dyspnea, wheezing, and coughing and not for the nonallergic bronchial lesions producing similar respiratory symptoms. . . . Asthma is a disease entity with known etiological factors that can become complex with chronicity and lead to death" (p 3). This allergic disease involves the bronchi and bronchioles with an increased production of tenacious mucus, edema of the mucosa, and bronchospasm. Therefore, the airway is reduced. Since there is a combination of large and small airway obstruction, air is trapped and hyperinflation of the lungs occurs. The lungs become larger and the vital capacity decreases; breathing becomes more difficult. Alveolar ventilation is decreased as well as arterial oxygen tension with an increase in arterial carbon dioxide tension. Early treatment is essential (Fig. 2).

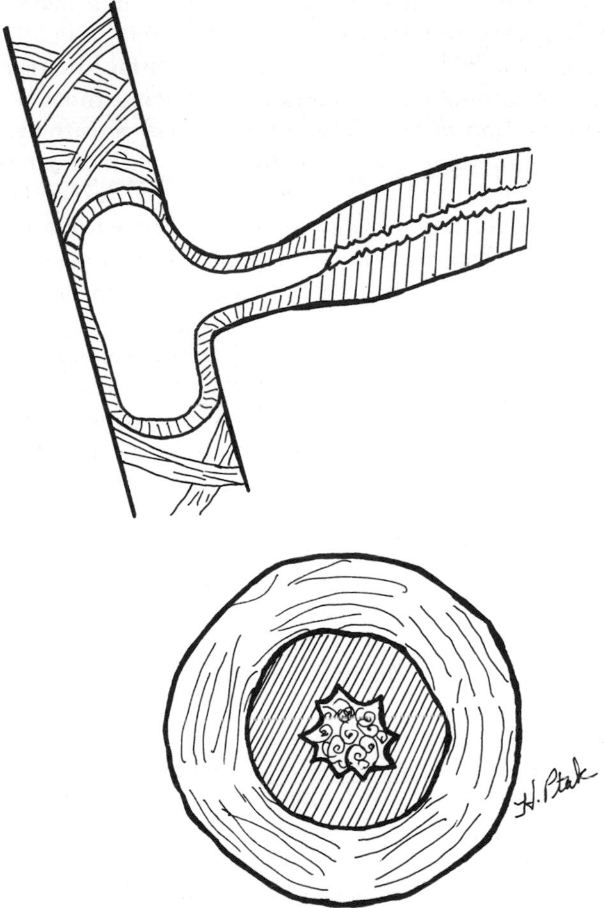

FIG. 2. (Top) Longitudinal section of bronchiolar obstruction. (Bottom) Enlarged cross section of obstructed bronchiole.

Bronchial asthma may be due to extrinsic causes such as inhalants, foods, or drugs. In some instances, it is associated with bacterial or viral infection. At times, there is a combination of an extrinsic cause, such as food, and an intrinsic cause, such as infection.

In the acute asthmatic attack, the severity of symptoms depends on the inflammatory reaction of mucosa, the amount of bronchospasm, and the degree of obstruction of airways and distended alveoli.

When proper allergic management is provided, the effects are often reversible. In the long-term cases, response to medication may be poor due to changes that have taken place in the bronchi and alveoli resulting in lowered vital capacity and deformity of chest cavity.

The infant may fail to thrive or have vomiting, diarrhea, excessive mucus, or other respiratory manifestations. When asthma is diagnosed in infancy, the condition is often the result of food sensitivity. This is one reason why it is important to teach mothers to introduce one new food at a time, especially when there is a history of allergy in the family, so that reactions can be evaluated over a two- to three-day period. A skin rash may be observed rather than respiratory symptoms. In reviewing charts of older children with asthma, it can be seen that infantile eczema was often recorded in the history.

Although there is considerable difference of opinion among physicians as to which foods tend to cause allergic reactions, milk, wheat, eggs, and citrus juices are usually among those listed to be eliminated. Peanut butter is often also listed as an offender in preschool or school-age children.

When foods are being eliminated, a hypoallergenic diet is usually instituted. Milk is usually replaced in the diet by a soybean preparation. Rice, oats, or barley cereal are also used in the diet. Meat (such as lamb) is added later. The restricted diet is usually supplemented with synthetic vitamins. After a week on a regimen, one new food may be added at a time and the infant observed for any reaction. A simple log should be kept by the mother with comments relating to tolerance of foods or symptoms noted. Later, when foods are reintroduced, the physician may add milk, wheat, and eggs. A written diet, clearly stated—including foods to avoid—is important for the mother. For example, although milk was not given, a cube of cheese containing milk might be offered by the mother if she is not cautioned about the milk content in other products. Reading of labels for content should be stressed. The term rotary diet was described by Rinkel in 1934. The diet contains foods which can be eaten one or two days a week or only one time in ten to fourteen days without return of patient's symptoms resulting from food allergy. A modification of this concept is used by some practitioners in feeding infants. The mother is instructed to select three or four cereals, vegetables, and fruits which her infant has never or seldom eaten and rotate them every four days. If the mother finds one food that is not tolerated, then it is discontinued. This provides a more varied diet and avoids the practice of feeding only soybean and rice cereal daily for fear of an allergic reaction. The initial diet history is most important to elicit food patterns that the parent or caretaker has been using. Upon return visits to office or clinic, the nurse should review logs recorded by the mother and use the opportunity for teaching and counseling.

For older children, a menu may be offered omitting some of the foods most apt to cause allergic reaction. If improvement is noted, over a two-week period, foods are reintroduced which were omitted. If symptoms return then offending food is identified. Clinical trials and accurate recording of offending substances will assist in interpreting the results of dietary studies.

This regimen may seem difficult for a mother to accept. She may become discouraged when the infant refuses to eat the food which he is allowed. This reaction should be anticipated and ways suggested to modify the diet within the restrictions. The refusal of food may also be due to deceleration of the growth rate. Force-feeding should be avoided and there should be acceptance of the fact that appetite will vary from one meal to the next.

As the child grows, *inhalants* take on a more prominent role and may be responsible for respiratory symptoms, although dust can be a problem in the infant age group.

The allergic history will be the initial step in diagnosis. The nurse in the clinic or office may observe that on the visit following the initial workup, the mother may share additional important information that she did not recall on the first visit.

The nurse should provide an explanation of what to expect on the physical examination, laboratory tests, or special pulmonary function tests. With a young child, the mother can play an important role. Techniques for examining infants, such as having the mother urge the child to puff on her hand or a plastic windmill may permit auscultation. Children often become distressed when undressed completely, even with the mother present. Removal of clothes from the upper half and replacement after head, neck, and chest examination may avoid this reaction. Enlistment of the aid of an older sibling helps on occasion to serve as a model of what to expect. The use of distraction is often effective in dealing with toddlers. For example, a toddler, clothed in pajamas, resisted standing still on the scale. He clung to the shaft and screamed loudly. His pajama bottoms began to slip. The nurse suggested he hold his pajamas up. He removed his hands and held onto his pants. His weight was secured without further resistance.

Environmental contacts, such as dust, flowers, animal dander, and feathers, may need to be eliminated to study the effect that they have on the child's condition. Although this may seem like a reasonably simple request, the family may need a nurse to visit the home to provide the necessary assistance to complete this task. Sleeping arrangements should be explored. Realistically, it is the child's bedroom on which special emphasis is placed. The need to remove a favorite pet from the household can become a tragic request in the eyes of the entire family. Resentment could be directed toward the child with the allergy by other siblings. A free guide distributed by A. H. Robins is available in many physician's offices or upon request. Considerations are included which assist the family in controlling dust and other allergenic articles (Fig. 3).

When expensive articles must be provided, such as Kapok pillows and

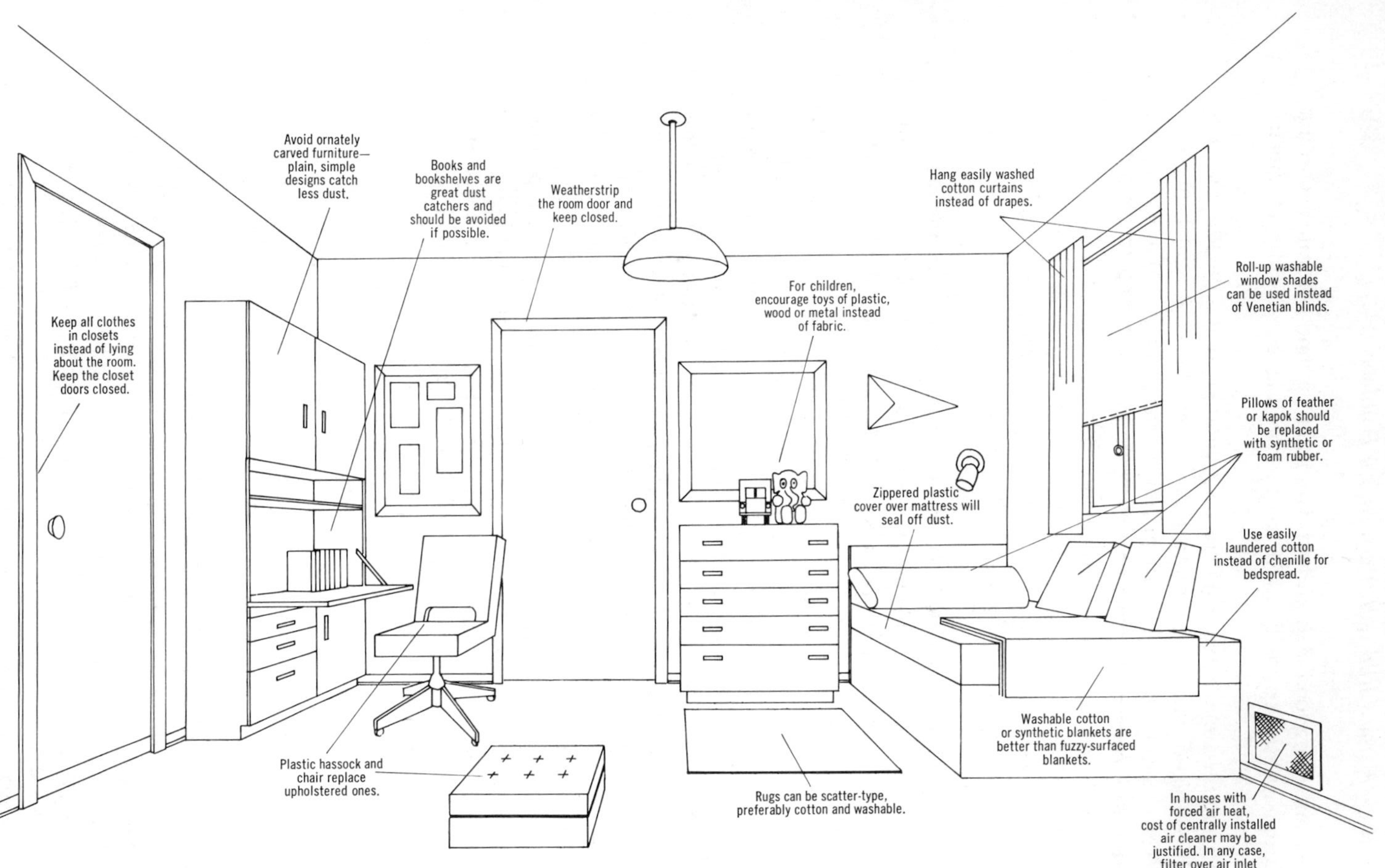

FIG. 3. How to "desensitize" a room. (Courtesy of A.H. Robins Co., Richmond, Va)

mattress covers, or when the use of a special air cleaner, air conditioner, or humidifier is suggested, the family budget may not be flexible enough to facilitate the acquisition(s). The problem may require assistance from the welfare or social worker. Articles used by other family members, such as powders, perfumes, and scented tissues, may be offending substances. Ways to protect the child from exposure to them will need to be explored.

Emotional Aspects of the Disease. Psychiatric studies of children with asthma have indicated that the onset may follow the death of a close member such as a grandparent or parent. In some children, emotional upsets may play a major role in onset of symptoms. Although these situations do not cause the asthma, they do aggravate it.

The child's liabilities should be assessed to determine what action can be taken to reduce the child's disability. The nurse should observe the child's behavior as to how he approaches living with a disability and how he cooperates with those offering treatments or other help. Failure to cope with the disease may lead to the use of inappropriate psychologic defenses. The goal of treatment should be shared with the child and involve him in the plan of care.

The values held by the child will likely determine his attitude toward his disability. For example, a five-year-old will view limitation of diet very differently than will an adolescent. On the other hand, to an adolescent, one's cosmetic effect assumes central importance, and this limitation may not be so significant to a younger child. The mother's acceptance of the illness may affect the extent to which the child will accept it. Most of the children on a pediatric unit find a certain amount of solace in the attention provided by the staff. However, a few may appear to need and enjoy dependency and exaggerate helplessness. The nurse should be alert to this and a team conference may be indicated to help the child become more independent. Chronic or severely handicapped children are unable to express aggressive impulses through physical activity used by healthy children in acts of play. Self-esteem may be affected as a result of some limitations. Other types of activities should be identified that will still involve the child with his peers, such as serving as score keeper, being the assistant in charge of checking equipment, or engaging in a similar activity that is an important contribution to the school or team effort. In general, children are permitted to participate in activities according to their capability.

Hospitalization. Many acute attacks of asthma can be managed at home, but admission may be necessary when the child has failed to respond and respiratory insufficiency continues. In some instances, there is an inability of the family to cope with the illness; hospitalization may be required to provide an opportunity for diagnosis or may be an emergency admission with status asthmaticus. The child's response to admission must be considered and reassurance may be needed by the parents. Their main concern is often that the nurse will not be with the child if and when another attack occurs, or that the patient will not make his needs known. The attitude of the nurse on admission can indicate an understanding of their concern and a beginning sense of trust can develop. Encouraging the parents to call later in the evening means a great deal when they wish to return home but are reluctant to leave.

Some hospitals have considered development of a special unit for allergy in their construction programs. Air conditioning and hypoallergenic bedding and furnishings are provided. For those not acutely ill, kitchen facilities and a dining room are available as well as a play area. Oxygen and resuscitation equipment is built into the walls. Children wear their own clothes, and the staff—made up of pediatric allergist, nurse, nutritionist, medical social worker, and psychologist—utilizes the team approach in providing comprehensive care. The team is highly skilled in the art of observation and assessment. Home visits are also included in the management regime.

Residential centers for children with asthma are available in at least ten states. Some children seem to improve after separation from family and environment. Some physicians prefer partial separation and select a facility fairly close to the child's home.

The Nurse in the Outpatient Clinic. Since the incidence of allergy is high in the pediatric population and the number of allergists is limited, the allergy clinic is usually one of the busiest clinics in the hospital. Following the precise history, physical examination, and laboratory tests and/or x-rays, the patient is skin tested. These tests are done by a scratch or intradermal method usually on the upper arm. To complete the series, depending on the number ordered, it may take three or four visits. The approach of the staff is important initially, so that anxiety and fear of "shots" can be alleviated. Some allergists do not order skin tests to determine food allergens since they believe the best way to avoid food phobias and to detect reaction due to foods is to put the child on a strict elimination diet and have the mother keep an accurate diet chart.

Clinical Example. The following is a description of an allergy clinic which was changed to facilitate improved patient care. When the clinic was first instituted, the house officers in the pediatric clinic interviewed the patient and family, wrote the orders, and administered the injections. Because of their rotations through the service, changes were frequent. Therefore, the child and his family had to relate to several physicians.

It was decided to assign one nurse to the allergy clinic (Clinic A) and she gave the injections on written order of the house staff. During "hay fever" season, over 100 children, some requiring three injections each, were seen in the clinic.

The next change that was instituted was to assign half of the allergy clinic population to the nurse who had been giving injections only, so that she assumed more responsibility for interviews, injections, and follow-up. A guide provided by the physician was used to determine dose of injections. A house officer and staff nurse continued to be assigned to the other half of the patients, in Clinic B. It was observed that the children assigned to the nurse in Clinic A looked forward to greeting her and to observing the preparation of their injection. Children assigned to Clinic B were unhappy because a new person was assigned to give their injections. They resented this at first, but adjusted to the change. They still returned to visit the nurse in Clinic A, who had previously been their nurse. What was it that appeared to make the difference in attitude of the children in the two clinics?

Mrs. S., nurse in Clinic A, consulted the allergist in the clinic when necessary and referred patients to be seen by him. She tried to recall something special about each child, jotting down personal notes on a small slip of paper on the chart. Upon the return visit to the clinic, it was not unusual to hear her say, "How did you make out in the school play?" or, "You decided on long hair!" or,"Who won the game?"

When a new child or one who becomes upset over injections has an appointment, his injections are prepared prior to entering the room to avoid waiting, watching, and worrying. Soon the child adjusts and he is able to watch preparations as well as other youngsters receiving their injections. By the third or fourth visit, there are no more tears. Needle-play is another alternative for decreasing the child's fear of injections. The nurse assembles the equipment and teaches the child to draw up the solution, usually water. The child follows the injection routine and injects a doll to relieve some of his anxiety. By helping the child to express his hostility through therapeutic play, the nurse helps the child to develop the ego strength he needs to cope with future painful experiences.

Now that the role of the nurse is being exended to make better use of her/his educational preparation toward improved patient care, she/he reviews with the parents the list of allergens, foods, and other factors that should be eliminated and discusses the plan that has been identified for management.

School problems and requests for excusal from gym are not uncommon in this child population. On 10-year-old wanted to be excused from school in order to be at the clinic at 1:00 in the afternoon rather than 3:00 so he could meet his friends. Some preadolescent girls wanted excuses from gym which were not reasonable because this condition did not warrant being excused. They were attempting to use their chronic condition in an unhealthy way. The philosophy of the clinic's staff in relation to activity is that children are allowed to participate according to their individual capability and individuals are not excused unless their physical condition warrants it. Most excuses are written "to participate as tolerated."

Use of oxygen. Anticipation of respiratory emergency and knowledge of location of emergency equipment cannot be overemphasized regardless of the respiratory condition. An important consideration in administration of oxygen is a low flow rate. The reports of the blood gases are evaluated. Careful observations of the patient's response to oxygen by the staff, are vital, since severe respiratory acidosis may develop in patients with severe asthma who receive high inspired oxygen concentrations. This results from continued airway resistance and not because of poor ventilation. If oxygen is administered at higher levels, hypoxia results due to the rise in alveolar carbon dioxide tension.

When oxygen is ordered by croupette or tent, it is the responsibility of the personnel and family when opening the tent to do something for the patient, to leave the patient with the canopy tucked in and the oxygen and motor turned on before leaving the bedside; otherwise the patient is without therapy. In high-humidity tents, 70 to 100 percent humidity can be provided. The child who cannot see through the fog of the tent or whose clothes are supersaturated may resist the tent and need more frequent attention.

As the infant or child responds to therapy, one of the early indications that the tent is no longer required may be determined by observing the behavior of the child. A toddler may be observed sitting at the foot of the bed breathing "normally." Nurses must utilize judgment in carrying out their responsibilities. Evaluation of color, cough, and respiratory effort during the bath or at feeding time should be carried out. A trial period without the croupette or tent may be indicated to determine progress. On the other hand, a tent that has been discontinued may need to be reordered if the child's respiratory status deteriorates.

Parents are often concerned that the child will be afraid in the tent. It is helpful for the admission nurse to remain at the bedside until the patient is settled in the tent. Children tend to receive relief quickly from the treatment and will begin to settle down. Parents should be permitted to remain with the child. It is important to have a light by the bed of any child in an oxygen or other special tent in order to assess respirations and color frequently.

Medications. Medications play an important role in relief of asthmatic symptoms. It is important for the nurse to know the nature of drugs, such as bronchodilators, aerosol sprays, expectorants, or tranquilizers, in order to assess symptoms and take appropriate action. Self-prescribed medication should be discouraged. Most intractability is caused by medications and not by psychologic or environmental factors. Some consideration is currently being given to recommending the prescription basis for buying hand nebulizers. It is important to include demonstration of the use of nebulizers, mask, or mouthpiece when this type of therapy is recommended for the first time at home. The patient's chart should be properly tagged or flagged, if there is a history of specific drug sensitivity. Strong sedation is usually avoided. Pediatric doses of tranquilizers have been used when the child is extremely restless. Antibiotic therapy is usually ordered when an infection is present.

Epinephrine is a most effective drug in treatment of allergic conditions. Proper dosage is vital so that an effective response will occur. Many physicians will be very specific in instructions to the parents and may not teach or permit parents to administer this drug in the home. Their rationale for this decision is related to concern about causing an "adrenalin-fast" patient and they believe that the patient should be seen by the physician to evaluate management. Overdosage is noted by increased pulse, elevated blood pressure, headache, and increased apprehension.

Aminophylline suppositories are effective when the proper dosage is used; 5 mg/kg of body weight is listed as an effective dosage. The parents should be instructed that suppositories have been ordered and how and where to insert them. This may seem obvious; however, one mother who was told that the nasal symptoms her child was experiencing would improve after this medication, returned to the clinic to report that "the medicine was too big to put in Johnny's nose." If vomiting or restlessness occurs, the drug should be stopped. When half of a suppository is ordered, it should be sliced longitudinally so that the medicine is equally distributed between the two halves of the suppository.

Bronchodilator aerosols contain agents to relieve bronchospasm. Some incorporate isoproterenol with corticosteroid. This type of therapy is preferred by some authorities for adults with chronic asthma for relief of bronchospasm rather than for children. Several reasons are given for this stand: (1) the side-effects, such as dependency or addiction, result from increased use, as well as toxic symptoms; (2) they lead to intolerance to other medications used in the treatment of asthma; (3) pulmonary complications; and (4) sudden or unexpected death may result.

According to Fontana (1969), "in the asthmatic child with uncontrollable chronic disease or life-threatening, acute respiratory failure, the steroid drugs are most useful in conjunction with, but not as a replacement for the standard allergic management procedures. The general management procedures including: hydration, expectoration, tranquillization should certainly be tried for a period of time before steroids are prescribed" (p 57). Steroids are usually continued for a seriously ill child who has already been treated with them. Saturated solution of potassium iodine may be used to activate proteolytic enzyme, which acts on secretions. Administration with fruit juice or milk with each dose lessens gastric irritation.

Aerosol therapy may be ordered for a young child or infant to decrease mucosal edema and to relieve bronchospasm. This therapy may be in the form of cold steam, mucolytic agents, antibiotics, enzymes, or oxygen. Some ultrasonic equipment provides much finer particles with dense concentrations. When the infant is treated with aerosol therapy that utilizes ultrasonic equipment, daily weights should be taken to evaluate water retention. The effects of excess water include convulsions, edema, and circulatory failure. Bronchospasm seems to develop more readily from any agent that might irritate the bronchial tree when the patient is dehydrated. Therefore, hydration is very important before aerosol agents are instituted. The simplest way to reduce sputum viscosity is to keep the patient well hydrated. The child should be encouraged to drink liquids frequently.

Recent developments in the field stimulated one community to attempt to break down the resistance of parents and clients to participation in physical exercise, particularly strenuous exercise. A family asthma program was developed with the goal of educating both the child and the family about exercise and to encourage the family to treat the child in as normal a way as possible. Physical activity had often been limited unnecessarily due to fear on the part of the parent and/or child. Six weekly sessions were provided for the child and his parents to work with a health team, including a nurse practitioner, respiratory therapist, psychologist, and physician. The children were involved in physical activities with volunteer instructors and the respiratory therapist. Breathing exercises, calisthenics, and games were included in a gym setting. The swimming ability of one girl improved to the point where she qualified for a Red Cross beginners swimming card. The objective of parent sessions was to discuss the disease and share concerns as a way of alleviating their fears.

With the advent of Cromolyn Sodium, activities which were once thought to be out of the question, can now be included if judgment on the part of the parent and or child or adolescent is utilized. Cromolyn Sodium—Aarane or Intal—is a drug that can be used to prevent attacks rather than to treat them. It is not a bronchodilator nor a bronchial mucus liquifier. It is thought to prevent attacks by interfering with the release of tissue autocoids during an antigen-antibody reaction. This drug permits the child to exercise and to participate in normal activities with peers without difficulty. It can be used prior to anticipated emotional stress such as participation in a school play or examination, exposure to Christmas trees, dust or pets, and while on vacation.

Each capsule contains a powder which is inhaled. The capsule is not swallowed. A special container (spinhaler) pierces the capsule so that the powder is spun out. The child must tip the inhaler upwards, breathe very deeply and hold his breath before exhaling. Inhalation of one capsule is usually recommended one hour prior to exposure and every three to four hours, up to four times a day, during the period of exposure.

This has changed the restrictions that many children have had to endure. Parents and clients can be instructed in the proper use in order to handle and control exposure. Activities can be undertaken within reason.

For example, skiing would not be recommended on a bitter cold windy day. However, participation in this activity is possible under more favorable conditions.

TUBERCULOSIS

The development of an individual throughout the course of his life time is dependant on a complex interaction between genetic components and environmental factors (Whaley, 1974). Tuberculosis is an infectious disease due primarily to environmental factors. In reviewing the statistics related to tuberculosis in children, it is evident that the disease is still an important health problem. Tuberculosis-control programs attempt to prevent the spread to the pediatric population. Casefinding to prevent contact of infected individuals with those who are healthy is important. In 1974, 30,210 new cases of tuberculosis were reported in United States—a decline of 2.9 percent. Certain segments of the population have a higher incidence. Social and environmental stress play a significant role. Susceptibility to tuberculosis is greater during the periods of infancy and puberty.

Since few patients with tuberculosis are hospitalized today, one might question including this condition in this discussion of the implications of long-term respiratory problems for nursing. However, child-health nursing is no longer confined to the hospital but extends to homes, schools, and clinics. It is often through health supervision or the ambulatory service that the condition is found. In the majority of cases, primary tuberculosis infection is an asymptomatic process.

Tuberculosis is highly contagious and is usually spread by droplets containing the viable tubercle bacilli. When children are in contact with an individual with the active disease, they are very susceptible. Often it is difficult to trace the contact that is the host for the infection. The infection usually occurs as a result of inhalation of droplets of sputum sprayed by coughing, sneezing, or talking. Discussion will be confined to primary pulmonary tuberculosis, although extrapulmonary tuberculosis occurs.

The pulmonary lesions in children may be seen in any part of the lung, with some tendency to be localized near the periphery. The site is more likely to be in the lower part of the lungs. At the site of the initial focus, there is an accumulation of polymorphonuclear leukocytes followed by proliferation of epithelioid cells which surround the tubercle bacilli, creating the typical tubercle formation. Lymph nodes are usually involved at the time of the initial parenchymal lesion in children. There is a strong tendency in children for these lesions to heal by calcification.

Since more individuals reach maturity today without having acquired the disease, there is an increase in the primary infection in adults. Primary tuberculosis infection has been referred to as the childhood type of tuberculosis. The course of primary tuberculosis is benign in the majority of cases. Most complications such as tuberculosis meningitis result from hematogenous spread from the primary focus. Chronic tuberculosis occurs as a late involvement in individuals infected earlier with bacilli tubercle.

The diagnosis is often made in retrospect after the tuberculin test has changed from a negative to a positive reaction. Tuberculin tests play an important role in the diagnosis and are recommended by several authors to begin at six to nine months of age and be administered at school entry and in early adolescence. The purpose of the test, how it is administered, and the significance of the reaction should be explained to parents in the clinic. There are certain limitations to the test, but a positive reaction in the tuberculin test indicates the presence of tuberculosis infection that is allergic or hypersensitive to its protein. Although the degree of activity cannot be determined, further procedures, such as chest x-ray and examination of gastric contents, may be ordered. False-positive and false-negative tests can occur for various reasons. Mantoux test is considered an accurate reliable skin test. Old Tuberculin (OT) solution or Purified Protein Derivative (PPD) solution can be utilized.

A stabilized Tuberculin PPD Solution is now commercially available for the intracutaneous Mantoux Test.* It is no longer necessary to use the tablet form and dilutent. The potency of this new form has been extended and it is stable up to 12 months when stored between 35 to 46 F. The skin of the forearm is cleansed with alcohol or acetone and allowed to dry. The initial test dose consists of 0.1 ml of First Strength PPD injected intracutaneously on the flexor surface of the arm about 4 inches below the bend of the elbow. The PPD test is read 48 to 72 hours after administration of the tuberculin. The widest diameter of distinctly palpable induration should be recorded. Presence of redness, edema, or necrosis should also be recorded. A positive reaction (greater than 5 mm of induration after two or three days) indicates a sensitivity to tuberculin, which may be the result of a previous infection with mycobacteria. This infection, likely due to mycobacterium tuberculosis, may have occurred years ago or may be of recent origin.

Clear instructions should be given to the parents when the test is administered on an outpatient basis. A small drawing or picture is helpful to give parents, and the parent is either contacted or requested to call the clinic for the report. It may be necessary to repeat the test.

There are two multiple puncture tests: the Heaf test and the Tine test. The Heaf test is administered with a Heaf gun with disposable cartridges making multiple simultaneous punctures of the skin through a layer of con-

**Manufactured by Connaught Medical Research Laboratories, University of Toronto, Ontario, Canada. U.S. Distributor: Panray Division, Ormont Drug and Chemical Company, Englewood, New Jersey.*

centrated PPD (Figs. 4 and 5). Three to seven days later, the test is read. A positive reaction is indicated if four or more papules appear. The tuberculin Tine test is an inexpensive, newer test and consists of a sterilized disposable unit with four tines which have been predipped in Old Tuberculin concentrate (Fig. 6). Two millimeters or more of palpable induration around one or more puncture sites is equivalent to five millimeters or more by the standard intradermal Mantoux Test. This may be considered positive.

Regardless of which type of test is used, the child may express fear or apprehension because a puncture of the skin is involved. When the test is administered to a young child, the child should be held on the lap, holding the arm gently and distracting the child with conversation to allay fear. The wheal on the skin can be compared to a mosquito bite to a preschooler. A child who knows how to count can be encouraged to count with the nurse to see how long it takes for the test. This technique is quite effective.

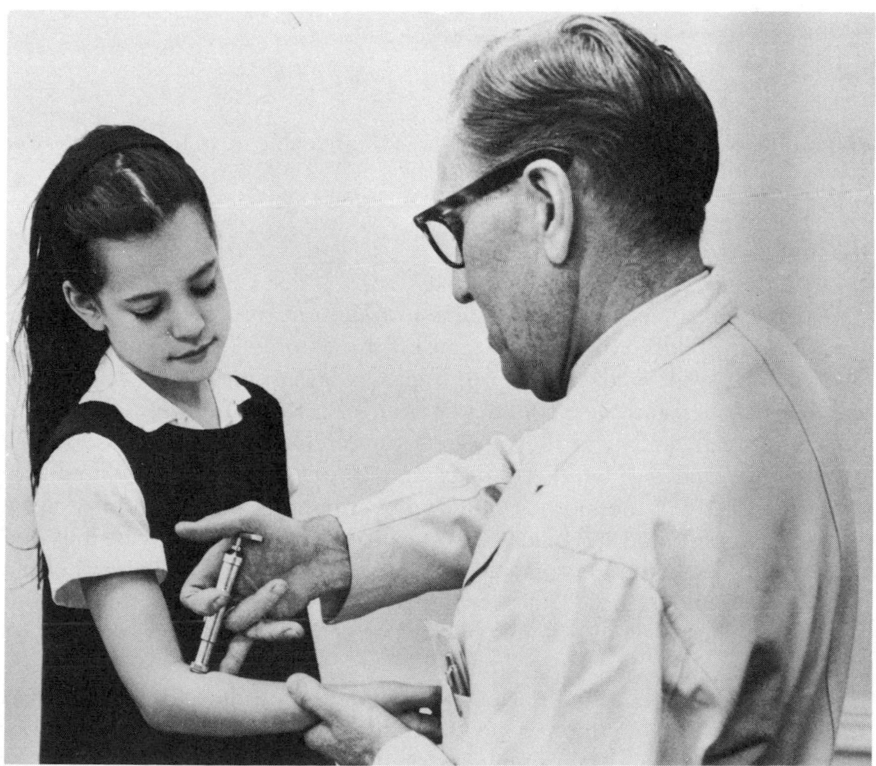

FIG. 4. Physician administers the Heaf Test to Adrian. (Courtesy of Panray-Parlam Corp., Englewood, N.J.)

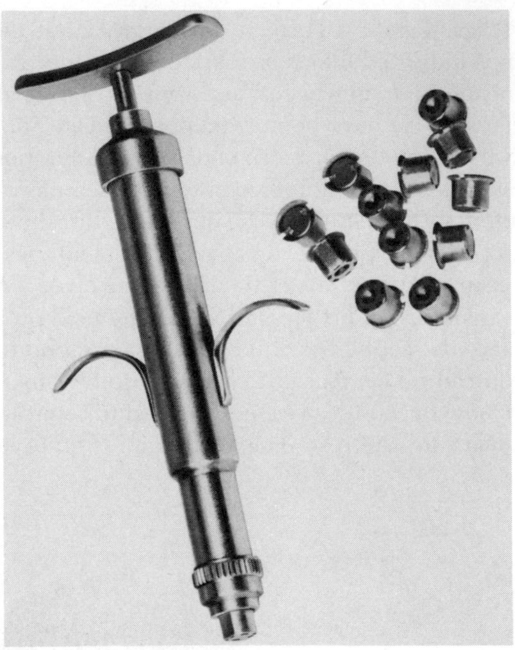

FIG. 5. A close-up view of the Heaf gun with disposable cartridges. (Courtesy of Panray-Parlam Corp., Englewood, N.J.)

Gastric Lavage

It is difficult to obtain a specimen of sputum to recover the tubercle bacilli from children because organisms from lung lesions reaching the pharynx are swallowed. Therefore, a gastric lavage may be ordered. The number of bacilli and the frequency of positive cultures recovered by gastric lavage is small, and it is therefore recommended that the procedure be carried out each day for three successive days. Gastric lavage should be performed early in the morning after an overnight fast. The contents of the stomach are aspirated and placed in a sterile container. This may be followed with 60 ml of sterile water, and this is aspirated and added to material in the container (Kendig, 1972). This procedure may be carried out by the nurse or physician. The specimen should be sent directly to the laboratory for culture.

It is not my intent to describe the complete procedure for lavage but to comment on a few important aspects. In infants and young children, proper restraint is necessary. A mummy restraint is usually most effective so that the procedure can be carried out safely and as quickly as feasible. The

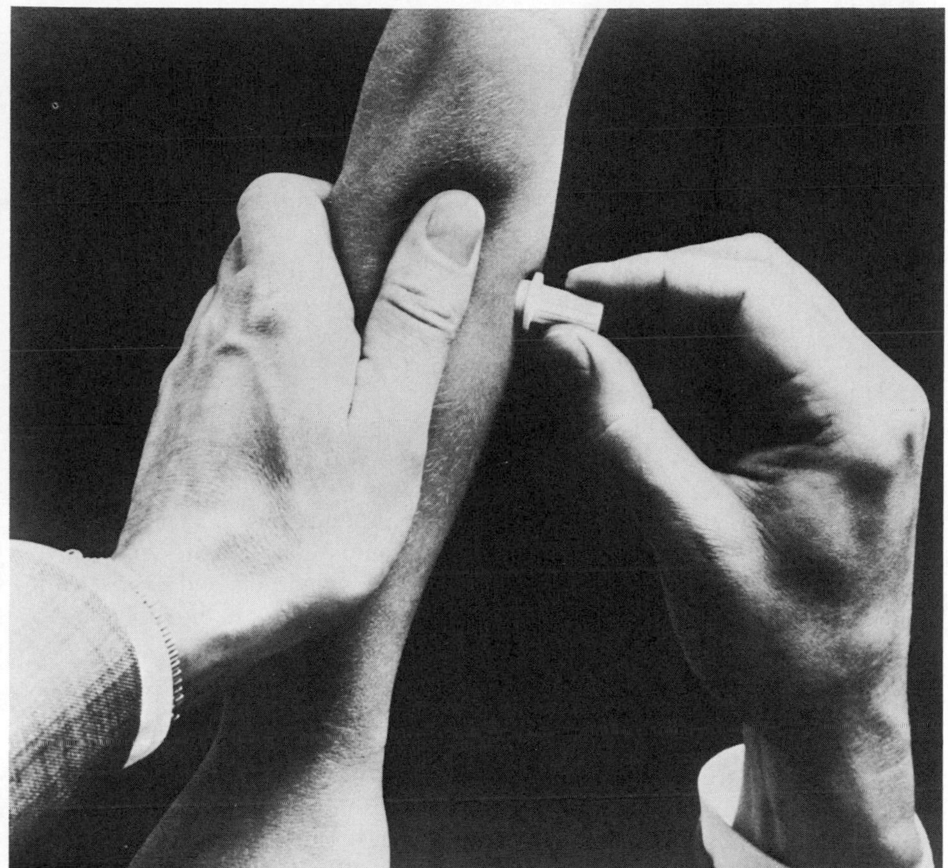

FIG. 6. Administration of the Tine Test used in tuberculosis detection. (Courtesy of Lederle Laboratories, Pearl River, N.Y.)

attitude of the nurse and the manner in which the restraint is applied make a difference: for example, "I am doing this to make it easier," rather than an attitude such as, "I'll wrap you up so you can't move." Nonverbal communication speaks louder than words. When a catheter is inserted, coughing, difficult breathing, or cyanosis may indicate insertion into the larynx. If such a reaction occurs, remove the catheter at once. For confirmation of proper placement of the catheter in the stomach, gastric contents can be aspirated. The size of the catheter is determined by the child's age. As with any pediatric procedure that is uncomfortable, the nurse should hold the infant, or in the case of an older child spend a few minutes with him, for reassurance after the procedure.

Treatment

With the advent of antimicrobial drugs, such as para-aminosalicylic acid, isoniazid, and streptomycin, mortality rates in tuberculosis were greatly reduced. Therapy is initiated as soon as a diagnosis of tuberculosis is made.

Isoniazid is given usually orally by tablet or syrup. Side effects to be watched for include neuritis and convulsions. These are more common in the adult or adolescent than in younger children. When this drug is given to young children, it should be crushed and the taste disguised through the use of puréed fruit or preserves. It is usually ordered in divided doses at the morning and evening meals. Pyridoxine is administered in association with INH to prevent peripheral neuritis.

PAS (para-aminosalicylic) is sometimes administered with isoniazid to provide a higher blood level, since PAS competes with isoniazid for acetylation in the liver. Gastrointestinal symptom may be a sign of toxicity.

Dihydrostreptomycin is more likely to produce eighth cranial nerve deafness. Streptomycin sulphate is given intramuscularly. Toxic symptoms include: disturbances of vestibular function, fever, vomiting, and a variety of skin eruptions. Personnel as well as parents should be alert to the problem of deafness. Observe how the child responds when his name is spoken or to conversation, as well as the degree of loudness of the radio or television.

Unless there is some specific reason, children are usually checked monthly while on medication. Periodic x-rays are ordered. Annual checkups should be stressed after therapy is completed.

Children, and adolescents in particular, cannot appreciate the importance and effectiveness of the antimicrobial drugs. These drugs may be given over a long period of time. Charts, logs, or any other creative methods may act as a necessary stimulus to assist the child in taking his medication. Protection should be provided to prevent intercurrent infections so as to avoid lowered resistance. Exposure to communicable diseases should be reported at once to the physician. Household contacts of a reported case of tuberculosis are skin tested and chemoprophylaxsis is advised. Other methods used to prevent tuberculosis include: isolation of those adults with infectious tuberculosis and use of BCG vaccine (used mainly for children exposed to an individual in a home or in a high-incidence population).

Older individuals can appreciate the changes that have been brought about in the therapy for tuberculosis. Years ago there was considerable stigma attached to tuberculosis. Parents or grandparents of the child involved may still recall the sanitarium, the mountain climate, and the elaborate isolation technique carried out. These attitudes could be easily transmitted to the adolescent. Members of the health team should be sensitive to the concerns and attitudes of the family toward the disease. Whichever member is in the best position at the time to handle these concerns should do so. It may be the nurse, physician, or social worker. What is important is that they be handled.

A diet high in protein, with adequate calories to promote growth, is furnished. If the child is asymptomatic, limitation of activity is not required. In those children who are symptomatic, prolonged bedrest is rarely used after therapy has been instituted as it may lead to further complications. The guide generally used for activity is the comfort level of the patient. Excessive sunlight should be avoided.

Suitable toys and activities should be provided to amuse preschool children when activity is limited. School-age children may be more restless. Painting, books, crafts, felt boards, puzzles, and records may help to pass the time. New hobbies should be promoted. The school-age child or adolescent should be encouraged to talk about his concerns related to the illness so that guidance can be provided. He should understand the goals of treatment and be involved in the plan for his care when possible. Contact should be maintained with peers through letters and phone calls until visitors are permitted, or he returns to school. Children with primary tuberculosis return to school when they are asymptomatic. A conference with the teacher in the school may be indicated to clarify any questions she may have about the child's ability to attend school and engage in activities permitted.

The role of the nurse in the office or clinic is an important one. The quality of the initial history and subsequent interviews during health supervision plays a significant part in diagnosis, management, and prevention of this disease. Identification of contacts and referral for tuberculin testing is essential. The pretreatment work-up including laboratory tests and x-rays requires explanation. The nurse is in a unique position to provide support and teaching during this stressful period for the client and/or family. The child or parent should record the child's daily temperature. Upon return to the office or clinic assessment of the child's general condition, evidence of weight loss or gain, history of malaise and any special concerns should be noted. Throughout the course of the disease there are many instances in which an explanation or response to questions is required. The family will usually want to know information about the impact of the significance of the change from a negative to a positive tuberculin test in an infant or young child as well as subsequent investigation that is required to establish a positive diagnosis.

CYSTIC FIBROSIS

Cystic fibrosis was selected for inclusion in the chapter on nursing care in long-term respiratory problems of children because it is recognized as one of the more common chronic diseases in children today and it is considered to be the most serious lung problem of childhood. It is an inherited disease of children in which there is a dysfunction of all or most of the exocrine glands. The incidence is thought to be one in 1000 or one in 1600 live births. This condition can range from a very mild form of the disease, with good nutrition and no respiratory involvement, to the severe form, with extensive pulmonary obstruction and marked malnutrition that imposes very limited activity.

Dramatic changes have been brought about in the past 20 years through study and research resulting in improved management of the disease. The prognosis is often dependent upon the degree of pulmonary involvement.

Early diagnosis and aggressive therapy have been responsible for survival of infants and younger children into adolescence or adulthood. Presently more children are surviving to later years. The highest incidence of death from the disease occurs between the third and ninth month of life. It is reported in a recent article by Shwackman et al (1975) that out of approximately 2500 patients, 90 of their patients have survived beyond 25 years of age and the oldest patient is 43 years of age.

Patients who manifest symptoms of the disease are homozygotes. Some authorities feel that if heterozygotes for the mutant gene could be detected, counseling these individuals against marrying each other could play an important role in future prevention in the high incidence areas.

Characteristic symptoms in children with all the clinical manifestations of this disease are due to involvement of three areas: the pancreas and other abdominal organs, lungs, and exocrine sweat glands. Most of the clinical manifestations are secondary to obstruction of some of the organ structures due to secretions which behave abnormally. Bronchial obstruction leads to bronchopneumonia. Pancreatic duct obstruction leads to pancreatic insufficiency. In hot weather or in febrile episodes, excessive loss of sodium chloride in sweat leads to dehydration, reduction of extracellular fluid volume, and then cardiovascular collapse. Hyperthermia, coma, and death may follow rapidly. When one reviews charts of patients with diagnosis of cystic fibrosis, it is usually found that repeated respiratory symptoms were reported in infancy and early childhood. Rectal prolapse and nasal polyps occur and are difficult to explain. Frequent bulky, foul, fatty stools arouse suspicion of the disease, as well as failure to gain weight without anorexia.

Diagnosis is usually made from the family history and after the following tests: (1) sweat test to determine electrolyte content (in cystic fibrosis there is a marked elevation of sodium and chloride levels, two to five times above normal); (2) test for absence of pancreatic enzymes by aspiration of duodenal secretions (the viscosity of pancreatic fluid is increased and there is an absence or deficiency in pancreatic enzymes—namely, trypsin, lipase, and amylase); and (3) pulmonary function tests (the degree of pulmonary involvement is important in determining the severity of the disease and the prognosis).

The child may be already hospitalized for respiratory symptoms and the disease suspected, or the tests may be ordered on an outpatient basis. In either case, the nurse has an important role in explaining the tests and supporting the child during the tests, carrying them out skillfully, comforting the child after the tests, and providing adequate responses to parents' questions or concerns.

When meconium ileus occurs in the newborn, surgery is usually required to relieve the intestinal obstruction. The lumen of the small intestine is plugged with puttylike meconium near the ileocecal valve, which is inspissated. Abdominal distention and vomiting occurs.

Postoperatively, a high protein formula is offered and pancreatin supplement is initiated. A work-up for cystic fibrosis is performed after the infant has recovered from surgery.

The discovery of increased sodium chloride in the sweat of children with cystic fibrosis was of real value in the advent of improved diagnosis of cystic fibrosis. Parents may report the infant tastes salty when kissed. Several methods have been used for the sweat test. The "bag method" was used extensively until the last few years. This method was not the safest. The skin was washed to remove surface chloride and a plastic bag was used to wrap the child and additional blankets used to stimulate sweating. The temperature was recorded rectally before the test and at least every 30 minutes by the axillary method during the procedures, as well as after the test was completed. At least 0.5 ml of sweat was required.

The most reliable and safest method today to collect sweat for chemical analysis is the pilocarpine iontophoresis technique, which can be used even on newborns. A dilute solution of pilocarpine is introduced into a small area of skin on the forearm, with a weak direct electric current, to stimulate local sweating. The sweat, collected on a small gauze pad, is analyzed for sodium and chloride concentration. This test is much easier for the child to accept and is less traumatic.

Duodenal intubation is a direct approach to examine enzymes. The procedure should follow a fast of at least six hours. Some sedation may be ordered about one half hour before the test. The nasogastric tube is inserted, and if secretions are tested with litmus paper, the paper should indicate an alkaline reaction, which confirms the presence of pancreatic juices. Secretions aspirated must be kept cold and analyzed without delay in the laboratory.

Insertion of any tube is an uncomfortable, frightening experience for the child. In the case of an infant or toddler, restraint will be required. Sometimes the procedure is lengthy. The use of distraction, such as reading a story or using an animated toy, will help. A preschool child will often offer resistance when the tube is inserted, but once the test is under way he may relax. A nurse should remain with the child. After the removal of the tube, the patient may be fed, and special attention for a few minutes will help the child regain his composure.

It is important to know what pulmonary function tests will be carried out so that explanations can be provided as to what to expect and how to cooperate, if the child is old enough. Pulmonary function in children over five years of age can be more completely evaluated than in younger children. No single, simple pulmonary function test accurately depicts pulmonary function in cystic fibrosis patients. Personnel who assist with these tests require special training, and must be selected for their ability to work with children.

Treatment of bronchial obstruction, when it occurs, is considered of vital importance. A great deal of the team effort is devoted to this aspect of care. The abnormal viscid secretions in the lungs of these children are a continual process which results in bronchial obstruction and requires vigorous measures. Normal cleaning mechanism by which dust and bacteria are removed is impaired. Accumulation and stagnation of secretions results in chronic bronchial and bronchiolar infection; partial bronchial obstruction, producing patchy emphysema; and complete bronchial obstruction, producing atelectasis (Figs. 7 and 8).

As a result of infection, pulmonary obstruction is increased and further impairs the normal cleansing mechanism. This creates a vicious cycle (Fig. 9). The purpose of therapy is to liquify the secretions and to promote and maintain pulmonary drainage. Methods which will be discussed include: aerosol treatment, mist tents, postural drainage and breathing exercises.

Therapeutic Measures

Bronchopulmonary Hygiene. Nebulization therapy is utilized to moisten and thin respiratory mucous secretions and to disperse the appropriate agent, such as bronchodilators, antibiotics, or mucolytic agents onto the mucous membranes of the tracheobronchial tree. The aim of nebulization therapy is the provision of particles of water, or of water-containing medication, for deposition in the respiratory tract at the site of the disease process. The size of the particles deposited is determined by the nebulizer used as well as the solution and humidity of the air used for nebulization to provide the mist. In order to produce very fine particles for the smaller bronchioles, ten percent propylene glycol may be used in order to reduce vapor tension of the nebulized solution. It is important that an adequate amount of water or medication is inhaled and deposited for the treatment to be effective. The child should be encouraged to breathe slower and deeper so more deposition can take place. Compressed air rather then oxygen is usually used with a croupette or standard oxygen tent. Cooling measures assist in maintaining the tent temperature under 80 F.

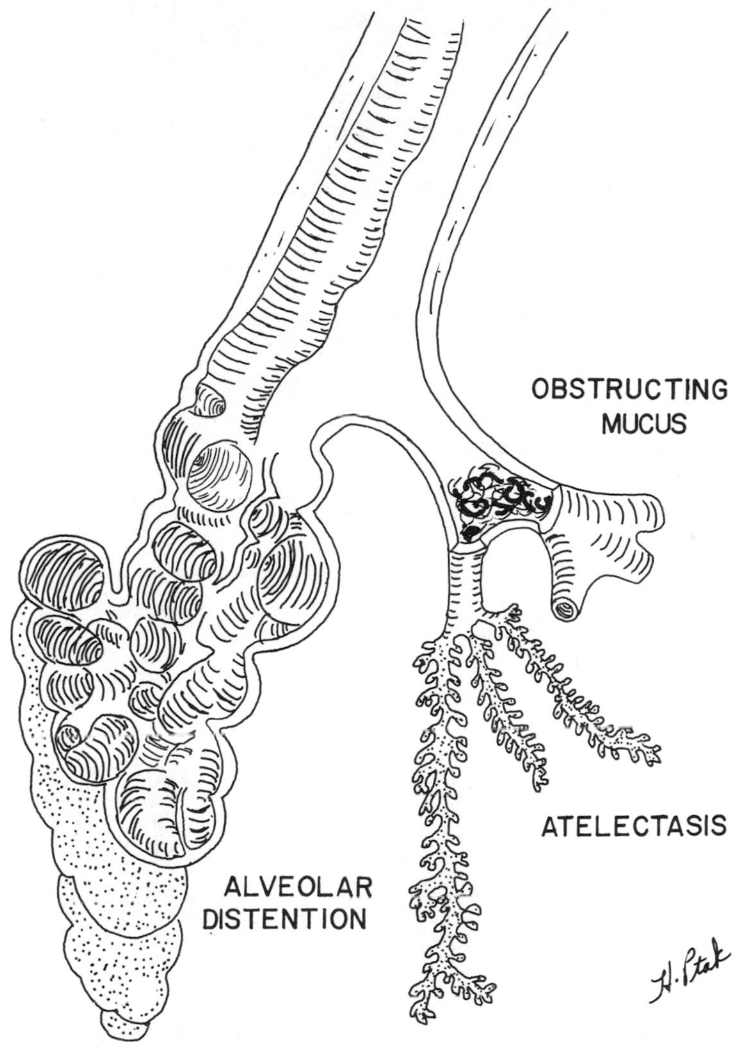

FIG. 7. Schematic representation showing pathology resulting from accumulation and obstruction.

Mist Tent. Mist tent therapy is used to provide longer periods to thin tracheobronchial secretions. Many physicians who have had considerable experience with treatment of patients with cystic fibrosis, now begin prophylactic mist therapy as early as possible, regardless of absence of pulmonary symptoms. The tent is utilized during sleeping hours. This applies to the adult as well as the infant or child.

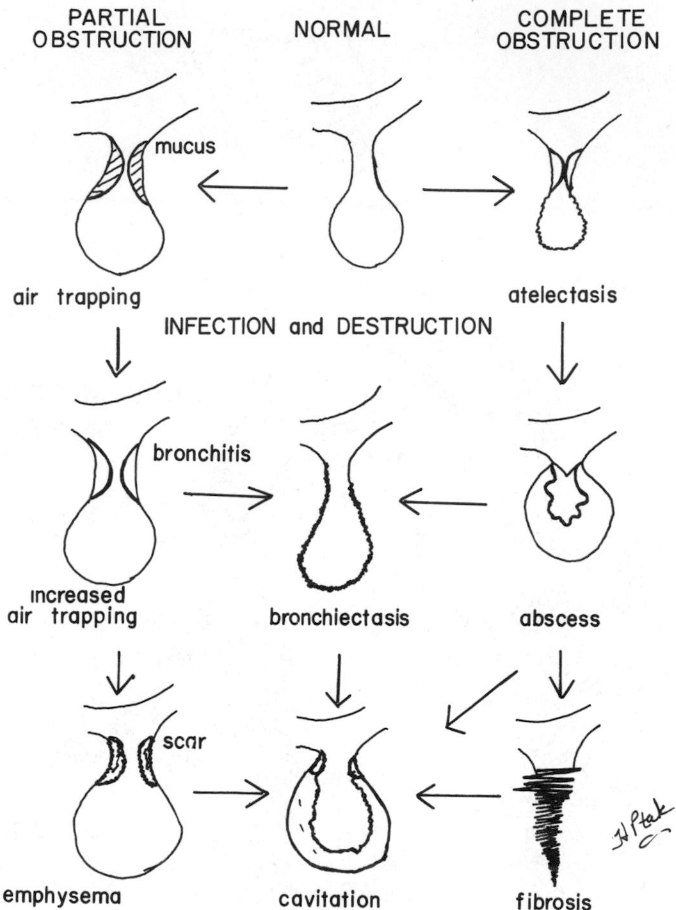

FIG. 8. Pathologic physiology of cystic fibrosis.

Equipment consists of a croupette or regular oxygen tent and nebulizers powered with compressed, filtered air from a portable compressor or from a cylinder of oxygen. The mist should be dense so that it is difficult to see the individual in the tent. The ultrasonic type nebulizer is used for the child when the solution must be provided to the periphery of the lungs (Fig. 10). The type of solution used will depend on the type of nebulizer and the patient.

When the mist tent is used therapeutically rather than prophylactically, it is ordered during the initial hospitalization to provide intensive therapy or for subsequent acute flare-ups. The patient will remain in the tent for the majority of the 24-hour period (Fig. 11).

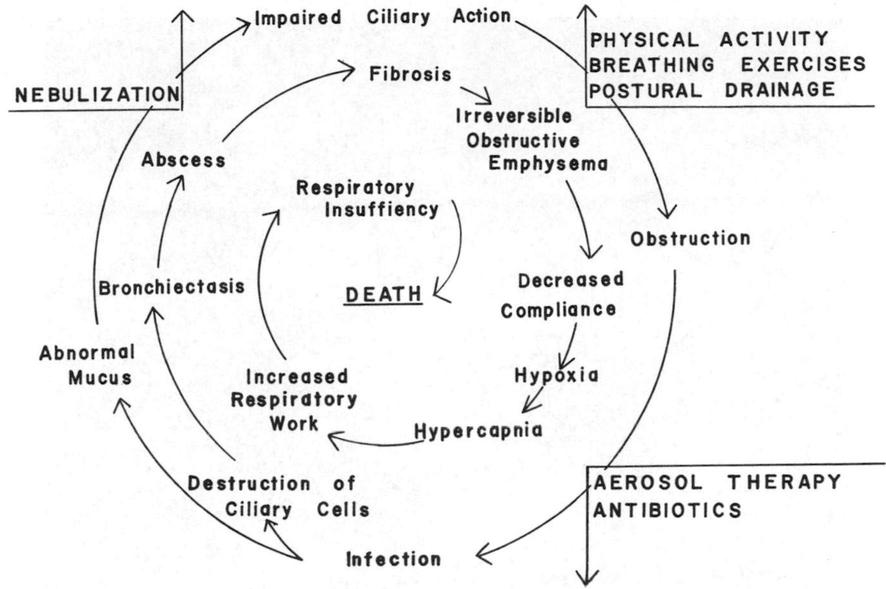

FIG. 9. The vicious cycle of cystic fibrosis and complicating infections can be broken by effective therapy.

When the therapy is first instituted, the nurse must remember that large amounts of thinned secretions may be evident and intense bronchial drainage must be provided. Careful and frequent observation should be provided by the nursing staff. Suction may be required. The length of continuous therapy will depend on signs of response to treatment. It may be as long as 10 to 14 days.

Intermittent Aerosol Therapy. A face mask or plastic mouthpiece is the type of equipment used with a nebulizer for intermittent aerosol therapy. It provides administration of smaller quantities of prescribed solution than the mist tent. Some children will use intermittent therapy in the day time and the mist tent at night.

For the infant or young child, holding the child on your lap with the face mask held near the face provides for an effective treatment. Distractions which are planned through the use of a toy or making a game of applying the mask gains the cooperation of the toddler. The acutely ill child may remain in bed with the use of the nebulizer attached to the croupette or tent. Positioning of the infant is most important. He should be placed on his side as well as alternately elevating and lowering the head of the crib.

Postural Drainage. Postural drainage is utilized with inhalation therapy to promote hygiene for the tracheobronchial tree. Techniques used

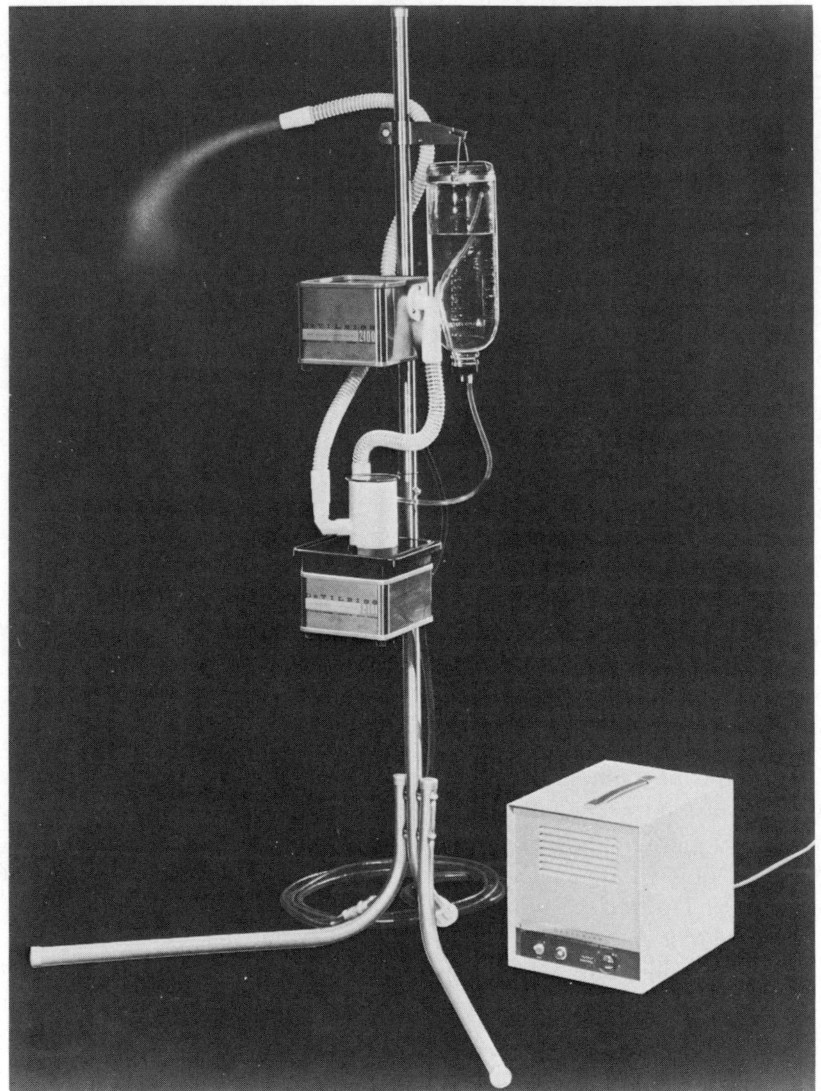

FIG. 10. DeVilbiss ultrasonic nebulizer designed specifically for home mist tent therapy. (Courtesy of DeVilbiss Co., Somerset, Pa.)

are not complicated and should be learned by the nursing staff, whether hospital- or community-based, and the family. The physical therapist, today, is usually responsible for this function and he is an important member of the health team. The staff nurse may need to provide therapy during part of the 24-hour period when the therapist is not available. The community health

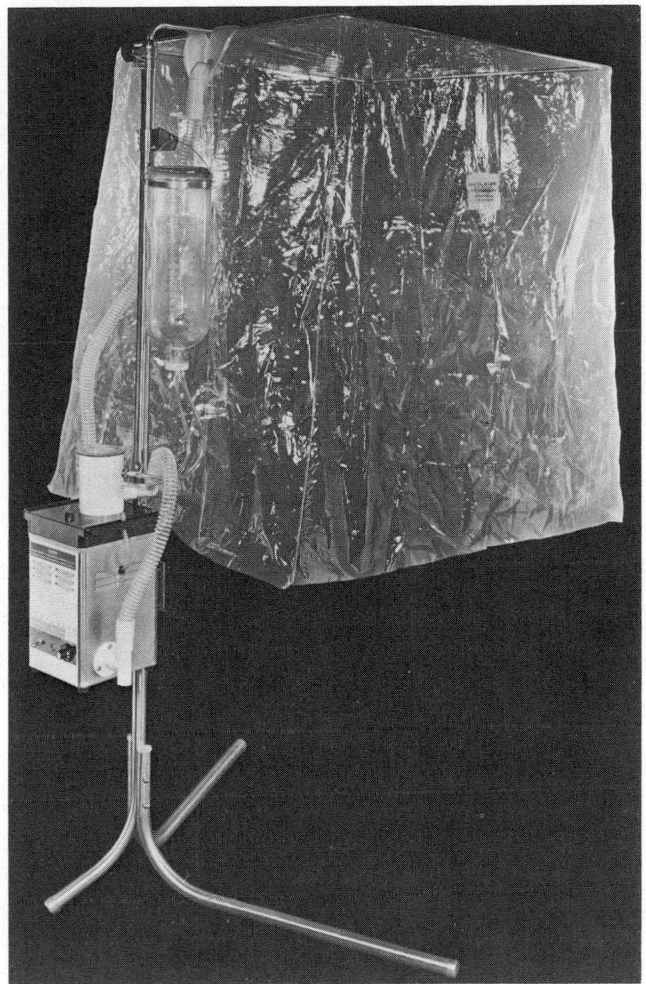

FIG. 11. DeVilbiss ultrasonic nebulizer with frame and canopy. (Courtesy of DeVilbiss Co., Somerset, Pa.)

nurse will need to evaluate the program in the home. A referral may be indicated to the physical therapist upon return to the clinic.

The various positions utilized will be determined by the area of the lung involved (Fig. 12). One particular lobe is drained at a time. Clapping or vibration of the chest wall is carried out during expiration, while in the postural drainage position. The best time is usually before breakfast and before retiring. Each position is assumed for at least two minutes.

Rapid clapping is best carried out with cupped hands on the uppermost

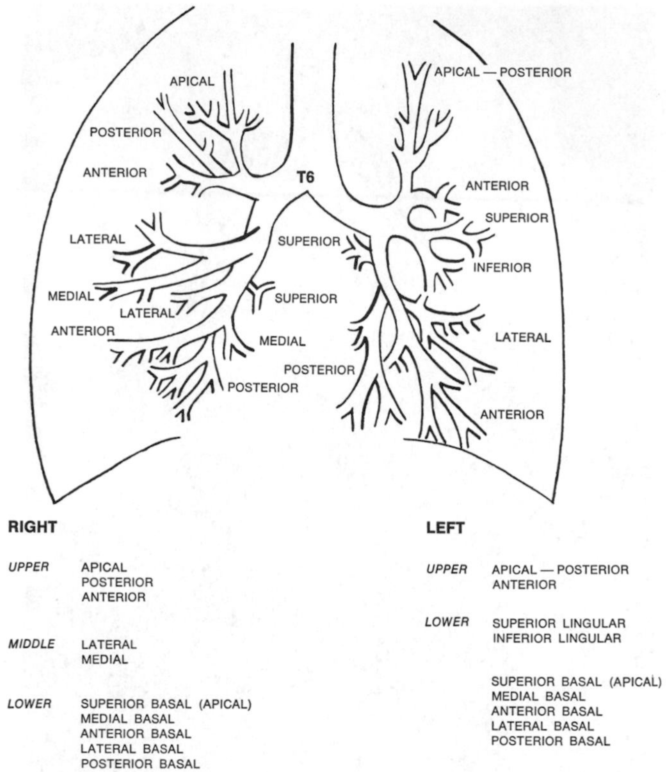

FIG. 12. Segments of the bronchial tree. (Courtesy of the Children's Orthopedic Hospital and Medical Center, Seattle, Wash.)

area. Air is trapped between the hand and the chest wall. At the same time, the patient is urged to exhale and cough to raise sputum.

Vibration through the hands follows this by tensing the upper area and shoulder muscles. Vibration is applied during slow exhalation with slight pressure over the area to be drained. Coughing and expectoration is again urged.

Practice in each of these techniques will provide skill. The therapist usually demonstrates it and the mother participates over a period of time until she feels comfortable in her performance. It is helpful if another member of the family can also be trained (Fig. 13).

The physical therapist will also teach the child and parent breathing exercises in order to increase expiration and strengthen the diaphragm for improved ventilation.

General Management. Infants receive low-fat, high-protein formulas. Soybean protein is not absorbed as well as protein in cow's milk and is not used in cystic fibrosis. The dietary management for older children includes high-protein diet, high-caloric snacks, and moderate restriction of fatty foods. Although undigested fat and proteins as well as calcium and fat-soluble vitamins are lost with the stool, the voracious appetite of these patients lends to a large intake of food, so that absorption of as little as 50 percent of the ingested material may be adequate for satisfactory nutrition.

When enzyme preparations are instituted, the voracious appetite de-

UPPER LOBES
APICAL SEGMENTS
RIGHT AND LEFT UPPER LOBES
RIGHT AND LEFT UPPER LOBES
SITTING, LEAN BACK 20°. CLAP AND VIBRATE OVER COLLAR BONE ON BOTH SIDES.
SITTING, LEAN FORWARD 20°. CLAP AND VIBRATE OVER BOTH SHOULDERS.
ANTERIOR SEGMENTS
LEFT UPPER LOBE
RIGHT UPPER LOBE
LYING ON BACK, PILLOW UNDER KNEES, CLAP & VIBRATE JUST BELOW THE COLLAR BONE HALFWAY BETWEEN THE NECK AND SHOULDER ON BOTH SIDES.
POSTERIOR SEGMENTS
LEFT UPPER LOBE
45° — 18″
RIGHT UPPER LOBE
LYING ON RIGHT SIDE ¾ TURN TOWARD FACE DOWN, (PLACE 3 PILLOWS UNDER LEFT SHOULDER AND HEAD TO LIFT 12 INCHES OFF BED.) CLAP AND VIBRATE OVER LEFT SHOULDER BLADE.
LYING ON LEFT SIDE, ¾ TURN (ON TO PILLOW) FACE DOWN, CLAP AND VIBRATE OVER THE RIGHT SHOULDER BLADE.
LINGULA
LEFT
Tip bed 12″
MIDDLE LOBE
RIGHT
Tip bed 12″
LIE ON LEFT SIDE, ROLL ¼ TURN BACK ON TO PILLOWS, CLAP AND VIBRATE OVER RIGHT NIPPLE AREA.
LIE ON RIGHT SIDE, ROLL ¼ TURN BACK ON TO PILLOWS, CLAP AND VIBRATE OVER LEFT NIPPLE AREA.

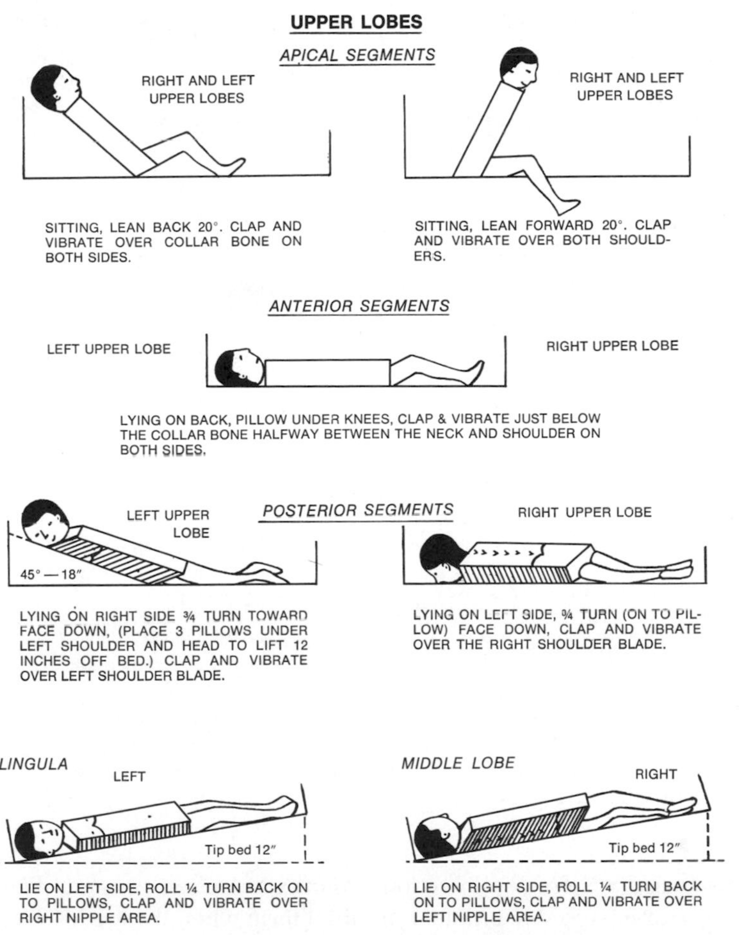

FIG. 13. Instruction sheets provide aid in teaching parents procedures to be done at home. Part I. (Courtesy of the Children's Orthopedic Hospital and Medical Center, Seattle, Wash.); Part II, [Lower lobes]. (Adapted from design and material by Eloise Draper, LPT., available from Pediatric Department of University of Louisville Medical School, Louisville, Kentucky.)

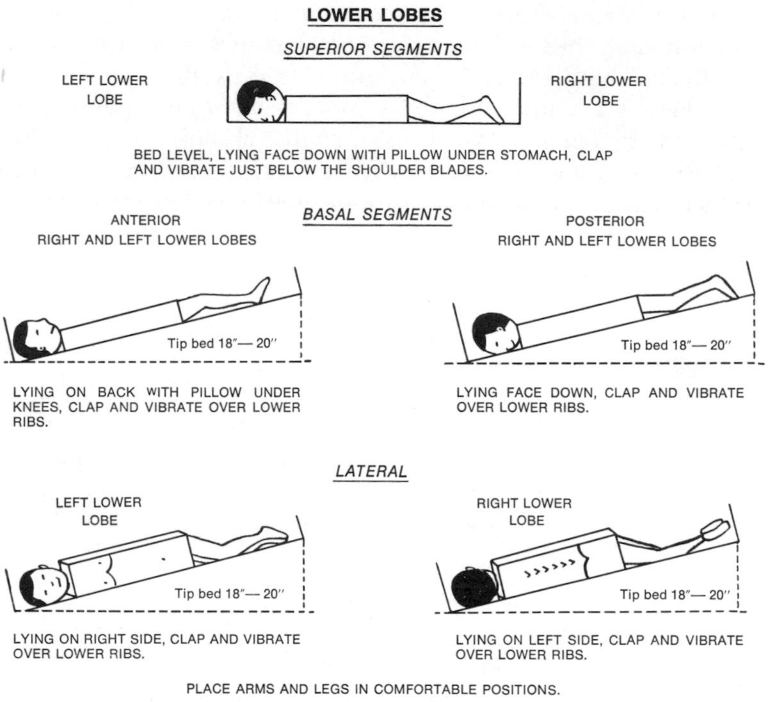

LOWER LOBES

SUPERIOR SEGMENTS

LEFT LOWER LOBE

RIGHT LOWER LOBE

BED LEVEL, LYING FACE DOWN WITH PILLOW UNDER STOMACH, CLAP AND VIBRATE JUST BELOW THE SHOULDER BLADES.

BASAL SEGMENTS

ANTERIOR RIGHT AND LEFT LOWER LOBES

Tip bed 18"— 20"

LYING ON BACK WITH PILLOW UNDER KNEES, CLAP AND VIBRATE OVER LOWER RIBS.

POSTERIOR RIGHT AND LEFT LOWER LOBES

Tip bed 18"— 20"

LYING FACE DOWN, CLAP AND VIBRATE OVER LOWER RIBS.

LATERAL

LEFT LOWER LOBE

Tip bed 18"— 20"

LYING ON RIGHT SIDE, CLAP AND VIBRATE OVER LOWER RIBS.

RIGHT LOWER LOBE

Tip bed 18"— 20"

LYING ON LEFT SIDE, CLAP AND VIBRATE OVER LOWER RIBS.

PLACE ARMS AND LEGS IN COMFORTABLE POSITIONS.

PROCEDURE FOR POSTURAL DRAINAGE

1. CLAP ABOUT A MINUTE IN EACH POSITION
2. VIBRATE DURING 5 EXHALATIONS; REST ON INHALATIONS
3. COUGH
4. REPEAT PROCEDURE IF SO ADVISED BY DOCTOR
5. DO 3 TIMES A DAY (UNLESS OTHERWISE ORDERED BY DOCTOR)
   A. MORNING — BEFORE BREAKFAST — DO UPPER, RIGHT, MIDDLE, AND LEFT LINGULA LOBES.
   B. MID-DAY — BEFORE LUNCH OR AFTER SCHOOL — DO RIGHT MIDDLE, LEFT LINGULA, AND LOWER LOBES.
   C. EVENING — BEFORE DINNER OR BEFORE BED — DO UPPER AND LOWER LOBES.

FIG. 13. *(cont.)*. Instruction sheets provide aid in teaching parents procedures to be done at home. Part II. (Adapted from design and material by Eloise Draper, LPT.; available from Pediatric Department of University of Louisville Medical School, Louisville, Kentucky.)

clines. During respiratory infections, anorexia is often present. Pancreatic extract is administered in granular or tablet form when the food is eaten. The dosage is adjusted according to the appearance of the stools; for example, unformed bulky, floating stools indicate more pancreatin is necessary. If excessive pancreatin is administered, anorexia and constipation may result. Skim milk is often advised until later childhood. Adolescents require less dietary restrictions as a whole. Fat-soluble vitamins in water-miscible base are required so that absorption can take place.

In hot weather it may be necessary to add extra salt to the diet. In emergency, saline solution may need to be administered intravenously.

Antibiotics are ordered by some physicians for treatment of a specific organism involved in an infection. Some authorities prefer intermittent intensive therapy. There is agreement that respiratory infections should be treated adequately and long enough to be effective.

An expectorant, such as saturated solution of potassium iodide, may be ordered. Codeine and similar cough suppressants are counterindicated.

Oxygen therapy is used with discretion. It may be required for hypoxia. If used with mist tent, concentration should be less than 40 percent and blood gases monitored.

Problems for the Family

What does the diagnosis of cystic fibrosis mean to the family? In the family in which this is the first case, it may be overwhelming or it may mean very little at first. The reaction will be dependent on their exposure to information through television, radio, newspapers, magazines, yearly drives to assist handicapped children, or experience with a child of a neighbor, friend, or relative with the disease.

For the family who does not realize the impact of the disease, the nurse should expect questions and concerns after the physician has talked with the family and after they have read about the disease or talked with relatives or friends.

For the nurse to appreciate the meaning of this illness to the family, one would have to consider the items below.

Present mortality statistics. If this child is diagnosed early and medical care and a health team are available for supervision and management, the outlook is brighter.

Effect of child's therapy on routine of the household. Learning what is involved in the treatments and acquiring skill in preventing or treating bronchopulmonary obstruction is necessary. Clapping and vibration is usually carried out four times a day before each meal and at bed time. For a mother with other children this is very demanding on her time and it affects household routine. This is only one aspect of the therapy that is time-consuming for her; it requires a great deal of energy and patience.

Need for special or improvised equipment in the home. The family must know how to maintain it and where to have it repaired.

Effect on sleeping arrangements. If space is limited, the mist tent and compressor may present special problems.

Sleep disturbance for other family members. This may particularly affect the mother who may listen for the cough or sleep lightly in order to hear the child if he calls.

Effect on visitors in the home. Whether it is relatives, neighbors, peers of the other siblings, or friends of the child involved, concern will be present in relation to problem of infection. Respiratory infection, pertussis, and measles in particular can prove very serious for the child with cystic fibrosis. The mother may need assistance so that visitors are not eliminated entirely. Stools are foul-smelling and incontinence may occur. Suggestions which will assist in control of odor of stools include: changing the infant's or toddler's diaper as soon after defecation as feasible; the use of a product available on the market for deodorizing the bathroom. Solutions are available to use in the water tank of the toilet which are automatically dispensed after flushing, for control of odor.

Effect on family outings. This may involve visiting relatives, weekend excursions, or yearly vacation plans. Now special equipment may need to be transported or planning ahead to know which city has a pediatrician or facilities available if needed in an emergency. In many instances, the family may eliminate these trips due to expense.

Effect on husband-wife relations. Concern over hereditary aspects, possible future pregnancies, as well as family budget may occur.

Willingness to accept financial assistance. Assistance may be necessary from welfare or state aid, if necessary, for special diet, cost of medicines, and equipment. One should consider the family's ability to accept services from the local chapter of the Cystic Fibrosis Research Foundation, if available in their community, or to acquire such services if in a small town.

Problem of travel. If medical facilities and special clinic are at a long distance from home, travel for the parents and obtaining a babysitter for other siblings can impose additional burdens.

Problem of finding a babysitter. They will need a babysitter who can manage the child and be trusted to make the right judgment so that parents can have an evening out together.

Perhaps this is only the beginning of the list, and you could add many more items.

Some points to remember in assisting the family from the beginning to begin to cope with the following factors.

Each member of the health team has a contribution to make. Each should be alert for cues about denial or acceptance of the disease. The clergyman may have an important role in assisting the family in terms of concern over mortality or guilt in relation to heredity.

Education and preparation for discharge begins early after admission. Begin slowly, provide demonstration and repetition. Continue presence of a skillful person at hand to take over in the beginning when necessary until parents are confident that they understand the regimen. The personality of each parent may determine the best approach.

A home visit by the nurse from the clinic or the community health nurse to assist in transition from hospital to home. It is becoming a more frequent practice for the community health nurse to come to the hospital prior to home visit to meet the child and to review the needs of the child and plan of care. Information should be shared with her to assist in planning.

Listening carefully to the parents to identify cues that will furnish insight to areas that need further discussion. For example, if the mother will tend to be oversolicitous, or if concern over the acquisition of infection is going to create a crisis in the household.

Knowledge of community facilities and services available to family. The nurse may need to refer the parents to the social worker or may acquire information needed from the social service agency and handle the problem herself. Another example is knowledge of some babysitting service often provided by nursing students or college students so that parents may have an evening out.

Keep channels of communication open between members of the health team. This is necessary so that needs of the child and family are being met to the extent possible. Parents may need assistance with other siblings. It has been observed that parents often are unwilling or unable to discuss the implications of cystic fibrosis or the disease itself with other children. Behavior problems can result due to emphasis on needs of the affected child.

Problems for the Child

The age of onset as well as the degree of pulmonary involvement will affect the problems for the child and his ability to cope with this chronic disease.

Considerations and activities that should be included in nursing care plan in the hospital or the home are noted below.

Provision of good oral hygiene. Saliva is more salty. With expectoration after postural drainage, oral care will provide comfort. Teeth may also become discolored from antibiotics and current studies on this matter are being carried out in dental schools.

Help the child accept the need for medications. Make them palatable when possible. Explain the purpose of each, if the child can understand. Use dolls for demonstration of the injection or the use of the space mask for inhalation if he is a preschooler. Iodides are more palatable if administered in grape or orange juice or a cola drink.

Sites for injections are always rotated. This is most important due to wasted gluteal muscles and decreased amount of adipose tissue.

Anorexia may be a sign of depression. This should be assessed carefully. History of likes and dislikes can provide some choice within the limitations of the diet. Eating with a group in the playroom may aid appetite. Effect of medications on appetite may need to be evaluated.

Weight loss. Weight loss and increased anterior-posterior diameter of the chest is a clue to progress of the disease.

Odor of stools. This should be combatted so that patients or other visitors do not make comments that would offend or embarrass the child and his family. Staff should air the room and request housekeeping to provide deodorizer. Aerosols or special deodorant products are available on the market that are effective for the household. In case of an infant or toddler, change the diaper as soon after the stool as possible. Care of the skin in the diaper area is important. Ointments should be applied as indicated. Bony prominences may need protection.

Temperature. If the temperature of the room is lower at night, the mist tent is more comfortable. Hyperthermia can result from the use of a mist tent in a hot room.

Shampoo is required frequently due to mist tent. The hair becomes sticky from various aerosols.

Increased oral fluid intake. This acts as an expectorant and should be included in the plan as a very simple tool to improve respiratory problem.

Repeating instructions. When instructing the child, keep in mind the short attention span of the younger age group. Repeat instructions to the child about breathing and coughing with a rhythmic approach.

Use of word games or funny stories. This makes the time seem shorter for the child during therapy for bronchopulmonary hygiene. Games for two, such as Old Maid or Parcheesi, are fun. Laughter helps the child breathe more deeply. Wind instruments are also effective.

Somersaults, hand stands, tumbling. These activities are appropriate to provide pulmonary drainage and are more attractive to the young child. In the hospital, a bicycle or work-out on a mat in the playroom or in physical therapy will provide needed activity for the child. Running and swimming are allowed as tolerated.

When the child returns to school, the teacher will need to understand the nature of the child's problem, the reason for his cough, and the problem of exposure to infections. If the cough is severe in the morning at home, the child may be absent until noon. Chill should be avoided. If there is a fire drill, a coat should be made available. Outdoor clothing should be put on just prior to leaving school to prevent overheating and perspiration. The nurse in the school or community can serve as liaison between home and school.

It should be pointed out to the teacher that physical activity is an important aid to preventing the accumulation of secretions in the lungs. Running and active play are more effective in raising sputum than any other form of therapy. Activity should be encouraged during recess period. If a large amount of mucus is present and coughing is severe, the child can be positioned on a straight chair which has been turned upside down and padded so that the child's head is lowered. A tilt board in the gymnasium is also effective. A supply of tissues and paper cups for expectoration of sputum should be available. The child should remain at home when coughing is excessive so that therapy can be evaluated.

The developmental needs of the child should be considered whether one is dealing with an infant, toddler, school-ager, or adolescent. Physical, mental, emotional, and social needs must be considered. Hobbies that will promote satisfaction within the limitations imposed by the disease will meet an important need. Music through use of records provides pleasure for many age groups.

Information about the Cystic Fibrosis Foundation should be provided. (A new pamphlet "Living with Cystic Fibrosis," a guide for the young adult, is now available as well as other material.) Through the local chapter of the Foundation, parents will have an opportunity to meet with parents of children with the same problem as well as to receive information about the disease and research being conducted.

A mother at one of the local meetings suggested that percussion and postural drainage be accompanied by music from a record player or radio. The rhythmic beat made the activity less tiring. Another suggestion for the older girl who is embarrassed when her friends ask her about the mist tent consists of using a four-poster bed with a canopy and draping long sheets of plastic to provide a tent.

Follow-up clinics for patients with cystic fibrosis provide the family with an opportunity to discuss problems with members of the health team as well as the reassessment of the therapy. These clinics also provide a source for teaching students in the health field. Treatment continues over an indefinite period and encouragement and support must be provided.

A Home Care Evaluation sheet provides a method of recording pertinent information so that the therapeutic plan can be studied and modified if necessary at the next clinic visit. This would be used after return to home after the first hospitalization or it may also be requested if the child was having recurring respiratory and gastrointestinal problems. There is hope for even greater improvement in the outlook for cystic fibrosis patients as the diagnosis is made earlier and effective treatment instituted. Continued research may also furnish new information for more effective management.

CASE PRESENTATION AND STUDY QUESTIONS

Barbara, ten years old, was admitted with status asthmaticus. Dyspnea, coughing, and wheezing were evident. Her orders included: arterial blood gases, correction of acid-base balance, steroid therapy, oxygen, and Isuprel by nebulizer. Barbara has been hospitalized previously on this same unit.

Consider the following questions in providing nursing care for Barbara:

1. What are some of the immediate actions of the nurse upon Barbara's admission?
2. What considerations should be given the immediate environment in Barbara's hospital room?
3. What types of play activity would be appropriate to provide after recovery from the acute stage?
4. What might the psychologic effects be of prolonged steroid therapy on a ten-year-old?

BIBLIOGRAPHY

Anderson CM: Long term study of patients with cystic fibrosis. Mod Probl Pediat 10:344, 1967

Barnett HL (ed): Pediatrics, 16th ed. New York, Appleton, 1977

Caplin I: The Allergic Asthmatic. Springfield, Ill, Thomas, 1968

Cole RB: Essentials of Respiratory Disease. Philadelphia, Lippincott, 1976

Di Sant' Agnese PA: Clinical findings and research in cystic fibrosis. Mod Probl Pediat 10:10, 1967

Falliers C: When to hospitalize the child with asthma. Hosp Pract 3:24, 1968

Fontana VJ: Practical Management of the Allergic Child. New York, Appleton, 1966

Gallagher JR, Heald F, Garell D: Medical Care of the Adolescent, 3rd ed. New York, Appleton, 1976

Holschaw DS: Common pulmonary complications of cystic fibrosis. Clin Pediatr 9:346, 1970

Horesh AJ: Allergy and infection. J Asthma Res 6:147, 1969

Horowitz L: Chronic obstructive bronchopulmonary disease in children with asthma. J Asthma Res 6:211, 1969

Howe PS: Basic Nutrition in Health and Disease, 6th ed. Philadelphia, Saunders, 1976

Johnson ME, Fassett BA: Bronchopulmonary hygiene in cystic fibrosis. Am J Nurs 69:320, 1969

Kendig EL (ed): Pulmonary Disorders, 2nd ed. Philadelphia, Saunders, 1972

———: Disorders of the Respiratory Tract in Children. Philadelphia, Saunders, 1968

Krause M, Hunschler M: Food Nutrition and Diet Therapy, 5th ed. Philadelphia, Saunders, 1972

Matthews LW: Morbidity and Mortality. Weekly Report, 24:78, 1975

———, Doershuk CF: Inhalation therapy and postural drainage for the treatment of cystic fibrosis. Bibl Paediatr 86:297–314, 1967

Rapaport HG: An allergist looks at chronic disease. J Asthma Res 7:3–6, 1969

Rapp D: Allergies and Your Child. New York, Holt, 1972

Robbins S, Angel M: Basic Pathology, 2nd ed. Philadelphia, Saunders, 1976

Rodman M, Smith D: Clinical Pharmacology in Nursing. Philadelphia, Lippincott, 1974

Rowe A: Food Allergy Its Manifestations and Control and the Elimination Diets. Springfield, Ill, Thomas, 1972

Scipien B, Howe P: Comprehensive Pediatric Nursing. New York, McGraw-Hill, 1975

Shwachman H, Khaw KT, Kowalski SM: The management of cystic fibrosis. Clin Pediatr 14:1115–18, 1975

Silver H, Kempe CH, Brwyn HB: Handbook of Pediatrics. Los Altos, California, Lange Medical Publ, 1975

Tempel CW: Tuberculosis prevention: the child-centered program. Am Fam Physician 37:99–104, May 1968

Travis, G: Chronic Illness in Children—Its Impact on Child and Family. Stanford, Calif, Stanford University Press, 1976

Vaughn V II, McKay RJ (eds): Nelson Textbook of Pediatrics, 10th ed. Philadelphia, Saunders, 1976

Wasserman, E, Slobody L: Survey of Clinical Pediatrics, 6th ed. New York, McGraw-Hill, 1974

Whaley LF: Understanding Inherited Disorders. St. Louis, Mosby, 1974

Wohl T: Current concepts of the asthmatic child's adjustment and adaptation to institutional care. J Asthma Res 7:41, 1969

SHIRLEY STEELE

8 Nursing Care of the Child with Congenital Anomalies and Developmental Disabilities

Improved health care supervision of childbearing women has resulted in earlier detection of problems. The high-risk pregnancy is now monitored by a variety of means such as sonograms, Oxytocin Challenge Tests (OCT), amniocentesis, and urinary excretion tests for estriol determination. This intensive surveillance of a pregnancy may result in the parents developing fears that the child will not be "normal." These fears were probably not as common prior to the institution of these techniques to study the fetus' progress in utero. The parents may develop realistic fears concerned with whether the pregnancy is of too great a risk to the woman or fetus to warrant its continuation. Each test that is done may be anxiety-provoking and the anxiety may be heightened or lessened by the test results. A test result that signals fetal distress may cause the woman to begin grieving for the "normal" child she hoped and planned for. A woman whose pregnancy has been progressing normally may have a sonogram late in the pregnancy to determine fetal size or position and learn that she has a placenta previa that is presently asymptomatic but is clearly diagnosed by the sonogram. This discovery helps with the monitoring and management of the pregnancy, but it will probably cause disbelief or dismay to the potential parents.

Whether the pregnancy was considered of high risk from conception or evolved as high risk during the process, many of the treatments are the same. There will need to be changes in the woman's lifestyle that will help to promote the best possible outcome from the pregnancy. She may need to make alterations in the amount of activity she can have, alter her dietary patterns, make changes in employment or recreational activities, make revised arrangements for other children, alter her relationship with her sexual partner, or make arrangements for the possibility of additional financial considerations. The way the woman is able to cope with these changes in her lifestyle will be assessed by the nurse so that she/he can help to support the woman through the immediate crisis and help to enable her to manage the potential crises that may occur such as a premature delivery, a surgical procedure, or an infant born with a disability or inability to survive.

Because many of the children who have congenital anomalies or developmental disabilities are the result of premature births, a short discussion of this topic will now be presented.

When labor begins prematurely, the family is not prepared. Depending on the length of gestation, the early delivery predisposes the infant to potential hazards. The hospital staff and family are faced with the situational crisis which surrounds the birth of an infant before its expected date of arrival. Aguilera and Messick (1974) state,

> Researchers have identified four phases or tasks the mother must work through if she is to come out of the experience in a healthy way.
>
> 1. She must realize that she may lose the baby. This anticipatory grief involves a gradual withdrawal from the relationship already established with the child during the pregnancy.
> 2. She must acknowledge failure in her maternal function to deliver a full-term baby.
> 3. After separation from the infant due to its prolonged hospital stay she must resume her relationship with it in preparation for the infant's homecoming.
> 4. She must prepare herself for the job of caring for the baby through an understanding of its special needs and growth patterns" (pp 67–68).

Caplan (1964) suggests that the mothers who were more distressed when the infant was in danger were actually dealing with the stress in an effective manner. The mothers who were less concerned were actually the ones who were closer to a crisis situation.

According to Aguilera and Messick, a crisis is defined as the point at which a person cannot solve a problem using his established coping mechanisms. As a result, his anxiety is heightened and tension is aroused. He finds himself mentally upset and unable to problem solve. Crisis intervention is essential to aid the person in his return to a normal equilibrium. Crisis intervention is viewed as short-term, inexpensive help focused directly on the problem that precipitates the crisis. The reader is referred to the original book for the excellent in-depth explanation of the process of crisis intervention. An understanding of the process is essential to the nursing process.

The stress or crisis of prematurity is a major problem for the mother to solve. If it is broadened by the child being disabled, it poses a potentially greater crisis. The increasing emphasis on establishing support systems for the family is based on the knowledge that these two situational crises can be potentially devastating to the family. In addition to the effects on the mother, there is evolving evidence that fathers are indirectly affected by these situations as there is a higher incidence of divorce in families with handicapped children. It is important to facilitate the early mother-child and father-child bonding by allowing interaction as early and as frequently as possible.

"It is the mother who 'produces' the infant, it is she who 'gives' it birth. If the 'product' turns out to be defective (a term used here to include all defects in the child, whether physical or intellectual), the mother perceives this as a defect in something she has produced" (Ross, 1964, p 56). The mother who delivers in the hospital may have her feelings of defeat reinforced by the hospital staff. The maternity unit is generally considered a "happy" unit. Fortunately, most of the events taking place here result in a new life and a fulfillment of a goal for the child's parents. The child with a defect is not an ordinary part of the unit and, therefore, the staff's care for this child is not ordinary. Joyful overtones are not appropriate at this birth. As a result, the staff frequently withdraws and does not give the mother the support she needs to cope with the birth of a child with a defect.

"The mother is thrust into the stark reality very soon after the birth. The father, because of his less active role in the birth and immediate post delivery period can deny the situation longer than the mother. The father also is able to fall back on the defensive fantasy that the child is not really his own" (Ross, p 56).

The nursing personnel in the delivery room have a vital role to play in the beginning of the coping process. The nurse must be especially careful of her/his facial expressions. Even the forehead above the surgical mask can give nonverbal clues that something is wrong. Withholding the infant from the mother's sight is another way of saying that your child is "less than expected." If the mother has actively participated in the labor and delivery process, she will be most anxious to view the child immediately after birth. It is only fair to prepare her for the child with its defect and show her the child, briefly. The silence which frequently prevails during this crisis period is most anxiety-producing to the mother. She may very well imagine a much more severely handicapped child than her infant. This needless anxiety may influence the future mother-child relationship. In addition, it may lead to the mother's mistrusting the medical and nursing personnel in whom she will need to have confidence during the long-term care of the child.

In some hospitals, the doctors prefer to talk with the father prior to telling the mother about the child. If this is the chosen plan, the mother must be given close nursing supervision to make her feel personally comfortable. At least, this physical comfort will help her to relax. The sooner the mother is told, the easier it will be to begin to help her plan for the child in a constructive way.

After the announcement has been made to the parents, many different defense mechanisms may be utilized by the parents. The mother is usually more subject to them than the father. Some of these defense mechanisms are described by Ross (1964) and are summarized briefly here. She may choose to repress the incident, trying to keep the handicapped child out of her conscious awareness. She may utilize projection, trying to treat the child as though it had its source outside herself. She may utilize sublimation whereby she represses the impulse until it can be changed from a socially objectionable to a socially valued outlet. She may use intellectualization whereby she controls affects and impulses through thinking about them instead of experiencing them. Another possibility is displacement which can involve aggressive impulses against the self. Another mechanism is controlling; this allows her to interfere with suggestions or attempts of others, or allows her to comply without thinking. Denial is a very commonly utilized mechanism; it allows the mother to keep threatening perceptions from coming to the surface. Withdrawal is a mechanism which may occur as a temporary and immediate response to threat and usually lasts only until she is able to bring another defense mechanism into play.

An understanding of the possible mechanisms the mother can use will help us to plan nursing intervention effectively. The mechanism of withdrawal is frequently utilized immmediately after delivery. It can be expressed by desire to sleep. This can be very beneficial for the mother. There is no need to try to talk her out of it. She needs rest following the labor and delivery. She also needs sleep to aid in developing strength to deal with the resultant stress produced by delivering an infant with a disability.

It is important to remember that the use of defense mechanisms aids our daily living and their usage is normal during crisis periods. The assistance the mother receives can turn these defense mechanisms into useful tools for coping with the unique problems she will have to face. The use of denial, for instance, is not abnormal at first. However, its persistence can be abnormal. How, then, can the nurse help the mother to relinquish the use of denial? One way is to show the infant to the mother early. The infant should be exposed to the mother while the nurse is available. The mother should explore the child slowly and carefully. She should be encouraged to ask questions. The nurse must watch the mother closely to interpret her tolerance level. If it is evident the mother cannot benefit from further time with the infant and nurse, then the session should be terminated. A new time should be set up for the mother to see the infant again. Perhaps viewing the child in the nursery can help to prepare the mother for the next visit. Rooming-in should not be discouraged unless the infant is severely handicapped and needs vigilant observation. The less severely handicapped infant may benefit greatly by being close to his mother's side so that when she feels the urge to see and handle the infant, she can do so. The policies governing many maternity areas sometimes interfere with the optimum times at which the mother feels ready to have her child. Rooming-in can circumvent this problem. The concept of family-centered maternity care is being implemented slowly.

Following the birth of an infant, the mother undergoes a period of time when she relates to the infant in terms of who he looks like. This is a short period of time that aids in the mother's task of establishing maternal identity. It is hypothesized that mothers of infants with defects are hampered in their process of establishing maternal identity. It is felt that these mothers have a decreased ability to cope with an infant if there is any kind of stress during the pregnancy or during the child's early life. A child with a defect is frequently a product of a stressful pregnancy and is an additional source of stress at birth. Mothers have reported shock, anxiety, and hostility towards their children with defects. These reactions interfere with the mother's ability to establish ties with the infant.

To help alleviate denial, the mother must learn to love the infant first and then to cope with the accompanying defect. Acceptance of the defect is an extremely difficult process. Therefore, to learn to cope with it is a more realistic goal.

The more natural the periods of time the mother and infant spend together, the easier the process of adjustment will be for both of them. Special care necessary for the infant should be introduced slowly. The mother cannot be expected to assume responsibility for these procedures until she has had appropriate orientation and practice. When the mother finally is able to assume the responsibility for these procedures, her denial of the infant's condition is usually lessened or alleviated.

Ross (1964) states that "religious attitudes" may offer rationalizations whereby the child with a disability comes to be viewed as a special sign of grace, for only the most worthy of mothers would be "entrusted" with the care of a handicapped child. This is but one variable that can influence the mother's reaction to her infant. The verbal responses of the mother may give clues to her real feelings regarding the infant. However, her verbal responses may be conditioned by her background or her family rather than by her true feelings. Let me illustrate by examples. The mother may have religious beliefs that all children are a gift of God. As such, she feels she must be satisfied with her infant despite her disappointment. Her statements might be, "It is God's will," or "If God has chosen me to raise this baby, I will."

Another conditioned response might be in relation to old wives tales such as, "I expected the child to be affected because I was scared during a thunderstorm." This comment not only indicates an attempt to find a reason for the handicap but also represents a conditioned response elicited by family and acquaintances. The mother's true feelings are not unleashed in the statements. A nurse's response might be, "It is difficult to understand the reasons for an infant being born with a handicap. It is also normal to be disappointed." It is probably not the appropriate time to deal with misconceptions about the old wives' tales at this moment. This can easily be handled during future interactions.

The impact of this birth is extremely personal and individaulized and no set plan of care will meet the mother's needs. The nurse needs to be alert for clues and to act appropriately. For instance, the mother may ask the nurse if she has ever seen another infant with this defect. The nurse needs to show her/his concern for the infant and then to answer the question. An example would be, "I know you are concerned about your infant's cleft lip and I can certainly appreciate your concern." The rest of the response depends on the nurse's past experience. If the mother seems to need assurance that other infants have had the condition, the nurse can reply that she/he has studied the condition but has not had any personal experience with it. She/he can also refer the mother to someone who has had the experience.

Thus far, the discussion has focused on infants that will be expected to survive the immediate postdelivery period. In keeping with this category, mention needs to be made of the guilt a parent feels for the birth of an infant with a defect. In addition, the mother begins a mourning process for the normal child she expected to deliver. This mourning process progresses from the initial phase of numbness and disbelief, to the dawning awareness of the disappointment and feeling of loss with the accompanying affective and physical symptoms, to the last stage of the grief reaction in which intense reexperiencing of the memories and expectations gradually reduce the hypercathexis of the wish for the idealized child (Solnit and Stark, 1961).

This mourning process is a very important part of the postdelivery period. Mourning is a strenuous process and it leaves very little energy for the person to deal with other activites of daily life. The timing of this is crucial as it happens right after the stress situation of birth. The imposition of too many crisis situations at the same time makes it extremely difficult for the person to regain equilibrium. It should also be noted that this mother is now extremely vulnerable. It will take less to upset her than it would ordinarily. Her ways of handling past stress situations will also play a big part in her adjustment to this crisis situation.

The mother needs time to work through her own feelings. Frequently, a medical social worker can be instrumental in helping her with this process. The social worker will also be a welcomed member to the professional team during the period of long-term care. Caplan (1959) states that it is a very difficult thing for a family, particularly for a mother, to deal with a child who has a congenital anomaly or a birth injury. If she is left on her own she is very likely to develop a disturbed relationship with the child and so compound his difficulty. In keeping with this same concept, I believe it is extremely important to have a community health nursing referral made immediately after the birth. This will give the community health nurse the opportunity to visit the hospital, talk with the mother, and consult with the professional staff. The interdisciplinary team is needed to help the family get the very best care and guidance for the child.

DISCHARGE

Mother and Infant

The trend toward early discharge of maternity patients lessens the period available for the mother to adapt to her situation prior to discharge. This early discharge can be beneficial in reuniting her with her more normal home situation. However, it also means that responsibility for normal tasks can be added to her already overburdened backlog of emotionally charged tasks. The community health nurse can plan visits to give the mother an opportunity to talk. The visit usually provides the mother with an excuse to sit down and relax. As time passes, the mother is usually in a better position to begin to manage the problems which will result from the child's disability. All of the information given the mother during her confinement will probably need to be reviewed. It is natural that she will be able to ask more intelligent questions as she begins the normal care of the child. She may need encouragement to bathe the child and handle him. Her normal maternal instincts to care for the child may be overshadowed by her fear of the defect. If the defect necessitates a change in bathing techniques, the nurse can demonstrate the altered bath. An example of this might be a child discharged with an untreated meningomyelocele. With her other children, the mother has used a small plastic bath tub. The baby seemed to enjoy being bathed in the shallow water. With her handicapped child, she is hesitant to use this comfortable method, so she does not bathe the infant. The nurse demonstrates proper handling of the child and bathing with a sponge or washcloth. A protective shield is placed below the meningomyelocele. A small piece of plastic or saran wrap can serve this purpose (Fig. 1). During the bath demonstration the the nurse emphasizes the need to prevent pressure on the sac. She/he tells the mother to observe for drainage and to report it to her doctor. She/he demonstrates the proper positioning after the bath, placing the infant on its abdomen rather than its back. If the lesion is very large the sac may need support by sandbags on each side of the infant. The infant's head should be turned to the side and the usual precautions taken to avoid suffocation. This is especially important as the infant may have a decrease in motor control. Care of the child with a myelomeningocele is covered in greater detail later in the chapter.

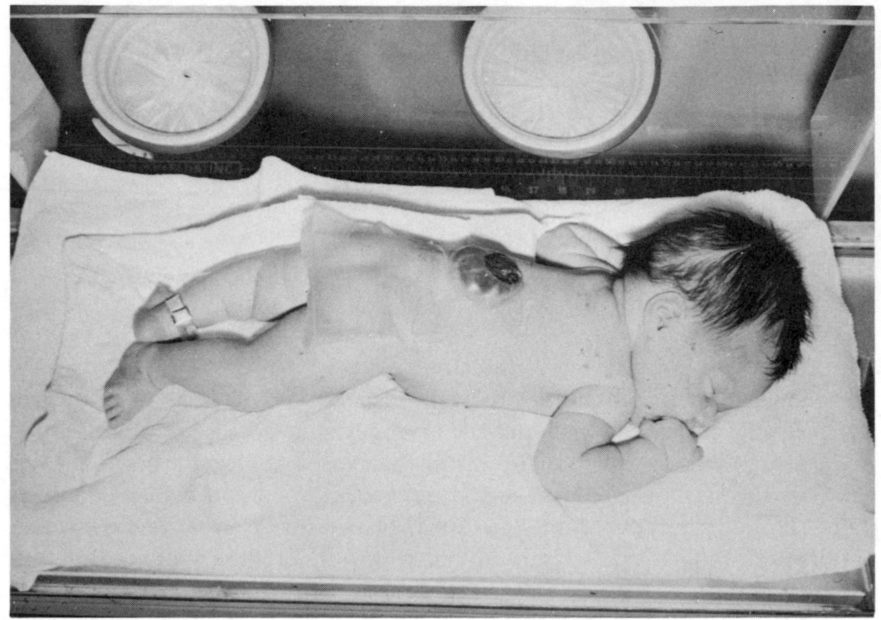

FIG. 1. Protective shield placed below the meningomyelocele of an infant.

The reactions of others to the infant will influence the mother's reactions. It is very difficult to form positive feelings when everyone else seems repelled by the situation. The nurse is in a perfect position to provide one positive response. In order to be most effective, the nurse needs to work through her/his own feelings regarding the defect. There is no guarantee that she/he will not be repelled by the situation. The nurse should view the infant alone before viewing it with the mother present, if this is possible. Then she/he will have an opportunity to "see beyond the defect" to view the infant as an individual. Focusing on the child as a person first and on his handicap later is an important part of learning how to cope with disabilities.

A situation involving the birth of a child with a cleft lip provides a good example to illustrate an appropriate positive response on the part of the nurse. When an infant is born, the cleft becomes a barrier to the normal tendency for the mother to kiss and hug the child. The nurse can demonstrate acceptance by warmly hugging the child. This close association accompanied by endearing words can be very reassuring to the mother. After cuddling the child and smiling warmly, the nurse can return the infant to the mother's arms. A statement such as , "You must be eager to know what the doctors can offer your baby" will be useful in determining the mother's readiness for information and need for support.

It is important to realize that the extent of the defect has little bearing on the response of people. Even a very small defect such as an extra digit can cause grave concern. The nurse should not attempt to predetermine the amount of concern the family will have for any defect. The impact of any defect, no matter how small or large, can be determined only by direct association with the parent. Each parent will have an individualized reaction.

Mother Without Infant

Early discharge of the mother often necessitates the separation of mother and infant. The infant may not be ready for discharge because of the anomaly. This presents a different set of problems. A community health nurse referral is still essential. The nurse is then able to visit the mother prior to the infant's discharge.

The nurse is able to evaluate how the mother is coping with the separation from her new offspring. She/he is also able to start evaluating how the mother is readjusting to her family. The period prior to the infant's discharge can be effectively utilized to provide the mother with opportunities to grieve for the normal child she expected and to derive satisfaction from the child she delivered.

The nurse should refer to the child by name to emphasize to the mother that she has another child. The referral to the infant and the problems connected with the infant help to bring the infant into the mainstream of the family. If the infant is not included in the conversation, separation will provide the mother with an excellent opportunity to deny the existence of the problem and perhaps even the existence of the infant.

Separation can be effectively utilized to give the mother an opportunity to recover from the crisis, created by birth, prior to assuming the responsibility for the infant's care. However, the separation period should be enriched by regular visits to the hospital to see the child. The mother should be given the opportunity to hold and perhaps feed the infant. In this way, she will begin to know her child while someone else is assuming the primary responsibility for the child's care. The father should be encouraged to visit the child with the mother. The importance of the bonding process of the father and infant is only just beginning to be given consideration. In addition, he is usually able to provide support for the mother. At the same time, he will also begin to appreciate the added responsibilities he will have because of the infant.

The mother discharged without her only child may feel a real emptiness. She expects a reward for her labor and delivery. Going home empty-handed does not fulfill her expectations. She may long for her infant just to talk to. The nurse can help by visiting and breaking up the long empty hours. The mother who has young children may find her days less empty, but adult companionship is very important during trying hours. The other children are too busy with their own lives and regaining their mother's attention. They do not show concern for their new brother or sister, probably because they do not really realize the child exists. Even if they do, they may not want the child and they may be secretly delighted that the child did not come home.

It is very important for the mother to receive progress reports from the hospital. These reports can be given by the doctor, the nurse, or the clergy. All are in a position to offer the mother information from their own special vantage point. The doctor is obviously the one responsible for keeping her up-to-date in relation to the medical plans and the infant's prognosis. The nurse is in the best position to keep her informed of the infant's eating, his weight gain, how he is sleeping, and any developmental milestones he surpasses. Mothers appreciate knowing that their infant yawns when he is finished eating, or he sucks on his fist, or his one lock of hair curls. These are the very personal things which help the mother identify with the infant as a person. The clergy provides a dimension that none of the previous information grants. Somehow a clergyman has an "extended power" which gives solace to a person who "believes." When he calls and just says, "I saw Danny today," it provides a source of "higher" quality. His visit and his call are an important part of mother's readjustment to a normal routine.

If possible, a time should be arranged with the mother, by each of the professionals, so she does not get needlessly apprehensive when the phone rings. It is human nature to expect the calls from the hospital to be "bad news." If she becomes anxious by the ring she may not be able to benefit from the messages planned to reduce her anxiety.

The longer the infant remains hospitalized, the more difficult it may be to help the mother build a relationship with her infant. It is important to stress the positive aspects of the infant's being united with the family, as soon as possible. Otherwise the mother may begin to feel that the infant "would be better off in a home." This statement gives the nurse the opportunity to discuss the pros and cons of institutionalization. Depending on the seriousness of the anomaly, the nurse can discuss with the mother the benefits the infant will derive from being with his own family. She/he can also familiarize the mother with the agencies and institutions in the community that help with her particular problem. Parents must be the ones who decide whether the infant will be institutionalized and at what point in his development.

Children born with congential anomalies are born with varying degrees of handicap. The anomaly may cause severe interference with function or it may be so subtle that at first glance it seems insignificant. The handicap may be so subtle at birth that it is not recognized, such as minimal cerebral dysfunction. While the information in Chapter 3 applies here, there are also additional considerations when one is caring for the child born with a congenital anomaly or developmental disabilities. Some of these factors also apply to other long-term conditions, but they are included here as they have such a vital role to play with these conditions.

Olshansky (1962) points out that parents of children with handicaps have varying degrees of capability in handling the child over their lifespan. The parents' ability to handle the situation coincides with significant milestones in the child's development. The child born with cerebral palsy may be a great shock to the parents. The initial shock is cushioned when the child survives the initial critical period after delivery. The child learns to suck after practice and patience and begins to gain weight. The parents receive satisfaction from their child's physical progress. They begin to question whether the original diagnosis of cerebral palsy is legitimate. The parents have two older children and they have a fairly good memory about their development. When Barry does not sit up at six months, they relate this to his rough start. At nine months Barry still does not sit up and they become aware that he is much slower than their other children. At twelve months their disappointment is very evident. They are reminded of the diagnosis and they are made painfully aware of their child's problem. At this point in time, the parents are less likely to function as effectively as when a crisis is not present. At the next major developmental milestone they may again be reminded of the diagnosis. This continues over the child's life cycle. Some of the milestones may be more "pain producing" than others. These might be the milestones of going to regular school, or late adolescence when the child should be planning marriage.

There are other factors which may interfere with the parents' ability to cope with the handicap, such as the repeated "threats" of surgery or the fear of progression of the condition.

The professional personnel should be alert to these check points and make themselves readily available to the parents. It may only take a talk with the social worker or the listening ear of the nurse to help the parents over these hurdles.

Parent Education

Another important factor to remember in caring for children with anomalies is to be sure that the parent is considered as an integral and vital member of the team. The parent needs to know exactly what they are or are not expected to do. Frequently therapies are provided and their lack of carry-over into the home is the result of neglect on the professional personnel's part to teach the parents what to do. The young child spends the majority of the time at home. The child with a severe anomaly spends an even greater amount of time in the home. To guarantee maximum function for the child, the home must provide the milieu to learn and grow.

A reassessment of the needs of parents and infants with disabilities resulted in a movement to establish early stimulation programs. Early stimulation programs must focus on strengthening the mother or parenting role. The curriculum includes developmental assessment, feeding techniques and behavior, nutritional guidance, techniques for developing sensory and motor skills, and behavior shaping techniques. The early institution of programs capitalizes on the most significant period of growth. (Godfrey and Eddington, 1975). A significant benefit of these programs is that the child is not developing poor habits that are difficult to break by the time he would reach the age when he would normally be entered in school.

Children with severe anomalies also need periodic reevaluation so the parents have an up-to-date report of their assets. The parents also need help in determining when to push for new developments. The child with cerebral palsy may have gross motor deficiency. The mother learns to expect the child to be slower than her other children. She continues to feed the child without reevaluating to see if the child is maturing enough to begin the developmental task of self-feeding. During the occupational therapy or nursing reevaluation, the child is fitted with a feeding device, the involuntary movements of the other extremities are controlled by especially prepared weights, the child is placed in a comfortable chair with a feeding tray, and a bib is applied. The child is given pureed food and encouraged to feed himself. His efforts are rewarded and encouraged by praise. He is allowed to continue feeding himself until he seems to be tiring or becoming too frustrated. A little frustration is healthy to encourage learning in the child with a disabled body as well as in the child with an able body.

After the reevaluation of the child, the parent is given specific realistic goals to achieve before the next clinic visit. In the interim, the mother is encouraged to telephone when she has a question.

School: Regular or Special?

Most of the discussion surrounding children with handicaps is to "mainstream" them in regular classrooms.

The question posed in this section is probably too narrow a consideration for this edition. The question should have been posed as a philosophical one, "Is education a right for all human beings?" Goldberg and Lippman (1974), remind us that the idea of the right to education was expressed by Horace Mann in 1864. Despite legal milestones to encourage this movement, many children with serious handicaps are still being excluded from the formal educational process. Goldberg and Lippman view education as a "continuous process of developing life skills (or physical, emotional, and social survival skills) needed for effective coping with developmental tasks and demands, as well as with the environmental tasks and demands" (p 330). They state, "The process of education, so defined, takes place through some structured or deliberate efforts and some accidental teaching-learning situations and through educational agencies in our society other than schools" (p 330). They caution that if education is a basic right then children, adolescents and probably some adults who were previously excluded because they did not have academic potential or the ability to learn basic skills of daily living will be admitted into special education settings. Goldberg and Lippman hypothesize that the entry of such persons into the system will result in an interaction of special educators with, "More desperate and confused families of the severely handicapped than we knew before" (p 332). The charge to special educators and their health professional colleagues will be how to normalize the life space of these families who have seriously handicapped members.

In order to achieve this normalization goal, well-defined goals will have to be developed by the team utilizing the school and home to provide quality education at the child's level of development.

The answer to the question of school for the child with an anomaly is not an easy one. The teachers will need to be fully aware of any special needs of the child. The child with more severe handicaps will probably attend a special school for the handicapped. Some school systems do not have special facilities available and the children will have to be bussed long distances. The children may even have to be transported by the parents, which places an additional strain on the family.

Children who attend special schools have the benefit of competing with other children with handicaps (Fig. 2). However, this does not realistically prepare them to function in the more diversified society at large. It is true that some of the children with more severe handicaps may never be capable of competing at this level. Their potential for achievement may well be restricted to "sheltered workshops" or living within a family or in an institution. The special class may adequately prepare them for these roles.

When the special classes are all located in the same building, the teachers have the benefit of sharing teaching methods with one another. When the classes are spread singly or in some clusters in several areas, the teachers may find it more difficult to share teaching ideas with other teachers of the handicapped. There is one other complicating item inherent in special education; that is, when children are cast in a particular mold, their achievements are frequently based on the expectations of that mold. Frequently, this decreases the amount of stimulation the child receives.

The child who attends a regular class may be so different from the other children that he is given special privileges. Or he may be laughed at or ridiculed by the other children who do not understand the child's differences. Being an outsider can severely hamper his opportunities to learn.

Architectural barriers may determine where a child can attend regular

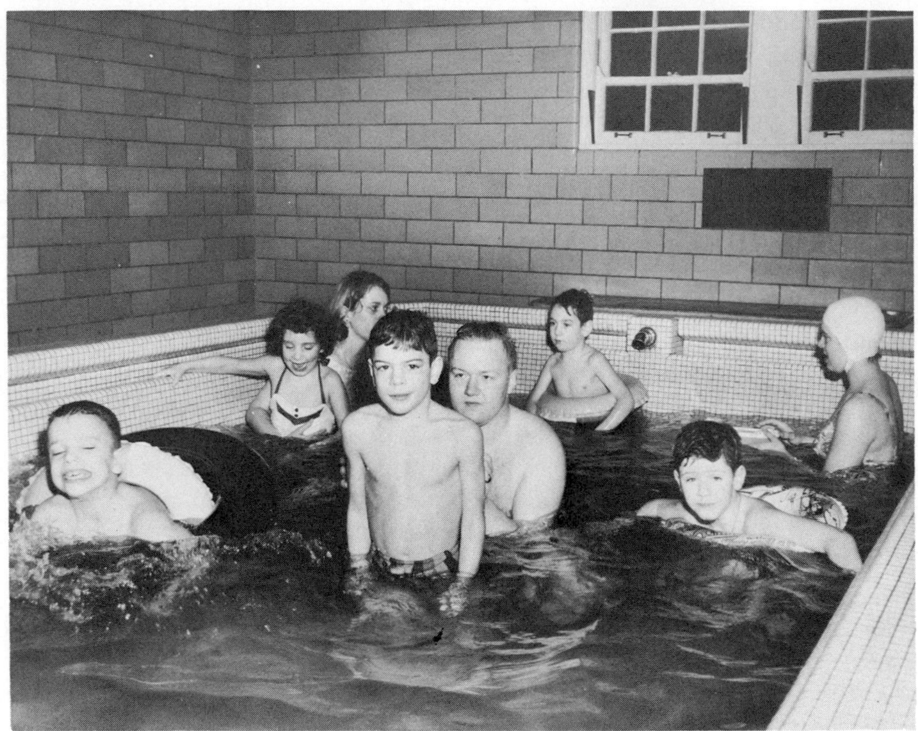

FIG. 2. These handicapped children enjoy the swimming pool at the Children's Rehabilitation Center, the Children's Hospital of Buffalo, N.Y. They are assisted by college student volunteers, all future teachers of exceptional children.

school. A child with two lower-limb prostheses may have to attend a school for the handicapped because he cannot sufficiently negotiate the many stairs in an old school building. If the stairs were not so steep, a regular school placement would have been far superior as the child would be given credit for his assets rather than focusing on his defects, which are adequately corrected. Programs focusing on removing architectural barriers are springing up around the country.

Human Sexuality Education

The early nurturing process sets the stage for positive early education in the area of human sexuality. The parents are role models for their children. They begin fostering healthy concepts about human sexuality by showing positive responses to each other and by their responses of love and affection toward their children.

During the childhood years the child is encouraged to take on increasing independence in thought and action. His questions regarding sexuality are answered simply and honestly. He is inquisitive about the growth process including questions about pregnancy as well as the end of life. He must be given factual information about the differences between the sexes. During the school years he is presented information about his potential body changes with special emphasis on the physical and emotional changes which he will have to cope with. The child will need special emphasis on any adaptations which will have to be made due to his or her disability, such as special considerations for menstruation in a girl with paralysis of the lower trunk.

The child who has received consistent information and has developed a good self-concept will be well prepared for the adolescent period when the needs of human sexuality may include the selection of a wife or husband and the special sexual responses of that relationship. If the adolescent does not choose to marry, he still requires the same information, so he can make intelligent decisions about his sexual experiences.

The sexual experiences of the disabled individual are worthy of considerable attention by the health professionals responsible for their care. Depending of the degree of disability, they may have to use methods other than sexual intercourse as alternate means of sexual gratification. They need to be presented with information about themselves that will help them to understand why the alternatives are necessary. Alternatives that may be suggested are oral-genital sex or caressing and petting. They should be given sources for obtaining vibrators and stimulators and materials that deal factually and pictorially with their situation—books, for example, that illustrate how to adapt the human sexual experience so as to achieve a mutually positive experience for themselves.

A much greater emphasis is being placed on meeting the sexual needs of disabled persons. In the past, they have been encouraged to ignore their desires for sexual gratification. Now they are being encouraged and facilitated in their desire to have similar sexual experiences to their able-bodied peers. The way they will respond to these new challenges will depend a great deal on how society responds to their actions. Many people still ignore or cannot accept the idea that disabled individuals should have the same rights as themselves. They tend to feel that their sexual drives should not be encouraged but should be discouraged. Listening to individuals with disabilities discuss the value of a positive sexual relationship with another caring adult only strengthens the position that they should have the type of experience that best meets their desire to fulfill a productive life. As beautifully stated by one person with a serious physical disability, "I deeply value each sexual experience as they do not come easily to me. From my vantage point I cannot understand how anyone can take the sexual response of another adult lightly."

The newer trend toward sexuality will lead to the nurse assuming the responsibility of knowing how to respond in a variety of situations. A male child with an ileal conduit may ask if he can ever get married. His question is probably much broader than that. He may wonder if anyone with a "rose bud on his belly" can show this to anyone of the opposite sex or if he can have intercourse when his penis is not used to urinate. A girl, paralyzed in an auto accident, may wonder how she will know when she is in labor if she gets pregnant or what type of contraceptive to use. An adolescent with cerebral palsy may wonder how to have a positive sexual response when his muscles are so spastic. A mother may ask how to tell her child with developmental lag that she cannot undress for a male stranger who makes advances at her without at the same time suggesting she can never share in a sexual relationship with a man. An adolescent preparing for marriage may ask how to do "a stuffing procedure" for his limp penis to penetrate his wife's vagina despite his lower trunk paralysis.

The best way to be prepared for these situations is to first come to grips with your own sexuality. It is then possible to feel comfortable in discussing other people's sexual needs. One cannot help another person if one is uncomfortable and tense talking about the subject. It is also important to understand your own limitations and to seek assistance from others and the literature when you are in doubt. It is valuable to keep in touch with persons with disabilities and have them help by explaining how they have satisfactorily achieved their human sexuality goals. It is well to keep counseling sessions on a professional level and to discourage joking or self-demeaning comments and examples. The concerns of the patient must be dealt with so that they will not interfere with their potential for self-actualization. In addition, they must be helped to realize that even though they desire an active sex life, it may not be easy to obtain, just as it is not always attainable by their able-bodied peers.

As with the able-bodied individual, the disabled find the act of masturbation a pleasurable experience. They will benefit from knowing that many parts of the body can be stroked, touched, and manipulated to provide pleasurable sensual experiences. The parents are frequently very distressed by their child's discovery that masturbation is a satisfying experience. The parents need to be helped to understand that much of the stigma surrounding this activity has been removed. Most of all they need to know that masturbation is not harmful and there is "nothing wrong" with their child if he explores his own body to help bring himself sexual gratification.

The sexual capabilities of the child with developmental lag deserve special consideration. The process will focus on helping the child deal with his feelings. Many of these children are prone to outbursts of temper and negative behavior. Their acting out results in reprimands or punishment. The child is helped to develop good feelings about himself through positive experiences with other children and adults. When he does not respond in appropriate ways he is shown alternative ways of responding. One modality for teaching these children more acceptable ways of handling is behavior modification which is covered in the chapter on emotional conditions of childhood.

The child with developmental lag has been described as being without sexual drives or, at the other end of the spectrum, to be over-sexed. These descriptions have served to malign the person with this disability. They frequently have the same requirements for positive human responses, but they are less mature developmentally in expressing their sexuality.

The mother who is developmentally retarded will have special needs that relate to her own sexual requirements as well as to the nurturing needs of the child. The mother will need counseling and guidance to be certain that she is not using the child only to meet her own needs. She frequently sees the child as a means to satisfy her own sexual drives and to decrease the loneliness which is often associated with the adult who is developmentally retarded. This is more likely to be prevalent in mothers who are not living with their spouses.

The goal of human sexuality education should be to provide warm interpersonal relationships consistent with the client's maturational level. The sexual experiences should be viewed in the broadest sense as any experience which is related to womanliness or manliness. To be most beneficial the education will continue throughout the life span. The human sexuality requirements of the physically and mentally disabled are best summed up in the title of a magnificent film on the subject, "Like Other People."

EXAMPLES OF DEFECTS AND NURSING INTERVENTION

Other chapters in the book also deal with possible congenital or acquired defects. Therefore, the areas of heart, diabetes, and cystic fibrosis will not be included in this chapter. The magnitude of these problems necessitates chapters dealing specifically with the topics. Further, I will not attempt to cover all the conditions which require long-term care but rather some of the more common conditions.

Hypospadias

> Hypospadias is a relatively common congenital anomaly of the penis, occurring once in 2,400 live male births . . . Hypospadias is an abnormal opening of the urethra, frequently on the underside of the penis. It may vary in degree from a minor shift in the opening to such a complex malformation that the sex of the child is questionable. The penile shaft distal to the hypospadiac meatus is angulated ventrally. This aspect of the deformity is termed "chordee" (King, 1967, p 1097).

The impact of this condition on the parents can be almost devastating. The reproductive organs of the male child are usually a highly emotionally charged subject for the parents. They may possibly have some knowledge of this condition from past experience. Although the condition does not follow a strict Mendelian inheritance, it does run a familial pattern in families.

The defect makes it impractical to circumcise the infant. This may be very upsetting to the parents, especially if they belong to the Jewish faith, in which religious ritual is connected with circumcision.

The nurse in the newborn nursery can easily detect the variance in voiding pattern. It is her/his astute observation regarding frequency of voiding, amount of voiding, and difficulty in voiding that may alert the physician to additional defects.

Although fathers are usually able to conceal their concern for children with defects until school age, it has been my experience that they are very concerned when their son is born with a hypospadias. They frequently ask the question, "Will he be able to marry and have children?" The mother may ask more immediate-type questions, such as, "Can it be repaired?" and "What did I do to cause it?"

After a period of observation, the infant can be discharged home without any specialized care. The time for the surgery will vary with the physician. The surgical procedures are done to straighten the penis by release of chordee, and subsequent operations to construct a cylinder of buried skin to serve as a urethra. This may be accomplished in one or more stages (King, 1969, p 1099). The opinion concerning optimal age of the child for repair also varies with physicians. It is usually planned to try to complete the repairs before school age. This will permit the child to void in the normal standing position, if the condition was severe enough to interfere with this normal process. If the repair is to be done in more than one stage, six months are allowed to elapse before the second stage is done. In spite of careful attention to surgical technique and postoperative care, the two-stage operation results in urethral fistulas in about 40 percent of patients so treated (King, p 1102).

One child who had seven surgical procedures to try to repair the defect was asked why he was hospitalized. He threw back the covers from the bedcradle, exposing himself and said, "See I just wasn't put together right!" This child benefited by water play in the bathtub. Prior to putting the child in the bathtub, his Foley catheter was clamped off. He was taken twice a day to the tub by a nurse and appropriately supplied with toys. At first, he merely used the tub to bathe. Then he began to act out. His first change in attitude occurred when he splashed the nurse accidentally." He eventually became able to ask, "Why do I need this tube?" He then teased, "I'm going to pull it out!" The soothing bath plus the close relationship of water to his problem, allowed him to express his true feelings which he was not able to do in his bed or wheelchair. The use of the bathtub varies with different physicians as some prefer not to have the child take tub baths. If this is the case, a bath basin is the second best idea. Boats and sponges can be used in a small basin. However, the child does not get the added benefit of the feel of being submerged in the water.

Immediately postoperatively the child may have a dressing. The dressing is utilized to help alleviate edema and to reduce the tension of the suture lines. This dressing should not be removed, as it is used for pressure. If there is an unusual amount of drainage—some is to be expected—the physician should be notified. The parents need to know that the dressing is a necessary part of the repair, so they will not be tempted to move it so see how the incision looks. The indwelling catheter may be a source of concern to the parents, especially if immediately postoperatively the urine is a little pink-tinged. Any serous drainage mixed with urine looks like a larger amount than it is. The parents must be assured that the child is not hemorrhaging and that this situation will clear. They should also be told the optimal positioning of the catheter for draining. Parents frequently move it to facilitate playing games. I have seen the catheters draped up over the bed cradle by an unknowing parent.

An overbed cradle is frequently utilized to keep the pressure of the bed clothes off the area. The child is also left without pajama bottoms. To guarantee privacy, the sheet must hang freely over all sides of the cradle. The school-age child is especially modest and will appreciate the excess sheeting. I do not approve of using diapers anywhere on the child's bed. A diaper is a degrading object to any child who has outgrown them. When the child's dressing is removed, anywhere from two to five days postsurgery, pajama bottoms or a sheet are usually allowed to cover him when he is up in the wheelchair. The use of the bed cradle is usually continued until the sutures are removed.

In a two-stage procedure, the second stage is frequently more anxiety-producing to the parents, as its success or failure determines whether more surgery will be indicated. If parents have prepared themselves for two stages, the addition of another may produce another crisis situation. It may decrease their hope that the child will ever have a successful repair. The child may be more concerned with the pain from the procedure rather than the results of the surgery.

I feel there are a few addtional things which need to be considered by nurses. First, it is not consistent with our culture to focus as much attention on the genitals as is necessary during the postoperative period. Therefore, observations of the genitals may be deemed necessary only by the physician. If the catheter has to be irrigated, every care should be taken to guarantee privacy. Discussion of the drainage and emptying the urinary drainage bag should not take place in the corridors, playroom, or other public areas. It is better to take the child to his room for the short time needed to complete this task. Children are frequently self-conscious of the drainage tube and bag, so this material should be placed as inconspicously as possible. The child may fear the removal of the Foley catheter as he fears voiding. After the Foley is removed, the child may need to be encouraged to void by the usual methods of increasing fluid intake, running the water in the sink, and providing privacy in the bathroom. The child may feel more comfortable with his mother present. She should be instructed to note the stream and where the voiding takes place. The child may choose to sit down on the toilet at first, as this has been the way he voided prior to surgery. Standing is usually accomplished readily by just showing him that this is the way other boys void. The need for him to be like his peers is very great at the school-age period.

The aim of the surgical procedures should be to obtain correction with the smallest amount of emotional shock possible. The effects of hospitalization can be lessened by the parents and the medical personnel being as truthful with the child as possible. The child should be an active participant when the results of the surgery are known. If future surgical procedures are indicated, he must be helped to understand the reasons for the operation and not just made to conform.

Tracheoesophageal Atresia

In contrast to the previously discussed condition, tracheoesophageal artresia necessitates fairly immediate surgery. The long-term care begins soon after birth. The condition is rather easily diagnosed by passing a catheter through the infant's nose into the esophagus. If there is an obstruction, the catheter will coil in the pouch. It is usually routine to pass a catheter soon after the birth of the infant, while he is still in the delivery room. If this has been omitted, the parent or nurse who feeds the infant the first time will find the infant regurgitating the formula as it cannot get past the defect. In addition, the infant may have a great deal of mucus and if this is not aspirated, he will become cyanotic. There is a tendency for these infants to drool or secretions may bubble from the nose. The excessive mucus is caused by the infant's inability to swallow his own saliva. The respirations become coarse if the secretions enter the lungs. Cyanosis may also result from laryngospasms due to the accumulation of saliva in the pouch. The excessive secretions spill over into the larynx and causes the laryngospasm and resultant cyanosis. It is imperative that proper suctioning be done to remove the saliva.

The size of the infant is a major factor in relation to the surgical risk The improved techniques in surgical procedures, pediatric fluid therapy, and the use of local anesthetics have greatly increased the survival rate of infants born with this condition. A significant number of infants having tracheoesophageal anomalies are also premature. An attempt is usually made to have the infant reach 5 pounds prior to the surgical correction. However, a gastrostomy may have been done to decompress the stomach and to decrease the possibility of aspiration pneumonia prior to the time of the surgical correction.

If the infant has to be transferred to another area of the hospital or another hospital, it is imperative that the mother see the child first. The mother should even be allowed to hold the infant. This will help her to work through her grief if the infant dies. It will also decrease the fantasies she has of the handicapped child. She may even benefit from seeing the infant having slight respiratory difficulty or bubbling mucus. I vividly recall one mother whose full-term infant was having respiratory distress and was kept in an isolette. The mother had a real desire for her infant to get well. She could not imagine what was wrong with the infant. The explanations from her husband, doctors, and nurses did not provide her with a vivid picture of the infant's condition. She was finally taken to the intensive care nursery to view the infant. She took one look, saw the infant gasping for every breath, saw the deep retractions, and immediately knew the infant was in critical condition. Although she was upset, she now stated she understood what we were trying to tell her about her infant. The infant died and she was left with the feeling that there was nothing that could have saved the life of her infant. She experienced much relief from knowing this. I do not want to leave the impression that the majority of these infants will die. However, seeing the infant early and frequently can also help the mother during her long separation from the child. It is at least a slight reward for her months of waiting and her labor and delivery period.

Preoperatively the infant is usually kept in an isolette to maintain body temperature. The infant is usually placed in a semisitting position to minimize the possibility of aspiration and prevent reflux of gastric juices into the lungs. A 30 degree elevation of the chest is suggested. The use of oxygen and humidity follow the suggested plan for any premature infant. Conscientious suctioning is carried out. Fochtman and Raffensberger (1976) suggest as an alternate to hand nasopharyngeal suctioning: the use of constant suctioning by a small tube (Replogle tube) that is inserted into the proximal esophageal pouch through the infant's nose. "The sump draws air through the second lumen and prevents obstruction of the suction tube" (Fochtman and Raffensberger, p 39).

The postoperative course will depend on the type of congenital malformation. (Fig. 3). Figure 3B illustrates the most common anomaly and therefore the postoperative nursing care described here will be based primarily on this type.

Immediately postoperatively the infant is returned to a warmed isolette

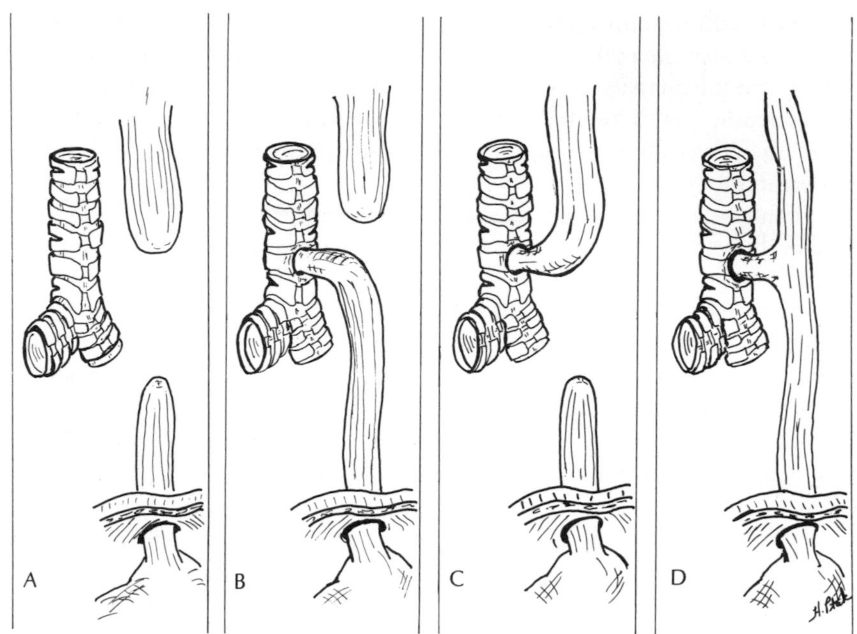

FIG. 3. View A, Esophageal atresia without tracheoesophageal fistula; **View B,** Esophageal atresia with tracheoesophageal fistula with distal segment; **View C,** Esophageal atresia with fistula between proximal segment and the trachea; **View D,** H-type tracheoesophageal fistula without atresia.

with humidity. The isolette does not preclude the mother from touching the infant after appropriate handwashing and gowning, if gowning is required in the particular agency. To decrease the effects of isolation in an isolette, music via music boxes or musical toys or by commercial music programming companies is now being introduced into isolettes. Patterned or designed sheets are also being used and toys are no longer out of bounds. Mobiles are most appropriate.

Another postoperative nursing function is the conscientious nasopharyngeal suctioning. This is done to prevent the infant from aspirating secretions and developing atelectasis or pneumonia. It should be done unless contraindicated, as the suctioning can cause undue irritation. The infant's facial expression will signal the need for suctioning. They exhibit the anxiety of anyone who is deprived of oxygen. If the airway is not opened, the respiratory rate will increase. The soft plastic catheter should be marked so that it is not inserted too deeply, causing pressure on the sutures. The pressure used for suctioning should be as low as possible to adequately remove the tenacious material.

When oral feedings are started, they must be given slowly and cautiously. Sometimes a medicine dropper is used. Difficulty with the feeding is reason to stop the feeding and notify the physician. Continuing to feed may further complicate the situation. The most competent nurse should be assigned to this infant for his feedings. The oral feedings are usually started after the fifth postoperative day. However, this will be determined by the physician based on the infant's progress. The infant will want more feeding than the esophagus can tolerate. Despite his eagerness to eat, the feeding must only be done as prescribed. The suction equipment should be close by during all feedings.

Some infants will have gastrostomies performed. This facilitates feeding when oral feedings cannot be accomplished. The nurse will begin the gastrostomy feedings when ordered. They are given by gravity with use of the glass or plastic funnel of an Asepto syringe. The tube is elevated up through the hole in the top of the isolette. After the feeding, the tube can be left open and any postfeeding vomiting will be allowed to pass freely up the tube. Care must be taken not to put tension on the gastrostomy tube when one is turning or bathing the infant. The feedings should be sterile and prepared as carefully as any newborn feeding. The gastrostomy tube is left open after the feeding so that any regurgitated fluid and air will pass out the tube without putting pressure on the suture line. The open tube prevents gastric distention.

Despite the infant's innate desire to suck, pacifiers are frequently omitted as they increase the production of saliva. It is important to know if the surgeon allows pacifiers. If he does, a sterile nipple filled with sterile cotton should be utilized as a pacifier for the infant during feeding times. This will help to satisfy the required sucking needs of the infant and encourages use of the jaws and facial muscles. It can also be used to soothe the infant who is not getting the ordinary handling and cuddling. Some surgeons prefer the infant to be moved very little immediately postoperatively and therefore nursing procedures are planned to minimize contact. Others prefer the infant be moved from side to side and stimulated to cry every half hour to promote expansion of the lungs.

The infant is frequently kept in the isolette until a couple of days before discharge, to decrease the possibility of infection. The nurse should check with the physician to see when it is permissible to take the infant out of the isolette for feedings.

When the infant is able to take the whole feeding by mouth, the gastrostomy tube is clamped. If the total repair has been accomplished, x-rays are taken to be sure there is no leakage. If the results are adequate, the gastrostomy tube is removed.

Depending on the severity of the anomaly, the surgical corrections may take a long time to complete. Each surgical procedure causes a separation of the mother and infant. These separations are during the period most important for the infant to be with his mother. The severity of the condition necessitates doing surgical procedures at the poorest time, developmentally speaking, for the child. As there is no way to safely delay surgery with its long hospitalizations, other things must be done to help compensate for the surgery.

Maintaining the mother-infant relationship should have top priority in the nursing care plan. Some infants will be discharged with the gastrostomy. The mother is prepared for the discharge by learning how to feed the child, care for his skin, react in an emergency, and when to contact the physician. The nurse spends time explaining to the mother and also listening to the mother. She/he demonstrates procedures and has the mother return the demonstration. She/he also provides explanations to other family members if they are available. A successful discharge will be based on thorough preparation.

Meningomyelocele and Hydrocephalus

> Meningomyelocele is a nervous system anomaly of the newborn. The protruding pouch contains meninges, neural tissue, and spinal fluid. The condition is accompanied by hydrocephalus in 75% of the cases. . . .
>
> The lesion may be located anywhere along the spinal cord, however, the most frequent are in the lumbar region, 40%, and then the lumbosacral region, 30%, (Amador, 1969, pp 1206–7)

The child born with meningomyelocele is one of the more dramatic examples of children with long-term illness. With the advent of antibiotics, infections have been amenable to control and the children frequently survive.

Immediately after delivery the child is kept warm as the interference with the neural system gives the child a poorer temperature regulation mechanism than the normal newborn. Frequently, an isolette is utilized. It is generally accepted practice to place the infant on the abdomen with his face to the side. A plastic strip is usually applied below the meningomyelocele over the rectal area (Fig. 1). The mildest form of adhesive should be used to keep it in place. Disposable plastic urine collectors with their mild self-adherent can be easily applied. Saran Wrap, which has a tendency to adhere to skin surfaces, can be tried. The shield will help to protect the lesion without the necessity of covering the area with dressings. The lesion itself usually is treated by exposure to air.

Positioning is imperative to prevent the infant from developing contractures. The infant frequently has associated bony abnormalities and every attempt should be made to prevent the development of additional ones. A physical therapist should evaluate the child early, and also a physiatrist to determine the child's muscle potential. Early surgical correction is now beginning to be more widely used. It is believed that early correction helps to prevent more serious muscle involvement and neural deterioration. The surgical correction of the lesion is frequently preceded by a shunting procedure for the hydrocephalus. The shunt is done to control the increased cerebrospinal fluid pressure which may result from repairing the sac.

There are several types of shunting procedures referred to in the literature. Three of the most common types of shunting procedures are the ventriculoauricular, ventriculovenous, and ventriculoperitoneal. The positioning of the infant postoperatively will be determined by the type of shunting procedure, the meningomyelocele, and the postoperative evaluation of the fontanelles. "Valve systems are usually inserted and they are pumped frequently post-operatively to remove small pieces of matter which may find their way into the tubing and valve systems" (Amador, p 1220). Hospitals vary in their practice as to whether nurses and parents are taught to pump the system. In any event, the nurse can evaluate the child to help determine if there is an obstruction in the system. The fontanelle becomes full or tense when there is an interference with the flow of cerebrospinal fluid. The child becomes listless, may fail to feed or begin vomiting, and is irritable and fretful. He does not respond to voice or touch as quickly when there is an obstruction. If the obstruction becomes extensive, the child may develop respiratory problems and progress into coma. Early recognition of symptoms will allow the physician to investigate the obstruction and to do a revision if necessary. Over a long time period, the shunt will need revisions due to the growth of the child. The child may dislodge the tubing from its site as he grows. To date, no tubing has been found that can successfully "lengthen" with the child.

Following the shunting procedure, the meningomyelocele is usually corrected—although, as previously stated, some physicians prefer to close the meningomyelocele first and to insert the shunt later. Again, after closure of the sac the positioning of the infant depends on all the contributing factors. A general principle is to keep the infant off the operative sites. Changing of position is especially important to prevent respiratory complications. Feeding the infant is usually done in the crib or isolette until healing begins to take place. The best position is usually to place the infant on the side opposite the shunt. Burping must be done cautiously depending on the location of the meningomyelocele lesion.

As soon as the infant's condition is stabilized the mother should begin to feed the child. She should be taught the signs to note in relation to the shunting procedure. She should be given explicit directions for bathing the infant with special emphasis on the operative sites. She should be given directions for passive exercises to the lower extremities, if indicated. The parents need to become aware of the necessity and value of close medical follow-up for their child. The parents should also be aware of the complications which might result from the decrease in circulation to the lower extremities, including such factors as keeping the infant dressed warmer and preventing pressure. Decubitus can develop from bed clothes which are tucked in too tightly. The infant's limited ability to turn himself should be explained so the parents will turn the child periodically.

The urinary system also needs close supervision. The paralysis caused by the neural damage frequently results in urinary dribbling. The use of Credé is usually indicated in order to manually express the urine. Credé is the application of pressure over the bladder area. It is easily accomplished by gentle pressure of the palms of the hands. The mother is taught to express the urine manually at definite intervals to help empty the bladder. As the child gets older, he can be taught to do the Credé himself. The process can be facilitated by using toys to help the child put pressure on the bladder. Such toys as balloons, horns, bugles, or plastic bubbles can all be utilized when the child is sitting on the potty chair or toilet. The older child, who has outgrown these toys, can be taught to pucker up his cheeks with air and then blow slowly through his closed lips. Additional pressure can be made by using the hand to cover the lips and therefore create more resistance. This procedure may also depend on the preference of the physician. Even when it is utilized, the infant is usually wet more frequently than the child who does not have a disability. The skin of the child is especially prone to breakdown as it has poorer nourishment and less adequate temperature control. Frequent diaper changing and cleansing of the area is necessary. If a rash begins, exposure to the air should be tried. Occasionally it is necessary to apply an ointment, such as A&D or Desitin, to help alleviate the rash. If skin breakdown occurs, the mother should be cautioned to call the doctor for directions. An alternate approach to Credé is intermittent catheterization.

The severity of the kidney involvement usually increases with time. It is one of the most challenging aspects of the long-term case. The child is prone to frequent urinary infections and they are usually difficult to control with medications, as the child develops resistance to them. The child who dribbles all the time is usually diapered to keep her* outer clothing dry. This diapering provides an excellent media for bacteria to multiply when it is wet for long periods. The diaper is usually covered with a plastic panty that further adds to the warmth, and the warmth contributes further to the bacteria formation. When the child is old enough to enter school, it is important to plan times for her to go to the bathroom or nurse's office to change the diapering. If there is a space available, diapering can be brought

**Here I use the pronouns "her" and "she" because the urinary problem is more difficult to control in girls. In boys, there are urinary appliances which are fairly successful. However, boys should also be given time to go to the bathroom. They must empty the appliance and wash and dry the penis to protect it from excoriation due to continual contact with the urine.*

in once a week and stored. If there is not a space available, the child should bring adequate daily supplies. Bringing the supplies in a child's lunch box or small doll suitcase will lessen the child's resistance to taking the supply. A definite time should be established for the child to go to the bathroom. She cannot feel wetness and frequently the odor of urine is more noticeable to others than to the child herself.

Depending on the severity of the accompanying handicaps and the facilities available, the children may need help to complete their personal care. Handrails help a great deal especially if one is placed near the toilet and another near the sink. It is also convenient to have a table available near the sink so they can place their supplies on it.

If the child has a urinary diversion and is wearing a prosthetic device, it is very important that he also be given specific times to use the bathroom. The urinary appliances also have a tendency to develop odors. This can be fairly well controlled by washing the appliance frequently, airing it on a routine basis, using deodorant or vinegar in the wash water, using deodorant tablets in the pouch, and keeping the child's skin clean and dry. The child should have at least two appliances so they can be alternated and aired adequately.

There are several different varieties of appliances used. One utilizes a leg bag for collecting the urine, another has a pouch. The one with the leg bag is made of a soft rubber and is easy to keep clean. The advantage of the appliance is it creates less pressure on the stoma. Occasionally pressure from an appliance can cause the stoma to herniate. The disadvantage to this appliance is that the leg bag shows with girls and they are embarrassed. The bag fits under the trousers of the boy so it is not as much of a problem (see Figs. 4 and 5). The one with the pouch has the advantage of being easily concealed under clothing. But it is more difficult to keep odor-free if it is neglected (see Figs. 6 and 7).

Both types of appliances are better connected to a urinary collection bottle at night. This facilitates better drainage. It also allows the child to move around freely without putting pressure on a bag of urine. The skin surface near the appliance must be washed with soap and water and dried thoroughly. There is a tendency for skin irritation to develop. This may be due to the skin reacting to the cement used to apply the device or due to urine leakage. At times the skin problem becomes severe and the appliance will have to be left off so the skin can be exposed to air and light treatment.

The bowel incontinence associated with myelomeningocele is more easily regulated. A program is established individually for each child. A convenient time for utilizing the toilet is essential. In large families this can be a problem. The child frequently needs extra time to complete evacuation. Suppositories are helpful in getting the pattern established. After a while, the child will usually evacuate without the suppository. The success of the

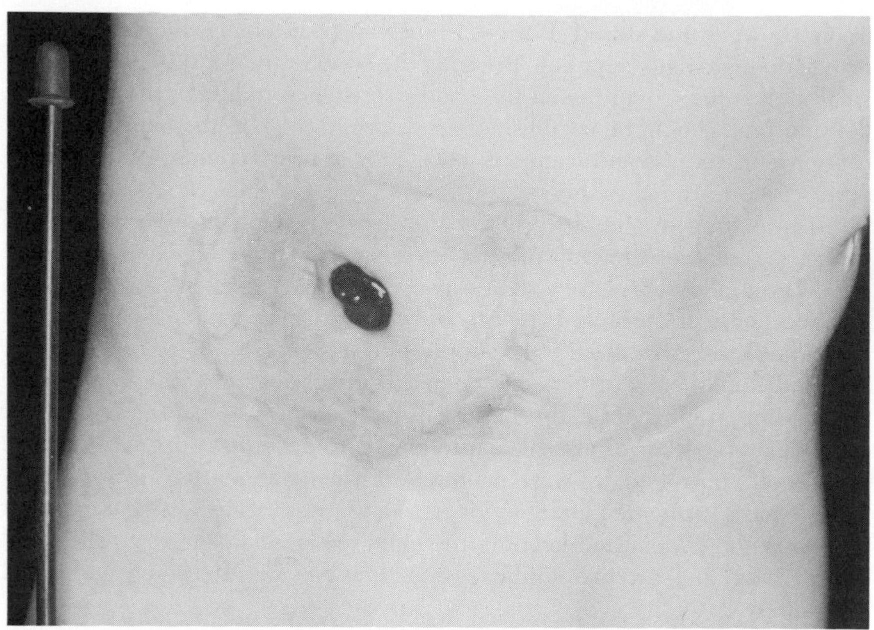

FIG. 4. A healed stoma. The skin area around the stoma demands excellent care.

bowel training may also be directly related to the dietary and fluid intake of the child. The mother and child should both be aware that any drastic change in the dietary intake may interfere with evacuation and cause incontinence during the day. The bowel evacuation may be more successful if scheduled for evening. The morning hours may be too hectic in the household. Occasionally suppositories, an adequate diet, and good timing are not sufficient for evacuating the bowel. It may be necessary to resort to enemas. This is not a complicated procedure with the commercial enemas now available. The least amount of solution should be utilized to stimulate the movement. Again, the pattern of establishing a time, consistent from day to day, will cut down on the incontinence.

The bracing of the child will also contribute to the nursing responsibilities. The braces must fit properly if the child is to utilize them effectively. Also, the joints must move freely. Dust collects in the joints and must be removed. Oiling is also necessary. The child's skin should not have pressure marks from the braces. The leather parts should not be cracked. The leather can be preserved by the use of saddle soap. The braces must be checked frequently especially during growth spurts. The child's lower limbs do not grow as consistently as the rest of his trunk; however, he may gain weight and the braces may be too tight. The child should be encouraged to use his braces. It is often easier to push him around in a wheelchair but this does not help him in his future adjustment to life. The emphasis should be on making the child as self-sufficient as possible.

The nurse will also play an important role in counseling the parents and the child. The parents usually have many questions relating to growth, education, employment, finances, and so forth. Frequently the parents know the answers to many of their questions but they need an opportunity just to talk with someone. The children may need much more help in dealing

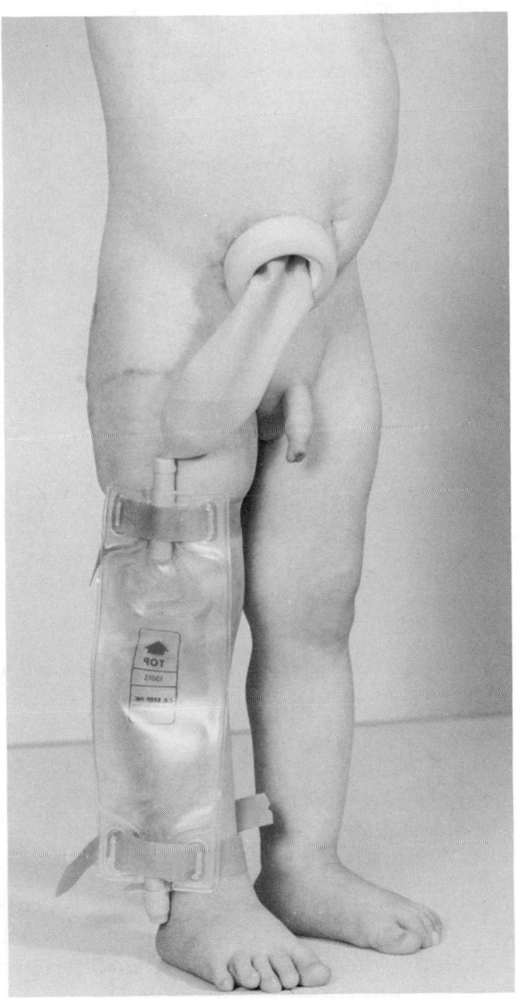

FIG. 5. Ileal appliance with leg bag for urine collection.

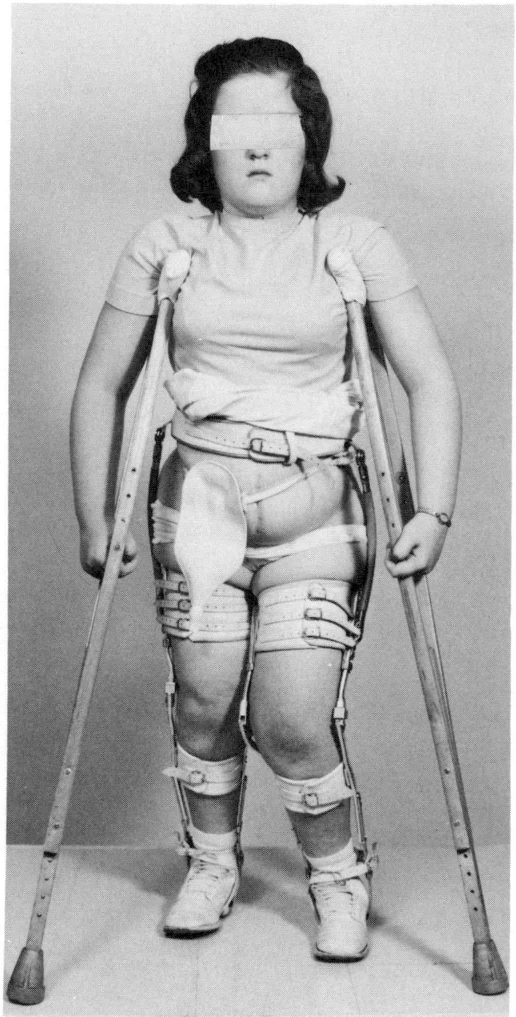

FIG. 6. Mary is 13 years old. She has a repaired myelomeningocele, arrested hydrocephalus, repaired bilateral dislocated hips, and ileo conduit. She is an outstanding student and gets around well with the use of crutches and long braces.

with their questions. Their limited understanding prevents them from getting satisfaction from many of the answers given them. They find it very difficult to live in a world where their peers are so different from themselves. The child needs to learn to appreciate what he has and to focus less on his deficits. The child may fantasize that his body is not disabled and this interferes with his understanding. If the child becomes too involved with fantasy he may need the help of a psychologist or psychiatrist.

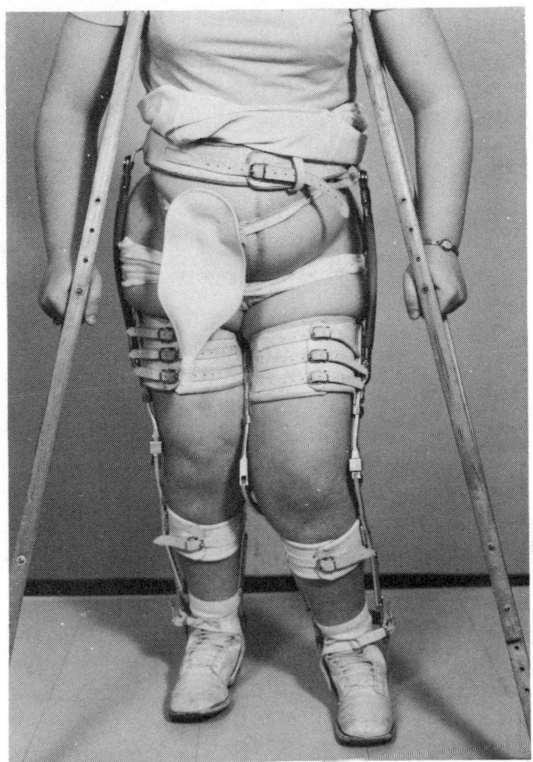

FIG. 7. Here Mary illustrates the wearing of her urinary drainage appliance. The waist belt can be removed and washed or replaced. The bag is washed, dried, and deodorant tablets inserted. Note she does not wear a leg bag and this appliance is completely covered by her dress.

Deformities of Limbs

A number of anomalies can be found in relation to the extremities. They may be obvious anomalies such as a missing limb or limbs or less noticeable such as a dislocated hip. The duration of care is frequently dependent upon the time lapse between discovery and therapy. For instance, a dislocated hip discovered in the nursery and treated immediately, will usually require only short-term therapy for correction. If the condition is not detected until the child is walking, the medical therapy will usually span a long period of time.

The child with a missing limb will require long-term care to guarantee that his prosthesis is functioning effectively. The skin areas also must be watched closely to prevent breakdown due to the added stress produced by the prosthesis.

Let us first consider the child with a missing or severely deformed upper extremity. The newborn clenches his fists. The infant also sucks on his fists. The missing limb is important because of its absence. The infant may irritate the skin of the only limb. It may be useful to supply a pacifier to the infant to help compensate for the missing limb. As the infant grows he is ambidexterous. The infant with the missing hand is forced into a preference early unless a prosthesis is fitted to aid the child. The infant is able to use the prosthesis to assist with toys and later in learning to crawl and sit. The prosthesis helps to stabilize the body and provides the weight lost by the missing limb. The prosthesis becomes imperative when the child's neurological system begins to mature. He is capable of doing all types of two-handed activities and needs the prosthesis to complete his tasks. The early prosthesis has an uncomplicated design. As the child grows he needs a prosthesis that can bend, grasp, lift, pull, and so forth. The early prosthesis demands much less care than the more complicated type. The infant and child prosthesis should be worn over a tee shirt to protect the child's skin from excoriation. The straps must be kept clean and in good repair. The child's prosthesis will also need attention to the rubber bands, the joints, and the cables. All parts must be in excellent condition in order to provide maximum function.

In addition to checking the prosthesis for functional ability, the nurse needs to encourage the parents and child to use the prosthesis consistently. The more uniformly the child uses the prosthesis, the more secure he will feel. The child who is permitted to go without the prosthesis for indefinite periods will develop one-handed skills and may resist using the prosthesis. As he develops the one-handedness may become a disadvantage which he cannot easily correct.

At this point in time, the hook is far more functional than artificial hands. The child usually will want an artificial hand to alternate with the hook for more formal occasions.

Lower-extremity prostheses are usually more readily accepted than upper extremity prosthesis. This is due to the almost impossible task of getting around on one leg. The length of the affected limb may influence this. One child with an almost perfectly formed leg refused to wear the prosthesis which provided him with a foot. The prosthesis slowed down his gait. He preferred to play sports without the prosthesis and consequently frequently injured the tissue at the end of the limb.

Injury to the tissue of the remaining limb is a critical problem. The prosthesis must be left off during the healing process. This necessitates an inconvenience to the child. It is wise to have a pair of crutches available in case this happens. Then the child will not have to miss school during this time. Care to the stump is best achieved by the use of a soap such as Dial. The area should be rinsed thoroughly and dried. In the hot weather powder may reduce itching. A stump sock made of virgin wool is placed next to the skin. This sock should also be washed daily. The sock should fit smoothly. The prosthesis fits over the sock. There is a tendency for stumps to shrink with time. The child should not attempt to remedy this by adding extra socks or stuffing cotton or the like in the prosthesis. The prosthetist should be consulted for all repairs or revisions to the prosthesis.

The school nurse should play a key role in introducing other children to the prosthesis. The child may be asked to demonstrate how he uses the prosthesis. The children need to be cautioned about pushing or shoving the affected child. They should understand that the affected child may need more time to master certain sports. They need to know that at times the child with a lower prosthesis will use crutches instead of his prosthesis. This introduction will help to erase the unknown element and help the children to appreciate the handicap.

The nurse should also talk with the teachers to help them understand the implications of the prosthesis. One important factor is that the child may tire more readily due to the added energy needed to use the prosthesis. The child may need a short rest period after gym, before beginning ordinary school activities. The teachers should try to treat the child as "normally" as possible but not to completely dismiss the possibility of fatigue. Gym should be encouraged, as well as swimming. An upper-extremity prosthesis may have to be removed during contact sports to protect the other children from accidental injury. Unless a special lightweight prosthesis is available for swimming, the regular prosthesis is removed and the child is taught to swim with one lower limb.

Much of the adjustment the child has in later life is dependent on his early experiences. Therefore, it is worth the extra effort in his early years to have the child adjust to his prosthesis. Even with much patience, it is not unusual for the adolescent to rebel against the prosthesis and the reasons for his anomaly. Every effort must be made to help the adolescent understand. If he has been given honest answers all along, it will be easier during his adolescent period. He may become quite hostile to the medical personnel providing his care or to his parents. Venting his feelings may be all that is necessary to make him feel better. He may need a period to talk over problems with others with similar anomalies. The adolescent may need help when he realizes that it is more difficult to achieve some of the developmental milestones, such as dating or getting a job. Too many failures may lessen his self-image. With the right professional counseling, the adolescent should be able to make an adequate adjustment.

In addition to the ways already spelled out, nurses can be helpful to children with prosthesis in the following ways:

1. The mother may need help in adjusting clothing to compensate for the prosthesis. Instead of disappointing the child because a garment does not fit, snaps or a zipper may be inserted in the side to accommodate the prosthesis. The use of Velcro strips on clothing can also be suggested.
2. When the child is hospitalized, the nurse should be sure the child wears the prosthesis whenever his condition warrants it. Failure to encourage

the child to wear it may further his dislike for the prosthesis. He may get the idea that the nurses, too, think it is useless.

3. During hospitalizations make a place available for the child to wash his stump socks and to hang them up to dry. If the child is able to assume this chore he should be encouraged to do so. If not, the nurse should assume this for the child. The socks should not be sent to the laundry as the harsh detergent is not good for them.
4. The school nurse should check the gait of the child with a lower-extremity prosthesis. She may be the first one to detect an ill-fitting prosthesis or an irritation to the tissue. Children will frequently try to hide these facts so they do not have to go to the doctor.

The nurse's role in relation to any of the disabling conditions of childhood is dependent on the setting and the other professional personnel responsible for the child's care. As a member of an interdisciplinary team, the nurse has an excellent opportunity to share her/his expertise with other health professionals.

The majority of cases of missing limbs are amenable to the use of prosthetic appliances. However, there are anomalies of the extremities which cannot be improved by prosthesis. Some children are born with severely deformed hands. For various reasons the hand may not be amputated to permit a prosthesis to be fitted properly. The nurse now has a more complicated role to play. She/he may be involved in devising appropriate utensils to teach the child to feed himself (Fig. 8). Hopefully, an occupational therapist will be available to do much of the initial training. The nurse will then visit the home to see that the adaptations are being effectively utilized. Encouragement needs to be given to let the child feed herself. The nurse can help the mother protect the floor by using newspaper under the child's chair. The mother must realize that this may be a long and tedious process, but the end results will be worth the additional effort.

Other adaptations which may help the child to achieve successful self-feeding are the use of a deep dish with sides and a suction cup on the bottom of the dish. This will help the child by keeping the food on the plate and the plate on the table. The hand appliance then has a back edge to aid it in getting the food on the spoon. The suction cup on the bottom keeps the dish from moving out of the child's reach (Fig. 8). The use of a "cobbler-type bib" will decrease the chances of the child soiling her clothes. When the child is ready to drink from a cup, the training cup with the cover and spout will be useful. The wide cup without the handle will adjust to the deformity of the hand. The child will then grasp the cup on each side and raise it to his mouth. If the cup drops it will not spill much because the cover is on securely.

When the deformity does not lend itself to prosthesis application or an appliance, the child is taught to eat by the less socially acceptable way of holding the utensil in his toes. However, it is acceptable to the child as it helps him to be more self-sufficient.

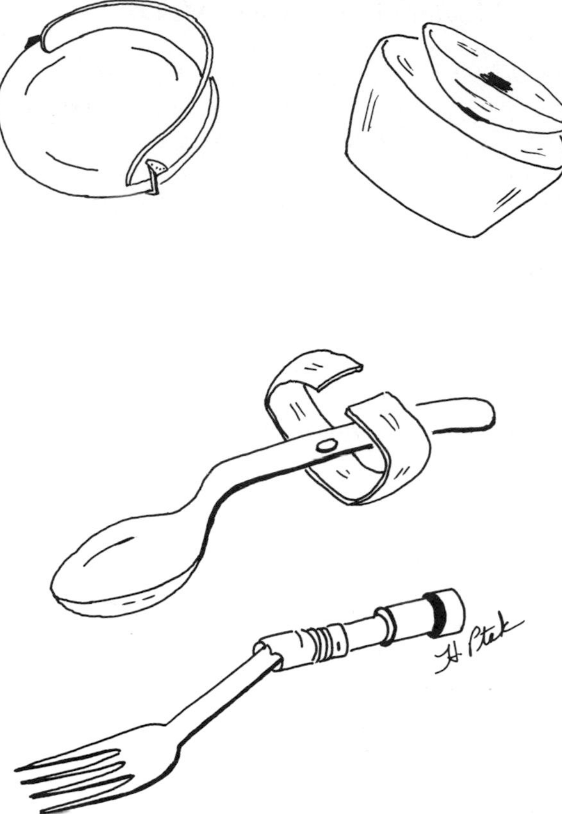

FIG. 8. Utensils adapted for use with children who have deficient hand function.

There are several other types of congenital anomalies which have been omitted as they are more short-term in nature. The scope of this book is to focus on the ones that ordinarily require long-term care. According to Bramley (1963), regardless of the nature of the disability, it cannot be overstressed that very few children will have severe emotional problems when the attitudes of the parents are essentially healthy ones:

> We should remember that the child almost invariably mirrors the fears and the attitudes that his parents have about him and that, in general, the child will be a much happier individual when the parents regard him as a normal youngster, similar in his feelings to other children of comparable age and background (p 310).

I would also like to add that the child will be better adjusted if he can also trust and accept the health professionals responsible for his care.

Minimal Cerebral (Brain) Dysfunction (MBD)

This section will be concerned with the understanding and nursing care necessary in meeting the needs of children with hyperkinetic syndrome, sometimes called HLD (hyperkinesis learning disabilities); that is, those children who have difficulty with perception, conception, and/or a behavior problem; in other words, children who are not primarily mentally retarded, or who do not have cerebral palsy or a severe convulsive disorder. Children who have learning disabilities as their major problem may, of course, also have these conditions as a complicating problem.

Cantwell (1972) stresses that only a small minority of children with hyperactivity actually present with hard evidence of brain damage. Therefore, the terminology of cerebral or brain dysfunction may be misleading. Further research in the area may result in a better way to describe the syndrome.

Over the years, many different names have been given to children with this syndrome. Doll (1932) and Strauss (1951) referred to them as brain-injured and distinguished them from generally mentally-retarded children. Basara (1966) refers to them as perceptually handicapped. I am certain that additional names can be found that have attempted to describe more accurately the syndrome which manifests itself in a number of overt ways.

Before I identify the signs, I should like to first point out that not every child will have all of these signs. He may have only two or three, or he may have many or all of them. In the book, *Helping the Brain Injured Child*, Siegel (1962) addresses himself to the following characteristics (not listed in order of importance):

1. talkativeness
2. awkwardness
3. poor speech
4. destructiveness
5. animism
6. distractibility
7. hyperactivity
8. impulsiveness
9. perserveration
10. irritability
11. guilelessness
12. aggressiveness
13. social immaturity

Such an extensive list would indicate that almost any child could be classified as having this syndrome at periodic intervals.

When the brain is damaged, there is a complex field of forces disrupted, and this disruption makes it difficult for the child to interact, in the usual way, with his environment. The extent to which this happens will be dependent on the extent and the locus of the damage. In a study by Schulman et al (1965), it is stated that the only variable that approached unequivocal support as a correlate of brain damage, regardless of extent or location of damage, was distractibility. No evidence in their study supported the hypothesis that hyperactivity is a correlate of brain damage. They also found that autonomic lability may not be a direct correlate of damage, but rather that it may be related through its association with performative lability. I bring this out at this point as I believe that much of the literature in relation to these children has focused on symptoms which may not be the result of the brain injury itself, but rather may reflect environmental factors which might be controlled or manipulated to intervene before the child exhibits many of the behavioral signs listed by Siegel (1962).

In addition, we must consider that the response patterns of the child with H-LD will also be influenced by the psychologic defenses utilized by the child. It becomes evident that we are dealing with a complicated reciprocal interaction between the biologic defect and the psychologic and environmental structures of each child. In order to understand the outcomes of these reciprocal interactions, one must evaluate thoroughly the biologic, environmental, and psychologic factors.

While many of the injuries are present at birth, there are others that are the result of an injury after birth. The child's progress prior to the injury should be evaluated to ascertain what progress he had made both psychologically and physically before the injury and what environmental support he received at the time of the injury. Generally, the earlier the injury occurred on the developmental scale, the greater is the potential for behavioral or psychologic defects. The biologic defect may affect three main areas: (1) normal maturation is interrupted, with the possibility of retention of primitve patterns, and/or a delay in acquiring new functions and abilities. Therefore, the child may exhibit behavior patterns of varying age levels. (2) The next area is in relation to perception and manifests itself as an interference with initiative and control of impulses. (3) Another common result is a "predisposition to anxiety."

Feingold (1975) presents evidence to link the rise in H-LD with food additives such as coloring and artificial flavorings. He stresses that these additives have no nutritional value and they have caused disturbances to most body systems. Feingold suggests that in infants he studied who had symptoms of restlessness, head banging, sleeplessness, and crib rocking there was a history that the child received artifically colored and flavored pediatric vitamin drops. The nutritional aspects of the syndrome will be discussed in more detail later.

For the remainder of this section, I shall refer to these children as children with minimal cerebral dysfunction. I have chosen this term as it clearly identifies to me that the child will have areas of normal functioning and areas of abnormal functioning depending on the part of the brain involved, and also that this damage may be minimal in nature—which permits a more optimistic outlook on the future for the child.

The nurse in the nursery has an increasing responsibility to identify early signs of brain injury. A good indicator of a problem is the infant's cry. The cry of the newborn normal infant is easily elicited by painful stimulation. The newborn with brain damage needs to be repeatedly stimulated to cry and the cry is weak, strained, and at times barely audible. A brain-injured child at one week of age may exhibit a cry with short abrupt bursts which have a shrieklike quality. These variations in cry should be quite evident to the nurse in the newborn nursery, who is in a good position to get early attention for this child.

As a child grows, his cry begins to have variations in pitch and rhythm with speechlike sounds intermingled. The brain-injured child's cry has a flat quality and lacks the speechlike sounds. Frequently the cry is gutteral in nature and seems to be forced rather than spontaneous. It is sometimes high-pitched and frequently shrieklike. These clues, evidenced by cry, should not go by without receiving adequate attention. The nurse's role is especially important in relation to charting the character of the cry and reporting this to the physician. She/he may be instrumental in getting the physician to listen to the cry. When the physician examines the infant he may not hear the cry so an attempt must be made to elicit a cry response. The delay in response and the amount of stimulation needed to sustain the response can be very striking.

The way the child feeds is another early cue to difficulty. The child with a brain injury is generally referred to as a "poor feeder." To be more concrete, the child does not suck well and must be stimulated frequently. He needs larger, softer nipples than normal infants the same weight. He seems to lose parts of his feeding as he does not grasp the nipple and milk flows out the sides of his mouth. As the child gets older, he seems to drool a great deal of the time. When it is time for him to be tried on junior foods he is unable to chew meats.

The latter problems can be easily identified by the nurse when the infant is brought for well-baby supervision. In addition, she/he can check for other signs, such as the prolonged Moro reflex present in children with neurologic disturbances. The hands are a good indicator of disturbances in infants. Infants ordinarily prefer to clench their fists. The infant with fingers spread apart should alert the nurse to a possible problem. As the child matures physically, the developmental milestones are evaluated and deviations from the expected are evaluated to determine if they are biologic or environmental in nature. Suggestions for altering environment to enhance developmental achievements is indicated. If the changed environment does not help, then biologic conditions are probably the cause. Again, this is not a black or white thing, and a combination of biologic and environmental factors is very common.

An example of changing the environment to enhance development might be observed in a child of seven months who is not sitting with support. You learn from the mother that she has never put the child in an upright position. The child spends the majority of the day in bed or lying in a play pen. The child is encouraged to be quiet so the mother can get things done. It is imperative that before the child is labeled retarded in developmental achievements he be given the opportunity to sit up with help and that he is stimulated by toys, voice, and other means to sit up for increasingly longer periods. In addition, the mother is encouraged to foster development and shown how to stimulate the child toward the next developmental goal if he achieves sitting before the next visit.

Earlier diagnosis puts new demands for treatment at an early age. The child with minimal cerebral dysfunction will need special educational considerations. He will need consistent handling at home. The earlier the special education is begun, the sooner the child may be able to transfer to regular classes.

Let us consider, for a moment, the handling of a hyperactive three-year-old. His daily pattern consists of running around the house, disrupting furniture, pushing the other children, destroying toys, and crying easily. His mother reacts with frequent outbursts of anger which tend to make the child more hyperactive. In advising the mother, the nurse should emphasize several points which may tend to lessen the frustrations. The child with minimal cerebral dysfunction finds it difficult to filter out stimuli. Therefore, he tries to react to them all at once. If he is watching TV and the wind blows the window, he tries to react to it and gets up and attempts to run to the window. His poor perception does not tell him the TV is in his way, and he runs right into it. His mother reacts by yelling a command, "Be careful," thus introducing another stimulus and further confusing his filtering mechanism. A therapeutic environment, for this child, would be one that controls stimulus. The more "nude" the environment, the better. In fact, this child often does much better completely screened off with just one thing to concentrate on. Instead of TV, he should be given simple block forms to work with or toys that are used to develop other senses and thus help to make his visual sense more dependable.

It is very desirable to have fairly strict routines established as they tend to make the child feel more secure. He needs a definite sequence of events as he does not change easily from one activity to another. What could be considered a highly undesirable environment for a normal three-year-old may be the best environment for a three-year-old with minimal cerebral dysfunction.

In exploring the reasons for broken toys, it is frequently found that the child does not want to break the toy but he does not know how to use complicated ones. If the toy has wheels he may spin them until they fall off or if the toy has headlights he may become so entranced he pulls them out. Things that go around seem to fascinate him. Fewer and less complicated toys will tend to lessen the breakage problem.

The child with minimal cerebral dysfunction frequently pushes or physically irritates other children. This may be caused by poor perception or it may be partially due to the poor body image the child has of himself. The child frequently feels the need to reach out and touch others and in our society touching others is not always considered appropriate.

The child also changes easily from one mood to another. He frequently cries and may almost seem to laugh and cry at the same time. He frequently gets scolded for his many unacceptable behaviors and crying seems to be his only way out. The nurse should try to help the mother see that the child who meets many failures during the day may feel very distraught. She must try to be sure to praise the child when he makes small gains, as the praise will help him to develop some self-worth. He needs praise desperately and his day will be much brighter if his failures are interspersed with some success.

In helping the mother to set limits and goals it is important to assess the child's assets rather than his deficits. His assets frequently get buried beneath his deficits and the child, as well as the parent, does not make sufficient use of them. Trying to find his strengths and building on them should be the goal of intervention. Frequently, the child is gifted verbally because he finds less confusion with this method of communication. He has learned by repeated failure that his motor performance is frequently not acceptable. Therefore, education should include introducing things to help him with his verbal knowledge such as carving letters out of wood for him to trace as he says words, or showing him pictures to reinforce his words. Asking him to write the word "ball" may result in failure whereas spelling it verbally may result in success.

It is easy to predict that a three-year-old who exhibits these tendencies will not readily adjust in a regular classroom situation when he gets older. Some authorities feel that medication may help to quiet the child and make it easier for him to pay attention. The reaction to the medication is not always favorable and frequently the child has an adverse effect producing exaggerated behavior. The parents and the child should know this is a possibility and they should realize that sometimes several medications will be tried before they find one that helps the child. They should also know that sometimes medication is not indicated.

Proper classroom placement is still not available for all these children, or even for a major portion of them. This means that many of them get into regular classes where they are a disrupting factor and their educational needs are not met. The teacher describes their behavior very nicely when she states they are in "constant motion," swinging their legs, tapping their pencils, destroying books, and seldom completing an assigned task. The teacher must be helped to give the child simple, direct instructions. If she/he punishes him by putting him in the corner facing the blackboard, he frequently does much better. She/he needs to know that it is not his reaction to the punishment that improved his output, but rather the decrease in stimulus. Also, the child with minimal cerebral dysfunction will need periods during which he can release his excess energy. After this release he is better able to return to work.

The school nurse should be aware that these children react poorly to minor stresses such as a toothache or a cold. Such a child may be unusually difficult to control and perhaps he would be better at home during these periods when additional stressful situations should be kept to a minimum. Other associated problems which may present themselves in school are the child's tendency to not step high enough and trip up stairs, or his seeming lack of knowledge that there is a step—so he falls down. He frequently misjudges and walks into the sides of doors. He may have difficulty getting his coat as he cannot reach high enough. If some of these things are kept in mind, intervention can be given which will aid the child and tend to cut down on his sudden outbursts which occur when he becomes frustrated.

In addition to the regular classroom work the child will benefit by "motor therapy." This is a conditioning process in which he learns to step down or step up. This can be done as a game making all types of obstacles for him to get over. At first these obstacles should be very simple, and then increased in complexity as he achieves and he masters a step.

Such children will frequently need help with reading as they see letters backwards and sentences seem to run together. The nurse can interpret to the parent and child his need for additional help. She/he may also help the parent to understand that it is not good to push the child to read at home because his reading skills are developed under very special conditions. Parents frequently find it difficult not to push the child as he looks so "normal" and they cannot understand why he does not progress like other children.

Since 1972, Feingold (1975) reports that there are several investigators who have found positive results from using diets free from synthetic flavors and colors. The best results have been reported with the younger children. Approximately 50 percent of the children placed on a strict elimination diet have a loss of the hyperactivity, aggression, and impulsiveness tendencies. Following these improvements, there is an improvement in the child's motor ability. He states that disturbances in cognition and perception are usually the last areas to show improvement by the diet therapy. The dietary management of these children can be facilitated by the nurse helping the mother to identify and eliminate foods containing additives without nutritional value.

The Hospitalized Child. When the child with minimal cerebral dysfunction is hospitalized, he often disrupts the entire unit. This is easy to understand when we take a minute to listen and watch the day and night happenings on the unit. His easy distractibility will make the hospital almost unbearable. Every attempt should be made to decrease stimuli. A private room, if available, can be very soothing. In contrast to the other children, treatment may be easier to do in his own room—where it is familiar, where he does not see myriads of equipment, and which is away from the mainstream of activity.

Even though we consider the hospital to be very "routine," it can frequently lack the consistency the child needs. A late breakfast may be intolerable to this child. A consulting physician may get greeted with hostility or the new nurse may get medications thrown at her/him. This child will frequently eat much better in his own room without all the usual things children like for eating time, such as music, dishes with pictures in the bottom, straws, and surprises. If the child wants to try eating in the group at another time, he should be given the opportunity. This does not guarantee that he will succeed but it does show him you know he is trying. If his behavior is completely disruptive to the entire group then this exposure should be discontinued. Types of disruptive behavior exhibited at meal time include taking everyone else's food, spilling the milk out of everyone's glasses, tearing up napkins, and throwing food on the floor.

Nap Time. Nap time may be a particularly trying time for the hyperkinetic child. Many parents have complained that these children are in constant motion all day and although they may appear exhausted, they never give in to a nap. Then they come to the hospital where a rest period is planned and they cannot tolerate the confinement. Putting them in bed may increase their irritability and may cause temper tantrums. When they are in bed they frequently rock, bang their hands, or shake the siderails. This activity can be best tolerated in a single room. The crib may need padding to protect the child from injury. It would be wise to have an understanding adult sit next to the child's bed during nap time.

Heights. The child also has difficulty judging heights. When he is outside he falls down because he cannot judge curbs. In the hospital the nurse must be cautious in using bedside stools to assist the child when getting up. He will not be able to judge the distance and will fall the same as he does when he meets a curb outside. This factor also is important when the child tries to negotiate stairs. He is extremely awkward and will need a nurse's hand as assistance.

Helping the Child Understand Himself. The hospitalization provides the nurse with an opportunity to help the child to understand himself. Frequently he is frightened by his sudden outbursts; he is lonely and he feels isolated from the rest of the world. It takes a nurse who is not personally hurt by cutting remarks to work with this child. It also takes a nurse who can accept the idea that the child will have good and bad days and many more bad than good. She/he also needs to know that at times he will seem to regress and all her/his efforts seem to be in vain. She/he can introduce the school-age child to the book by Gardner (1966), which was specifically written to help the child learn to understand himself, and read sections with him. The book should be only a supplement to her counseling and not a replacement for it. The parents should also be introduced to the book. The parents should know which sections are currently being discussed with their child. The parents may appreciate knowing some of the child's responses to the book.

One of the most frequent reasons for hospitalizing this child is for diagnostic evaluation. This may be a very difficult period for the child as he is exposed to so many new things and people, frequently without proper preparation. The hospitalization may be extremely stressful for the parent, as they are anxiously awaiting a decision on just what is causing the hyperactive behavior. Many parents seem relieved when something is found to be organically wrong, as this then seems to somewhat justify the child's unacceptable behavior. A careful interpretation of findings is necessary so the parents know what the findings indicate. For instance, the parents may be told the EEG is normal and they think this means there is no brain injury. Other factors may be so much more relevant, such as the scatter performance on psychologic testing and not the IQ number itself. Minor neurologic deficits and history of behavior are also more significant than getting an abnormal EEG. There may be other parents who cannot accept the fact that their child is brain-injured and after a period of denial they may very well need a reinterpretation of what this means.

The EEG. An EEG (electroencephalogram) is a diagnostic assessment frequently used in relation to neurologic conditions. The procedure is used in conjunction with other diagnostic measurements and is not an independent assessment for making a diagnosis. The EEG is a recording of the brain wave activity of the child. It is done to determine electrical abnormalities which may be present. It is an especially useful procedure for determining seizure activity.

Preparation of the child is paramount to decrease the anxiety which may accompany being taken to a strange room. The room is usually constructed to eliminate any distractions and therefore is usually very plain and isolated. The child should know about the room and the people that will be responsible for his care. There is usually a technician to do the EEG's.

The EEG can be done with the older child sitting in a chair. For younger children, it can be done lying down. Young children may need sedation in order to get an adequate reading because crying and excessive activity make a reading impossible to obtain. In older children maintenance medications such as phenobarbital and dilantin (anticonvulsants) are usually ordered to be withheld for 48 hours prior to the recording. This will provide a more accurate picture of the normal brain wave pattern for the particular child.

After the child is positioned, electrode compound is applied and electrodes are placed on the child's scalp. The child needs reassurance that these electrodes will not hurt him. The child may fear the unknown and also make self-explanations drawing on his limited body of knowledge. He may think he is being electrocuted and become unnecessarily alarmed. This is especially true of the child with minimal cerebral dysfunction. Each step must be explained very simply and the procedures done slowly. The nurse needs to help the technician understand the child's proneness to hyperactivity and overreactions to tests. If the child gets too upset, it may be necessary to postpone the procedure until another time.

After the child is adequately prepared, the technician asks the child to sit quietly while the recordings are taken. This may be very difficult for the child with minimal cerebral dysfunction. Rest periods when he can move around should be liberally interspersed between quiet periods to help decrease the child's frustration. After the recordings are completed, the nurse should remove all the electrode compound and be sure the child's hair is combed.

The Parents. Probably the best advice that can be given the parents is that they should try to see the child first and the hyperactive behavior second. While this may be difficult, it does provide for a better parent-child relationship. The parents should be encouraged to praise the child for very small successes. They should be encouraged to reward appropriate behavior as soon as it occurs otherwise the frequent inappropriate behavior may overshadow the child's small accomplishments and go unrewarded.

It is interesting to note that in a study by Cantwell (1972) there were more psychiatric problems in the parent population of children with hyperactivity than in a control group of parents whose children were not affected. In the subject group, there were significantly more fathers with histories of alcoholism and sociopathy as well as psychiatric hospitalizations than in the control group. In the subject group there were significantly more mothers with histories of alcoholism and hysteria than in the control group. There was also a high incidence of alcoholism, sociopathy, and hysteria among the relatives of children with hyperactivity.

This study also showed that ten percent of the parents of hyperactive children were also hyperactive themselves as children. Cantwell suggests that his findings indicate that the syndrome of hyperactivity may be a precursor to alcoholism, sociopathy, or hysteria in adulthood. Cantwell states that his findings are consistent with those of a previous study done in St. Louis. Drawing on the evidence from the two studies, Cantwell suggests that the hyperactive child syndrome is a familial syndrome which passes from generation to generation. His study does not clarify whether the tendency is genetic or environmental. Additionally, a study by Weiss et al (1971), reported that 25 percent of hyperactive children had a history of antisocial behavior at follow-up evaluations.

These studies suggest that it may be difficult to get parent participation in the care necessary for these children to develop their maximum potential.

A case history of a family situation will illustrate the degree of family instability that may be present with these children.

Kim was four years old when he was diagnosed as having minimal cerebral dysfunction. I was asked to visit the home to give him an enema as he had not had a bowel movement for two weeks. Kim was not toilet trained. It took a great deal of effort to give him an oil retention enema due to his hyperactivity and inability to respond to verbal explanations. After a period of time the enema was successful and Kim seemed relieved to be free of the distention and discomfort caused by his impaction.

Kim's family history was significant. His father was an alcoholic and his mother worked nights as a bar maid to support the family. His mother tried very hard to follow through on suggestions regarding Kim's care, but was always too tired to be successful. In addition to Kim, she had three active school-age children. At one point, the family was offered the opportunity for family counseling, but they refused to accept the help.

The supervision of the family was scanty since they moved frequently without leaving forwarding addresses. After a period of years we learned that Kim's father had shot himself to death in front of Kim.

In retrospect it is hard to say what could have been done to help this family accept more professional help. They were not ready to accept it and their wishes were respected. The consequences were great.

Developmental Lag

Developmental lag is the term which is currently being used to describe the child who was formerly called mentally retarded. Miller (1968) quotes Farber's seven stages of family development. Family development begins with the family with no children, then it is a family with infant children, progresses to the family with preschool children, then to the family with elementary school children, with college-age children, and with children out of the home. He suggests that each stage of family development has its particular stresses and rewards and anticipatory preparation for the next stange. The family with a child with developmental lag finds itself frozen in one of the early stages of family development. The stresses of the stage are intensified and the rewards of the particular stage are less or nonexistent.

Miller suggests that a first born child is special to the parents, as they perceive the child to be a replication of themselves. If the child has impaired developmental function, it makes the parents feel particularly sad. He suggests that a family that is more solidified is better able to cope with a child with developmental lag. He suggests that coping with the outer reality of the child who is handicapped and the inner reality of the feelings associated with the loss of the desired child requires a great deal of mental effort.

The three stages of parental adjustment suggested by many authors and spelled out by Miller are as follows:

1st stage: Shock and disorganization. Complete inability to deal with the reality of the situation. Denial is the chief coping mechanism used by the parents. The parents are so involved with their emotional response that there is little or no energy left for coping with other situations in the environment.

2nd stage: Adjustment begins. During the second stage the parents are suffering chronic sorrow. They vacillate between partial acceptance and partial rejection of the child's handicap. They seek for someone or something to blame for the child's condition.

3rd stage: Reintegration. A stage that few parents are able to obtain. The parents would be able to successfully integrate this child into their family and be able to distribute their parental attention appropriately between or among their children.

The parents of children with disabilities are very concerned about the future for their child. This is especially prevalent in parents of children with developmental lag. They have concerns about school, work, self-care, and institutionalization. Many of their concerns seem premature as parents of children without disabilities seldom have the same degree of urgency to discuss the distant future of their children. The counseling of these parents should help them to set goals for the immediate care of the child and lessen their need to predict the child's entire future.

The needs of the child with developmental lag are similar to the needs of any child. They need constant and loving parenting. They must be stimulated to achieve the developmental milestones. Difficulties arise when the child is given frequent reminders of his inability to succeed. MacMillan and Keogh (1971) studied children with developmental lag and concluded that these children have a high expectancy for failure. The children tended to blame themselves for failures. This blame is probably related to the way adults have responded to them. Instead of encouraging them to develop, these children are frequently told that they cannot achieve and that they are not trying. These reminders convince the child that he is at fault and tend to lessen his self-concept and desire to achieve.

Two early indicators of developmental lag are the cry and sucking responses. The cries of children with brain injuries are different from the cries of normal newborns. They have been described previously. The nursery nurse can assess the quality of the cry, the spontaneity of the cry, the length of the cry, and the consistency of the cry. Infants with brain injury tend to need more stimulating to begin crying. The amount of stimulation given should be recorded on the nurse's notes.

In addition to the cry, a poor sucking reflex is a sign that the infant has some deviation from expected. Many children with developmental lag feed poorly. It will take patience to provide the infant with the necessary nutritional intake. If the infant tires he may become irritable and refuse the bottle or breast. If he has not received adequate intake, he will not sleep soundly or for long periods of time. His dissatisfaction with the feeding process encourages him to be irritable and can be interpreted by the mother as failure on her part. This reciprocal dissatisfaction can have lasting negative effects on the mother-child relationship.

The nurse must assist the mother with finding adequate ways to have the feeding experience less traumatic. A variety of feeding methods may have to be tried before an appropriate one is found. The child may go through periods of choking and gagging during this exploration time. This is not uncommon with these children. In addition, they may let the fluid just flow out of their mouths as quickly as it goes in. The chin may need to be supported in order to decrease this. Different positioning should also be tried. The use of padding or bibs to protect the child's clothing and decrease the amount of clothing that will be soiled in the process is helpful. During the feeding the mother should be encouraged to talk to the infant and cuddle him. She should know that her facial responses are important to the infant. If she grimaces all the time the child will begin to realize that she is uncomfortable in the situation. It is difficult to help parents understand that even though the infant does not make eye contact with them, that they must still attempt to elicit this response. It is so easy to give up with these children.

The child with a developmental lag will not begin to play as spontaneously as a child without a disability. Before he will use a toy it must be placed in his vision, it must be rubbed gently on his body, and he must be supported in a comfortable position so he can utilize it when he has learned to pay attention to it. A variety of toys will need to be given to him at periodic times so he will be stimulated and want to reach out to his environment. It will take longer for the child to learn to imitate peek-a-boo, patty cake, and other hand games. But when counseling the mother it is well to point out the value of her persistence in helping the child to master the task.

The child with developmental lag will be slower to develop language skills. The mother should know that encouraging vocalization will foster this process. She should talk to the infant or child when she is diapering and bathing. She should respond to any sounds that the child makes with delighted vocalizations of her own. Humming and singing little tunes will help to simulate the child. Times when she is playing with him or tending to his physical needs are opportune times for this activity.

As the child grows it is good to associate words with items, such as saying "button" when fastening one and "hat" when putting it on. Then the child should be encouraged to say "hat" and encouraged to point to it. The nurse can demonstrate these activities to the mother to be sure she understands what you are suggesting for her to do. In addition, toys which stimulate language development are useful. A wind-up toy that makes music will encourage the child to respond with coos of delight. The child is praised for his vocalization by saying things like, "Oh you tell such a pretty story," or

"Good boy!" or by clapping the hands in delight. The positive reinforcement will help in the teaching-learning process.

The framework in the chapter on growth and development is valuable in relation to children with developmental lag. However, these children will progress at a slower rate and more emphasis will be placed on adapting the environment to meet their special needs. More attention will be focused on getting the child to pay attention to what you are demonstrating. These children tend to have altered attention spans and limited ability to initiate experiences on their own. If left to their own resources, they may be willing to spend long hours in a playpen lying on their backs or lying motionless in a crib. Due to their slow motor development they may not explore the environment even if they are left on the floor to facilitate movement and exploration. Parents are encouraged to move the child to new areas, put him at varying heights, use swings, and other mobility toys to give him the feel of motion even if he cannot produce it himself.

The nurse takes time to explain to the mother about the value of her role in the nurturing process. She suggests that the other family members can play a vital role in helping with the stimulation process. Just as the child deserves positive reinforcement for his gains, so does the family. They should be praised for assisting the child in his progress, through statements such as, "You interact very well with Johnny, listen to how he coos in response to bouncing him on your knee" or "Johnny has come a long way since your last appointment, you really are doing a fine job."

The nurse serves as a role model to the mother. During visits to the home or during clinic visits, he/she spends time talking to the child and using play to stimulate his attention. In addition, he/she evaluates his development and then demonstrates the next tasks which can be encouraged. Guides such as the Denver Developmental Assessment are valuable tools for visually helping the mother to plan for the child's next activities. After the nurse charts the child's development, she/he shares the chart with the mother and encourages her to focus her attention on stimulating the child and he/she suggests appropriate ways to accomplish the stimulation.

The nurse's role will be partially determined by the setting where he/she is employed. Professional teams have found that many professionals are capable of giving the same service to children with developmental lag. This does not mean that the nurse's role is any less significant. He/she adapts the role to compliment the role of other health team members, sometimes serving as team member and sometimes as a team leader. The goal of habilitation must be to help the families avail themselves of resources and services which will benefit their particular situation. Referrals will be made to assist the family when appropriate. The school will take on added responsibility for the child's development when he is old enough to enter. The key role of the school in relation to children with developmental lag has changed the focus of care of these children from a medical model of care to an educational model. Under the educational model, these children have made significant gains toward independence and autonomy. The nurse with preparation in the teaching-learning process and health education is in a strategic position to contribute to the care of these children following the educational model.

BIBLIOGRAPHY

Aguilera DC, Messick JM: Crisis Intervention. St. Louis, Mosby, 1974

Amador LV: Congenital anomalies. In Swenson O: Pediatric Surgery, 3rd ed. New York, Appleton, 1969, Chap 74

Amundson MJ: Nurses as group leaders of behavior management classes for parents. Nurs Clin North Am 10:319–27, 1975

Barnard KE, Erickson ML: Teaching children with Developmental Problems, 2nd ed. St. Louis, Mosby, 1976

Basara SC: The behavioral patterns of the perceptually handicapped child. Nurs Forum 5:24–39, 1966

Bean MR, Bell BJ: Nursing intervention in the care of the physically handicapped child. Nurs Clin North Am 10:361, 1975

Blakeslee B (ed): The Limb-Deficient Child. Berkeley, University of California Press, 1963

Bleck EE, Nagel DA: Physically Handicapped Children. A Medical Atlas for Teachers. New York, Grune & Stratton, 1975

Bramley GL: The handicapped child–his attitudes and behavior. In Fishbein M (ed): Birth Defects. Philadelphia, Lippincott, 1963

Bruce SJ: Reactions of nurses and mothers to stillbirths. Nurs Outlook 10:88–91, 1962

Cantwell DP: Psychiatric illness in the families of hyperactive children. Arch Gen Psychiatry 27:414–17, 1972

Caplan G: Mental Health and Consultation. Washington, DC, U.S. Dept of Health, Education and Welfare, 1959

Clemmens RL: Minimal brain damage in children. In Rudick E (ed): Pediatric Nursing. Dubuque, Iowa, Brown, 1966, pp 82–90

Cohen PC: Impact of the handicapped child in the family. Social Casework 48:137, 1962

Connors M: Ostomy care: a personal approach. Am J Nurs 74:1422, 1974

Cormay RB: Returning special education students to regular classes. Personnel and Guid J 48:64, 1970

Debuskey M (ed): The chronically ill child and his family. Springfield, Ill, Thomas, 1970

de la Cruz FF, LaVeck GD: Human sexuality and the mentally retarded. New York, Brunner/Mazel, 1973

Eddington C, Lee T: Sensory-motor stimulation for slow-to-develop children: a home-centered program for parents. Am J Nurs 75:59, January 1975

Feingold BC: Hyperkinesis and learning disabilities linked to artificial food flavors and colors. Am J Nurs 75:797, May 1975

Ferrer JM: The esophagus. In Barnett, HL (ed): Pediatrics, 14th ed. New York, Appleton, 1968, pp 1519–25

Fochtman D, Raffensberger JB: Principles of Nursing Care for the Pediatric Surgery Patient, 2nd ed. Boston, Little Brown, 1976
Frankenberg WK, Dudds JB: Denver Development Screening Text Manual. Denver, University of Colorado Medical Center, 1970
Galloway KG: The uncertainty and stress of high risk pregnancy. Mat Child Nurs 1:294, 1976
———: Placental evaluation studies: the procedures, the purposes and the nursing care involved. Mat Child Nurs 1:300, 1976
Gardner R: The Child's Book About Brain-Injury. Association for Brain Injured Children, 1966
Gearheart BR, Weishahn MW: The Handicapped Child in the Regular Classroom. St. Louis, Mosby, 1976
Gendel ES: Sex education—learning about human sexuality. In Knotts GR, McGovern JP (eds): School Health Problems. Springfield, Ill, Thomas, 1975
Godfrey AB: Sensory-motor stimulation for slow-to-develop children. Am J Nurs 75:56, January 1975
Harmon V, Steele S: Nursing Care of the Skin: A Developmental Approach. New York, Appleton, 1975
Heisler V: A Handicapped Child in the Family: A Guide for Parents. Grune & Stratton, 1972
Holmberg NJ: Serving the child with MBD and his family. Nurs Clin N Amer 10:381, June 1975
Holt JL: A long-term study of a child treated for hypospadias. Pediat Clin N Amer 4:27, 1969. Philadelphia, Saunders
Jackson PL: Chronic grief. Am J Nurs. 74:1288, July 1974
King LR: Hypospadias. In Swenson O (ed): Pediatric Surgery, 3rd ed. New York, Appleton, 1969, Chap 66
Kini J, Scahill M: The institutional setting: innovations in nursing care. Nurs Clin N Amer 10:393, June 1975 ·
Klaus MH, Kennell JH: Maternal-Infant Bonding. St. Louis, Mosby, 1976
Lehtinen LE: The brain-injured child: what can we do for him? Dallas Med J (Special edition):15, 1959
MacMillan DL, Keogh BK: Normal and retarded children's expectancy for failure. Dev Psychol 4:343, 1971
Marlow DR: Textbook of Pediatric Nursing, 3rd ed. Philadelphia, Saunders, 1969, pp 107, 173–75
Martin L et al: Nursing care of infants with esophageal anomalies. Am J Nurs 66:2463, 1966
Mathews ES, Ransohoff J: Hydrocephalus. In Barnett JL (ed): Pediatrics, 16th ed. New York, Appleton, 1977
Mattson A: Long-term physical illness in childhood: a challenge to psychosocial adaptation. Pediatrics 50:801, 1972
McCollum AT: Coping With Prolonged Health Impairment in Your Child. Boston, Little, Brown, 1975
Mercer RT: Mother's responses to their child with defects. Nurs Res 23:133, 1974
Miller LG: Toward a greater understanding of parents of the mentally retarded child. J Pediatr 73:699, 1968
Newcomer BL, Morrison TL: Play therapy with institutionalized mentally retarded children. Am J Ment Defic 78:727–33, 1974
Olshansky S: Chronic sorrow: a response to having a mentally defective child. Social Casework 43:30, 1962
Owens C: Parents' reactions to defective babies. Am J Nurs 64:83–86, 1964

Parad HJ, Caplan GA: A framework for studying families in crisis. In Parad HJ (ed): Crisis Intervention. New York, Family Service Assoc of America, 1965, pp 53–72.
Passo SD: Positioning infants with myelomeningocele. Am J Nurs 74:1658–60, September 1974
Pattullo AW: The socio-sexual development of the handicapped child. Nurs Clin North Am 10:361–72, 1975
Rose MH: Coping behavior of physically handicapped children. Nurs Clin North Am 10:329–39, 1975
Ross AO: The Exceptional Child in the Family. New York, Grune & Stratton, 1964
Rothschild BF: Incubator isolation as a possible contributing factor to the high incidence of emotional disturbance among prematurely born persons. Psychol Abstr 42:537, 1968
Scahill M: Early intervention with newborns. In O'Neill SM, Newcomer B (eds): Sixth National Workshop for Nurses in Mental Retardation, March 20–22, 1974, Cincinnati, Ohio
Schulman JL, Kaper JC, Throne FM: Brain-Damage and Behavior. Springfield, Ill, Thomas, 1965
Schulman K: Meningomyelocele. In Barnett HL (ed): Pediatrics, 16th ed. New York, Appleton, 1977
Smith ED: Spina Bifida and the Total Care of Myelomeningocele. Springfield, Ill, Thomas, 1965
Solnit AJ, Stark M: Mourning and the birth of a defective child. Psychoanal Study Child 16:523, 1961
Steele S: Children with amputations. Nurs Forum 7:411–23, 1968
———: The nurse's role in the rehabilitation of children with meningomyelocele. Nurs Form 6:104–17, 1967
Stogdill CG: School achievement, learning difficulties and mental health. Canada's Mental Health 48 (Suppl):1–7, 1965
Strauss AA, Kephart NC: Psychopathology and Education of the Brain-Injured Child. New York, Grune & Stratton, 1955
———, Lehtinen LE: Psychopathology and Education of the Brain-Injured Child, New York, Grune & Stratton, 1947
Strother CR: Discovering, Evaluation, Programming for the Neurologically Handicapped child. National Society for Crippled Children and Adults, 1963
Sugar M, Ames MD: The child with spina bifida cystica. Rehabil Lit 26:362, 1965
Swenson O (ed): Pediatric Surgery, 3rd ed. New York, Appleton, 1969, Chap 29
von Schilling KC: The birth of a defective child. Nurs Forum 7:424, 1968
Zieman HF: The neurologically handicapped child. Am J Nurs 69,2621, 1969

CAROL REN KNEISL

9 Nursing Care of the Troubled Child

There is no doubt but that troubled children constitute a target population and a social problem of considerable magnitude in the United States. The material presented in this chapter will provide the knowledge base on which to plan nursing intervention for these troubled children.

Historically, the field of child mental health care services owes its emergence (1) to twentieth century psychoanalysts who began to focus on personality development and deviation and (2) to courts and correctional institutions that began to call attention to the need for prevention, treatment, and rehabilitation of juvenile delinquents. Out of these efforts the first child guidance and child treatment centers in the United States were established in New York, Boston, and Chicago.

Consequently, larger numbers of persons from many disciplines became involved in this field. The interdisciplinary range of child care workers is varied and includes nursing, psychiatry, pediatrics, psychology, social work, speech and hearing pathology, neurology, sociology, anthropology, and many others who engage in a wide spectrum of activities with troubled or delinquent children. Earlier interests in the study of deviant or abnormal children turned to interest in the study of the well child or the normal child in the belief that one must understand normal development before one can understand developmental deviations.

Attempts to devise methods of bringing up children based upon understanding of growth and development have led to a number of absurd as well as common-sense or rational approaches. Historically, our beliefs about child care and parental responsibility vary along a continuum with the extremes of the continuum gaining the greatest attention from parents and professionals alike. For example, we have vacillated for a number of decades in our ideas about breast versus bottle feeding, parental permissiveness versus parental restraint, and demand feeding versus feeding on schedule. One of the most pragmatic helps available to parents concerned with child-rearing can be found in the beautiful prose by Dorothy Law Nolte entitled "Children Learn What They Live" (Fig. 1).

More recently, the emphasis is being placed upon the study of animals, particularly primates. John Bowlby, who spurred interest in maternal and emotional deprivation as the result of his monograph published by the

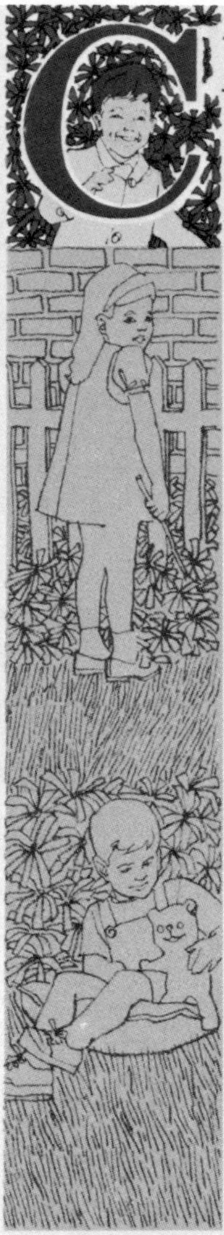

CHILDREN LEARN WHAT THEY LIVE

If a child lives with criticism, He learns to condemn.

If a child lives with hostility. He learns to fight.

If a child lives with ridicule. He learns to be shy.

If a child lives with shame. He learns to feel guilty.

If a child lives with tolerance. He learns to be patient.

If a child lives with encouragement. He learns confidence.

If a child lives with praise. He learns to appreciate.

If a child lives with fairness. He learns justice.

If a child lives with security. He learns to have faith.

If a child lives with approval. He learns to like himself.

If a child lives with acceptance and friendship,
He learns to find love in the world.

FIG. 1. Dorothy Law Nolte's "Children Learn What They Live." (Courtesy of Ross Laboratories)

World Health Organization of the United Nations in 1951, has presented the thesis that the study of animal behavior, particularly that of primates, has extreme relevance to human psychology (Bowlby, 1969), an attitude which has previously been ignored, doubted, or denied. It has been proposed that consideration of growth and development is based upon certain inherent biologic capacities through a long history of primate evolution combined with behaviors man shares with other primates and which is augmented through the use of a culture that is uniquely human (Morris, 1969). When considering the relationship of human behavior to primate behavior, one ought to keep in mind the fact that aspects of the uniqueness of human development are based upon infant behavior, which demonstrate not only intelligence but adaptability and flexibility as well. The strategies invented by the infant when working within his limitations are plainly different from those of other primates (Bruner, 1968). The film, *Rock-A-Bye-Baby* beautifully illustrates the nurturing aspects of primates and builds a convincing case for studying their behavior to help understand the nurturing process of human beings. And so the controversy continues in an attempt to refine and define those developmental characteristics and necessities which make for effective adaptation in living.

In 1961, the Joint Commission on Mental Illness and Health published the results and recommendations of their five-year study of mental health in America. While this report concerned itself mostly with adults and the establishment of community mental health centers, it did have some recommendations to make regarding children and their treatment in residential schools, clinics, and the community at large. The report noted the paucity of specialists in the area of children's mental health and recommended supplementation of state funds with federal funds in the training and education of professionals and lay people to augment the current number (Joint Commission on Mental Illness and Health, 1961). Impetus was given to these recommendations and to further study by the assassination of President Kennedy. President Kennedy's assassin, Lee Harvey Oswald, had been studied by the Bureau of Child Guidance in New York. However, their recommendations, regarding Oswald's treatment were never carried out.

One outcome was an amendment to the Social Security law introduced in 1965 by Senator Abraham Ribicoff which provided funds for the establishment of a Joint Commission on Mental Health of Children. This project was a three-year study undertaken by a large number of professional organizations concerned with the mental health needs of children. The results were made public in May of 1969 (Joint Commission on Mental Health of Children, 1969).

The Commission viewed as a national tragedy the lack of any unified or cohesive national commitment to children and youth. It called for drastic changes to bring about such a commitment and a "child-oriented society."

Some of the changes recommended consisted of federal assistance for research, training, and treatment at every level of society to ensure effective implementation of programs designed to be of assistance to children. By May of 1970, one year after the publication of its report, the Commission regretfully announced in the communications media that not one community in the United States had yet provided adequate services. The seriousness of the problem can be deduced from the knowledge that at least 10 million young persons under the age of 25 have an emotional disorder.

Some sense of the magnitude of the problem of troubled children in the United States can be appreciated upon review of the report of the 1970 White House Conference on Children. This report noted that:

> As of 1966 nearly two million young people were enrolled in special education programs.
> In 1968 approximately ten percent of the fifty million children of school age had moderate to severe emotional problems.
> There were serious emotional problems that required attention in fully one out of three children from poor families.
> Some children with severe reading problems were reported in ninety-two percent of all public elementary schools.
> The 682,000 children and their families who received mental health care in 1968 represented only a fraction of the children and families in need of it. (1970 White House Conference on Children)

These numbers mask an incredibly bewildering array of diagnostic labels—neurotic dysfunction, psychotic dysfunction, infantile autism, childhood schizophrenia, juvenile delinquency—and a continuum of problems ranging from the mildest behavioral difficulty to the most severe psychosis.

The use of such labels has come under increased criticism in recent years on the basis that labeling plays a crucial role in both the development and maintenance of deviant behavior. There is ample data to indicate that members of the helping professions readily assume the role of labeler (Ennis, 1972; Rosenhan, 1973; Cullen, 1974; Sayre, 1976). The effects on children have been specifically considered by Hobbs (1975), and his book with its helpful suggestions for professionals is heartily recommended. Because professional helpers can influence an individual's self-concept, it is absolutely essential to give careful consideration to the entire process of labeling.

Paradoxically, in order for mental health workers to communicate across disciplines and fulfill certain local, state, and federal regulations to obtain funding, it remains necessary in most instances that such labels be understood and applied—at least on appropriate forms. It is for these reasons that this chapter is organized around the labels that will provide the student with the necessary means for understanding the psychiatric jargon with which he or she will be faced. At the time of this writing, there are no psychiatric nursing textbooks which consistently provide a nonmedical model approach. However, one with a humanistic/interactionist perspective specifically designed to enhance holistic nursing perspectives will be available in the near future (Wilson and Kneisl, 1978).

MALADAPTATIONS AND NEUROTIC DYSFUNCTIONS OF CHILDHOOD

Neuroses or maladaptations of childhood were little recognized prior to the advent of psychoanalysis and the Freudian era. However, references were made in earlier centuries to the importance of child-rearing activities and the various thoughts, feelings and actions inherent in the parent-child relationship. The description of clinical cases concerning mental disturbance or disorder in children was treated as unique, highly unusual, and curious, perhaps more appropriate for "Ripley's Believe It or Not" than for consideration by the professionals of the time.

One development which encouraged the use of the term "neurosis" when applied to children was Freud's turn-of-the-century analysis of the horse phobia of Little Hans (Freud, 1936). In their study of hysteria, Breuer and Freud established the relationship between the experiences of living and neurosis, thereby drawing attention to the need to study childhood development (Breuer and Freud, 1936). The psychobiologic approach advocated by Meyer, who utilized both analytic and descriptive psychiatry, also emphasized the importance of biographic study of the patient including childhood development (Meyer, 1948).

Much of the knowledge concerning childhood neuroses comes from psychoanalytically trained therapists. Anna Freud's modification of the technique of psychoanalysis made it possible to study and treat children with neuroses (A. Freud, 1946). The play therapy techniques developed by Klein were analytically oriented and obviated the necessity for verbal confirmation required in the psychoanalytic treatment of the adult (Klein, 1932). Recently, professionals with varying orientations have been engaged in the direct study of children in child-study laboratories.

Some of the specifics that differentiate the child with neurosis and the child who is adapting follow. The child with neurosis fluctuates in behavior, and while he, at times, may respond appropriately in terms of age-expected behavior and reality, at other times he exists in a state of distress and has diminished capacity for testing reality. The child with neurosis exists in a state of conscious and subjective mental distress, discomfort, or anxiety. His ability to call upon adjustment mechanisms or defense mechanisms to come to his rescue is diminished and, therefore, he is easily irritated and considerably excited by stimuli which others would perceive as relatively minor, nontoxic, or innocuous. Fortunately, complete disorganization of the personality or mental function does not take place even when the child's behavior appears disrupted to the onlooker. The symptoms the child with neurosis exhibits indicate a self-orientation as, for example, is present in common signs such as daydreaming, masturbation, bed-wetting, fears, and neurotic compulsions and obsessions. One should not link such behaviors only to childhood neurosis, since both the quality and quantity of the behavior and/or symptomatology needs to be considered. What child has never been fearful? Or daydreamed? Although there are certain phenomena which can be unhesitatingly labeled neurotic (conversion hysteria is one), others need to be analyzed in terms of their frequency, severity, and duration.

It is difficult to assign any one single cause in the development of childhood neurosis. This difficulty has been well phrased by Cramer (1959):

> Neurosis in childhood is caused by social experiences which are traumatic; that is, inappropriate in respect to the capacity of the mental apparatus of *that* child at *that* moment to contain and integrate them in a manner consistent with the maintenance of normal development. Since normal means something different depending on where one is, and especially depending on how old one is, adaptive devices of the child's mind find different responses in different environments and at different ages. Thus, differences in what constitutes a noxious stimulus may depend on various cultural influences (p 800).

Traumatic experiences, parental attitudes, and constitutional makeup are among the variety of factors generally present in the neuroses of childhood. Life experiences which may prove traumatizing to the child include loss of one or both parents when accompanied by unsuccessful mourning or inadequate substitutive figures, physical illness, injury, neglect, and traumatic acts of fate. Specific traumatic life experiences, parental attitudes, and constitutional makeup will be considered in view of the various neurotic and psychotic developmental deviations noted in this chapter. Before continuing, the reader would do well to review sources on personality development and adjustment mechanisms as background material necessary to an understanding of the emotional disorders of childhood. The author assumes that the reader possesses this necessary basic knowledge.

Crying

When continuous, extensive, and unrelieved crying occurs in situations in which its presence seems unreasonable—that is, in the absence of physical pathology or physical discomfort—it serves as a signal denoting mental distress. Generally, parents learn to distinguish within the first few weeks of the infant's life between cries which signal hunger, pain, or bodily discomfort. They then require decreasing periods of time in which to diagnose and meet the unfulfilled need demanded by the infant. When crying persists beyond the point at which apparent needs have been met by the one who is parenting, the infant's experienced distress is likely to be mental rather than physiologic. Further evidence that the infant's distress or anxiety is subtly communicated from the parent and reflects anxiety regarding parenting duties, may be seen in instances when someone other than the parent is able to reduce the infant's tension and anxious cry. The difference between these two individuals in handling the infant has to do with the quality of response.

Sullivan, a psychiatrist who devoted most of his time to the psychotherapy of schizophrenic adults, conceptualized an interpersonal theory of psychiatry based upon the belief that the quality of infant's earliest interpersonnel relationship was a crucial factor in determining the infant's later adjustment to the trials and vicissitudes of life (Sullivan, 1943). If the parent or other nurturing person is insecure, unsure, anxious, she or he empathically communicates this to the child, who responds with a like anxiety. Out of such a pattern, a vicious cycle is born. The infant's increasing anxiety and discomfort adds to the anxiety of the other, which in turn escalates the distress the infant feels. The cycle is broken when the nurturing person feels secure, calm, and relatively nonanxious, thereby allowing the infant to experience similar pleasurable feelings. Crying infants do not become "spoiled" if they are picked up and held. During this stage of infancy children do not need, nor can they cope with stringent setting of limits and the delay of gratification. When their needs are met they will experience greater security, trust, and self-worth. Wise parents set limits, make demands, and impose restrictions when the child is able to handle delayed gratification.

Feeding Disturbances

Eating is one of the earliest meaningful experiences the child has and, concurrently, hunger is the most common cause of crying and discomfort in the newborn. The magnitude of the problem becomes evident when the review of the records of 110 preschoolers referred to the Child Development Center of New York City indicates that in 56 percent of the children, feeding problems were present, with the far greater majority present during the first year of life (Beller, 1962). Once physical disturbances such as allergy, pylorospasm, and inappropriate formula (which may account for feeding problems) are ruled out, emotional factors must be considered. Food refusal, colic, and vomiting are common disturbances of feeding. Less common disturbances are pica, obesity, and anorexia nervosa.

Kessler indicates that when feeding problems occur, parents may find themselves repeating the same ineffective behavior of their own parents while feeling increasingly anxious, angry, and guilty. This knowledge has focused more attention on the study of the parenting behaviors of the parents in an attempt to improve child-rearing techniques.

> This is but one example of the important general principle that parents have special conflicts in handling problems which are a repetition of their own. Whenever a parent has a blind spot, it is worth exploring for evidence of the same difficulty a generation earlier (Kessler, 1966,p 105).

Food Refusal and Vomiting. With food refusal and vomiting, eating is associated with experiences of discomfort, as food often becomes the battleground in the parent-child relationship. What the infant is communicating is that he prefers the unpleasant state of hunger if his only other choice is to tolerate the interpersonal and intrapsychic discomfort which feeding brings.

Sometimes the problem is relatively simple. The parent simply needs to learn what to expect from the infant in terms of feeding and to readjust expectations. The mother or father who responds with rigidity in terms of the amount of food that should be eaten as well as the appropriate time in which to do so, is likely to be faced with an unhappy infant who is forced to vomit because he has been overfed, or has waited too long, or cried too hard, and is unable to eat when the "magic hour" finally arrives. Resolution of some of these conflicts can oftentimes be reached through parental reeducation.

Sometimes, however, feeding problems may be indicative of deep-seated hostility toward the child. A parent may rationalize the need for a strict schedule, thereby forcing the infant to wait for the gratification of need, or may overfeed in an attempt to compensate for or to deny the resentment felt. In this case, an attempt is made to convert the gift of food into a gift of love. The person who refuses to play this game through the rejection of food, which is the offered but dubious gift, is the child. For example, in one situation a mother actually force-feeds her daughter when she refuses to eat. The child is placed on her back on the floor and is fed from a spoon while the mother sits astride her to keep her arms and legs flat. Needless to say, in this household mealtime has become battletime. Rational and logical explanations to the mother regarding her own behavior have had no effect. It is likely, in such a situation, that an irrational and unconscious motive prompts this mother's actions. Her child is a candidate for more severe emotional disturbances in the future.

Colic. Sharp intestinal pain accompanied by loud crying, flexion of the legs, and abdominal distension is the generally accepted definition of infant colic. Holding or carrying the infant does not relieve the pain.

Colic usually ceases by the third or fourth month of life. It may be classified as an eating disturbance because of some of the curious factors which surround it. For example, the infant seems to be most uncomfortable for three or more of the early evening hours, although he appears to be relatively comfortable during the remainder of the day. Most pediatricians and child psychiatrists believe that colic is likely to result from a combination of two circumstances: an immature digestive tract and disruption of the interpersonal relationships in the family.

Colic is distressing not only to the obviously uncomfortable infant but also to his parents, who become more and more frustrated when their well-meant intentions and attempts to alleviate the infant's discomfort are unsuccessful.

Infants who are colicky are often found to be more hyperactive than other infants. They are often called tense, vigorous, lusty, and easily stimulated and startled. This may be an indication that the role of inborn constitutional differences may be important in producing colic.

The correlation between infant colic and its appearance in the evening hours may be the arrival home of the father who has been absent during the day while at his job. It is likely that the father's appearance alters the mother-child relationship. For example, the immature man may resent the time his wife spends with the child, or his return and the need to prepare dinner for the family realistically takes the mother away from the child for a longer period of time, or perhaps the mother does not look forward to her husband's return home in the evening. Any one of these factors is bound to disrupt the child-parent relationship, particularly if anxiety is an accompaniment.

Because of the distressing nature of infantile colic, parents inevitably embark upon the search for a solution which often takes them to the pediatrician's office in search of alterations in the formula. Occasionally, formula alterations can be helpful when an immature digestive tract is present. Unfortunately, formula alteration is not always helpful and some parents may request formula changes every few days or may even embark upon the search for a pediatrician who will be able to offer some sort of "cure."

As such behavior continues, the relationship between the child and his parents becomes more frustrating and unrewarding and fraught with anxiety. At such times, both parents and infant deserve a respite from each other, a vacation, if you will, to interrupt the escalation of dissatisfaction. The empathic nature of anxiety becomes more evident when colic cannot be attributed to physiologic problems or constitutional defects.

Attempting to soothe the infant may be temporarily helpful and at least offer some relief to both parents and child. At the same time, they could be encouraged to become aware of the pattern of colic and attempt to correlate it with their activities and the environment in the home. They perhaps may be able to determine events that increase their own anxiety communicated to the infant, and thereby alter their behavior or the environment.

Pica. Pica, the ingestion of substances generally considered inappropriate, such as clay, plaster, charcoal, and wax among others, is not unusual until approximately one year of age. During this first year of life every child who explores and tests the world around him is likely to have eaten a variety of unusual and generally unappetizing substances. The child who purposefully seeks out certain objects to eat, such as sand or paper or whatever, and remains persistent in his efforts evidences a feeding disturbance. Environmental and cultural conditions seem to play an important role in the development of pica.

Numerous research studies have been carried out in attempts to determine the influence which such factors as socioeconomic status, race, intelligence, and nutrition have in cases of pica. The results of the investigations are oftentimes contradictory. For example, some studies have indicated that children with pica are often severely retarded and almost always of subnormal intelligence, while other investigations conclude that pica has no relationship to level of intelligence. The influence of nutrition is also unclear. While some children who eat plaster have been found to have a calcium deficiency, others have not. Dietary lacks have not consistently correlated with the presence of pica. In her study of pica, Cooper (1967) indicates a higher incidence of pica among blacks and in lower socioeconomic groups. Among these groups, pica may be considered a somewhat natural state of affairs since of the more than 700 mothers interviewed, 171 reported it upon questioning while only one mother spontaneously offered this information. Cooper's results have been corroborated by others (Gutelius et al, 1962).

Physical environment may be an important factor since the active child who does not have an interesting and constructive way in which to release his energy may well turn to chewing furniture, clothes, or windowsills. Consistency is absent here since children who are stimulated and even overstimulated have developed this particular feeding disturbance. This may indicate that relationships between the child and the significant persons in his environment need to be investigated further in an attempt to determine etiologic factors.

Although pica generally disappears by the time a child is about six years old, there are numerous instances of pica in school-age children and adults, particularly in pregnant women.

Anorexia Nervosa. Anorexia nervosa, which occurs most often in females, is a condition in which food is perceived as revolting and inedible. The patient with anorexia refuses food, or regurgitates food which has been taken, resulting in excessive weight loss and malnutrition which can proceed to the level of starvation.

The patient with anorexia seems to be caught up in a power struggle with those persons who are attempting to cajole, persuade, threaten, or punish her into eating. According to a variety of points of view, anorexia nervosa may be an unconscious method by which the fear of sexuality, or anal aggressiveness toward the self or others may be expressed. When it is part of a psychotic disturbance such as schizophrenia it may relate to withdrawal from the unsafe, external world to a safer, internal one.

Certain commonalities have been identified as present in children and adolescents who are anorexic. One factor is that food has a special importance and meaning to the child's parents who often eat or drink to excess. In addition, food and eating is not newly important to the patient herself since the developmental history frequently indicates earlier power struggles with parents over food in various forms. The child has often been overweight before this symptom developed and engaged in bouts of compulsive eating. Third, there seems to be evidence of unwillingness to grow up, mature physically and become heterosexually oriented (Kessler, 1966).

Case Presentation. These commonalities were evident with Margie, a 14-year-old girl who was hospitalized when she was near starvation. Margie refused all food and when force-fed by one or both parents would regurgitate. She was extremely emaciated and so weak that she was unable to walk.

Margie's mother drank heavily on a rather sporadic basis, and when she did, she was in no condition to prepare lunch or dinner. It was often up to the child herself to assume responsibility for preparing food for herself and a younger brother and sister. The mother's drinking bouts coincided with the father's absences from the home for business reasons. Margie's mother questioned his absences and suspected that her husband was interested in extramarital relationships.

Before the onset of these symptoms, Margie's mother described her as "fat, sloppy, and unattractive." She often berated her daughter for her appearance and compared her unfavorably to other children who lived in the neighborhood. Margie often heard her mother say that she would "give anything to have a daughter I could be proud of." Suddenly after one of the mother's alcoholic periods, Margie refused to fix lunch or dinner for herself or the other children, and refused food prepared by others.

The day she was admitted to the hospital, Margie wore a pullover sweater. It was only since her excessive weight loss, her mother said, that Margie would consent to wear sweaters. She previously refused to wear them and often commented that "my bust shows up too much." Margie expressed joy over the fact that she had not had a menstrual period for months.

Initially, Margie was given intravenous feedings since the malnutrition was at a critical level at which irreversible damage could take place. Although one does not want to be caught up with the patient with anorexia in the power struggle over food, intravenous feedings may be necessary as a life-preserving therapy. In addition to medical management, psychotherapy was instituted with Margie and her parents. While Margie was being treated by a child psychiatrist, her parents' psychotherapy took place in a marital couple's group led by a clinical specialist in psychiatric nursing. Eventually

Margie consented to chewing fruit-flavored gum and proceeded from there to eat one soft-boiled egg daily. As both Margie and her parents began to work through individual and mutual conflicts, Margie's symptoms abated and she began to gain weight. The last time that staff members saw Margie they found her to be a "a little thin but cute." She informed them that her mother had agreed to her request to remain late after school one day a week to take ballroom dancing lessons, an exercise that was now possible not only because she was consuming a more adequate nutritional intake but also because her increasingly positive self-view permitted greater social and interpersonal contact with others.

The prognosis is not so favorable when anorexia nervosa is only one of many symptoms which are present in a child with psychosis.

Sleeping Disturbances

Disturbances of sleep seem to have to do with the fear of being left alone. The child, who is totally dependent upon his parents for his survival, needs to experience feeling secure and wanted and knowing that his needs will be met and his discomfort eased. Such security comes about through experiencing gratification, time and time again, in the meeting of needs. The child who is not sure whether his needs will be met will exist in a state of uncertainty and apprehension and will experience difficulty in learning to trust. Such a child will be fearful of being alone and in the dark, for it brings with it a state of uncertainty since the child's expectations of what will, or will not, happen to him are not clear.

Many times disturbances of sleeping, as well as the other neurotic disturbances previously mentioned, are encouraged by parental beliefs that meeting children's needs will "spoil" them, and so they purposefully delay the child's gratification. What the child will learn from such experiences, however, is that people cannot be trusted and that he cannot depend upon others. He will constantly feel threatened for his own safety and well-being, since the persons his physiologic and emotional survival depends upon have proven themselves to be untrustworthy.

Young children with problems of sleep are often fearful of their own aggressive impulses and loss of control associated with sleeping. These fears can generally be linked with the child's developmental stage and the current difficulties and stresses he faces. Nightmares reach a peak between the ages of four and six and are infrequently reported by younger children. When sleep disturbances are severe and chronic in nature they can be deemed pathologic and indicate that the level of anxiety experienced by the child cannot be reduced by the mechanisms known to him. In such instances, psychotherapeutic treatment is useful and generally effective within a short period of time.

Thumb-Sucking

Thumb-sucking is an important method of self-gratification enjoyed by the infant. Generally, after the first year of life, thumb-sucking decreases and loses its fascination for the child. When it remains a persistent behavior and chief source of gratification it can be considered a sign of mental conflict. Attitudes toward thumb-sucking are as polar as the extremes of a swinging pendulum. In our society a rather permissive attitude toward thumb-sucking exists. Relatively few parents continue with earlier forceful measures in attempts to suppress or prevent thumb-sucking in their children. Parental indulgence or permissiveness has not negated the need for thumb-sucking and in this sense it is as much a failure as bandaging the child's hands or coating them with an unpleasant-tasting liquid. The reason is that thumb-sucking, while partially or temporarily relieving the anxiety associated with intrapsychic or interpersonal conflict, does not cure or resolve the child's troubles.

Thumb-sucking may be considered more serious when factors of age, quantity, and association with other symptoms occur. The older child who sucks his thumb persistently and frequently while indulging in other symptoms indicative of immaturity or neurosis is certainly in greater emotional difficulty than the child who regresses to thumb-sucking upon the advent of a critical event, physical trauma or boredom. Temporary regression usually reverses itself when the critical event or physical trauma assumes a less threatening nature or the boredom is relieved. In the case of the immature child or child with neurosis whose thumb-sucking occurs in conjunction with a multiplicity of dysfunctional behaviors, psychotherapy and parental education may be required.

Phobias

Like sleep disturbances, phobias in childhood are common and are regarded as developmentally normal when they occur at an early age, and when they are transient in nature. However, phobias of children at the age of five and older can be disabling to the child when they are severe in nature. When the child is preoccupied with the situation, event, person, or thing he fears so that he seems to be existing in a constant state of dreaded anticipatory anxiety the phobia is considered to be severe in nature.

Although numerous theorists attempt to explain the cause or causes of phobias, most include the onset of a frightening experience which arouses anxiety and guilt which is repressed. A phobia gives the child something tangible to fear and, as frightening as it may be, is not so intolerable as the uncanny dread experienced during anxiety, an inner event.

The most frequent childhood phobias are of animals, transportation, and schools. Although horse phobias such as that of Little Hans, reported by Freud, are rare, dogs and insects seem to be leading contenders. The phobic object gives a clue to the unacceptable thought, wish, or impulse being repressed by the child. For example, according to psychoanalytic interpretation, insects are often feared because of their association with dirt, horses are feared because they are equated symbolically with the father, and the fear of snakes indicates the projection of sexual feelings.

Phobias involving transportation interfere more significantly with family life. It is for this reason that treatment is more often sought and needed than in the case of an animal phobia.

School Phobia. School phobias are those which present the greatest concern and problem for the child, his parents, and school personnel. Since legalities are involved, a child's frequent and prolonged absence from school cannot be ignored. For this reason, school phobias are those most often discussed and treated by parents, educators, school psychologists, and others.

Although school phobias may occur at any age, they are generally associated with the lower elementary grades and with transient somatic symptoms such as vomiting, diarrhea, or headache which diminish once the child is assured that he does not have to go to school. The interesting phenomenon that children with clear-cut learning difficulties, or those in real danger of failing, do not develop school phobias has been noted (Kessler, 1966).

School phobia is another instance of the empathic communication of anxiety between parent and child, specifically, a fear of separation. This mutual dependence forces the child into a rather strange role—that of meeting another's needs while striving to have his own met. The child's unacceptable thoughts of aggression and hostility are believed by some to account for his regression to an earlier stage of dependency.

The treatment of children with school phobia must also include the family and the school in a collaborative process. It may include a variety of methodologies in the psychotherapeutic process ranging from psychoanalysis to play therapy to behavior modification.

Problems in Speech and Language Development

Difficulties in speech and language development are not at all uncommon among children referred to child guidance clinics. Many of the problems of enunciation and articulation are treated solely by professional speech pathologists. Such difficulties as stammering, or stuttering, and the delayed speech often present because of organic causes or functional psychoses are those which are most often brought to the attention of mental health professionals in the area of child psychiatry.

Stuttering. Stammering, or stuttering, indicates a disturbance in the flow of speech due to muscular contractions or spasms and is most often observed in male children. The onset generally occurs between the ages of two and four.

The most problematic feature of stuttering is the social alienation that frequently results as the stutterer bizarrely attempts to control his speech through facial grimaces, slapping himself, using unusual body gestures, and substituting other words or phrases for those originally intended.

Many researchers have focused upon the identification of personality characteristics of the stutterer and to date have not been able to pinpoint a special personality type. There seems to be general agreement, however, that the interruption of the flow of speech displays conflict and indicates withholding rather than giving. Theories as to the nature, origin, and identification of this conflict are varied and run the gamut. Basically, physiologic views are those which consider the cause of verbal difficulty to be related to a constitutional predisposition in which stuttering is believed to be a miniature epileptic seizure or the result of a metabolic disturbance. Most theorists now allow room for a psychogenic variant which either stands alone or is associated with a somatic one. The widely accepted theory of mixed cerebral dominance propounded in the 1920s and 1930s has fallen into disfavor. This theory held that an existing physiologic rivalry between the two cortical hemispheres, if one was not sufficiently dominant, accounted for a poorly synchronized speech musculature which resulted in stuttering (Travis, 1931). However, more recent studies have indicated that children who stutter are not particularly ambidextrous, or left-handed, or have had their handedness changed by parents or teachers (Bloodstein, 1959).

Psychologic views of stuttering often focus on the intrafamilial relationship. Stuttering has been attributed to disturbances in the mother-child relationship (Wyatt and Herzan, 1962), an approach-avoidance conflict (Sheehan, 1962), a conflict of gratification of instinct according to the psychoanalytic view (Fenichel, 1945), and undue parental criticism which fixates the symptom by calling attention to it (Johnson, 1955).

Children who stutter and are anxious about it often need the direct help which psychotherapeutic treatment offers. Behavior shaping based on learning theory has been found to be effective also, as has speech therapy with a professional speech therapist. Parental education is important for the attitude of the parents can serve to either increase or decrease the child's anxiety and his stuttering. A well-written pamphlet which ought to be recommended to the parents of children who are beginning to stutter was authored by a speech pathologist, Engel, and a clinical psychologist, Helfand. Entitled "Stuttering is a Family Affair," it is available through the Cleveland Hearing and Speech Center, Cleveland, Ohio 44106.

Problems in Toilet Training

Problems in toilet training often reflect an interpersonal battle between parents and child and in this way are similar to feeding disturbances. The toilet, anus, and genitals are often sources of taboo and constraints imposed by parents in their attempt to acculturate their young in a way that will make them hygienically clean and acceptable members of human society at large. Because of the importance placed upon the bodily functions of micturition and defecation a child's refusal to play by the rules of the game can result in intrafamilial havoc.

Eneuresis. Eneuresis, or wetting, when occurring occasionally and at night in children younger than eight is considered usual and of little consequence. As with stuttering, there has been no identification of a consistent personality type or behavior associated with eneuresis, although it is seldom found as the only sign or symptom of emotional disturbance or emotional immaturity in a child. In fact, these children are often found to be thumb-sucking, masturbating, nose-picking, nail-biting, and so forth, for longer periods in their lives than the majority of children.

Kanner, who makes the point that symptoms of emotional disturbances and emotional immaturity were generally present in eneuretic children categorized them as follows (Kanner, 1957, p 448):

Aggressive, fighting, mischievous, cruel	8%
Whining, complaining, moody, irritable	32%
Restless, overactive, fidgety, excitable	21%
Disobedient, impudent, spiteful, stubborn	14%
Timid, shy, bashful, seclusive, unusually quiet	8%
Listless, indifferent, apathetic	5%
Overconscientious, serious-minded	3%

Kessler has regrouped Kanner's categories to focus on the way the child handles aggressive impulses. She notes that the first four categories, or 75 percent, include aggressive children, while the second four, or 25 percent, include children who have turned the aggression inward against themselves (Kessler, 1966, p 120). She has also identified what she believes to be common dynamic patterns in children with eneuresis: regression as a response to separation from the significant person originally responsible for toilet training, confusion and/or ambivalence over sexual identity, and "revenge eneuresis" as a way of expressing felt anger toward the parents (p 122).

Attempts to explain eneuresis as a purely physiologic event have met with little success. Children who have eneuresis do not have EEG patterns that differ from those of children who do not have neurosis, they do not have smaller bladders, nor do they wet their beds because they sleep more soundly. Children have been eneuretic on occasion for a variety of physiologic reasons, and certainly bladder infection and its accompanying symptoms may encourage nighttime bed-wetting. However, these instances are the unusual rather than the usual. Unfortunately, when parents or significant others subject their children to a variety of diagnostic urologic procedures which focus upon the genitals, it often adds to their fearful fantasies regarding differentness and genital mutilation.

Helpful measures for the child with eneuresis include environmental changes which realistically encourage the child to assist himself. They may include a night-light for the child who fears walking to the bathroom at night, removing diapers and/or rubber pants which set up the expectation that the child will wet and is unable to control his bladder, and firm but kindly encouragement from the parents.

Behavior modification principles and approaches are found to be particularly effective as a means of reducing eneuresis and encopresis in children (McDonagh, 1972). Nurses are becoming increasingly involved in training parents for intervention in the natural environment of the child. In these situations, psychiatric nurses provide consultation for parents whose goal is to facilitate the growth and development of their children (Hyde, 1976).

Encopresis. Encopresis is the term used to indicate soiling with feces. Although it may occur through anatomic defect, impairment of the nervous system, or in the child with developmental lags who is not toilet-trained, it is considered a severe neurotic symptom when it occurs in physiologically normal children who have passed the stage when toilet-training should be successfully achieved. As with many of the feeding disturbances, disturbances of toilet-training take place on an emotionally invested battleground. The struggle of child against parent or significant other and vice versa may subvert and minimize all other aspects of the adult-child relationship while the war over power and control takes place. It often brings to the fore the latent and not-so-well-hidden hostility of both the adults and the children as each autocratically attempts to rule the other. For example, an acquaintance asked what she ought to do about her five-year-old, Tessa, who continued to soil herself and withhold feces even if on the potty seat for hours on end. When I asked the mother what she had done so far she responded with: "Everything I can think of. I've spanked her, I've shouted at her, I've embarrassed her in front of her playmates, I've sent her to bed without supper. I've even rubbed her face in her soiled diaper and refused to change it all day, but even that doesn't help. I've tried everything!" It seems to me from what she continued to say that this mother had not tried affection, increased attention, or attempted to diagnose the basis for Tessa's behavior and her own responses to it. Instead of making these points evident to Tessa's mother, I asked her if she had any ideas about what she might do next. When she said that she was planning on phoning a child psychiatrist for an appointment, I encouraged her in her wise decision and attempted to prepare her for the visit. To have chastised this mother for her behavior toward Tessa would only have increased her guilt and anger.

When combined with withholding and eneuresis, soiling takes on a more pathologic form and calls for psychotherapeutic treatment. In such instances it may signal nascent antisocial disturbances or psychoses. However, when soiling occurs because of training failure or is regressive in nature, as upon the birth of a brother or sister, it often resolves itself when the significant persons in the environment recognize the child's temporary, albeit increased, needs for love and attention.

Ritualistic and Stereotypical Behavior and Thinking (Compulsions and Obsessions)

Ritualistic and stereotypical behavior and thinking, or compulsions and obsessions, exist together—although one may be a predominant mode of expression over the other. Obsessions take the form of recurrent unpleasant or anxiety-producing thoughts, while compulsions are ritualistic acts designed to reduce the anxiety to a level that can be tolerated, at least temporarily.

Obsessional compulsive symptoms may be present during the process of normal growth and development. For example, it is not at all unusual for children about the age of two or three to be greatly worried about preventing messiness or dirtiness or to insist upon changing clothes as soon as they become soiled. The child is simply over-responding to his newly learned rules and regulations and superego restrictions resulting from toilet training. School-age children in their efforts to attain and maintain perfection in self-control will often engage in ritualistic behavior such as that identified by Spock (1963, p 390):

> The commonest is stepping over cracks in the sidewalk. There's no sense to it, you just have a superstitious feeling that you ought to. It's what a psychiatrist calls a compulsion. Other examples are touching every third picket in a fence, making numbers come out even in some way, saying certain words before going through a door. If you think you made a mistake, you must go way back to where you were absolutely sure you were right, and start over again.
>
> The hidden meaning of a compulsion pops out in the thoughtless childhood saying, "Step on a crack, break your grandmother's back." Everyone has hostile feelings at times toward the people who are close to him, but his conscience would be shocked at the idea of really harming them and warns him to keep such thoughts out of his mind. And if a person's conscience becomes excessively stern, it keeps nagging him about such bad thoughts even after he has succeeded in hiding them away in his subconscious mind. He still feels guilty, though he doesn't know what for. It eases his conscience to be extra careful and proper about such a senseless thing as how to navigate a crack in the sidewalk.

However, when obsessions and compulsions are allied with phobias, tics, and hysteria, the child finds himself severely limited and handicapped in relation to other people, his environment, and even himself. In these instances it has been found that many children with this combination of symptoms have been mistakenly diagnosed as psychotic (Despert, 1955). Because of the extremely limiting nature of obsessive compulsive neurosis with its resultant restrictions upon the maturing child who should be exposed to new and different learning experiences, individual therapy is the recommended method of treatment in an attempt to assist the child in relaxation of his superego controls.

Hysteria

Hysterical symptoms occur when the attempt to repress forbidden wishes, desires, or impulses fails and the previously repressed thoughts begin to come to the surface and are more available to consciousness. They take various forms such as sudden uncontrolled outbursts that border on panic, conversions such as hysterical blindness, dissociative reactions such as amnesia and sleep walking, multiple personality made famous by the case of "the three faces of Eve," tics, and even hallucination. Fewer cases of hysteria in childhood are seen today. Some ascribe it to the fact that the repressive child-rearing practices of the Victorian era have given way to overindulgent and permissive practices more likely to encourage hedonism, pleasure-seeking, and character disorder rather than hysteria (Wallder, 1960). It has also been suggested that hysterical reactions are responses to extreme inconsistency between word and action particularly when parents link their children's sexual feelings with evil and punishment while at the same time encouraging them through their own seductive behavior (Proctor, 1958).

Because persons with hysteria are so suggestible and easily influenced, a symptomatic cure can generally be quickly obtained in psychotherapeutic work. Maintenance of the "cure" may depend upon a continued relationship with a therapist to prevent either a relapse or the appearance of a different hysterical symptom. To resolve the tendency to acquire new symptoms may require intensive psychoanalytic treatment.

PSYCHOTIC DYSFUNCTIONS OF CHILDHOOD

It is always much more difficult to talk about the psychotic dysfunctions of childhood because of the constant controversy over etiology, treatment, diagnosis, and nomenclature that rages in professional circles. While some of the emotional disturbances discussed in this section may be considered more severe than neurosis in both quality and quantity, others may not be considered along the same continuum and may be viewed as entirely separate.

Despite the fact that psychosis is relatively rare in childhood, approximately 2000 volumes concerning these severe disturbances have been written within the past 30 to 40 years; in comparison, the literature is relatively scant regarding the less severe and more frequent maladaptations discussed earlier. Perhaps the reason may be found in the fascination which childhood psychoses hold for the researcher, the clinician, and the theoretician, and the startling uniqueness often presented in the case studies of such children and their families.

Psychotic dysfunctions in childhood differ significantly from those which make their appearance later in life. In adulthood, the most common form of psychosis is schizophrenia, followed in frequency by the affective psychoses and organic psychoses. Although classical schizophrenia may appear during adolescence, the childhood psychoses discussed here are those with onsets by the time the child is five years old. Symptoms often begin to be observable within the first year of life when the child responds to and communicates with others in a strange and often bizarre way. The signs which Kessler (1966) has identified in behavioral terms are the following:

> . . . the most important single sign is a severely disturbed relationship with people. This may take the form of a lack of interest in, or awareness of people (i.e., autism) or it may take the form of an inability to separate from another person (i.e., symbiosis). From this distorted relationship with people arise difficulties in communication . . . inability to imitate or to engage in normal play, extraordinary preoccupations with inanimate objects, and clinging to a mechanical, routinized, compulsively repetitious mode of living. Neurotic children, of course, also have disturbed relationships with people, but not to the same extent and without side-effects which encroach upon every aspect of their functioning (pp 263–64).

Children who fit into these categories will be considered in the sections dealing with hospitalism and anaclitic depression, autism, childhood schizophrenia, and symbiosis. A separate section on behavior disorders and delinquent behavior follows. The author wishes to avoid a lengthy discussion of nomenclature and semantics which she believes serves only to cloud the issue rather than to illuminate the student's understanding of the severe and psychotic dysfunctions of childhood.

Hospitalism and Anaclitic Depression

Effects of emotional and social deprivation have historically aroused the curiosity of others. The literature and nonfiction of old include tales of the study of children found roaming the countryside or living in forests supposedly being reared by wild animals. In colonial America and in Victorian times, children who were reared in attics, closets, or secluded rooms because they were "possessed," retarded, or illegitimate have also been studied. The interest in the study of such deprived children continues today since a reawakening of interest in the 1940s when a number of child psychiatric workers began studying the effects of maternal separation on children being raised in institutions such as hospitals and orphanages, in particular.

In 1940, Lowrey, an American psychiatrist, reported upon his observations of children who had spent the first three years of their lives in orphanages (Lowrey, 1940). He described a clinical syndrome consisting of self-centeredness and an inability to give and receive affection coupled with aggressive behavior and speech impairments. Interestingly, he did not find this behavior pattern occurring in children who entered the orphanage after the age of two or three. His observations were supported by Ribble (1941), who emphasized the personality disorganization and its relative irreversability which occurred through deficient mothering. In addition, Goldfarb's (1946) study of children reared in an orphanage indicated that those deprived of family life in early childhood were less intelligent, had poorer memories, and showed marked impairment in language development and school adjustment when compared with children who had been fostered out as soon as they arrived at the orphanage. Another early investigator who reported the results of his studies of emotionally deprived children was René Spitz. The results of his studies were the identification of two clinical syndromes in infancy that he called hospitalism and anaclitic depression.

He described hospitalism as a condition in which the infant is physiologically and socially deteriorated as the result of long confinement in an institution. In his first and now classic study, Spitz studied 164 children in two institutions—a foundling home where infants were cared for by staff members and a nursery in a penal institution where infants were cared for by their mothers, who were incarcerated there. Spitz (1946) demonstrated that infants cared for during their first year of life by the mother, even in such an unfavorable setting, surpassed the infants cared for in the foundling home in a number of ways. For example, they were more agile, active, vocal, and physically healthier, while the infants in the foundling home were more prone to illness, sustained a great mortality rate, and lagged behind developmentally in a number of ways. It should be noted that in the foundling home, for "ease of care," the children were isolated from one another and adults by covered crib sides and received almost no stimulation except at feeding time. Since they received food, medical care, and housing to the same extent as did the children in the penal institution nursery, Spitz concluded that their developmental lag and general deterioration was the result of a lack of mothering. His follow-up study two years later supported his original conclusions (Spitz, 1946). He found that the children in the foundling home continued to deteriorate in a number of ways. Not only was the earlier deterioration present but they also failed to adapt to toilet training, were underweight and undersized.

Anaclitic depression, on the other hand, is a specific reaction of the infant to separation from the mother occurring once an established interpersonal relationship, particularly a good one, between mother and infant is disrupted or discontinued. Such infants develop a severe mourning response to the loss of the mother which progresses to depression, withdrawal, physical debilitation, and severe disturbance in relationships with others. Spitz described this syndrome in 1946 when he found 19 severe and 26 mild cases of anaclitic depression among 123 infants in an institution (Spitz, 1946a). He also found that the syndrome developed only in infants whose mothers assumed the full care for them until between six and eight months of age when they were removed from the child for a period of at least two to three months. These infants wear a constant sad expression on their faces, become rigid, insomniac, withdrawn, apathetic, and eventually apprehensive and fearful of human contact to the point at which the infant screams at the approach of another human being. When the mothers are restored, the infants seem to recover and become happy again. When the mothers are not restored the deterioration and depression continues through apathy, to a catatoniclike state, and often to death within the year.

Research still is incomplete, however, for not all infants deprived of mothering develop anaclitic depression. In addition, separation from the mother before the age of six months does not result in this syndrome. This seems to indicate measures which might be taken to prevent and reduce cases of hospitalism and anaclitic depression among infants. For example, other studies have indicated that the critical period seems to be between six and eighteen months of age and therefore, that it is possible for institutional staffs geared to the recognition of the emotional needs of children to provide adequate substitute mothering and intellectual stimulation at this particularly critical time (Rheingold, 1956; Rheingold and Bayley, 1959; David and Appell, 1961).

Another researcher whose work substantiates the detrimental effects of maternal deprivation is Bowlby. An early study by Bowlby in 1946, which concerned itself with juvenile thieves, demonstrated that out of the total 44 youngsters studied, 17 had undergone early or prolonged separation from the mother or mother figure during the first five years of their lives; this was a much higher percentage than that of a control group of children being treated at the same clinic. In addition, these children had been described with many of the same adjectives used in the description of children with behavior problems, delinquent behavior, or sociopathic and antisocial tendencies. Bowlby spurred further interest in research in maternal and emotional deprivation as the result of his monograph published in 1951 and his more current work dealing with the infant's dependence on its mother (Bowlby, 1969).

Since Bowlby's early work, large numbers of researchers, theoreticians, and clinicians have been interested in the effects of separation as a basis for child-rearing and social welfare practices. The result has been that until recently, the opinion was that any mother is better than no mother at all and the tendency has been away from group care of children. More recent work in the Israeli kibbutzim and in group-care homes in other countries may be indicating that the advantages of group care when mothering is absent, negligible, or hostile have been unfortunately discounted in the past (Bettelheim, 1969; Wolins, 1969). Other eminent authorities have begun to sternly criticize the group care offered in settings such as kibbutzim, which they believe hamper the initiative and creativity essential for fostering future leadership abilities.

Although the unfortunate results of hospitalism and anaclitic depression are generally understood to be the result of emotional and maternal deprivation, the questions which remain to be answered revolve around the best means of prevention and effective treatment modalities. At this time, the pros and cons remain unresolved.

Autism and Childhood Schizophrenia

The clinical entity of autism was first described in 1943 by Kanner, who used the term early infantile autism to describe children whose behaviors seemed to constitute a unique syndrome that he believed to be a form of childhood psychosis. Prior to Kanner's definition and identification of the syndrome of autism (from the Greek word for self), most doctors believed that these children were mentally retarded and most often recommended that they be placed in an institution for the mentally retarded to receive the custodial care given at that time. Kanner believed that the condition was innate and probably incurable, while noting that parents of autistic children were highly intellectual but tended to be emotionally cold. In fact, Kanner labeled them "refrigerator parents." This belief and similar beliefs are still held by many experts in child psychiatry regardless of their theoretical orientation or their ideas regarding treatment. Others believe that such attitudes have only served to saddle parents of autistic children with useless and harmful guilt; these workers note that some of the symptoms of autism or differentness become noticeable in infancy even before strong parental influence upon the child's behavior is regarded as likely. Indeed, approximately 11 years ago an organization called the National Society for Autistic Children was founded by a group of parents of autistic children in order to give one another moral support, to provide education for themselves and the public at large, and to stimulate research into the cause of autism—focusing particular attention on the biologic causes. Many hope that autism will turn out to be similar to cretinism and PKU phenylketonuria. A predominant belief in Great Britain is that some heretofore undiscovered biochemical abnormality of the brain, based upon hereditary factors, lies at the root of autism (Wolff, 1969). Increasing numbers of child care experts seem willing and eager to avoid the label of blame and the etiologic roots of autism in an attempt to concentrate on helping the child with autism and his family.

Many children with autism are not identified or do not receive treatment before the age of two, at the earliest, and more usually not before the age of three or four, when the signs of autism are readily recognizable even to the casual observer. Some advice given to family doctors on recognizing the child with autism is helpful and merits repeating here:

> The child does not speak properly for his age, or at all.
> He has no awareness of his identity.
> He is pathologically preoccupied with a particular object.
> He resists change around him, struggling to maintain or restore the familiar.
> He is excessively anxious without any apparent reason.
> His emotional relationships are grossly impaired.
> He may twirl, rock, walk on tiptoe, or remain rigid for sustained periods.
> He appears to be seriously retarded but has flashes of normal or exceptional intellectual function.*

However, parents quite often report instances of strange and bizarre behavior in their children before they reach this stage and while they are infants in cribs. As infants they may be described as never cuddly or smiling, seemingly uncaring about whether mother or father is in the room, never physically reaching out to be lifted, hugged, or touched, contented in being left alone without apparent distress over separation, and failing to imitate gestures such as waving goodby, or participating in early games such as peek-a-boo and patty-cake.

In addition it seems evident that children with autism are much more object oriented than they are people oriented. For example, they may be fascinated for months on end, to the exclusion of all else, with toys or objects which spin, reflect light, or can be rolled, manipulated or twirled in some way. However, they seldom relate to gestures or verbal cues from persons to the extent that many are suspected of being deaf and are often referred to hearing and speech clinics for evaluation and/or treatment. When thwarted in their desires, children with autism may resort to primitive atavistic behavior such as screaming and tantrums which, with their frightening consequences of hurting the self or others, may result in parental responses in-

**From: Breaking through to the autistic child. Med World News, October 28, 1966, p 92.*

tended to end or suppress the primitive behavior. Some parents have reported being autocratically controlled by their child to the point at which they have to stand guard over the child or his environment in order to protect him. In this way, many children with autism are despots in their demands, and essentially have unyielding control over the lives of others in their environment.

It is not unusual to hear experts say that autism is a rare illness. In fact, such a statement may be found in almost any textbook concerned with child psychiatry. Such statements seem inconsistent with the findings of a survey which indicate that between four and five out of every 10,000 children are autistic (Lotter, 1966). It is alarming to note that the frequency of autism in children is greater than that of blindness and almost as great as that for deafness. Labeling autism as rare seems to minimize its seriousness and frequency. No one yet seems to be able to explain the additional fact that four out of five children with autism are boys.

Whether such a condition as childhood schizophrenia exists or not is a moot question. While some authorities classify autism and symbiosis as varying forms of the overall rubric of childhood psychosis, others consider childhood schizophrenia a separate category and often reserve it for children who seem to develop symptoms after the age of five years or in children whose disordered behavior appears after an initial period of normal development. Many liken the illness to a juvenile form of adult schizophrenia. In speaking of childhood schizophrenia most authors quote Bender who classified numerous organic as well as emotional disorders under this general heading. Her methods of diagnosis and statements of observed signs are couched in physiologic terms in accordance with her belief as to cause (Bender, 1947). She includes withdrawn and autistic behavior as only one of many signs of childhood schizophrenia. Others, such as Mahler et al (1959) do not acknowledge childhood schizophrenia as a separate category. Although they include both autism and symbiosis, their third category of more benign childhood psychoses is composed of a syndrome in which children may alternate between autism, symbiosis, and the neurotic states discussed earlier.

Symbiosis

Another subcategory of the overall rubric of childhood psychosis is symbiosis, which was not so defined until Margaret Mahler's now classic publication of 1952. The symbiotic child, in contrast to the child with autism, experiences extreme difficulty in separation from his relationship with the mother. The closeness of his association with his mother and the extent of the dependency is demonstrated by the fact that even brief and temporary separations such as mother's walking into another room may produce panic.

Children with symbiosis are seldom conspicuously disturbed as infants. Symptoms manifest themselves between the ages of two and five with a peak at four years of age. The behavior of the child appears to be an attempt to reestablish the mother-infant-as-one phase before the developing ego assists the child in separating himself from others and coming to understand the "me." In the course of normal development infants naturally undergo a state of symbiosis. In fact, the unprotected infant must indeed rely upon his parents for his life. When he becomes a toddler at about 12 to 15 months of age, his growing sense of ego identity assists him in his gradual separation from mother as he begins to gain some independence. He can tolerate going away from mother because he knows she will come back. This has been termed the beginning of the separation-individuation phase of personality development which has been described as a kind of second birth (Mahler and Gosliner, 1955).

It can be noted that the environment of the child with symbiosis cannot generally be said to encourage gradual separation from the mother, emergence of the ego, and establishment of interpersonal relationships with others. Although the possibility exists that constitutional predisposition may be a factor in determining symbiosis, there is little evidence at this time which would support such a belief. Mothers of children with symbiosis have often been identified as overprotective, however. It remains to be determined whether the mother is simply responding to the needs of a dependent child with symbiosis, or if the response of the mother encouraged symbiosis. Overprotection includes excessive contact between parent and child, prolongation of the stage of infancy, and the prevention or suppression of independent or autonomous behavior. Dynamically, maternal overprotection is closely related to maternal rejection. A number of researchers have found that mothers who were rejecting before the birth of the infant underwent a reaction-formation against their unconscious hostility and responded by being oversolicitious, compulsive, and smothering in the care of their infants. In fact, such maternal overprotection has also been linked to pervasive learning disorders in children (Buxbaum, 1964).

Children with symbiosis have often been described by their mothers as extremely sensitive infants who were frequent criers. The symptoms of psychosis become more readily identifiable in critical developmental periods which have to do with increasing independency. To the child with symbiosis, these periods are not viewed as milestones to be surpassed with delight, but as cruel and unwanted crises. Bergman and Escalona (1949) have described unevenness of growth and extreme vulnerability to frustration as some of the unusual sensitivities demonstrated by the child with symbiosis. For example, parents often report unusual reactions to small failures to the point that the child may give up locomotion and all attempts at locomotion for months because of a fall or bump in the learning process. Perhaps part of this response may be explained by the fact that locomotion might serve to take the child away from, as well as to, the mother.

Some authorities now believe that the child with symbiosis who finds his state of continual panic at the thought of separation unbearable regresses to the use of autistic behavior in an attempt to arrive at a solution through a form of secondary retreat (Mahler et al, 1959).

ASOCIAL, ANTISOCIAL, AND DELINQUENT BEHAVIOR

The term juvenile delinquency is generally not applied to children below the age of adolescence. While younger children are often labeled as asocial, antisocial, or having behavior problems or conduct disturbances, the dynamics are similar to those seen in the older child or adolescent.

Delinquent behavior has been a social problem throughout recorded history. Writings on papyrus and cave walls tell of community and individual concern with the problem behavior of youth. It was not until the eighteenth century, however, that children were treated differently than were criminal adults. At the present time, most persons view asocial, antisocial, and delinquent behavior as behavior opposed to or detrimental to the beliefs, attitudes, and laws held by society at large and our culture in particular.

This section will consider the individual delinquent—the youth whose behavior is intrapsychically or interpersonally determined—and the gang delinquent, the youth whose behavior is sociologically or culturally determined. Kessler, who believes that disorders of the superego cause juvenile delinquency, classifies the causes as follows:

1. The absence of a superego because of early neglect, deprivation and failure to establish meaningful relationships at the earliest level (also called the "psychopath" and the "unsocialized aggressive").
2. Identification with socially inadequate models, incorporation of antisocial values, inability to achieve satisfaction in socially acceptable ways because of either deficiencies in ego functions or lack of opportunity, or both (the "normal delinquent"; the "socially delinquent").
3. Imperfections in superego development resulting from the conscious sanctioning by the parents of behavior which they pronounce to be wrong.
4. Weakness of the superego in coping with instinctual desires (eg, as in the narcissistic, hysterical person who "does it now, regrets it later").
5. Abeyance of the superego because the delinquent behavior is an unconscious means of expressing aggression toward the parents or of acting out a special unconscious fantasy, or is a way of obtaining punishment for an unconscious sense of guilt ("neurotic delinquency") (Kessler, 1966, p 303).

Attempts have frequently been made to align delinquency with any one of various causes, predispositions, or tendencies. For example, in the early part of the twentieth century much attention was paid to the morphologic and anatomical differences which were thought to characterize persons with various mental disorders and delinquency. It was thought that the cranial structure of the criminal might be different as well as the general musculature, which was termed mesomorphic. Age and onset of puberty have been linked with criminal and antisocial behavior, the belief being that decreasing age of puberty may be a factor contributing indirectly to the increase in juvenile delinquency, particularly among females. More recently, the idea that a person's genetic make-up may be responsible for his committing acts of violence has found favor with the identification of the XYY chromosomal constitution. Rather than the usual XY chromosome composition in the reproductive cells, this person has an extra Y chromosome, which is thought to elevate aggressiveness potential. Since 1965, studies of men in penal institutions have tended to support this belief. Recently, researchers have begun to criticize the validity of some of these studies and propose that chromosomal differentness as a solitary factor is insufficient grounds for the suspicion of violent or aggressive behavior. It is difficult to think about problems of research methodology when examination of persons who have committed violent acts indicates the presence of the XYY chromosome, as in the case of Richard Speck, the convicted murderer of eight nurses in Chicago in 1966.

The Gang Delinquent

Sociologists and cultural anthropologists are highly concerned with gang delinquency which, although viewed as deviant behavior, may only be an expression of the accepted pattern of behavior of a subcultural group. In such a circumstance, while the child is considered delinquent by the larger society, he is considered normal by the smaller society that comprises the environment in which he exists (Miller, 1958).

Since gang delinquency is primarily a working-class phenomenon, it has been connected with lower socioeconomic class neighborhoods, which are more prone to a lack of social unity and organization (Cohen, 1955). In addition, some believe it to be a reaction-formation regarding the unattainable middle-class standard (Cloward and Ohlin, 1960). It is a way for the gang to outwardly turn against those values and standards that it covets. This suggests that the discrepancy between what lower-class youths want and what is available to them accounts for difficulty in societal adjustment.

In terms of treatment, it is important to determine whether a child's delinquent or antisocial behavior fits within this category since the treatment approach varies from that of the individual delinquent and his parents.

Problems of gang delinquency are problems for the community at large and all of the resources of that community must be mobilized for a broad-base community attack if it is to be effective.

The Individual Delinquent

The individual delinquent who fits into Kessler's first, third, fourth, and fifth categories is one whose intrapsychic conflicts (neurotic or psychotic) or interpersonal conflicts indicate a psychopathologic or emotionally disturbed bent either within the child himself or within the framework of his family. A review of these categories indicates the involvement apparent in the parent-child interaction.

Individual delinquency has often been ascribed to maternal deprivation and rejection in the early years, as well as paternal rejection in the later years. Many now believe that after dozens of years of emphasis on the importance of the mother in the development of the child, the pendulum is finally beginning to swing where it belongs—with a focus on both parents or parenting figures.

Treatment of the individual delinquent has a greater focus upon psychotherapy and counseling in attempts to resolve the conflicts present in both the child and other family members. Approaches range from family therapy to group therapy to individual therapy, either on an outpatient basis or in residential facilities where staff can work toward reeducation of the child and/or family.

Whichever the method of approach for either of these two types, most experts today agree that incarceration within penal institutions constitutes punishment and not treatment or rehabilitation. In the very institutions ostensibly designed to protect society and the child, the child unfortunately learns to improve his criminal "skills" and emerges a hardened and wiser criminal and consequently societal problem.

TREATMENT APPROACHES

A wide variety of professional disciplines in a variety of settings are engaged in work with troubled children and youth. In many areas of the country the traditional child mental health workers are still considered to be psychiatrists, psychologists, and social workers. Child psychiatric nursing as a specialty is a relative newcomer to the field, particularly since the care of troubled children is moving out of the psychiatric hospital setting and into the community. There may be reluctance at times to utilize child psychiatric nurses in facilities other than inpatient services. Some of the reluctance may be attributed to professional jealousy and insecurity among mental health workers. Most of the reluctance, however, can be attributed to two factors—the lack of child psychiatric nurses prepared at comparable educational levels (master's and doctoral degree holders) who can communicate with other professionals by sharing the same universe of discourse, and the willingness on the part of nurses to retain the comfort of the safe hospital setting in the assumption of managerial rather than clinical skills. The role of the child psychiatric nurse clinician will be discussed in the next section.

Having read the earlier data in this chapter, the reader should be well aware that psychiatric treatment, if it is to be effective, cannot focus only on the individual identified as the patient. Indeed, treatment of whole communities for their social ills may be necessary. Programs of treatment and education are particularly important for the parents and siblings of the child who is troubled. The need for a focus on parents in terms of the parent-child interactions previously described should be particularly apparent. Knowledge of growth and development makes apparent the need to focus our attention on the siblings of the child who is troubled. One hopes for a future in which preventive psychiatry will reduce the incidence, duration, and prevalence of mental disorder as well as the resulting impairment.

The Psychotherapies

Psychotherapeutic treatment may take place in a variety of ways in a variety of settings. Treatment of the child may be dependent on an individual relationship with a therapist, or a relationship with a therapist and a group of other children, or a relationship between the child, his family, and a therapist.

Child analysis or psychoanalytically oriented psychotherapy is based upon the achievement of insight for the child as well as change in the lifestyle and psychic structure of the child (A. Freud, 1946). Although psychoanalytic techniques vary with the age and abilities of the individual child, they are geared toward an intensive relationship requiring sessions with the child analyst as much as five times weekly. Child analysis is predicated on the ability of the child to relate verbally with the analyst. Although the medium of play may be introduced within the psychoanalytic relationship, its use and effectiveness in analysis is determined by verbal consideration of the conflicts expressed by the child (Klein, 1955). This indicates that psychoanalysis is certainly not the treatment of choice for children when certain pragmatic considerations are taken into account. For example, the child with autism who does not relate at the required verbal level would not be an appropriate candidate, nor is the prohibitive cost of three to five weekly sessions with an analyst within the financial means of the great majority of parents.

Group psychotherapy with children offers multiple stimuli. Rather than an intensive relationship with one therapist it offers a variety of relationships with others. In a group, children learn from one another; therefore, a mix between children who are aggressive with those who are passive and/or withdrawn offers opportunities to all to incorporate the positive aspects of the other and to receive pressure to change regarding their own negative behaviors (Slavson, 1952).

Family therapy is group psychotherapy with the members of the family, based upon the belief that the origins and stimuli toward emotional disturbance lie within the family system. Whether this is determined to be so or not, there is no doubt that emotional illness in one member of the family affects the others and, in the view of Ackerman (1958), is an expression of family pathology. In many situations, a combination of techniques may be used. A number of workers may engage themselves therapeutically with various members of the family in an individual relationship which is enhanced through the use of family therapy as an additional treatment modality.

Another approach utilizes the learning principles originally identified by experimental psychologists and based upon the premise that neurotic and even psychotic behavior is learned and therefore can be unlearned (Eysenck, 1960; Ferster, 1961). Societal norms or behaviors which are considered socially acceptable are emphasized. Generally, it requires a consistent environment in which all staff carry out measures designed to eliminate the unwanted behavior. For this reason, behavioral techniques are frequently employed in residential treatment centers.

Play therapy may also be used as a treatment modality, employed by itself or in combination with other forms of treatment. The particular theoretical approach of the therapist will determine the manner in which play therapy is instituted and utilized, and will vary according to the situation. Play as a nondirective therapeutic means which focuses on the relationship between child and therapist as the crucial factor in the outcome of the therapy is discussed by Axline (1969), who emphasizes the naturalness and spontaneity of the technique, whereas Kleinian analysts may use it for symbolic interpretation of unconscious conflicts (Klein, 1932).

The Somatotherapies

The somatotherapies or physical treatments for mental illness are all but discontinued in the treatment of children with emotional disorders except for the occasional use of medication which may be helpful in some cases to a lesser extent than in the adult. One strange paradox of drug treatment for children involves the child whose hyperactivity poses a learning problem for him in school. Such children have their hyperactivity diminished through treatment with a central nervous system stimulant which has entirely the opposite effect in adults. As with most somatotherapies, this too has been abused and is undergoing intensive reconsideration and study.

In the late 1940s and the early 1950s electroshock therapy was employed in the treatment of children with emotional disorders as was psychosurgery such as lobotomy. Fortunately, these methods employed in the treatment of disturbed children in the psychiatric hospitals of the time have been discontinued based on sound evidence that they are unwarranted methods.

The Sociotherapies

Sociotherapeutic or milieu therapy approaches may be employed in residential treatment facilities when it seems essential to treat the child away from his natural environment. The trend seems to be toward a greater application of therapeutic environment in the treatment of the child although there still are in existence a number of facilities which serve simply as places to live rather than as treatment facilities.

This form of treatment requires that everyone in the milieu contributes to the therapeutic effort so that in an institutional or residential setting efforts must be made to help maids, janitors, cottage parents, and secretaries become, if not milieu therapists, then at least therapeutic manipulators of the milieu. Kessler's excellent chapter, entitled Treatment Away From Home, is a recommended reading for those interested in the influence of milieu (Kessler, 1966).

THE CHILD PSYCHIATRIC NURSING CLINICAL SPECIALIST

The pattern of specialization in clinical nursing is one of the most important and salient patterns in professional nursing today. Although the term specialization was used as early as the mid-1930s, it signified the nurse who provided the bedside or administrative and management care for patients whose illnesses fell within the classification accorded certain diseases, conditions, or ages. More often than not, a nurse was considered to be a "specialist" in an area of patient care by simple virtue of the fact that the agency or institution which employed her was restricted to the care of tubercular, psychiatric, obstetric, medical, or pediatric patients. The longer the nurse cared solely for the patient with tuberculosis, for example, the more of a "specialist" she became as job-related experience became equated with specialization.

Today, the pattern is changing. The committed professional nurse who is a master practitioner actively engaged in the provision of excellence in patient care has been identified as the clinical nursing specialist.

Clinical expertise in psychiatric nursing focuses upon the subrole of counselor or psychotherapist. The nursing subroles of mother-surrogate, technician, manager, socializing agent, health teacher, and counselor or psychotherapist were identified by Peplau, one of the foremost psychiatric nurses in the United States. She identified the counselor-psychotherapist subrole as the emphasized one for the clinical specialist in psychiatric nursing. The remaining traditional subroles assume lesser importance for the clinical specialist, and remain chiefly within the province of other nurses who assume management and administrative duties or perform patient care under the guidance and supervision of the clinical expert.

In order to effectively carry out the expected functions inherent in rendering expert clinical patient care in the psychotherapeutic role, the clinician must have depth in theoretical knowledge and the skills of psychotherapeutic nursing process. Explicitly, she must be able to observe, assess, interpret, intervene, and evaluate in order to render expert direct and indirect psychiatric nursing intervention and to function as a change agent in the health care system. The functions have been specifically noted and defined for child psychiatric nurses by Middleton:

> Child psychiatric nursing may be defined as direct care to the emotionally disturbed child, usually within the matrix of his primary group—the family. The child psychiatric nurse is therapeutically involved in the exploration and resolution of the crises of childhood. The nurse directs her therapeutic influence on children, their families, and the settings within which interactions take place. She becomes involved with children who may have a variety of labels—"emotionally disturbed," "mentally ill," "behavior problem," "delinquent," "learning problem," or even "mentally retarded." Another way of describing child psychiatric nursing is that the nurse becomes involved with children who themselves may feel distressed or unhappy or who by their behavior cause distress to others. The involvement may occur in a variety of settings—the home, school, outpatient clinic, the pediatric ward of a hospital, or a residential unit in a treatment center or hospital for emotionally disturbed or mentally retarded children (Middleton, 1967).

The child psychiatric nurse clinician accomplishes these goals through a variety of modalities, which have as their core the nurse-child-family relationship. The nurse may utilize the one-to-one relationship, play therapy, sociotherapy or manipulation of the milieu, behavior-shaping based upon learning theory, and family or group therapeutic skills. Of additional importance is the necessity of collaborating with other professional and lay personnel who also contribute their skills to the therapeutic team.

As such requirements and techniques are spelled out, it becomes evident that experience alone no longer qualifies the nurse as a clinical expert in the area of child psychiatry. One is not fated to assume such a role from birth, although some individuals by virtue of their experiences in living

TABLE 1
NLN Accredited Master's Programs in Child Psychiatric Nursing

NAME AND ADDRESS OF UNIVERSITY	CURRICULUM OFFERINGS	LENGTH OF STUDY (approx.)
Boston University School of Nursing 635 Commonwealth Avenue Boston, Massachusetts 02215	Clinical specialization in psychiatric mental health (adult and child)	3 semesters
	Teaching of nursing with a major in psychiatric–mental health (adult and child)	3 semesters
New York University Division of Nursing Education Washington Square New York, New York 10003	Delivery of nursing services with concentration in child psychiatry	3 semesters
	Teaching of nursing in associate degree and baccalaureate degree programs with concentration in child psychiatry	3 semesters
University of Cincinnati College of Nursing and Health Cincinnati, Ohio 45221	Advanced nursing practice: child psychiatric	6 quarters
University of Maryland School of Nursing 655 W. Lombard Street Baltimore, Maryland 21201	Advanced Nursing Practice: psychiatric–child	3 semesters

University of Missouri-Columbia School of Nursing Medical Sciences Building Columbia, Missouri 65201	Teaching of nursing: psychiatric (children) Management of nursing care: psychiatric (children)	4 semesters 4 semesters
University of North Carolina School of Nursing Chapel Hill, North Carolina 27514	Advanced nursing practice: psychiatric (including community and child)	4 semesters
University of Utah College of Nursing Salt Lake City, Utah 84112	Clinical specialization: psychiatric (adult and child-adolescent)	6 quarters
Wayne State University College of Nursing Detroit, Michigan 48202	Administration–nursing education: child psychiatry Administration–nursing service: child psychiatry Teaching: child psychiatry Clinical specialization: child psychiatry	5 quarters 5 quarters 6 quarters 6 quarters

assume the role with greater ease than do others with like academic and professional experiences. Some of the experiences in living which are especially significant for the child psychiatric nurse are those concerning punishment, limit-setting, authority, sex, and competiveness. Therefore, in addition to depth in theoretical knowledge and the skills of psychotherapeutic nursing she must engage in preceptory or clinical supervisory relationships with a more experienced and knowledgeable clinical nursing specialist, to assist in the identification of conflicts and the resolution of anxiety.

The combination of these three essentials can be found in graduate programs in psychiatric nursing which lead to a master's degree. The reader is referred to Table 1 for the list of NLN accredited Master's Programs in Child Psychiatric Nursing.

BIBLIOGRAPHY

Ackerman NW: The Psychodynamics of Family Life. New York, Basic Books, 1958

Aichorn A: Wayward Youth. New York, Viking, 1935

Axline V: Play Therapy, rev ed. New York, Ballantine, 1969

Beller EK: The Clinical Process. New York, Free Press of Glencoe, 1962

Bender L: Childhood Schizophrenia. Am J Orthopsychiatry 17:40, 1947

Bettelheim B: The Children of the Dream. New York, Macmillan, 1969

Bloodstein OA: Handbook on Stuttering for Professional Workers. Chicago, National Society for Crippled Children and Adults, 1959

———: Maternal Care and Mental Health , 2nd ed. Geneva, World Health Organization, 1951

Bowlby J: Attachment and Loss. New York, Basic Books, 1969, vol 1

———: Fourty-four Juvenile Thieves: Their Characters and Home Life. London, Bailliere, Tindall, 1946

Breaking through to the autistic child. Med World News, October 28, 1966, p 86

Breuer J, Freud S: Studies in Hysteria. New York, Nervous and Mental Diseases Publishers, 1968

Bruner J: Processes of Growth in Infancy. Clark University Press, Barre Publishers, 1968

Buxbaum E: The parents role in the etiology of learning disabilities. Psychoanal Study Child. 19:xx, 1964

Caplan G: Prevention of Mental Disorders in Children. New York, Basic Books, 1961

Cloward R, Ohlin LE: Delinquency and Opportunity: A Theory of Delinquent Gangs. New York, Free Press of Glencoe, 1960

Cohen AK: Delinquent Boys: The Culture of the Gang. New York, Free Press of Glencoe, 1955

Cooper, M: Pica. Springfield, Ill, Thomas, 1957

Cramer JB: Common neurosies of childhood. In Arieti S (ed): American Handbook of Psychiatry. New York, Basic Books, 1959, vol 1, pp 797–815

Cullen AA: Labelling theory and social deviance. Perspectives in Psychiat Care 11:123, 1974

David M, Appell GA: A study of nursing care and nurse-infant interaction. In Foss BM: Determinants of Human Behavior. Ondon, Methuen, 1961

Eisenberg L: School phobias: a study of communication of anxiety. Am J Psychiatry 114:712, 1958

Ennis B: Prisoners of Psychiatry. New York, Harcourt, Brace, and Jovanovich, 1972
Eysenck HJ: Behavior Therapy and the Neuroses. London, Pergamon, 1960
Fenichel O: The Psychoanalytic Theory of Neurosis. New York, Norton, 1945
Ferster CB: Positive reinforcement and behavioral deficits of autistic children. Child Dev 32:437, 1961
Freud A: The Psychoanalytical Treatment of Children. London, Imago, 1946
Freud S: Analysis of phobia in a five-year-old boy. In Collected Papers. New York, Nervous and Mental Disease Publishers, 1936
Goldfarb W: Effects of psychological deprivation in infancy and subsequent stimulation. Am J Psychiatry 102:18, 1946
Gutelius M et al: Nutritional studies of children with pica: Part I, Controlled study evaluating nutritional status. II. Treatment of pica with iron given intramuscularly. Pediatrics 29: 1012, 1018, 1962
Hyde ND: Parental Counseling: The Psychiatric Nurse as a bahavioral consultant. In Kneisl C, Wilson HS: Current Perspectives in Psychiatric Nursing: Issues and Trends (Vol. 1). St. Louis, Mosby, 1976, pp 67–76
Johnson W: Stuttering in Children and Adults. Minneapolis, Minn, University of Minnesota Press, 1955
Joint Commission on Mental Illness and Health. Action for Mental Health. New York, Basic Books, 1961
Joint Commission of Mental Health of Children. Crisis in Child Mental Health: Challenge for the 1970s. New York, Harper & Row, 1969
Kanner L: Autistic disturbance in affective contact. Nerv Child 2:217, 1942/43
———: Child Psychiatry. 3rd ed. Springfield, Ill, Thomas, 1957
Kessler JW: Psychopathology of Childhood. Englewood Cliffs, NJ, Prentice-Hall, 1966
Klein M: The Psycho-Analysis of Children. London, Hogarth Press, 1932
———: The psychoanalytic play technique. Am J Orthopsychiat 25:223, 1955
Lapouse R: Who is sick? Am J Orthopsychiat 35:138, 1965
Lotter V: Epidemiology of autistic conditions in young children: I: prevalence. Soc Psychiatry 1:124, 1966
Lowrey LG: Personality disorganization and early institutional care. Am J Orthopsychiat 10:576, 1940
Mahler MS: On child psychosis and schizophrenia: autistic and symbiotic infantile psychosis. Psychoanal Study Child 7:286–305, 1952
———, Gosliner JB: On symbiotic child psychosis, In Psychoanal Study Child 10:215–40, 1955
———, Furer M, Settlage CF: Severe emotional disturbances in childhood: psychosis. In Arieti S (ed): American Handbook of Psychiatry, New York, Basic Books, 1959, vol 1, pp 816–39
McDonagh MJ: Behavior modification principles and the use of nursing approaches as a means of reducing enuresis and encopresis in children. In Fagin C (ed): Nursing in Child Psychiatry. St. Louis, Mosby, 1972, pp 105–25
Meyer A: The Common Sense Psychiatry of Dr. Adolph Meyer. Lief A, trans. New York, McGraw-Hill, 1948
Middleton AB: Introduction to child psychiatric nursing: the role of the clinical specialist. In Kalkman ME (ed): Psychiatric Nursing, 3rd ed. New York, McGraw-Hill, 1967
Miller WB: Lower-class culture as a generating milieu of gang delinquency. J Soc Issues 14:5, 1958
Morris D: The Naked Ape. New York, Dell, 1969
1970 White House Conference on Children, Profiles of Children. Washington, DC, Government Printing Office, 1972, Charts 43, 45, 121, 130

Rheingold HL, Bayley N: The later effects of an experimental modification of mothering. Child Dev 30:363, 1959
Ribble M: Disorganizing factors in infant personality. Am J Psychiat 98:459, 1941
Rosenhan DL: On being same in insane places. Science 179:250, 1973
Rutter M: Classification and categorization in child psychiatry. J Child Psychiatry 6:71, 1965
Sayre J: Alternative perspectives on deviance. In Kneisl CR, Wilson HS (eds): Current Perspectives in Psychiatric Nursing: Issues and Trends (Vol. 1). St. Louis, Mosby, 1976, pp 137–47
Sheehan JG: Projective studies of stuttering. In Trapp P, Himelstein P (eds): Readings on the Exceptional Child. New York, Appleton, 1962
Slavson SR: Child Psychotherapy. New York, Columbia University Press, 1952
Spitz RA: Anaclitic depression. Psychoanal Study Child 2:313–42, 1946a
———: Hospitalism: a follow-up report. Psychoanal Study Child 2:113–17, 1946b
———: Hospitalism. Psychoanal Study Child 1:53–74, 1945
Spock B: Baby and Child Care. New York, Pocket Books, 1963
Sullivan HS: The Interpersonal Theory of Psychiatry. New York, Norton, 1943
Travis LE:, Speech Pathology. New York, Appleton, 1931
Trieschman AE: Temper, temper, temper, temper, temper. The New York Times Magazine, April 12, 1970, p 99
Wilson HS, Kneisl CR: Comprehensive Psychiatric Nursing: An Interactionist Humanistic Approach. Reading, Mass, Addison-Wesley (in press)
Wolff S: Children Under Stress. London, Penguin, 1969
Wolins M: Group care: friend of foe. Social Work 14:35, 1969
Wyatt GL, Herzan HM: Therapy with stuttering children and their mothers. Am J Orthopsychiatry 32:645, 1962

SHIRLEY STEELE

10 *Nursing Care of the Child with Burns*

According to Cosman (1974) an estimated one million people below the age of 20 years in the United States are treated for burns each year. He cites a breakdown of age ranges in one study population. Two percent of the burn population were infants under one year, 20 percent were children under five years of age, and 36 percent were children under ten years of age. Burns are responsible for a significant number of deaths in children under five years of age. According to Donnellan (1969), in the United States alone, 2200 to 4000 children died per year from this painful injury during the decade reported on.

The toddler or preschooler, with his innate curiosity, explores everything. His curiosity can easily result in spilling hot liquids or igniting his clothing. It takes an especially conscientious mother to remember always to turn the handle of pots inward when cooking, to keep chairs away from the stove, or to put hot liquids away from the edge of the table. Despite the most careful attention to these precautions, children can still manage to burn themselves. They move chairs near the stove and climb up to explore the pots or they pull the overhanging tablecloth and hot liquid spills off the table.

In addition, there are the inconsistencies in the environment which confuse children. If they are allowed to touch the burners of the stove when they are turned off, then they are likely to try the same thing when the burner is on. If they are allowed to lean against radiators or space heaters when they are off, they are likely to do the same when these devices are turned on. Teaching has to be consistent for the young child who does not yet know the concepts of hot and cold or off and on.

Another contributing factor to this high incidence of burns is the variety of materials now used in producing clothing. Many of them are highly flammable and when they begin to burn they burn quickly; the child usually runs, which fans the fire. School-age children often burn themselves by playing with matches or fire.

The severity of the burn is usually determined by the duration of the exposure and the intensity of the heat. Other contributing factors are the way the heat was applied, the size of the child and the body surface involved, the age of the child and the protective aspects of his skin and vascular system, and the type of burn received.

Therefore, some of the initial questions that need to be asked when a child is admitted to the hospital include the following:

1. When did the burn occur?
2. What was the causative agent?
3. Approximately how long was the child exposed to the agent?
4. If the burn occurred in a closed area, were fumes and heat inhaled?
5. What was the child's last recorded weight?
6. Was the child in good physical health prior to the injury?

These questions will help to establish what the child's physical appearance and health status were prior to injury. This information is valuable in helping to establish the child's chances of recovery.

Other questions which need answering to permit adequate therapy are the following:

1. What first-aid treatment, if any, was given at the time of the injury?
2. Was any medication given (such as a tetanus injection or pain medication)?
3. Does the child have any allergies?
4. Has he had much pain from the burn?
5. Is he having pain now?
6. Does the child have any illness or medical condition (such as a viral infection or diabetes)?

This list of questions will help establish priorities for treatment. If the child has not had a tetanus injection, it will be included soon. If he has a concurrent illness, that will also be considered in the care plan.

CLASSIFICATION OF BURNS

Burns are commonly classified as first, second, or third degree according to the severity of the injury. First degree causes vasodilatation and damage to the epidermis and heals rapidly. Second degree burns, or partial-thickness burns, cause damage to the capillaries and involve the epidermis and upper portions of the dermis; there may be blebs containing fluid. Third degree burns, or full-thickness burns, destroy the epidermis and dermis layers, have thrombosed capillaries, and result in formation of eschar (dead tissue). See Figure 1 for the layers of the skin.

Calculating the extent of the burn can be a difficult process. It is possible to overestimate the severity of the burn and it is also possible to have second degree burns advance to third degree by bacterial infiltration. The "Rule of Fives" is usually used to assess the percentage of body area of the child which is burned. In this scheme, in children under five years of age, the head is 20 percent, arms 10 percent each, trunk 20 percent on each side, and legs 10 percent each. The child age 5 to 15 years is evaluated on the basis of the head being 15 percent, arms 10 percent each, trunk 20 percent each side, and legs 15 percent (Cosman, 1974). See Figure 2.

The care during the acute stages demands very skilled personnel as the child's recovery depends on proper replacement of fluids and electrolytes, prevention of infection, prevention of further damage to the tissue, and early recognition and treatment of complications.

The long-term care of children with burns may be directly or indirectly related to ministrations which are done to the child during the acute stage. Some of the long-term problems result because of omissions in care during the acute stages.

Many of the problems which demand long-term care are the direct result of the destruction of the skin; the child's natural defense against disease, his normal water evaporation barrier, his most obvious and largest organ of his body, and his visible sign of an intact body. The child's chances for survival are closely associated with the degree of destruction of the skin.

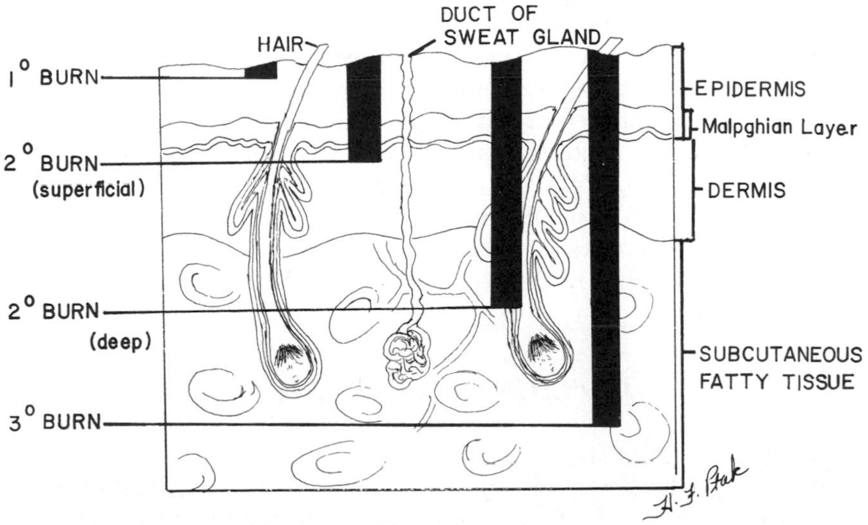

FIG. 1. Skin layers involved with first-, second-, and third-degree burns.

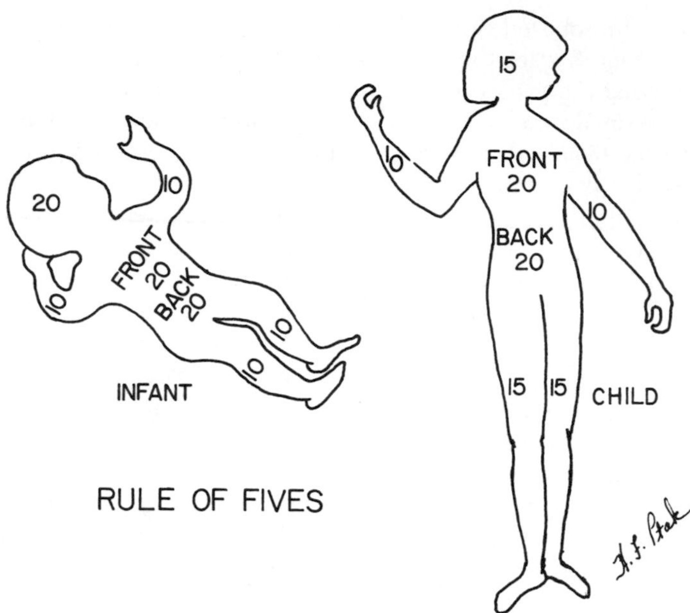

FIG. 2. Rule of fives used in determining the extent of burns in children.

See Figure 1 for the layers of the skin and a description of the involvement associated with each of the classifications.

When the skin is intact we tend to underestimate its value. As soon as the skin is destroyed it becomes very apparent that it is a valuable organ. If the child needs skin grafting during his acute care or long-term therapy, it becomes very evident that the child has limited sources for obtaining healthy skin to use as the graft. The smaller the child, the more difficult it is to obtain skin which is not damaged or skin which does not show when the child is dressed. During the acute stages, the need to cover the burned areas is paramount. Cosman (1974) states, "The longer the wound is open the greater the volume of scar tissue that will be laid down within it and the greater the extent of its contraction, with subsequent deformation and limitation. For these reasons speedy skin coverage is the fundamental goal of this period" (p 459).

IMPLICATIONS OF DIET

During the acute stages, the body is faced with meeting the changes produced by exchanges of electrolytes, hormonal changes, fluid changes, and destruction of tissue. During this period it is imperative to replace fluids and provide adequate nutritional requirements to cope with the insult. Initially, the fluid and electrolyte replacements may be adequately handled by the intravenous route of administration. This leaves the child free of the responsibility of accepting the medical routine. As replacement is established and the child begins to respond, he is given the responsibility for accepting the diet and fluids to restore him to optimal health. The effects of hormonal changes, as well as that of destroyed tissue and pain, may make this request seem unreasonable to the child. In addition, he is faced with decreased activity due to periodic bedrest, and frequently with isolation. He is not hungry enough or interested enough to want the food that is offered. His anorexia becomes a real challenge to the nursing personnel. Their interest in returning the child to wellness increases their persistence to get the child to eat. The condition created by lack of interest on the child's part in eating and increased interest on the nurses' part in getting the child to eat can be detrimental to the long-term care of the child. He begins to dislike the nurse who insists on his eating and to distrust the people giving him care. He misinterprets their interest as antagonistic to his well-being. Even after his appetite begins to return, he may dislike food as it evokes such unhappy remembrances for him. The slow healing process has been associated with long-term dietary impoverishment. Consequently, the medical personnel are very eager to have the child accept adequate nutritional requirements to support the healing process.

The problems of providing adequate dietary intake may be lessened by including the parents' participation. The parent is able to provide helpful hints about the child's likes and dislikes in relation to food. They are also helpful in providing supplemental foods. The parents are frequently amenable to preparing foods at home and bringing them in to the hospital. While we do not want to impose unnecessarily on the parents, their contributions cannot be underestimated. They can also provide nutritional requirements during periods when the hospital dietary facilities may not be operating. The child does not understand that he is supposed to get hungry at only the times that meals are scheduled. He may wake up during the night and request a hamburger. By working with the parents and the dietary staff, this request need not be impossible to meet.

Another implication to long-term care is the type of diet offered during the acute stage. It is usually high in protein, carbohydrates, calories, and some vitamins. To provide these requirements, nurses frequently resort to milk shakes and other high caloric liquids. The child may learn to like this very rich diet, and as his convalescence continues he may become obese. He may also develop eating habits which are much too expensive and selective for the family to provide. The best therapy is to have the child return to the normal family eating patterns, if they are nutritionally adequate, as quickly as possible.

IMPLICATIONS OF ISOLATION

Another area which needs exploring is the use of isolation for children with burns. Isolation has been readily accepted practice as it "cuts down on infection." It is now evident that isolation also cuts down on the child's interest in living. He is cut off from his parents by masks, gowns, and frequently by touch. He is also cared for by personnel who are silhouetted by gowned bodies, exposing only their eyes for him to receive nonverbal communication clues. He is frequently in an area where there are other acutely ill children who need similar demanding care. He may be in a sideroom and frequently has a cradle over his bed. He may even be on a Foster frame or Circulo-matic bed. He frequently has side rails up and often does not have a pillow. This bed is a far cry from the one he is used to at home. It isn't familiar, or for that matter, it may not even be comfortable for him.

Let us examine this isolation room. Despite his previous family conditions, the child is placed in a single room in a bed by himself. These two factors, a single room and a single bed, may be unknown to him—especially if he comes from a large or poor family. The stimuli in this room are medical in nature, and may very well be more depressing than stimulating.

He may be interested, at first, in the intravenous bottle or the equipment for checking specific gravity, or in listening to his heart beat with a stethoscope. These stimuli quickly change to boring ritualism, and the child becomes disinterested. The room may be air-conditioned and this provides an auditory stimulus for a short period. This noise quickly becomes agitating and tends to lead to disorientation over a period of time. The disorientation is further enhanced by the lack of clocks, calendars, and other daily reminders to the child of time and place. Reminders such as the school bell's ringing at 9:00 A.M., the factory whistle's blowing at noon, the mailman's coming in the morning, and the breadman's coming in the afternoon are all removed and the child's immature sense of time is destroyed completely. There are interruptions to his sleep patterns. He is use to going to sleep and not being awakened until morning. Now, just as he is able to fall asleep, he is disturbed for treatments or housekeeping activities that are scheduled during the night. These frequent interruptions during the acute stage establish a pattern of wakefulness that is likely to carry over into the long-term treatment. The child may be given sedatives or tranquilizers, but these do not provide him with the same restful sleep he knew prior to his injury. The periods spent in isolation are likely to be associated with sleep problems.

The isolation may indicate to the child that he is being punished. This connotation sets the stage for the child's feeling towards his burns and his revised body image. The child who is burned frequently feels the burns are punishment for his "wrongdoings," and the isolation serves to accentuate this feeling. The child who received his burns as a result of playing with matches or fire is especially prone to this reaction. He has probably been cautioned many times not to play with fire and he disobeyed his mother's wise counsel. Now he is receiving the punishment given to children who disobey their parents.

The child frequently displays regressive behavior during periods of isolation. This may be displayed in many ways such as his unwillingness to use a bedpan, or his whining and screaming when asked to participate in activities, or sucking his thumb for extended periods of time. The regression, if not treated, may become more serious with the child completely withdrawing from interest in his surroundings.

The isolation further adds to the separation of child and parent and nurse and parent. It puts a barrier on communicating in a usual manner. A frequent use of touch is utilized in normal adult-child relationships. The child learns early to cuddle and caress. He receives a great deal of gratification from this touch no matter how frequently or infrequently it is utilized in his early childhood. As he grows older, he relies less and less on this touch, but he frequently resorts to it in time of illness. The isolation, whether complete or partial, hampers the gratification the child receives from touch. *Complete isolation* is the term I use to describe when parents are forbidden in the room, and *partial isolation* is the term used when sterile gloves interfere with normal touch sensations.

Touch Deprivation

The effect of this isolation is that the child is deprived of the normal comforting sensation of touch. The touch he receives is usually only painful, as it is provided when turning the child. Turning can be a very painful experience for the child who is burned. Because the child learns to associate touch with pain he soon learns to prefer not to be touched. During the acute stage and during grafting, it is sometimes necessary to put mittens on the child or to use mild restraints as the skin is very itchy during these times. In an attempt to relieve himself of the discomfort caused by the itchy sensation, the child can inadvertently cause further damage to his skin.

During the long-term care it is necessary to help the child feel good about his body and to begin to get some gratification from touch. Depending on the severity of the trauma, the nurse can begin to reintroduce the child to kinesthetic sensations. She/he can utilize soothing lotion and gently rub it on the scar area. The soothing, relaxing motion with the warmth and tenderness of her fingertips can bring real joy to the child. At first, his tolerance may be extremely low, but it will increase with time. From this beginning she/he can then proceed to have the child apply the lotion himself, or to have his mother apply it and then the child. If the child is an adolescent, some of the cosmetic lotions can be utilized that mask some of the scar and have the same color tone as his skin.

The younger child may need to start by applying the lotion to the nurse. This gives him an excuse to get close and still does not threaten his will to be alone. The younger child might also enjoy applying the lotion to a doll.

A convenient method in reuniting the child with touch is established when the child is started on tub baths. In the tub it is perfectly acceptable to touch the child. As the child is being taken out of the bathtub, the nurse should lean over and make her/his neck readily accessible for the child to reach for support. The child reaches up and to his surprise finds the sensation satisfying.

Krieger (1975) describes a study that systematically evaluates the use of therapeutic touch with adult patients. She describes a statistically significant rise in hemoglobin rates of patients receiving touch therapy. Further studies of this nature may prove that a touch program is essential to the nursing process for children with burns.

Auditory and Visual Deprivation

The sensory confusion that can take place during periods of confinement is now being appreciated and explored further by health professionals. This sensory confusion is very relevant to young children because their sensory experiences are already limited by their age. They tend to interpret the sensory input on the basis of their limited exposure. This can result in very serious misinterpretations. The unfamiliar sounds in the hospital can be very frightening. The familiar sounds of childhood are missing, especially during periods of isolation. In addition, visual perceptions may be distorted. Shadows cast by night lights may cause moments of panic.

The auditory effects of isolation are usually reversed as soon as isolation is discontinued. They can, however, be prevented by providing music, radio, and normal voices during the isolation period. It is possible for young children to forget their parents' normal voices when separated from them for long periods. This is important to keep in mind, as the parents' voices may sound very different and foreign through a mask.

If it is not permissible for the parents to enter the child's isolation room, an intercom can be successfully utilized between the parent and child. Many children play with intercoms as toys, and they are well-known items to today's child. Intercoms can be bought very inexpensively if the hospital is not equipped with them. The value of getting a set especially for the child is that the parent can stand by a window so the child can see him as well as hear him. In some of the more progressive hospitals closed-circuit television is also utilized and the child can see and hear the parent who is located in another area such as the lobby.

This is also a means to have the other siblings communicate with the hospitalized child. The disadvantage is that the child is not able to answer back directly. This can be improved by having the child dictate his questions and answers to the nurse and have them delivered to the siblings. Cassette tape recordings are also a possibility for facilitating communication. The burned child may be very interested in asking his other siblings about his dog that was close by at the time of the accident. He may fear the dog is also burned. Or he may wonder about his friends or his toys during his absence. These are child-type questions and he wants an answer from another child who understands his concerns. This may be an example of the communication gap between adults and children, and the great satisfaction derived from communicating with children his own age.

Isolation may even occur when the child is simply subjected to long periods of hospitalization. He need not be in an "isolation technique" to be isolated. The isolation may be due to a decrease in normal developmental experiences. For instance, the child who is burned may have to be hospitalized during a very important spring. Spring to a toddler or preschooler is essential to introducing him to the rebirth of flowers, grass, and trees. The one-year-old child does not have the capacity to appreciate the buds. The toddler or preschooler does, and it is important to expose him to them at the time that he is developmentally ready for this experience. The nurse must provide substitute ways of providing the child with such an experience. Books with simple stories about spring are useful as a starting point. The stories can be read and then the books left with the child for his own exploration. A garden can be started in his room. He can plant seeds to watch the beginnings and various stages of growth. House plants which flower can de added for variety. In addition, the child should be placed near a window so he can see changes outside. Binoculars may be needed to bring things into closer focus. The family can be encouraged to take photographs of their yard and home during the season to keep the child up to date on his familiar environment. A bulletin board can be utilized to put up pictures which help to orient the child to time. Very appropriate pictures for display are those drawn by his peers or siblings. The bulletin board should be easily movable so the child can change it if he is old enough to participate in the activity. If he is too young the parents or health personnel must assume responsibility for updating it frequently. Other helpful items are pegboards, blackboards, magic slates, and drawing boards. All of these can be utilized to help cut down on the child's isolation and to nurture developmental progress. (See the discussion of play in Chapter 2 for additional ideas.)

Children's Views of Isolation

In a study by Pidgeon (1967), children were interviewed regarding their understanding of isolation. Pidgeon found that 71 percent of the 3.6- to 6.11-year-olds gave incorrect responses to her questions regarding the cause and effect and rationale for isolation. This high percentage indicates the real need for nurses to work with children to help them understand why they are isolated. The older age groups had a better understanding but still demonstrated the need for factual information regarding isolation. The younger age groups illustrated the idea that the cause of isolation was related to psychologic or moral issues. The school-age children were able to draw upon more experience and could identify physical aspects as the causative agents. In the adolescent age groups, 92 percent of the youngsters interviewed gave correct responses regarding their isolation. The findings suggest that a great deal needs to be done to help preschoolers understand isolation, while the school-age child and adolescent seem to need less professional help to supplement their other resources. The real challenge with children who are burned is to help them cope with the guilt that may exist. It is necessary for the child to be able to do more than just verbalize his knowledge. He must also be helped to deal with the information in a realistic way.

For example, John, a 10-year-old, was admitted with 35 percent of his body burned. He was placed on strict isolation in a sideroom. When asked if he understood the reasons for the isolation he gave this response: "I am being treated on open technique. I am isolated to cut down the possibility of infection." Initially, that response sounds like John thoroughly understands his isolation. However, after John feels more comfortable communicating with the nurse, he adds this statement: "I know why the doctors say I'm isolated, but do all kids get put in these rooms when they play with matches?" This additional statement opens the way for the nurse to explain that isolation is not punishment, that playing with matches is not the reason for isolation, nor is isolation used unless it is absolutely essential for the best possible care of the child. It is also helpful to explain that, as a nurse, you do not like to isolate children and you are willing to help children in any way possible to tolerate isolation. A question such as, "Is there anything I can do or get you which would make you feel comfortable while isolated?" Or, capitalizing on the child's imagination: "If you could wish for anything to have right now, what would it be?"

It is not always possible to provide the child with his wish but at least you can begin to find out how he feels and what he would like. You may even find that, by making some trade-offs, you can provide something which closely approximates his wishes without interfering with the isolation technique.

Parents and Isolation

The effects that isolation can have on the parents can be as detrimental as the effects on the child. The parent is placed in an awkward position by virtue of the child's being burned in the first place. Burns are referred to as preventable accidents in childhood. But the prevention is not as easy as prevention provided by periodic immunizations. It is prevention which requires almost constant supervision of the child. Burns may occur despite the most conscientious guidance, or, conversely, they may occur as the result of a battering parent. The wide range of causation behooves us to work diligently with the parents, from the onset.

Bright (1967) identifies an assessment tool that she used to record, assess, and plan care for the parent. I feel such a tool can be useful when isolation interferes with a close mother-child relationship. This is especially significant for children with burns as there is a high incidence of disturbed mother-child relationships in this pediatric population. What can the tool do? It can begin to identify the way the parent reacts and responds when isolation is a major obstacle to effective communication. It can also help to identify areas of concern which cause anxiety in the parent and further adds to the communication gap.

Recordings such as the following may help to identify ways the nurse can begin to help the parent and child to understand one another. One mother stated: "Jerry always does the darndest things! He's my trouble maker. He got what he deserves!" This statement, along with the following description of the mother, are recorded on the tool for use by the professional team.

Mrs. M. spoke with real feeling. She emphasized the words "he," "troublemaker," and "deserves." She maintained eye contact during the conversation and her facial expression was stern and determined.

From first glance, this information reveals a mother and child who may be temporarily helped by the isolation technique. It would not be beneficial to Jerry to hear his mother talk this way. The isolation also provided an opportunity for the mother to release these negative feelings to a helping person.

There is, however, much more to be done for this family. Parod and Caplan (1960) bring out the important fact that when one is dealing with families in crisis, it is possible to help them resolve the acute stress situation and at the same time to help them also bring satisfactory solutions to unresolved problems. They found that people can "rise to the occasion" and seem to find new strength to deal with the current crisis, and in the long run resolve other situations which have interfered with healthy family relationships.

The situation quoted would seem to need this type of intervention. How can we help the mother to see her responsibility to her child during this acute crisis and perhaps at the same time improve her feelings toward him when he is well? How can we minimize the effects of isolation to help meet our overall objectives? First, we must help the mother understand that her presence is essential despite her present feelings. A statement such as,

"I know how frustrated you must feel, but please try to believe that Jerry needs you." Or, "Isolation is only to prevent infection, we do not use it to separate the child and parent. We thoroughly believe that parents are the best therapy for their children."

Isolation is a barrier that interferes with the expression of motherly instincts when they are at their height. For instance, Mrs. M's first reaction might be to rush to Jerry and hug him and ask his forgiveness in an effort to release her guilt. Because he is isolated, she is deprived of this experience and must try to relieve her guilt without the help of her son. Despite a strained mother-child relationship prior to the insult, she might have benefited from this experience. Jerry might also have benefited by witnessing his mother being genuinely interested in his welfare and asking for his understanding. Each might have begun to see the other in a different light, but isolation blocked out this opportunity.

We can minimize the effects of isolation by helping the mother to verbally express her feelings to Jerry. The nurse might say, "Don't be afraid to tell Jerry how you feel. Let him know you are sorry he must withstand the pain." When working with Jerry you can help further by sharing with him his mother's desire to help despite the limitations created by the isolation. For example, "Your Mom would love to be able to come in the room. As yet, the doctors still feel it is best not to let her come in. Is there anything you want me to tell her?"

The success of intervention will greatly depend on the ability of the nurse to provide opportunities for the parent and child to interact in a meaningful way, despite the isolation, and to draw upon their hidden capacities to resolve conflicts that interfere with coping with acute stress.

IMPLICATIONS OF WHIRLPOOL

The use of whirlpool during the acute stages is a commonly accepted practice. The whirlpool helps to cut down on infection, reduces the odor from decaying tissue and stimulates capillary ingrowth. This very useful procedure has lessened the use of soaks to the burned area as it aids dressing changes and helps to remove the old antibiotic ointments. It can be an extremely soothing procedure. The way it is introduced to the child is most important and especially so if the child has been burned by liquid. The whirlpool may bring back uncomfortable memories for the child. If the original introduction to the procedure is handled correctly, the long-term use of the therapy is easy. Children innately enjoy water play and the whirlpool can be utilized this way. The use of squirt guns, boats, sponges, etc., help to make the therapy a treat instead of a treatment. The temperature of the water is usually 35 to 37 C and the hydrotherapy is usually prescribed for 15- to 30-minute periods. The temperature of the room should be regulated to decrease chilling to which the child is more prone with his skin barrier decreased. This factor is most important during the acute stages but should also be considered during the long-term care.

The trips to whirlpool should not be used as a bribe for good behavior. They should not be withheld for uncooperative behavior. This method of control interferes with the long-range satisfactory use of whirlpool in the child's care. Withholding whirlpool therapy may meet a short-term goal of care, but it really interferes with the long-term care of the child. In long-term goals, we want the child to appreciate and enjoy the whirlpool as a method of enhancing his grafting and promoting a return to health. As a part of the long-term therapy, we want it to have only positive connotations to the child.

CONTRACTURES

Cosman (1974) states that

> All body wounds close in part by contraction and the special formation of the special reparative tissue known as scar. . . . Contraction and scar formation continue as long as the wound remains open. . . . When wound contraction produces deformity of surrounding parts or limits function, it is said that a 'contracture' is present. . . . Contracture bands may form, especially on flexion surfaces. This use of the term refers to an elevated bow-string-like band of scar tissue. . . . The term 'contracture' also is used as a description of the stiffness of a joint mechanism consequent on the tightness and shortening of unused periarticular ligaments (p 466).

Contractures are a frequent result of burns. As described by Cosman some are the result of scar tissue while others are caused by lack of adequate protection during the acute stage. The prevention of all contractures is an impossible goal. However, limiting contractures is facilitated by proper positioning of the child with burns. The child has the tendency to put his body in the position which is the least painful. The position may cause a contracture or contractures and necessitate additional surgery. The key to good results is to place the body in good alignment, use a footboard, place pillows and sandbags as needed, use splints if necessary, and change positions frequently. These rules apply during the skin-grafting stages, also. It is equally important to control contractures during all periods of hospitalization. Frequently even during discharge periods, areas are splinted to keep them in good alignment. Even the smallest finger must be protected. A small splint made from a baby tongue blade can be used for this purpose. Splinting is especially useful if the child is unable to control and exercise the part involved. An arm that has been burned can be splinted with a padded arm board. Care must be taken to check for proper circulation.

The armboard is removed for whirlpool and exercises and then reapplied. Active and passive exercises are given to parts that are not immobilized by skin grafting. These exercises should be given during all hospitalization periods and taught to the mother for home use, if indicated. The exercises can be achieved through the use of toys that necessitate movement of the involved part. If it is a hand involved, throwing and catching a ball is useful, or playing pool in the case of an older child. If it is finer coordination, turning the pages of a book will suffice. Stretching the neck muscles can be achieved by placing the child's bed so he must turn to see TV or to see who is entering the room. The conscientious care taken to prevent contractures may save the child periods of being in traction or even surgical correction to release contractures. Most of this discussion related to contractures is associated only with joints. The other contractures will not be lessened by these techniques.

PRESSURE SORES

Fortunately, in the care of children we have fewer situations in which pressure sores are a problem. However, children who are immobilized due to the burns or grafting are good candidates for developing them. The positioning and turning done to prevent contractures will also aid in the prevention of pressure sores. If the child is immobilized for very long periods, an alternating-pressure mattress may be a helpful addition. Pressure sores are easily started on already destroyed tissues, such as burns, so close attention should be paid to the burned areas. Common sites for decubitus formation are the heels, sacrum, elbows and, in young children, the back of the head.

The treatment for pressure sores must be selected carefully. Routine care, offered in some hospitals, should not be instituted without checking with the physician. The application of a heat treatment with use of a light bulb can further aggravate the burn. The application of ointments can interfere with the therapy being given. The best treatment may very well be to keep the area clean and exposed to the air with additional consideration given to not putting pressure on the already involved area.

The child frequently likes to wear jewelry or clothing which may cause constrictions and result in pressure sores. Removal of all constricting bands will aid in circulation and help in prevention of pressure sores. If the constricting band is a "good luck charm," the child can choose another area in his room where it can be kept. He may want it taped to the foot of his bed, or hanging on a mobile. I have found that children will cooperate in removing such articles if they have been consulted in the decision rather than forced into it. Making a game of where the article can be placed is good fun.

A little child may even enjoy the magic of having the charm change places and guessing where it is, providing the charm is not kept out of sight too long. This same charm may reappear on every admission and the child will expect the same attention to be given to it.

DEPENDENCE ON ADJUNCT THERAPY

One of the concerns of long-term care with children who are burned is the dependence they may develop on measures taken to lessen their pain or help them progress. One of these measures is the use of narcotics. The older child quickly learns that the stick of the needle is worth the relief he gets from the medication. As the time passes, either on the first admission or on following admissions, it becomes necessary to evaluate the child's real need for the narcotic. This can be a real challenge. Each child's pain threshold is different and no one wants to expose the child to severe pain when it can be alleviated. The greatest adjunct to relief of pain is the alleviation of fear. The child who is afraid frequently requests pain medication so he can go to sleep and forget everything. I contend that providing means to lessen the fear will lessen the amount of medication needed, especially during convalescent periods. (Injections are considered again under the section on handling stress.)

To lessen fear, we must look at some of the things children fear and how they can be handled. Many children fear darkness. The use of a light in the room can take partial care of this. Close proximity to the nurses' station will allow him to see people when he wakes up. Some children fear being left alone. The use of volunteers or other roommates can lessen this fear. Some children fear unfamiliar noises. This is harder to control in a hospital. However, if each time a noise is made, no matter how familiar it is to the nurse, it is explained to the child, it will eventually become familiar and less of a threat. Some children fear unfamiliar voices. This is especially so when positioning keeps the child from seeing the person. The common courtesy of adults identifying themselves by name and function, when entering the room, can lessen this fear. Some children develop fears because the hospital does not conform to his home routine. If the child is used to sleeping with his door open, or with a radio playing, or with a favorite toy, the change in routine may cause him concern. Any return to normal conditions for the child will help to make him more comfortable.

The child will also fear the extent of the injury. The older child senses the severity of the involvement. They know how others have responded to them during and after the acute stages of their illness. Now during long-term interventions they begin to perceive that additional therapy is not going to eradicate all their problems.

One way to determine whether a child really needs a narcotic is to watch closely the times and conditions when the request is made. The child may request narcotics when he wishes to withdraw from a situation, such as when exercises are scheduled. He may request it when his parents visit. This request may be made because he wants them to know how painful the burns or surgical procedures really are. He may request them to make the parents feel guilty for his confinement. He may request them so he is conveniently asleep when the parents visit or when meals are served.

These types of clues can help you determine the use or misuse of the narcotic at a particular time. While it is certainly important to have the child as free from pain as possible, it is not fair to have the child become dependent on narcotics. Careful evaluation of the foregoing factors will help you make a more realistic evaluation of the child's need for the narcotic to alleviate physical pain. The emotional pain he has is more adequately treated by other methods.

It is also necessary to search for clues which might indicate that the child is having pain but will not request medication because he does not want another needle. The child must be told that after the "stick" he will soon feel relief of his pain. He should also know that at this time only a "needle stick" can be used to give the medication. He should know that you do not enjoy hurting him but you know that children do feel better after they get the medicine.

The parents will also need to know that narcotics are not used without jurisdiction. With the current emphasis on narcotic addiction by youth, they may have real concern about introducing the child to drugs. The parents should also know that occasionally a child may request narcotics when they cannot be given. They need to be assured that our aim is to make the child as comfortable as possible but also to assure safe delivery of medications.

Another adjunct to burn therapy, but one that is decreasingly necessary, is the use of tracheostomy, when the area around the face and neck are involved or when caustic inhalants are involved. The child can become very dependent on the tracheostomy. The longer it is utilized the more difficult it usually becomes to close it off and remove it. Partial "corking" can be attempted while the child is sleeping. During sleep it is easier to evaluate the child's need for continuance of the therapy. If the partial corking is successful, the next night complete corking is tried. When it is quite clear that the child can breathe with the tube corked, he can be introduced to the idea. This does not mean that the child will still not become anxious and develop respiratory difficulty, however. Very close supervision is still warranted and removal should be done when the child is calm. Occasionally repeated attempts at corking fail and removal is done under close supervision. The child should not be left alone during this time and sterile equipment must be close by in readiness for reinsertion.

It is sometimes necessary for the child to be discharged with the tracheostomy. The nurse is responsible for teaching the parents the proper care and danger signals. The child that tends to have difficulty swallowing liquids or food can be taught to flex his head forward. The mother should be taught that hyperextending the neck narrows the esophagus and food and fluid can easily flow into the trachea. Flexing the head allows the esophagus to open and the epiglottis closes facilitating swallowing (Weber, 1974). A referral to the local community health nurse is also indicated. The child should not be discharged until the equipment is in the home and the community health nurse has checked it for proper size and functioning. The community health nurse is able to check for outlets for the suction machine, evaluate home facilities for cleaning equipment, talk with the mother about her concerns, be sure that emergency telephone numbers are available near the telephone, and elicit the parents' understanding and willingness to assume the responsibility for the child's care.

BODY IMAGE

Case Study Presentations

My first meeting with Marty was momentary because it took immense concentration and stamina to bear the sight of him. Wearing a diaper and striped shirt, he lay in a bed on his back with his head held up, his legs and knees flexed and his right hand swathed in cumbersome bandages. He rocked back and forth, he wailed and moaned. Light brown hair on his head was sparsely interspersed with patches of scarred scalp tissue. As I dared to approach him he turned his head and looked at me. Mucus bubbled and streamed from his nose. Tears poured down his face although his sobbing abated as I drew closer. Reddened scar tissue encompassed his face, his features were twisted and taut, the masculature about his mouth was particularly puckered and tight. Could he open his mouth sufficiently to eat or to speak I wondered? His left ear was bent over upon itself, his right ear was whole but disfigured, then tissue tags adhered to both upper and lower eyelids near the inter-canthus of his eyes, there were eyelashes but only a resemblance of an eyebrow over his right eye (Slamar, 1967, p 212).

More attention is being given to the relevance of body image to the child. The child forms his body image in early childhood and the image varies as he grows and develops. The process has an abrupt interruption when the child is burned, especially if it results in deformity to a previously well-developed body part. According to Gruendemann (1975),

Body image in one's conceptual profile of his body ('I-ness'). It consists of conscious and unconscious feelings, facts, and perceptions about one's body. Its distinct identity is based on outward appearance, inner somatic sensations, and significant others' reactions to his body. . . . One's body image or mental picture of self may not be the same as the actual structure, function, or outward appearance of the body. Rather, body image is a representation or impression of the self, built around a particular body and its equipment, and screened through layers of personal, biased thoughts and wishes (p 636).

The child who is burned will need time to ventilate his feelings about his changed body. He will need the support of a helping adult to learn to understand his new appearance. Young children tend to use fantasy to help them cope with difficult situations. The child with severe burn scars may fantasize that his body is unchanged despite visible evidence to the contrary. He may spend time trying to wish back his former appearance. It may seem like the child is completely ignoring reality in his attempt to make himself into the person he was prior to the injury. The role of the nurse is to help to establish reality without stripping the child of all of his coping mechanisms.

Questions that can aid in the assessment of the child's progress are

1. How do you look?
2. Is the way you look today different than before you were burned?
3. How would you like to change yourself, if you could?
4. How do you think you will look to your brother (sister)?
5. When you get bigger, how will your body look?
6. Why is the doctor doing skin grafting?
7. If you could wish anything for yourself, what would it be?
8. What one word best describes how your body looks to you?
9. How do you feel when you say that (answer to question 8) word?

Utilizing some of these questions will help you to validate the child's progress. The assessment of his nonverbal responses is just as important as the assessment of his verbal responses. In fact, the younger the child, the more revealing his nonverbal responses will be.

For example, if you ask question 4, and the child's eyelids fall and his head lowers and he replies, "Fine" or "I don't know," the nonverbal response is interpreted as indicating that the child being very sad, not liking his body image, and still unable to express his true feelings in words. A response to this situation would be, "You seem very sad, can you tell me how you feel right now?"

The child's aspect during the day will also help to validate his progress. Does he smile and laugh spontaneously while in the playroom? Does he resist and cry when it is time for painful procedures such as dressing changes? Does he hide under the bed clothes and get very quiet and withdrawn during visiting hours? Does he talk to the other children on the unit? Does he whine all the while he has visitors? Does he refuse to brush his hair, clean his teeth, and dress attractively? Does he tend to act out frequently, such as playing the part of the unit's clown?

Specific time should be set aside to talk to the child. Otherwise he may not resolve his feelings about his changed body and develop a distorted body image. The art of active listening is vitally important in this process. The child must know that you are sincere and that you hear what he is saying. His messages should not be taken lightly or be underplayed. You must acknowledge his right to be disappointed and help him to see that he is still a special person who can live a fruitful life despite his disability.

Factors Influencing the Ways a Child Handles Stress

For this discussion, stress will be considered as being any situation or condition which is inherent in the environment and which poses a threat to the child's emotional state and causes him to make certain adjustments in order to cope with the situation. This stress may be of a minor nature or of major magnitude. The degree of severity is not necessarily proportionate to the response it causes.

Stress affects the psychologic as well as the physiologic functioning of the child. For instance, the child may be able to conceal his psychologic response to an incident but his physiologic response of a blushed face is readily evident. Or conversely, the child may scream loudly in response to stress but his bounding pulse may not be as evident to the nurse.

The way the child handles stress and the anxiety and tensions produced by stress are related to a number of factors. In planning nursing care it will be imperative to give attention to these influences. I will list a few: (1) the age of the child and the status of his personality development prior to stress; (2) his past ways of dealing with new and difficult situations; (3) the immediate emotional surroundings of his illness; (4) the nature of his illness and its acuteness, as well as the severity, duration, and type of symptoms; (5) the degree of discomfort involved in the diagnostic procedures; (6) the meaning of illness to the child and his preexisting feelings regarding health and disease; (7) his specific fears and fantasies; (8) the attitude of his family toward illness; (9) the child's relationships with physicians, nurses, and other hospital personnel, and their attitudes and feelings about children; (10) the nature of the hospital setting, and its policies and practices; and (11) the preparation of the child for the experience.

Injections. Students are usually painfully aware of their own stress in the clinical situation and therefore may be more atuned to the child's stress. I think this is especially so in relation to painful procedures which the student must do to the child. This awareness can help the student appreciate the need for paying special attention to the child after the procedure has been completed. However, the student is sometimes so relieved to have her/his own stress alleviated that she/he forgets the aftercare of the child.

This situation is prone to occur when giving the child with burns an injection (actually it applies when giving an injection to any child). The student frequently dislikes giving injections to children and she/he realizes that children fear receiving them. After the student mobilizes herself/himself to go to the child's bedside, she/he is aware that her presence increases the anxiety of the child (Torrence, 1968). This knowledge may also increase the stress of the student. After the child is prepared for and receives the injection his psychologic and physiologic states begin the return to his prestress level. The student is going through the same cycle. The fact that the student also receives relief can help her/him to gain confidence in her/his own ability to give injections to children. However, the same situation does not necessarily give the child any confidence and it may actually increase his anxiety regarding injections and serve to heighten his fears in the future. The next time the student attempts to give the same child an injection he may have an increased reaction to stress, which causes the student to lose some of her/his confidence. This reciprocal interaction tends to influence both the student and the child in relation to their stress responses.

What can be done to help lessen the child's stress with respect to injections? To answer this question it is necessary to consider many and quite complicated contributing factors. First, it is generally accepted from clinical evidence that all children dislike to receive injections. If you ask them what they dislike most about nurses, doctors, or hospitals they almost all reply "shots." The degree to which the child experiences stress from injections is not consistent, however. Even infants seem to recall receiving injections because they begin to cry when returning to the doctor's office or well-baby clinic where they previously received an injection. Their dissatisfaction with injections does not seem to be lessened by any type of preparation. It likewise seems clear that toddlers' and preschoolers' stress is not diminished by preparation for the injection. However, the school-age child and adolescent seem to benefit from the preparation which includes simple explanations of what the injection means to their bodily function.

According to Torrence (1968), the physiologic response of heart beat increased when the nurse entered the child's unit with the injection. The study was limited to children 3.2 years to 7.2 years, and specifically addressed itself to responses of these particular age periods. The information is valuable as it clearly identifies that stress is heightened as the threat becomes more intense. Although the study involves limited ages, clinical evidence supports that children of other ages may respond similarly when the threat of injection becomes inevitable. School-age children show signs such as clenching of lips, clenching of fists, facial grimacing, raising of shoulders, inhaling of breath with resultant rigid abdomen, tightly closed eyes, downturning of toes, tightly crossed arms, cracking of fingers, or hiding under the sheets. If these children were studied under similar conditions, they probably would have an increased heart rate also.

In light of this information, it would seem logical that injections should be given without unnecessary delay in order to decrease stress. A simple and quick explanation should be given followed by the injection. This method would be superior to entering the unit with the syringe and then delaying the process by attempting to decrease the child's anxiety by playing with his toys or attempting to engage him in a conversation.

Another factor which needs to be considered is the way the child perceives the size of the syringe and needle. If you ask the child to indicate how big the syringe is, he will usually give a size far too large to store in most drawers. His description of the syringe and needle may closely resemble the threat he feels from the injections. This fact is good to keep in mind, as nurses are sometimes tempted to show the child the small amount of solution in the syringe to try to convince him it will not hurt too much. The child sees the syringe and needle and the amount is not so significant to him as it is to the nurse.

After the injection is completed, the child can be helped to resolve the stress by being comforted by the nurse, by being allowed to act out his hostility, and by being protected from other stress situations before he has resumed his composure.

Injections might be better tolerated if they could be given at optimal time periods rather than on a regularly scheduled basis, as commonly ordered. For instance, the child with burns may be ordered to receive penicillin 300,000 units every 8 hours. The injection may be due when the child has just completed another painful experience and the child is poorly equipped to handle this additional stress. He reacts strenuously to this new stress and it is possible that this reaction is lessening his capacity for recovery. At a later time, the injection might possibly be less of a threat as the child has had time to recover and he feels less threatened by the same injection. If the injection is ordered only on a daily basis it is easier to vary the time of administration and to judge the optimum time for delivery.

The fact that any experience with a needle is considered as a "shot" by the child further adds to the confusion. The child who had a large amount of blood drawn after several painful attempts to find a vein, may remember this experience and expect it each time he gets an injection. His level of anxiety may go up in relation to that experience and expect it each time he gets an injection. His level of anxiety may go up in relation to that experience for a long time before he learns to adjust to what seems to be a lesser threat, that of a single injection. It is important to note, however, that the single injection may actually be as threatening as the more painful procedure and the child's anxiety may not be lessened.

There are other factors which could be added, but this list tends to illustrate the complexity of the situation and helps to identify the ways a nurse can be instrumental in helping the child cope with one of the many situations that he will face.

CASE DISCUSSION

Bobby

This patient required day-to-day brainstorming sessions to come up with creative ideas that would meet his needs.

Bobby was eight years old at the time he was transferred to our clinical area. His immediate care had been given in a small local hospital with a very small pediatric census. When Bobby was transferred, he was having nightmares and would scream out during the night or whenever he fell asleep. He had many fears of being left alone and these fears were interfering with his recovery tremendously. It was believed on the initial evaluation that Bobby would benefit a great deal by special nursing services. He had the good fortune to have a male nurse on the night tour of duty and Bobby gained a great deal from this relationship. After the really acute stage, when his condition varied almost minute-to-minute, the private duty nurses were released and Bobby was on floor care. At the time this decision was made, it was felt that Bobby's condition was such that he would not suffer from withdrawal of the nurses and that he might progress faster in a less dependent role. This was not the case and Bobby's condition worsened as he again felt very threatened by being alone.

With this in mind, a night nurse was assigned to Bobby and he was on floor care during the day and evening shifts. Bobby was particularly fearful of moving his limbs as the exercise program planned for him was quite painful. One of the things that helped Bobby tremendously was the nurse's convincing the physician that Bobby should be out of bed, riding a tricycle. This would stretch his contractors much more successfully than the exercise program. It was very rewarding to see this child, despite the pain and discomfort, "light up" and become very enthusiastic about his therapeutic plan of care when it was something that was so common and familiar to him as a tricycle. Bobby was also told that at the times he was scheduled for skin grafting, he would have to be separated from his tricycle. Although this was particularly difficult for him to do, he did accept it as reality.

Bobby showed one of the typical reactions of a child who has been severely burned, that of a great deal of antagonism, especially for the nurses who provide his care. These nurses do many painful procedures to the child. The child interprets these painful procedures as punishment—another punishment, in addition to the one he has already received—for what he thinks are his wrongdoings.

In reviewing the literature of burned children, especially children who have played with matches, as Bobby had, we see that frequently these children had some disturbed emotional development prior to their injury.

This was the case with Bobby. Bobby and his mother were having a real conflict with one another and on repeated occasions she told him not to play with matches. On this particular day he was playing with them and set his clothing on fire. His mother's immediate response to the injury was, "Didn't I tell you so?" This theme was carried through on the infrequent visits she made to Bobby. It was possible for his mother to protect herself from having to see him during his acute stages by just staying home. Because of her many responsibilities to her other children and because of the transportation problems, she was able to justify to herself her long periods between visiting. However, we were not able to justify them to Bobby. At times he would verbalize that he didn't want to see her anyway and this probably was very true. However, it was sometimes very evident that he wanted very much to see her despite their poor relationship.

Bobby had already experienced the uncomfortable feeling of people staring at his disfigured body. He could deduce that he would get a great deal of the same when he was returned home. He frequently would mention that he never wanted to return to school, that he hated other children, and that he would just like to stay in the hospital forever. One of my responses to such a statement was, "You do not like it when people stare at you, do you Bobby? I can understand why you would not like it." At first such a response would just bring a flood of tears from Bobby, but as he developed trust in me, he was able to say with a great deal of feeling and hostility, "No, I hate them when they laugh at me or stare at me." Over a period of time we were able to discuss how some of the surgery which he considered extremely painful could improve his appearance. While he did not like to go for skin grafting and reconstructive surgery because of its extreme discomfort to him, its end result was frequently an improvement in his outward appearance. We also discussed some of the clothing that he could wear to cover some of his more severe scars. We discussed, too, some of the things that could make him a very fine companion to other children despite his scars. Although I'm sure Bobby had many concerns to which there were no easy answers, and concerns to which he would not accept answers, the very fact that somebody was there to discuss some of his feelings seemed to relax him.

As stated earlier, much antagonism is exhibited by burned children toward the people who deliver their care, and it would not be humanly possible for the professionals not to feel some negativism in response. It would seem very important for a child with burns to have a consistent person in his environment; and this person should be one who has a great deal of maturity and insight. Even though he or she does not provide direct nursing care to the child, the person should be available to visit with the child each day. This person should plan to attend the team conferences relating to the care of the child and be able to present some of the things about which the child is thinking, and to do so without the feeling of breaking confidences with the child. He or she can contribute only those reactions of the child that will influence changes in the plan of care.

The way Bobby was reunited with his family is significant. We started by writing postcards to his family, and the other children in the family returned postcards to him. Then we advanced to the more personal contact of calling his home and allowing him to talk to his family. The nurse was working with his mother to encourage her to call Bobby. These phone calls were arranged at times when the phone would not be particularly busy and it would not inconvenience the staff to get Bobby to the phone. The mother also was encouraged to try to visit more frequently. While there were no treatments that were going to be her responsibility when she was home, she needed to become more familiarized with the very changed body of her child. There was not much overt evidence of changes in attitude between the mother and child before the discharge. However, we tried to achieve a beginning understanding before reuniting them. With the mother's consent a report was sent to the private pediatrician and a copy made available in case he wanted to send it to the local hospital where he had cared for Bobby. There was a possibility Bobby would be readmitted to the local hospital for more skin grafts in the future. This report had an extensive section by the nursing personnel documenting the fears that Bobby had when hospitalized and also some of his feelings regarding discharge. It was hoped that if Bobby was readmitted, consideration would be given to some of the factors that helped to make him feel more secure in the hospital setting.

Another thing that I have found consistently in relation to children with burn scars is that they misinterpret many of the things that we do to them, and one of the things that they frequently seem to misinterpret is the grafting procedures. I have had many children say to me, "You are skinning me alive," or, "Everytime you put me to sleep you take away my good skin." Postoperatively, I have seen more of them overprotect the donor sites than the recipient site and I think this is because of their misinterpretation. I think perhaps we should take a new approach to what we do to children and perhaps admit to them that some of the things we are doing are not for them but are done for us, such as, "I need to know what your blood pressure is and so I am doing this for my information." Or, "I need to know your blood pressure to be able to monitor your care." I think if we put more of the painful procedures on this basis, then the child would be more willing to accept some of the things that we do to him and not for him. Then, the things that we do specifically for him, such as provide him with play activities, would be more meaningful. He could see the direct relationship between what he likes and what he gets and what he dislikes and what he has to accept anyway.

Another area of concern is the one in which parents may be "overprotective." This term is rather broad and it has different connotations to different people. I shall use the term to denote a relationship which interferes with the child's ability to return to normal independence. Thus, a parent who does not allow the child to participate, at all, in his personal care is being overprotective. The nurse working with the child also needs to be working with the parent. She/he needs to set limits for the parent as well as the child. For example, "Mrs. G., John needs to use his hands to prevent contractures. He is capable of washing his own face." And, "John, your fingers need exercise. It may hurt a little to use them. Here, try washing your face with this washcloth!"

The nurse and Mrs. G. offer support to John during the procedure. If John is capable of doing more of his bath he is encouraged to do so. If he is not, Mrs. G. may finish the bath if she wishes to participate in this way. After the bath is completed recognition is given to John for his efforts. Praise is given only if justified. A word of encouragement for future participation is also given.

Then the nurse talks privately with Mrs. G. She/he gives her an opportunity first to express how she felt about the experience. Then the nurse explains to Mrs. G. that it is very important to John to help him to be self-sufficient. A statement such as, "It is painful for you to watch John try, isn't it?" or, "Does it hurt you to watch John try so hard?" is appropriate. It is also important to help Mrs. G. understand that with your nursing knowledge you will have to make decisions in the best interest of John. You explain that periodically you will discuss with her areas which will need revision in accordance with John's progress.

You attempt to establish an open line of communication so you can readily intervene if the child is being overprotected. This seems like a simple example and one which can readily be handled. The seriousness of it lies, however, in the results which may ensue. Early intervention may be the difference between functioning or nonfunctioning fingers. Another factor to be considered in whether to ignore early signs of overprotection is that frequently the problem grows in magnitude as the hospitalization continues. It is frequently easier to cope with the smaller problems than the larger ones which can follow. For instance, the mother may then wish to keep her child isolated from other children. If we have allowed her to overprotect him when it related to personal hygiene then why shouldn't she continue to overprotect him? If we have not guided her and shared our intellectual knowledge regarding the seriousness of overprotection in the past, then it is difficult to start interceding at this point. Periodic intervention helps to maintain an open channel of communication with the parent. If she is used to exchanging ideas with the nurse when things are going well, then she is less likely to be defensive or uncooperative when change is necessary. The well-being of the child is always of utmost importance. If our requests are centered on a more therapeutic environment for the child with emphasis on rehabilitating him to his maximum potential, parents will rarely disagree with the plan of action. The plan is further strengthened if the parent and child are included in its construction.

CASE PRESENTATION AND STUDY QUESTIONS

Amy is a six-year-old with 45 percent of her body covered with burn scars. Her burns were the result of getting too close to the stove in a flimsy nightgown. Amy comes from a family of two children. She has a sister two years older than herself. Mr. and Mrs. M. appear to be a happily married couple and show deep interest and concern for their family. Amy has been hospitalized on four previous occasions. She has a tracheostomy in place since the initial insult three years ago.

At the time you meet Amy she is in a rooming-in situation with her mother. She is admitted for release of contractures of both arms. Amy has had the surgery and is receiving postoperative physical therapy. When Amy is not at physical therapy her arms are restrained up over her head. She is allowed out of bed, walking 15 minutes per day.

Consider the following questions in providing nursing care for Amy:

1. What are the nursing considerations when a child is restrained in the described manner? How would you introduce the mother and child to the plan of restraints?
2. What types of intervention should be planned for the child's 15 minutes of ambulation? When should the plan be established? Who should be included in making the plan?
3. Who should assume the responsibility for the tracheostomy care? What factors will determine this decision? How should the child and family be prepared for removal of the tracheostomy of long-standing?
4. How can both Mrs. M. and Amy keep in touch with the other child and Mr. M.?
5. What types of activity are realistic for Amy after discharge?

BIBLIOGRAPHY

Ballack JP: Helping a child cope with stress of injury. Am J Nurs 74:1491, August 1974

Bernstein NR: Emotional Care of the Facially Burned and Disfigured. Boston, Little, Brown, 1976

Blake FG, Wright RH, Waechter EH: Nursing of Children, 8th ed. Philadelphia, Lippincott, 1970, pp 321–26

Bright F: Parental anxiety—a barrier to communication. A.N.A. Regional Clinical Conferences, 1966. New York, Appleton, 1967, pp 13–19

Campbell L: Special behavioral problems of the burned child. Am J Nurs 76:220, January 1976
Candle PR, Potter J: Characteristics of burned children and the after effects of the injury. Br J Plast Surg 26:63, 1970
Constable JD: Pre-injury emotional instability held clue to difficulties with many burned children. Pediatrics Herald, Sept–Oct 1968, pp 1–2
Cosman B: The burned child. In Downey JA, Low NL: The Child with Disabling Illness. Philadelphia, Saunders, 1974, pp 453–80
Donnellan WL: Burns. In Swenson O (ed): Pediatric Surgery, 3rd ed. New York, Appleton, 1969
Ducharme JC: Burns and pediatrics. Can Nurse 57:851, October 1961
Einhorn AH, Jacobziner H: Accidents in childhood. In Barnett HL (ed): Pediatrics, 16th ed. New York, Appleton, 1977
Gould M: A child with burns. Am J Nurs 61:101, December 1961
Gruendemann BJ: The impact of surgery on body image. Nurs Clin North Am 10:635, 1973
Harmon V, Steele S: Nursing Care of the Skin: A Developmental Approach. New York, Appleton, 1975
Krieger D: Therapeutic touch: the imprimatur of nursing. Am J Nurs 75:784, May 1975
Kueffner M: Passage through hospitalization of a severely burned, isolated school-age child. In Communicating Nursing Research, Batey MV (ed): WICHE, January 1975, pp 181–97
Little DE, Carvevali DL: Nursing Care Planning. Philadelphia, Lippincott, 1969
Long RT, Cope O: Emotional problems of burned children. N Engl J Med 264:1121, 1961
Parad HJ, Caplan JA: A framework for studying families in crisis. Soc Work J 25:3, 1960
Pidgeon VA: Children's concepts of the rationale of isolation technic. A.N.A. Regional Clinical Conferences, 1966. New York, Appleton, 1967, pp 21–27
Quinlan E: Dietary treatment of burns. Can Nurse 61:375, April 1965
Rubin M: Balm for burned children. Am J Nurs 66:297, February 1966
Seligman R et al: Emotional responses of burned children in a pediatric intensive care unit. Psychiatr Med 3:59, 1972
Slamar C: Behavioral interaction between a three-year-old child with burns scars and his nurse. A.N.A. Regional Clinical Conferences, 1967. New York, Appleton, 1968, pp 211–17
Stone NH et al: Child abuse by burning. Surg Clin North Am 50:1419, 1970
Talabere L, Graves P: A tool for assessing families of burned children. Am J Nurs 76:225, January 1976
Torrence JT: Children's reactions to intramuscular injections: a comparative study of needle and jet injections. Ohio, Frances Payne Bolton School of Nursing, Case Western Reserve University, 1968
Weber B: Eating with a trach. Am J Nurs 74:1439, August 1974
Woodward J: Emotional disturbances of burned children. Br Med J 5128:1009, 1959
———, Jackson D: Emotional reactions in burned children and their mothers. Br J Plast Surg 13:316, 1961

SHIRLEY STEELE

11
Nursing Care of the Child with Juvenile Diabetes

The importance of diabetes as a long-term illness of childhood cannot be underestimated. The disease has its onset in various age groups and includes the newborn period as well as adolescence. Advances in treatment have expanded the life expectancy. Diabetes is a hereditary disease transmitted by a recessive gene. The hereditary factor is responsible for some unique factors which contribute to the nursing care of the child and the family. These factors will be described in greater detail later in the chapter. Benoliel (1975) dramatizes the situation by noting that the disease interferes with the life-style of the family. She emphasizes that the immediate care of the child is within the domain of the physician. However, the care of the child is abruptly switched from the physician to the family at a given point in time. The family may not want or be able to provide this specialized care, but they have little or no choice in the matter. She suggests that the management of the child necessitates infringement on two very *personal* matters, the management of time and the uses of food.

Gorwitz et al (1976) quote estimates regarding diabetes in childhood in the United States. It has been estimated that there are 86,000 children under 17 years of age who have the disease, a rate of 1.3 per 1000 persons. There are more females with the disease, 51,000 as opposed to 35,000 males. The white population has a higher incidence than the nonwhite population, 74,000 to 12,000. These figures were questioned as the condition is not reportable. Therefore, Gorwitz et al (1976) studied the school-age population in Michigan and found a higher incidence, 1.6 per 1000. In addition to the more accurate estimates of the incidence of the disease, the Michigan study also found that 69.3 percent of the children were taking injectable insulin while 15.5 percent were not. The treatment regime for children not on injectable insulin was not determined.

A brief explanation of the clinical entity is essential to understanding the disease because nursing care in all of the age groups will be influenced by the pathology and the physiologic response of the body.

PATHOLOGY

Diabetes reflects a disturbance in carbohydrate metabolism. It is caused by a deficiency in insulin with a resulting hyperglycemia and glycosuria. The complicated process also results in an abnormal metabolism of proteins and fat. The pathologic process is aggravated by the loss of water and electrolytes by diuresis. These losses take place from both the extracellular and intracellular compartments. Hemoconcentration and dehydration occur as a result. Renal dysfunction occurs as a result of the dehydration and hemoconcentration (see Figure 1).

This situation is further complicated by tissue breakdown. The body is unable to utilize glucose, so protein and fat are utilized in an attempt to compensate. The increase in fat breakdown in the liver results in an overproduction of ketones. These ketones are released into the circulatory system and overload the excretory system. The accumulation of ketone bodies is of particular importance when the diabetes is out of control (see Figure 2). The above explanation is, of course, a simplification. For a detailed explanation the reader should consult a text on pathophysiology.

The etiologic process is usually abrupt in juvenile diabetes. In the obese adolescent the onset more generally resembles the adult response to the illness. Another variation of onset in children is one described as a latent phase of the disease (Weil, 1968). Weil describes children with hyperglycemia and glucosuria resulting from surgery, acute stress situations, or

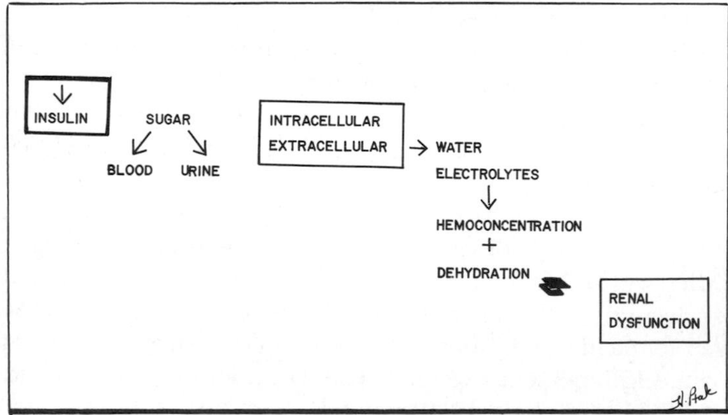

FIG. 1. Schema of pathologic effects of diabetes.

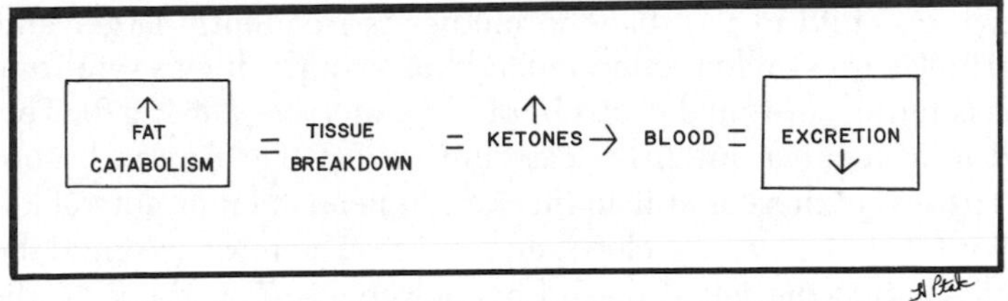

FIG. 2. Schema of diabetes resulting in an abundance of ketone bodies.

illness as being in a state of latent diabetes. He states that these children frequently become overtly diabetic in later years. The child is usually underweight as opposed to the adult patient who is generally overweight at the onset. The symptoms which are common in juvenile diabetes include loss of weight, increased thirst and appetite, and polyuria. The child may be seen in coma or stupor due to an acute infection. The symptoms which may precede the coma are flushing, drowsiness, dry skin or skin lesions, abdominal pain, nausea and vomiting, or generalized body pain (Nelson, 1960).

In an editorial in the April 1975 issue of the Journal of Pediatrics there is a suggestion that mumps virus may eventually be associated with juvenile diabetes. Early data suggests that juvenile diabetes has been found approximately three years after children have been exposed to this virus. With this preliminary data, scientific investigation continues to explore the possibility of a viral causation for this childhood disease.

The initial disbelief of the parents and the child is very understandable when a disease has such a rapid onset. The child may have a mild skin or throat infection and become acutely ill. He is admitted to the hospital and blood tests reveal juvenile diabetes. The child is treated vigorously and has a remarkable response to therapy. The parents are usually very relieved to see the dramatic improvement in their child. Their elation is short-lived, since they begin to realize the implications of the disease to their child and the family.

It is usually easier for the parents to understand the possibility of their child having diabetes if close relatives in the family have the disease. Even though it is easier for them to understand, this may not be a "plus factor" as they may have some misconceptions and fears because of their previous experiences with the disease. However, it is especially difficult for parents to understand how their child can be the "first" to have the disease. There are a substantial number of these "childhood firsts", as documented by the fact that "over a 20-year period of history-taking only 57 percent of the children with diabetes had a positive family history" (*Juvenile Diabetes*).

One of the reasons for the increase in reported juvenile diabetes in the United States is a result of better medical supervision of women who are pregnant and have diabetes and close supervision of their newborn infants.

"The newborn child of the diabetic mother is frequently larger and overweight. The face is swollen, often moon-like, as in Cushing's syndrome. The abdomen is tense, shiny and protruberant" (Anderson, 1964, p 6). The infant is placed in a neonatal intensive care nursery so that he can be observed closely. However, there is still an increase in neonatal mortality of infants of women with diabetes despite close supervision. The most accepted theory to explain this is that the infant dies of hypoglycemia. This theory is disputed by some and consideration is also being given to the respiratory and metabolic acidosis found in many of the infants (Gellis, 1960).

In addition to an understanding of the disease process itself, the reader needs to appreciate the prognosis and complications of juvenile diabetes. It is well to keep in mind that this disease is somewhat more difficult to control than the adult variety of the disease—hence the frequently used expression that the child is a "brittle" diabetic. Children are prone to periods of hypoglycemia and acidosis at any time. They are also prone to infections, neuropathies, and vascular changes. The degrees of control does not necessarily influence the onset and severity of these changes.

The reader needs to remember that the child is faced with a long-term condition that he is unable to forget for even one day. The administration of insulin at least daily and the frequent testing of urine are constant reminders of his disease process. In addition, he must pay more attention to his activity than the ordinary child. This is important as his insulin requirements will vary with his activity. The child's nutritional requirements must also be monitored more closely than the ordinary child. (Diet will be discussed in greater detail later in the chapter.) Great emphasis is also placed on good skin care. This may be particularly frustrating to the school-age child, who is very lax about his personal hygiene. If he slips, an infection may quickly develop. This is most unfortunate as the healing process is also delayed.

PARENTS' REACTION

According to Hughes (1967), parental acceptance, adjustment, and cooperation are hindered by several factors: (1) long-term nature of the disease; (2) dangerous immediate complications, arousing fear; (3) well-known later complications, causing chronic anxiety; (4) worries about future vocation; (5) thoughts of marriage and transmission of disease; and (6) monotonous problems of proper management.

While the list of six items may seem short, the magnitude and scope of the problems can present unlimited problems in gaining parent cooperation. It is easy to see why at certain periods in time, the parents will be able to cope with the disease more readily than others. For instance, when the child is of school age and has been controlled on a constant amount of insulin for a period of time, the parents may be comparatively relaxed. When the child reaches the preadolescent growth spurt and the insulin requirements are radically changed, the child is frequently absent from school because he feels sick. The mother becomes very anxious because the child is not well; she becomes impatient with the doctor because he/she cannot get the insulin adjusted; she worries about the child's falling behind in school work. The constant worry generated by the uncertainty makes the disease seem terrible. Her once relaxed attitude has been disrupted by this new need to focus on the disease. Her ordinary routine is disrupted and this can cause anyone to be impatient with the causative agent. Her anxiety influences other members of the family and particularly her husband.

Benoliel (1973) writes about the *fragility* of arrangements over time. She starts with the transition in roles of the parents and child with the onset of the disease and emphasizes that there are serious adjustments to be made:

> If tensions within the family are already high, the diabetes can serve as a focal point for the expression of unresolved conflicts and unmet expectations. . . . So, the potential for instability is always present in the changing symptomatology and social effects of the disease and treatment, and in the changing nature of the parent-child relationships. (pp 95–96)

The parents' reactions are of utmost importance because they have such a strong influence on the way the child accepts or copes with the disease. The child's emotional adjustment prior to the illness is another important element in the child's adjustment. If the child has a firm foundation to build on he is in a better position to make the needed adjustments. The basic emotional needs of the child are unchanged by illness. He still has a strong desire for parental love and acceptance. If the parents are too overwhelmed by the situation, they may be immobilized and unable to provide these basic needs.

PLANNING CARE

There are many aides in preparing to give care. Numerous pamphlets and guides are available for use in teaching. An example of this is the comic book supplied by Lily Drug Company entitled *Keith and Ellen Win a New Look On Life*. This is geared to the juvenile diabetic and offers a relaxed way for the child to learn about the disease. In addition, there are pamphlets prepared for the adult diabetic which can be adapted to meet some of the needs of the juvenile diabetic. A list is included at the end of the chapter.

The reader would also benefit by reading an excellent lay publication on juvenile diabetes. It is a chapter entitled "The Chirping of a Sparrow" in *Thursday's Child Has Far To Go*. The chapter will help you understand how a particular child and her family react when they are faced with the problem. It is written from a lay person's standpoint and probably more clearly identifies some of the feelings experienced than the majority of the professional literature does.

Nursing care for the newly diagnosed child with diabetes is somewhat more detailed than for the child with a history of diabetes. You will need to develop a plan of care utilizing what the child knows already, as repetition is particularly boring.

The newly diagnosed child with diabetes is usually taught a few simple facts about his disease, determined by the age of the child. A toddler may only be told that he has to get needles to help him stay well. It is very difficult for a toddler to understand this concept and he may think it is better to be sick than to get stuck every day. The preschooler can understand a little more but he is not any happier to get needles than the toddler. It may be helpful for him to talk to a school-age child with the disease and observe the other child also taking injections. The school-age child is usually the most cooperative in learning and assuming responsibility for his disease. However, he, too, will have periods when it becomes a drag and he will need assistance. During adolescence the child's natural tendency is to rebel and the disease receives its share. The actual degree to which the adolescent does rebel, however, does not seem well documented in the literature. Utilizing factors of normal growth and development we have assumed that the child will rebel—but, again, it is probably more related to each child's individual emotional makeup than to the adolescent group as a whole.

After the child has been told about his disease in a manner commensurate with his age, a next step is to have the child learn to test his urine. The school-age child or adolescent is ready for this task. He becomes quickly aware that urine specimens play a large role in his disease process. From the moment he is hospitalized people start asking him for specimens. Therefore, he should have some natural curiosity about what is being done with the specimen. It is necessary to prepare a place in the utility room and set up a teaching session. It need not be the time for a urine to be tested (Fig. 3). This will allow more time for teaching and discussion. The child should be taught to test his own urine and record the results. He should also be shown how to clean and replace the equipment. Teach the child never to use tablets which are discolored, out-of-date, or which have been exposed to moisture. Emphasize waiting the specified time period before reading the results. Each type of agent used for urine testing will have its own directions on the bottle or the box. Go over them carefully with the child and his parent. The parents should also learn this procedure as it will be their responsibility if for any reason the child is unable to assume the role. The toddler is too young to understand this procedure. The preschooler may be interested in seeing it done, but he is too young to do it himself. The parents of these younger

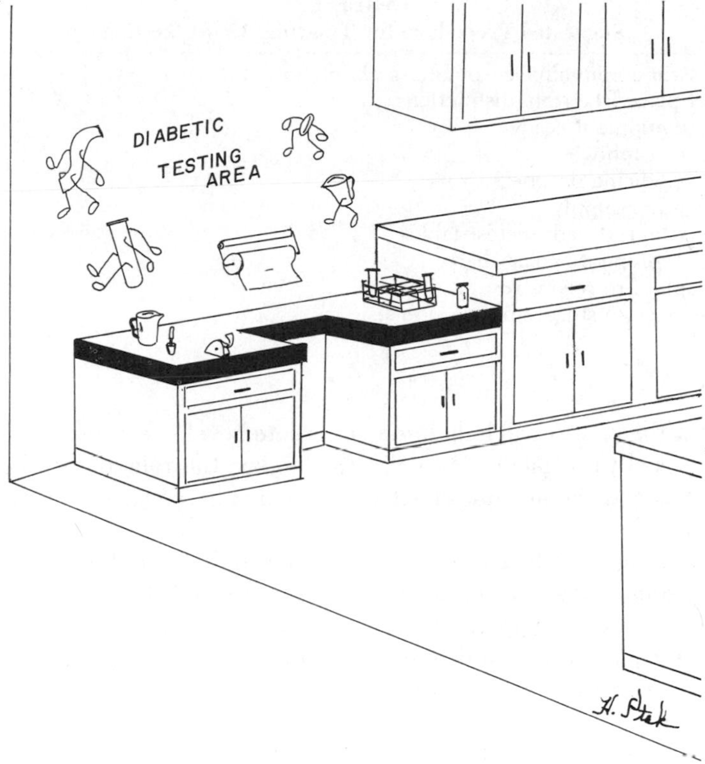

FIG. 3. A separate area should be set aside in the utility room for the child to test his urine. All equipment should be readily available.

children must assume total responsibility for the child's urine testing (Table 1).

At first, the child receives real satisfaction from achieving this task as it is new to him. It must be remembered, however, that the repetitive nature of the task may convert it to a chore and the child may lose interest. The strict routine of testing frequently should be replaced as soon as possible. In fact, there may be some value to the nurse's testing the urine while the child is hospitalized. This is, of course, debatable as some authorities believe the child should accept this chore as any other of his daily tasks. It must be remembered that even the brushing of teeth and washing are not done willingly by the child and one could question whether the child does indeed accept them as daily requirements.

Whether the child or nurse assumes the responsibility for the urine testing is not so important as what is done with the results. Talking with the

TABLE 1
Suggested Procedure for Teaching Urine Testing

Select time mutually acceptable to child and nurse
Select place free from distractions
Have equipment ready
a. test tubes
b. medicine dropper
c. water supply
d. Clinitest and Acetest tables
e. appropriate color charts
f. place to record results
Have place to store supplies after use

child about the results will help him to correlate how he feels when a urine is +4 as opposed to negative. He will begin to see the relationship between what he eats and the amount of activity in which he engages and the urine test results.

We here assume that the child is hospitalized during the initial stage. However, some physicians prefer to regulate the child at home. This allows for more accurate assessment of the child's activity as related to his insulin needs. The community health nurse will probably be the one to teach the child and parents the urine testing, or it may be done by the physician's office nurse.

If the child is hospitalized, there is usually sufficient time to space the teaching. It is not necessary to immediately begin to teach the child to give his own insulin. Timing is important in obtaining the child's cooperation. If he is feeling depressed from learning about his disease, he does not have enough energy left over to assume new tasks. After he has had time psychologically to internalize the disease, he is in a better position to proceed with teaching.

Again, there is not total agreement by medical personnel whether the school-age child should be expected to administer his own insulin. Utilizing the developmental factor that the child of this age has good eye-to-hand coordination, it is assumed that he is capable of the task. The decision would better be made on an individual basis, taking into consideration the way the child and parents feel about the procedure.

Assuming that the child is to take the responsibility for the task, a lesson plan should be prepared for teaching the procedure. The time allocated to teaching nursing students to give injections should be used to determine the time. Frequently, the nurse expects the child to learn this task in far less time than it took her/him to do it. The equipment utilized should be equivalent to the equipment that will be used at home. If disposable syringes will be used then it is realistic to use them in the hospital. If a glass syringe is to be used and boiled each time, then this should be utilized for teaching.

The principle of sterility may be an entirely new concept to the child. He may need considerable help in understanding it. Proper handling of a syringe is built on knowledge of what is or is not sterile. He can be taught to sterilize his syringe in the coffee basket of a coffee pot bought specifically for this purpose (Fig. 2). This method of sterilization cuts down on the possibility of the child's burning his fingers in boiling water. It also lessens the possibility of the water boiling over or boiling dry. The safety factors are of utmost importance with the school-age child, who probably has had limited experience working with a stove.

The community health nurse should also be utilized to be sure that the home situation can accommodate the procedure. Frequently, parents are too embarrassed to say that they do not have the necessary equipment at home. Or they may not realize what it is we are requesting. The parents need to know exactly what they will be given by the hospital and what is their responsibility to have purchased, prior to the discharge. If the child has not been hospitalized the home is probably better equipped as they have had to assume the full responsibility from the beginning (Table 2).

After the initial session, the child will need time to practice handling the equipment. He will need encouragement to transfer to his own person what he has learned using the orange (Fig. 4). A chart of the sites utilized for injection should be made available. The child is taught the necessity of rotating sites and he establishes a pattern for himself.

As soon as his insulin requirements are established, the child is given an explanation of the type or types he will receive and their expected action. He needs to know that regular insulin is quick acting and results begin in a half-hour. Its peak action is in 3 hours and its activity is over in 6 to 12 hours. Regular insulin is usually given in combination with a long-acting insulin such as Ultra-Lente or protamine zinc insulin (PZI). These long-lasting insulins have an effect 4 to 8 hours after injection. Two other frequently used intermediate-acting insulins are NPH and Lente. The child will be less confused if he is only introduced to the particular types he will be receiving. Just mentioning that there are other types available will be enough. He needs to know whether he can combine the long- and short-acting forms he will receive. Most of them can be combined, but PZI should not be combined with the short-acting type ordered. The child and parent will be taught to rotate injection sites (Fig. 5).

Another area of importance in teaching about insulin is the area of U40, U80, and U100 insulins. The child and parents must remember that a syringe calibrated with the appropriate markings must be used with their particular insulin prescription. An inaccurate dose will result from mixing

TABLE 2
Suggested Procedure for Teaching Insulin Injection

Prepare simple chart of role of insulin in body
Select time acceptable to nurse and child
Select place free from distractions
Assemble equipment
- a. syringe
- b. needle
- c. alcohol and cotton ball
- d. sterilization equipment (coffee pot)
- e. appropriate insulin
- f. orange

Explain each of the objects to the child
Demonstrate sterilization of syringe
- a. separate syringe and needle
- b. place in coffee basket
- c. put water in coffee pot
- d. place coffee basket with syringe in coffee pot
- e. place cover on pot
- f. place pot on burner of stove
- g. boil for 10 minutes
- h. let cool
- i. remove plunger of syringe by lifting near end
- j. remove barrel of syringe and place plunger inside
- k. remove needle by hub and attach to syringe
- l. draw up correct amount of insulin

Place syringe in appropriate spot to maintain sterility
Cleanse area with cotton ball saturated with alcohol
Inject insulin into orange
Pull back on plunger
Remove needle and cleanse area with alcohol sponge
Rinse syringe and return to appropriate storage place
Discard cotton ball
Free discussion

the wrong insulin with the wrong scale. The bottles are clearly marked and the differences in labels should be shown to the child and his parents.

Insulin must be stored out of direct sunlight and can be maintained at room temperature. The vials which are not being used on a daily basis should be refrigerated.

In helping the parents to determine whether to use disposable syringes, the cost factor is of utmost importance. Occasionally, the parents feel the cost is minimal compared to the convenience obtained. Some parents decide to use the glass syringe, but get a couple of disposable ones to have on hand for travel or in case the glass syringe breaks. Regardless of which type is chosen, more than one syringe should be bought so there is always one available (Fig. 6).

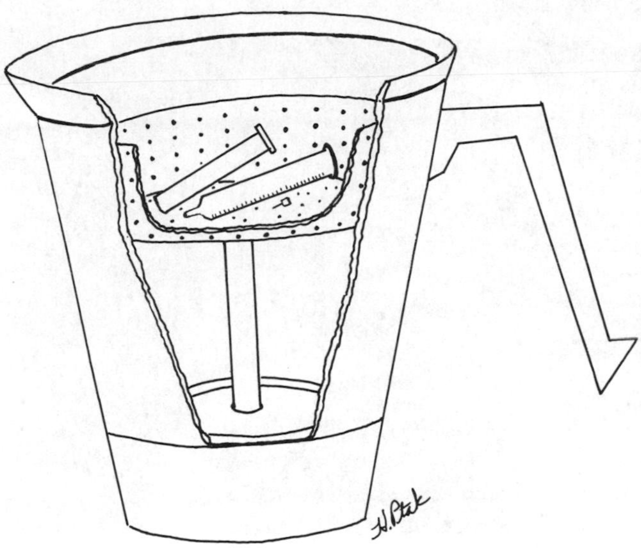

FIG. 4. An ordinary coffee pot can be used to sterilize the needle and syringe.

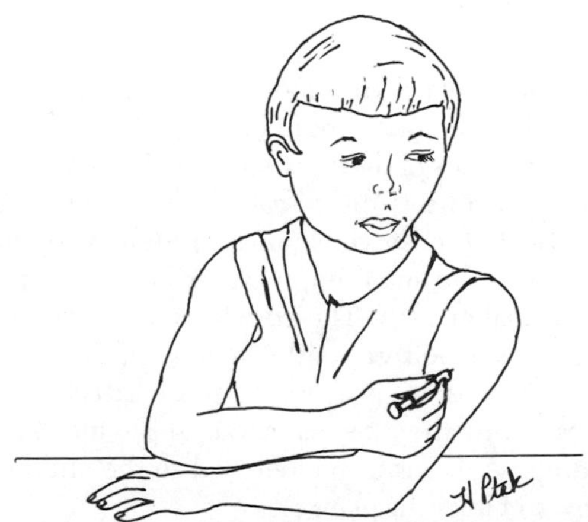

FIG. 5. The child learns to give herself insulin. The sites are rotated in a planned sequence.

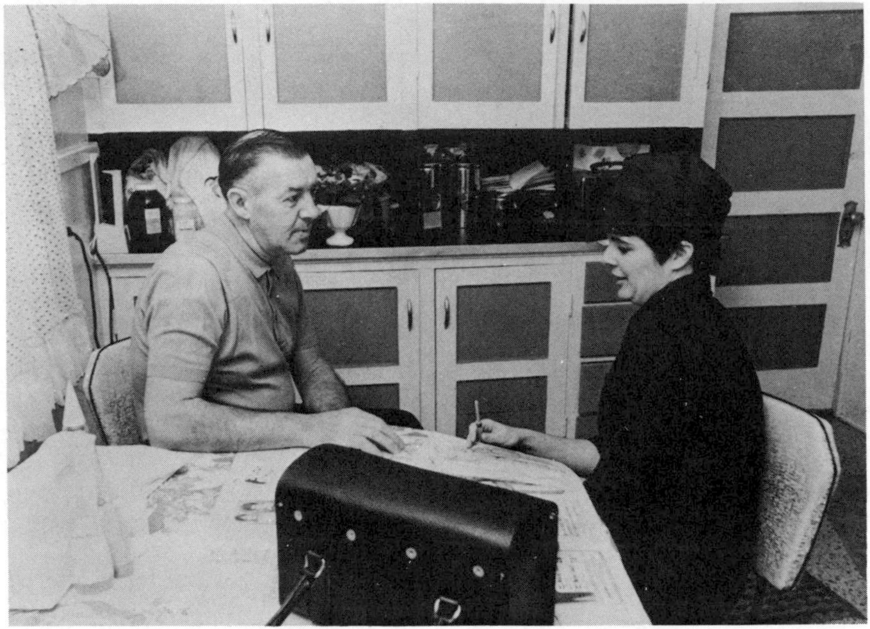

FIG. 6. A home visit by the community health nurse readies the father for the return of his son, with recently diagnosed diabetes.

DIET: FREE OR RESTRICTED?

The next area which plays an important part in the life of a child with diabetes is his diet. The dietician should be contacted to be a team member. There are basically two types of diets prescribed. The one receiving the most attention at the present time is the so-called "free diet." The other type is the restricted diabetic diet most well known to adults with diabetes. Regardless of which is chosen, the main emphasis is on supplying adequate nutrients to promote normal growth. The emphasis on supporting growth is the clue to why the diet must be frequently changed if the child is placed on a restricted diet. The "free diet" probably is more satisfactory to children as they are able to eat until they are satisfied. It should be established immediately which dietary plan is to be followed so the child does not have to be disappointed by a change in plan.

The "free diet" varies the least from the ordinary diet of the family. Therefore, dietary discussion will center around a good nutritional diet with avoidance of foods with too much carbohydrate content. Discussion of the ordinary dietary intake is necessary as many children have very poor dietary habits. A breakfast of potato chips and doughnuts will not do. However, some of the culturally determined breakfasts may be as adequate as the basic four requirements of the textbook diet.

The restricted diet will take more time to understand. The exchange lists are utilized in meal planning. The parents and child will need to study the exchange lists and check them against the diet served in the hospital. It is very important to elicit the child's likes and dislikes and include them in planning. This will cut down on the amount of replacements needed to supplement the food the child refuses to eat. From time to time the child's likes and dislikes change. He may also find that some of his favorite foods are not as palatable in the hospital. Reevaluation is an essential part of the diet plan.

It is generally believed that the less emphasis placed on the diet and its restrictions the better. The child should not feel that he has to steal food to have his appetite satisfied. Neither should he have to be laughed at or teased by his peers for being on a special diet.

The school nurse and teachers need to know the child has diabetes. They should know that the child may need supplements during school hours. The child should carry hard candy with him for periods when he feels weak. Also, if a snack is necessary during school time, it can be planned so the child does not appear to be getting special privileges.

An important consideration when one is planning the child's dietary intake is the amount of activity the child will be doing. In keeping the emphasis on a "normal life," adjustments will have to be made for increases in activity. On a day when the child has gym, he will need a decrease in insulin because of the increase in activity. His lunch may be changed slightly to include additional protein. This protein is valuable as it maintains the blood sugar level more adequately than do carbohydrates. A candy bar would give quick energy but it is rapidly metabolized and the blood sugar would drop quicker.

An appropriate way to teach the child about this requirement is to plan strenuous activities for him and have him compare how he feels and also to keep a record of his urine testing and the amount of insulin he received. He will soon be able to see the relationship between his activity and insulin requirements.

Another important aspect of the diet is to be certain that the child eats at regularly scheduled intervals. Children tend to eat sporadically unless supervised. They are too busy playing to come in to eat or the TV show is at an intense point and cannot be left. Depending on the lifestyle of the family, the regulation of time for the child to receive food may be a big hurdle to achieve. In some families, meals are seldom if ever prepared. The child assumes the responsibility for getting himself food when he is hungry. Under these conditions, the food restrictions and requirements will have to be discussed thoroughly and often with the parents and child. Trying to teach the mother who does not have an appreciation for the value of good nutrition to prepare nutritious meals is a challenge. In addition, she may feel these meals are a financial burden as well. In many families meal times are flexible. They are planned around busy people's variable daily schedules. This system of meal planning is likely to cause difficulty for the child with diabetes. The child may become weak or listless while waiting for his meals. His physiologic response may cause him to be irritable. To prevent this happening, the child may have to be fed before the rest of the family.

TEACHING ABOUT THE DISEASE

Thus far the teaching has been based on the tasks necessary to have the disease kept under control. This is only the beginning in helping the child and his parents understand the disease. A simple explanation of the "Three Ps," such as the one that follows, is essential:

1. Polyuria—increased amount of urine due to the sugar accumulation in the blood and ultimate excretion by the kidneys.
2. Polydipsia—increased thirst caused by the excretion of large amounts of fluid with the sugar.
3. Polyphagia—increased appetite due to the body's inability to utilize starch and sugars adequately.

The reader should consult a textbook on fluid and electrolyte balance for a more detailed explanation of the effects caused by the "Three Ps".

The parents and child also need to know the signs and symptoms of impending danger, such as light-headedness, sweating, restlessness, or rapidly beating heart, which are the result of too much insulin. Sugar should be taken immediately. Conversely, the child may have to actually experience some of these conditions before he really understands the states we are describing. The child also should be able to get to the "sugar" without too much disruption of his ordinary schedule during periods of hypoglycemia. This will decrease the chances of the child's using imaginary excuses to get special attention. An illustration would be as follows. The school-age child is frequently pressured by ordinary school routines. He is not allowed to escape from this pressure but rather he is forced to work under it and to cope with the situation. The child with diabetes could easily decide he is having an insulin reaction and leave the room to get his sugar supply. It is better to have the sugar in his desk or pocket and have him get it without leaving the room. Then the child is not tempted to try to use his disease as an escape valve when the going gets rough.

Skin Care and Foot Care

The exact importance of cleanliness has never really been proven. However, there is reason to believe that it is important for the child with diabetes to have clean skin. This is especially important as any child is prone to receive many cuts and scrapes which easily become infected if they are not kept meticulously clean. The healing process in diabetes is longer, and prevention is the best adjunct to care.

Foot care also is very important. Few people actually cut their toenails correctly. The child should be shown how to cut his toenails straight across and not rounded as is frequently the practice. Correct footwear is also imperative. If the child's shoes are too tight, his feet easily become prone to ingrown toenails and secondary infections. Well-fitting shoes will also cut down the number of callouses the child develops. If he does develop foot problems, he should get early medical attention before the condition has a chance to advance. Bathing of the feet with proper drying and an application of talcum powder is encouraged. The area between the toes should be given special attention. If the skin is dry it may be necessary to apply a soothing lotion. After daily bathing, a clean pair of well-fitting white socks should be worn. Because the blood supply to the feet is frequently diminished in diabetes, the child may feel more comfortable in a heavier sock than his peers wear. He may also need a slipper sock or loose woolen socks to wear to bed.

Hereditary Aspects

Studies of the genetic nature of the disease suggest that the occurrence of overt diabetes in certain circumstançes may be multifactoral, with different modes of inheritance (Weil, 1968). This statement clearly illustrates why it is so difficult to answer parents' questions in relation to "how their child got the disease." The nurse can only make statements which are general knowledge—such as the gene for diabetes is extremely common in our population. She/he should then refer the parents to their physician for a more thorough explanation.

The parents frequently feel a degree of guilt for the child having the disease. If they have questions regarding whether to have more children, they should be encouraged to speak to their physician or seek genetic counseling.

Additional Preparation for Life

The child with diabetes needs a consistent plan for living comfortably with his disease. The plan should include the normal things which children enjoy doing. The child should be encouraged to go to summer camp. If he is not accepted at a regular camp, there are specific camps for children with diabetes. The child may benefit from having contact with another child who has the disease. He should be encouraged to call this acquaintance when he needs answers to specific questions about coping with his disease. It is best to have as the older diabetic a person who had his disease during childhood so he knows what the child is going through. It is also important for the child to feel free to contact the people in charge of his medical supervision. The child is the best judge of how he feels and he can explain it best to the professional personnel. A simple phone call may be all that is needed and the child may be able to avoid missing school an entire day to go to the physician's office or clinic.

The child should also be given the opportunity to wear an identification bracelet or necklace describing his physical condition. He should also be offered a card to be placed in his wallet. These ideas are not always received kindly by the child. He does not like to be different and he frequently interprets these measures as overt examples of how he is different. They should be introduced by a person who is willing to spend time talking over the reasons for having such identification. The child can then make his own decision as to whether he feels they are essential.

The Need for Insulin

Another question that is frequently asked by child and parent is why the child cannot be treated with pills instead of injection; or when the child gets older, will he be able to switch to the pill instead of insulin? The explanation is fairly simple, but the child and parents may need to ask frequently as they do not want to accept what they hear. The juvenile diabetic is unable to be regulated orally because these agents' action is to produce insulin. The juvenile diabetic has no capacity to produce insulin so that stimulation by the outside agent is useless. The more intelligent child or parent may need additional information. They may need to know that the Islands of Langerhans are nonfunctioning and, therefore, it is impossible to stimulate production of insulin. This is not the case in the adult type of diabetes, and, therefore, the oral agents can be utilized effectively. The parent may know of another child who has received oral agents. This can be explained on the basis of the early management of diabetes, when insulin production is possible temporarily. However, if the parent checks further she will probably learn that the agent has decreasing effectiveness as the disease progresses and it is probably being used in combination with injectable insulin.

The parents and child should also be aware that as the child grows he will probably need larger doses of insulin. This factor will help them to understand that growth needs alone will necessitate close medical supervision. When the additional units are prescribed it may help to cut down on their anxiety regarding the condition's becoming "worse."

There is an early response to insulin which was not included in the section on teaching about insulin. It does not happen in all cases of diabetes but it still merits mention here. The new newly diagnosed child with diabetes may have some function of the pancreas. When the regimen of insulin injection is begun, the pancreas may temporarily recover the ability to secrete insulin. This ability makes it essential to monitor the child closely to prevent insulin shock. If the child is being regulated in the hospital, this reaction will be easily detected and allowances made for it. If the child is being regulated at home, the parents should be aware that this can happen and that its most common occurrence is around the second week of therapy. However, the response may not take place for six weeks after onset. The child's insulin will be adjusted accordingly and then the child's condition will usually remain stable for periods varying between two months and two years (Weil, 1968). The large variation in figures will help the parent to understand how individualized the plan of care must be for each child. The period of improvement should not be overemphasized as the parents may believe that their child is recovering from the disease. The emphasis should be on the long-range reactions, with this period as a small part of the overall course of the disease.

As we learn more about the transplants of organs, the outlook for juvenile diabetes may improve. However, at this point in time, it is safest to tell parents and children that they will have to take insulin daily in order to maintain and regulate their health.

Infectious Processes

Although we do not want to make the parents overly anxious regarding the disease, we must make them fully aware of the dangers of infection. As was stated earlier in relation to the onset of the disease, the child is prone to develop acidosis as a result of a relatively minor infection. This factor also holds true after the initial period. Children frequently develop infections which they do not call to the attention of their parents. Anything which does not incapacitate them is frequently ignored. A throat infection, in its early stages, is not evident to the parent. Unless the child makes it known, the parent considers the child well. In combating the infectious process, the body may develop a slight temperature elevation. This, too, can go unnoticed by the parent. This elevation influences the body's metabolism. When the metabolic rate is changed, the insulin requirements are also affected. The child needs additional insulin, if he is satisfactorily to combat the infection. The child's cooperation in reporting early signs of sickness is imperative. The parent then must seek medical advice regarding an alteration in insulin requirements, dietary changes, or changes in activity. The parents should be cautioned against altering insulin dosage on their own unless this is part of the management they have been taught.

In addition to early recognition of infection, parents should be cautioned about having the child unduly exposed to other children with infectious diseases. They should also be encouraged to have the child's immunizations kept up-to-date. Periodic review of the child's immunization is important as information in relation to current immunization protection emerges. It is also necessary as new immunizations are developed to have the child receive the benefit from them. The child will offer some resistance to receiving additional injections, but his objections should be overruled because of the benefits derived. If the child is exposed to another child with a severe infectious process it is also important to talk this over with the child's physician to see if prophylactic therapy is indicated.

During an infectious process urine testing is especially important. Urine testing may be relegated to a lesser position by the child when he is doing well. But during times of infection the urine must be monitored very closely. In addition to testing for sugar, acetone is also checked. The degree in normal variations is what is significant. Physicians differ as to what is the best maintenance for the child. If the physician prefers the child to have +1 sugar in his urine, then the deviation from +1 is what is significant. If the child has been maintained on negative urines, then the deviations of +2 will be more significant to this child. All children are maintained without acetone secretion, so any acetone will be significant. A physician should be called if acetone is present. One of the best suggestions to the parents regarding infection is, "When in doubt, call."

Eye Care

Another important consideration in treating the child with diabetes is the care of his eyes. It is well known that in older individuals there is a proneness to blindness. There is reason to believe that in juvenile diabetics there is a greater than normal possibility that they will have changes in vision. However, the onset of changes in vision is not well documented; neither is the relationship between the severity of the disease and the severity of the changes in the eye. The changes in vision may be of a temporary or permanent nature. The important aspect for the nurse is to remember that vision changes can be in direct relationship to fluctuations in the blood sugar; therefore, a child who is out of control may have blurring of vision which is only temporary in nature. The parent and child should both be aware of the necessity of having frequent eye examinations.

Other Complications of Diabetes

The child with diabetes is prone to other changes in addition to those affecting his vision. The degree to which the parents will be introduced to these possibilities is extremely individualized. In the beginning, the possibilities may not be brought up at all; however, as the child grows, it is important for the parent to be introduced to some of these additional possible complications. The introduction will be done according to what a physician thinks the parents should know at any given time. For instance, it is well known that the child with diabetes may develop arteriosclerosis. This concept may sound very simple to people in the medical profession but it is extremely foreign to the lay person. A very simplified explanation must be given, and one that the parent can utilize effectively. According to Engel (1962), "patients certainly, regardless of their level of education and sophistication, prefer to blame their illness on something they caught or ate or that happened to them, and consequently to think of disease as something apart from themselves" (p 241). An example would be insufficient insulin as the cause of (rather than the mechanism involved in) diabetes. Some of the other complications of diabetes are calcification of arteries, protein urea, hypertension, and other changes in the vascular system. Some lesser types of complications of diabetes are edema of the ankles, which corrects itself in the early treatment, and a proneness to an earlier menses. There is reason to believe that fertility is unimpaired in girls with diabetes, but the outcome of their pregnancy may be affected.

CONSIDERATION FOR AGE

The toddler or preschooler with diabetes will begin his medical regimen by having his parents take total responsibility for his care. This necessitates the parents' being fully aware of their responsibilities for the child and it requires that the medical personnel spend a great deal of time in preparing the parents. As the child grows older the medical personnel must assume direction along with the parents for getting the child to assume some of the responsibility for his care. As was mentioned in the discussion earlier, the school-age child may assume some of the responsibility for testing of his urine and giving of his injections, or he may even assume total responsibility for this care. The parents' role is then decreased in that they will not be assuming the tasks to be performed—but their responsibility will be increased in relation to supervision of the child in his own management.

As the child grows older the parent must be helped to relinquish control to make the child feel total responsibility for his own personal management. This is frequently very difficult when the parent has assumed all of the care for a large number of years. However, it is very important to have the child feel as normal as possible and normality requires that he begin to establish his own identity and responsibility for himself. The diabetic regimen should become part of the child's daily routine and should not necessitate a great deal of additional time to accomplish. It should not be treated so simply, however, that the child is not given credit for assuming the responsibility.

When the child nears adolescence it is hoped that he will be mature enough to assume the largest responsibility for his care. However, in relation to the rebellion that the adolescent is entitled to, we must make allowances and not be too critical when the child decides to rebel aginast his plan. The adolescent will also need additional information about his disease over and above what he was given in earlier stages. It is much easier for him to get medical information and his curiosity may stimulate him to read far in advance of what he is able to digest. The information should be discussed with the medical personnel responsible for his care so that he is able to understand the implications of what he reads. The adolescent who reads that most juvenile diabetics have early vascular changes may decide to give up as he sees his course becoming progressively worse. We must help him to understand the implications of what he reads and especially the implications to him personally.

Even though the parent has been told why the child cannot be treated with oral agents, the adolescent will need his own explanation. As he grows to adulthood it will be even more significant as he may talk to his fellow-workers and find someone who developed diabetes later in life and is being treated solely with oral agents. The importance of education cannot be over-emphasized. If he has an understanding of why, then he is more apt to be willing to go along with the regimen. In making the foregoing statement it is assumed that the personality development of the adolescent is commensurate with his age and that he has had a somewhat positive experience with his disease up until this time. It is also assumed that the reactions of his family have been such that he does not feel inferior for having the disease and that his disease has not been too debilitating to him over the years.

When more responsibility for care of the disease is given to the adolescent, outward or less overt signs of lack of interest in assuming this role should be monitored by the parent. Such signs as decrease in academic achievement, withdrawal from interaction with his peers, a need for self-gratification by such means as overeating, or an increase in aggressive behavior are all indicators that the adolescent is not ready to assume this increased responsibility. The adolescent may wonder about going to college. There is certainly no reason directly related to his diabetes why he should not attain a higher education. In relation to vocational planning, the adolescent with diabetes may have some limitations due to the fact that he is prone to having insulin shock. Such vocational plans as being a driver for a group of people may not be realistic, or a job which necessitates climbing on buildings or joining the ranks of policemen or firemen may be out of reach. However, most of the professional areas are now open to him—including the areas of medicine and nursing. The adolescent may be deeply concerned about the possibility of getting married. Here the hereditary factor plays an important role. This should be discussed frankly and truthfully with the adolescent. Both partners in the forthcoming marriage should be aware of the consequences of such a marriage and then be allowed to make the decision for themselves.

EDUCATION EXTENDED

Parents or Significant Others

Benoliel (1975) expresses the opinion that the role of the parents is substantially altered when they are given the added responsibility for carrying out the medical regime. They are now expected to socialize the child and to be surrogates to the physician. Their normal socialization process has to be transformed to include the behaviors necessary for maintaining control of the disease. This change in socialization procedure may be difficult to achieve especially if the parents do not fully understand their responsibility to the medical regime.

Parent education is a most significant segment of the overall plan of care of the handicapped child. It is particularly relevant to parents of children with diabetes in view of the hereditary aspects of the illness. Parent education can be achieved by many avenues. One is the large lecture approach. In this method, an expert is usually available to give a prepared speech describing the disease process. In addition, he may cover aspects of child care, implications of the disease to the family, information regarding services offered in the community, and perhaps a brief explanation of some of the current research in the field. From this lecture, the parent utilizes the process of *selective perception*. He filters out those aspects which are easy to accept, digest, and use and apply in his own situation. This educational approach is a good stepping stone to other processes which involve a greater participation of the parent. Lecture can also be supplemented by written information on the topic. Again, this written material lends itself to selective perception. The parent can easily ignore the pamphlet completely or skim it and find areas which enhance or support his knowledge of the topic. He is still able to avoid areas which may be particularly uncomfortable to him.

The smaller group meeting lends itself to another type of parent education. In this approach, the parent is afforded the security of a group to help him express his hostility, fears, fantasies, inadequacies, and expectations regarding the handicapped child and his family. The group provides a curtain of protection not generally found in the one-to-one relationship of parent and professional worker. This protection plays an especially significant role as the parent frequently fears alienating the professional workers who they inwardly feel they need for the care of their child. The small group eventually helps the parent to look at himself and to see the relationship of his own behavior to his handicapped child. The group can also be valuable in exposing the parent to new ways of handling the child and provide him with very concrete suggestions for day-to-day living. In addition, the parent has a healthy avenue for release of his feelings. He may feel freer to express his hostility about the cost of insulin to parents who also share the burden than to outsiders or even relatives who may see insulin as a life-saving factor and therefore feel the parent should be very thankful for its existence rather than complaining about its cost. The other parents, with similar concerns, are often able to pick up on the clues and expand the topic to get to some of the deeper concerns.

The need for parent education is readily accepted but the avenue for providing this education is not firmly established. Experimentation and research with different techniques and procedures continue in many areas and will eventually lead to a more scientific basis for determining individual needs. In the interim, many different approaches are being taken to meet the needs of parents and children. The foregoing are some of the values derived from group meetings. They must be considered along with other information to decide if a group meeting is an answer for a particular family.

Group Meetings

The organization of groups of children with similar handicaps and groups of parents of children with similar handicaps has received attention. The question of whether a group will be beneficial to a particular family is not an easy one to answer. The first consideration should be given to the leadership of the group. Intelligent leadership is of top priority. One parent may benefit from a group led by another parent, while another one might be more comfortable if a professional person is leading the group.

The goals of the group should be explored before suggesting that a child or parent attend the meeting. If the goal of the parent group is to raise money to support research, some parents may not be interested. If the goal of the group is to share common problems relating to rearing the child with a disability, the parent may be more interested.

Shostrom (1969) discusses groups in relation to sensitivity training. Some of his remarks are extremely applicable because the focus of many groups designed for children with disabilities or their parents really deal with the way the individual feels about the disease and the ways of coping with it.

The group frequently makes the individual focus on very "touchy" points. In this aspect, some groups can be destructive rather than constructive for some individuals. The points which seem relevant to this discussion are the size of the group, the leadership, timing of joining a group, and avoidance of a group composed of close associates.

Size of Group. To be fruitful, a group of less than six persons is not suggested. It is believed that a larger group is needed to work effectively with problems. A group of more than sixteen is considered too unwieldly for a leader to handle, even with assistance. Therefore, the parent or child should also use the size as a determinant in whether or not to join a particular group.

Leadership. Shostrom makes reference to a study by Margaret Rioch that found that "natural leaders," without benefit of group work, can be as effective as highly trained workers. This point merely relates back to my comments about leadership and discourages professional workers from "downgrading" a group simply because it does not have professional leadership.

Timing of Joining a Group. In relation to timing, Shostrom suggested that one should never join a group as a "fling, binge, or surrender to the unplanned." He suggests that a crisis (such as a handicap) deserves more consideration and planning and that a decision to join a group should get the same consideration.

Avoidance of Close Associates. Due to the nature of the group interaction, it is suggested that a person not join a group with a composition of close social or professional acquaintances. The nature of the discussions may be embarrassing under these conditions. Shostrom suggests that emphasis be placed on the confidentiality of the interactions in the group to guarantee the participants a measure of privacy.

Groups can be a most rewarding experience if utilized effectively. The parent or child should decide if the group meets his particular need.

Timing plays an important role in the adjustment of a parent or child to a group. He may not be ready for a group at the onset of the disability but may be ready for it after a period of adjustment. For instance, the school-age child may not benefit from hearing about another child's difficulties in getting regulated on insulin during the adolescent growth spurt if he is just learning to give himself injections. The other child's difficulties may be more anxiety-producing to him than beneficial, but this same child may benefit greatly by meeting with other adolescents with similar problems when he reaches adolescence.

In the same vein, a parent who is overwhelmed with the problems of adjusting to a new disability may find other parents' problems more than she can handle. As time goes on, she may receive satisfaction and consolation by knowing that other parents have had difficulties similar to her own and have been able to "get over the hurdle."

The personalities of the parent and child may also influence their interest or lack of interest in joining a group. Some people do not enjoy being a part of a group whereas others flourish with this type of activity.

As professionals, we should share with the parent and child the groups that are available and their functions. The decision to join or not to join should be made by the individuals involved.

Regardless of the type of intervention utilized, whether it be group or some other process, the aim should be to help the family or child gain a conscious appreciation of the crisis situation in order to problem-solve the situation creatively. This attempt at grasping the situation will help these people to achieve mastery of the difficult precipitating situation which resulted in the "crisislike" situation. By learning to cope with the precipitating cause, the child or parent may be able to prevent further crises from developing.

This does not mean that groups are indicated only when the situation has reached crisis proportions. I am merely suggesting that any situation that deviates from the parent's or child's "normal expectations" has the potential of resulting in a crisis situation. In an attempt to prevent crisis from occurring, help should be directed at the precipitant factors, identified by the parent or family.

CASE PRESENTATION OF INPATIENT, WITH STUDY QUESTIONS

John is a 12-year-old boy admitted to the hospital with an acute upper respiratory infection. He has been unable to retain fluids for the past 24 hours. He is a child with diabetes of two years' duration. He is admitted for parenteral fluids, treatment of his acute infection, and evaluation of his diabetic status.

After the initial history is taken by the nurse, a plan of care is designed. Additional information for consideration when one is establishing goals includes the following:

1. What is the meaning of the acute illness to John?
2. What is the meaning of the chronic illness (diabetes) to John?
3. What have been John's past experiences with hospitalization? On the nursing intake you have found that John has been hospitalized on four other occasions. Where was he hospitalized? Does he know this particular agency? What were the nature of the hospitalizations? Were they linked to his diabetes?
4. What cultural factors may be influencing the frequent hospitalizations?
5. Does the information regarding family constellation offer any clues which might need exploration?
6. How is John doing in school? Perhaps a call to the school nurse will be helpful.

7. How is John getting along with his peers? Have there been any recent changes in his living conditions? Perhaps a move to a new area?
8. What aspects of diabetic care need emphasis during this hospitalization? How much does John assume of his own special care?
9. What aspects of the acute illness need to be explored? Did the home atmosphere contribute to the illness? Are there other children in the family who are sick? Is the mother at home to care for the child or does she work outside the home?
10. What other members of the health team are needed to meet the objectives of comprehensive patient care?

Nursing tasks included in John's care will include the following:

1. Bathing
2. Skin care
3. Mouth care
4. Taking temperatures and administering specific therapy for elevations
5. Check of intravenous fluids; restraints as necessary for protection
6. Oral intake, if allowed
7. Providing warmth
8. Describe vomiting—amount, frequency, nature
9. Changing position while on bed-rest
10. Passive exercises to extremities
11. Record intake and output
12. Pulse and respiration: note variations
13. Note emotional responses
14. Provide appropriate play

After the acute phase, John's care will be changed to incorporate the medical regimen and plans for discharge. The dietician may be contacted to review John's dietary intake. She can make suggestions for changes, if indicated. The nurse will review John's knowledge of his disease and evaluate how he is coping with giving his own injections and testing his urine. The nurse will utilize information gathered to help the doctor decide on John's readiness for discharge. A follow-up report of John's hospitalization should be sent to the community health nurse.

To show how the history-taking forms can be adapted to other situations, I will use an in-patient nursing history-taking form to collect the information on a child in an out-patient setting. The example follows.

CASE PRESENTATION OF OUTPATIENT

Mary A. was referred to the school nurse by a substitute teacher in the exceptional education class. Mary is a ten-year-old child with developmental lag who was adopted as an infant. The possibility of diabetes and/or retardation were not discussed with the adoptive parents, prior to adoption.

Nursing Intake History

1. Appearance on first sight: Mary is a small, pale, and "dull-appearing" child.

2. Patient's understanding of illness: Mary had a limited understanding of her disease. She knew she received "shots" for "sugar."

3. Events leading up to referral: Mary is in an exceptional education class at a demonstration school. She was admitted to the school one year prior to the referral to the school nurse. The teacher in this particular class was "extremely efficient" and she did not use other professional members in meeting the needs of the children. Arrangements for the child's admission were made with the mother, teacher, and principal.

At the time of admission, the teacher told the mother there was no provision possible for testing the child's urine in school. Therefore, the mother sent a collection bottle daily for the child's noon specimen. The specimen was not refrigerated. The child took the specimen and the mother tested it when she arrived home.

4. Place in family constellation: Mary is an only child adopted by a middle-class white family.

5. Significant information relative to:

(a) Feeding. Mary is on a regular diet without a large concentration on carbohydrate. She has a bottle of orange juice in the classroom refrigerator. Mary's mother provides her with a half sandwich to eat on the long bus ride home. Mary feeds herself and likes most foods. She does not question why she does not have candy and desserts.

(b) Toileting. Mary is toilet-trained. Her training was delayed with complete continence being achieved only at age five.

(c) Sleep. Mary sleeps nine hours a night. She has a 15-minute rest period during school. She frequently requires a nap after her long bus ride.

(d) Play. Mary has limited experience with social contacts her own developmental age. In school, she was slow to socialize but this is improving with time.

(e) Language development. Mary also developed slowly in speech. It is easy to understand her but she communicates more like a five-year-old.

(f) Independent and dependent activities of daily living. Mary is completely dependent on adults for the management of her diabetes. However, she is able to dress and undress herself. She takes little interest in her personal hygiene or grooming and her mother assumes much responsibility for this.

6. What is important to this child to make her feel secure and comfortable in this situation? Mary's diabetic condition was simply explained to the class. The children are aware that Mary sometimes needs orange juice. The

children have been most willing to get this for her. Mary's previous teacher took the responsibility of getting Mary to the lavatory to obtain the noon specimen. Mary seemed to accept this procedure without question, and the other children did not seem aware of this special need. Mary seemed to be comfortable in the classroom. The advent of a new teacher was the precipitating factor for the referral to the school nurse.

7. What are the policies of this institution which interfere with or promote the well-being of this child? In this situation, the teacher had assumed a lack of provision for testing the child's urine. After the referral, the school nurse and physician saw the child. The mother was contacted to check the child's medical plan. The "assumed policies" were adjusted to meet the child's needs better.

8. What is the medical plan of care which will influence the nursing plan of care? The child was receiving Ultra-Lente and regular insulin daily. The mother adjusted the dosage in accordance with the urine results. The noon results were probably not accurate as the specimen was old. The new plan was for Mary to report to the school nurse each day and the nurse would test the urine. A weekly report of the results would be sent home. Mrs. A. was very eager to have the results and requested daily telephone reports until she was convinced Mary was "controlled."

9. What are the short-term goals for this child? Mrs. A. was interviewed and it was well-established that she thoroughly understood the disease process and its control. She was aware of "danger signals" and knew how to proceed if they occurred. Close contact with Mrs. A. by telephone was decided upon. This was at Mrs. A.'s request rather than because of an identified need. Mrs. A. was delighted that the urine would be tested at school. She was also appreciative of the additional professional interest in Mary.

10. What are the longterm goals for this child? The school nurse explored Mary's interest in testing her own urine. Mary did not seem interested but eventually urine testing will be taught. Health teaching will also be done regarding skin care, foot care, diet, and insulin. Due to the child's retardation, training for insulin administration will not be started for sometime.

Mary relates well with the school nurse and it is hoped that during her daily visits to the nurse's office she will begin to assume more of a direct role in relation to her health problem. The nurse will also work with the substitute teacher to help her with her anxiety over having Mary in her classroom.

The school nurse will also make contact with the medical source responsible for Mary's care and request a medical summary. Mrs. A. signed a consent for the release of this information. A telephone contact will also be made to the community health nurse in Mary's outlying district to familiarize her with the family. A formal referral will not be sent at this time, but Mrs. A. is interested in a resource close by in case of a future emergency.

Evaluation

The foregoing example points out the willingness of parents to accept help when offered. Despite a situation which was tolerable, more help was welcomed by the mother. A teacher's insecurity was responsible for revealing to the school nurse a child with a major health problem, which to this time she had no previous knowledge of. As there was no major precipitating crisis, it was fairly easy for the nurse to make a positive contact with the mother. The nurse was able to offer the help that the mother wanted and thereby establish a positive working relationship.

If a major crisis had precipitated the referral, it might have been more difficult for the nurse to establish a positive relationship. An example might be one in which a teacher suggested the child be excluded from class for health reasons. The nurse, who had no previous contact with the mother, might get a very negative response with this initial contact's being triggered by "unhappy news."

This situation also demonstrates that the person most qualified to be of help to the family is sometimes overlooked in delivering services. Even though the nurse is very effective in her position, there may be times when her expertise is not sought. This is more likely to happen when the teacher has been used to functioning without a full-time school nurse for a long period of time, which is the case at this school.

This case presentation also demonstrates the use of an outsider, in this instance a substitute teacher, to identify areas of concern which are considered routine by those in close proximity to the problem.

The use of the school nurse to do teaching in relation to the disease process will also help to gear the teaching to the child's readiness. The child was not ready for this teaching in the hospital. However, she may be ready before another hospital admission is necessary.

The school nurse can also keep the hospital's out-patient department up-to-date on the child's progress. The mother has not returned to the local medical doctor since Mary was hospitalized. However, Mrs. A. still wants a report to be sent to him. The school nurse will serve as a coordinator and leader of the team during the child's healthy periods and attendance at school.

BIBLIOGRAPHY

Andersson B: The crisis arising in pregnancy. Abottempo 2:4, 1964

Benoliel JQ: Childhood diabetes. In Strauss AL (ed): Chronic Illness and the Quality of Life. St. Louis, Mosby, 1975, pp 89–98

Dube AH: Diabetes—the three polys. Health News, Oct 1968, pp 1–8

Duncan G: Diseases of Metabolism. Philadelphia, Saunders, 1964, Chap 15

Engel GL: Psychological Development in Health and Disease. Philadelphia, Saunders, 1962, p 241
Fenske M: The endocrine system. In Scipien GN et al. Comprehensive Pediatric Nursing. New York, McGraw-Hill, 1975, pp 776–82
Gallagher JR: Medical Care of the Adolescent, 2nd ed. New York, Appleton, 1966, pp 216–34
Gellis SS: Infants of diabetic mothers. In Nelson WE (ed): Textbook of Pediatrics, 7th ed. Philadelphia, Saunders, 1960, pp 1214–15
Gorwitz K et al: Prevalence of diabetes in Michigan school-age children. Diabetes 25:122, 1976
Guthrie DW, Guthrie RA: Diabetic children: special needs, diet, drugs and difficulties. Nursing '73 3:10, March 1973
Hughes J: Psychodynamic aspects of chronic disease and childhood diabetic management. Report of the Fifty-first Ross Conference on Pediatric Research, 1965, pp 97–100
Isenburg PL et al: Psychological problems in diabetes mellitus. Med Clin North Am 49:1126, 1965
Jackson RL: Management of the young diabetic patient. Report of the Fifty-first Ross Conference on Pediatric Research, 1965, pp 101–9
Juvenile Diabetes. Upjohn, June 1967
LuKens K, Panter C: Thursday's Child Has Far to Go. Englewood Cliffs, NJ, Prentice-Hall, 1969
McFarlane J, Homes CC: Children with diabetes learning self-care in camp. Am J Nurs 73:1362, July 1973
Metheny NM, Snively WD: Nurses' Handbook of Fluid Balance. Philadelphia, Lippincott, 1967, pp 218–19
Moore ML: Diabetes in children. Am J Nurs 67:104, January 1967
Moss JM: Management of juvenile diabetes. Family Physician 15:46, 1968
Nelson WE: Textbook of Pediatrics, 7th ed. Philadelphia, Saunders, 1960
Parker ML et al: Juvenile diabetes mellitus, a deficiency in insulin. Diabetes 17:27, 1968
Schulman D: Tips for improving urine testing techniques. Nursing '76 6:23, February 1976
Shostrom EL: Group therapy: let the buyer beware. Psychology Today May 1969, p 37
Sultz HA et al: Is mumps virus an etiologic factor in juvenile diabetes? J Pediatr 86:654, 1975
Sussman KE (ed): Juvenile-type Diabetes and Its Complications. Springfield, Ill, Thomas, 1971
Tietz W, Vidmer JT: The impact of coping styles on the control of juvenile diabetes. Psychiatr Med 3:67, 1972
Weil WB: Current concepts juvenile diabetes mellitus. Medical Intelligence 278:829, 1968
———: Diabetes mellitus in children. In Barnett HL (ed): Pediatrics, 16th ed. New York, Appleton, 1977
White P: Childhood diabetes. Diabetes 9:345, 1960

PAMPHLETS USEFUL FOR TEACHING

A Handbook for Diabetics, Squibb
Clinilog, Ames Company

Diabetes and the Eye, No. 111, Commission for the Blind, New York, State Department of Social Welfare
Diabetics Unknown, by Groff Conklin, Public Affairs Pamphlets, No. 312
Foot Care for the Diabetic Patient, U.S. Department of Health, Education and Welfare, Public Health Service Publication No. 1153
Keith and Ellen Win, A New Look on Life! Vol 1, No. 1 Eli Lilly
The Three R's of Diabetic Care, Arlington Laboratories
You and Diabetes, Upjohn

SHIRLEY STEELE

12 Nursing Care of the Child with Cardiac Conditions

In developing a chapter in relation to cardiac conditions, one is immediately faced with the problem of what cardiac conditions still require long-term care. This question arises from the recent advances in cardiac surgery and pediatric anesthesia that make it possible to operate on children at a much younger age and get outstanding results. In working on such a chapter one then has to look at whether the cardiac surgery is palliative or corrective in nature. If it is only palliative, then one can say the cardiac surgery is but one phase in the therapy of the medical regimen for the child. The child, then, would require long-term medical care for his cardiac condition. The child with corrective repairs would fall into another category. With the current progress in cardiac surgery, some conditions such as patent ductus arteriosus would better fit into a text concerned with the nursing care of conditions requiring short-term care. However, many of the more complicated repairs require long-term supervision after the original surgical correction. The child frequently requires rehospitalization during some period of his childhood either for more surgery or for medical follow-up.

In this chapter, consideration is given first to cardiac surgery and then continues with the nursing care of a medical cardiac condition, rheumatic fever.

Most lay people have the idea that the heart is the most important organ of the body, and their emotional reactions to a diagnosis of heart impairment will be based on this idea. The initial reaction of parents to a diagnosis of congenital heart disease may be one of fear and anxiety. These two reactions do not necessarily diminish with time because the thought that the defect is still there is always in the parents' minds. Fear and anxiety may very well increase as the child shows signs of his illness. Such signs may be the appearance of cyanosis, becoming easily fatigued, inability for the child to drink his formula, periods of dyspnea, or overt fainting spells. These symptoms are periodic reminders to the parent that there is something wrong with their infant's or child's heart.

In a study of Glaser et al (1964), some interesting facts are brought out about the emotional implications of congenital heart disease in children. A key point was that the mothers seemed to live in constant fear that the child would die. This idea was strengthened by the slow and poor physical development of the child, the frequency of illness, and the somewhat undesirable personality of the child. The child was frequently negative, whiney, and irritable (see Figure 1). Despite his undesirable behavior, the mother felt unable to punish him because of the fear of aggravating the cardiac condition. Because of these findings, it is imperative to help the parent, and particularly the mother, better understand her responsibility to her child. The mother needs an explanation of the disease in simple terminology. She also needs assurance that sudden death is not a threat. The old idea of "keeping the child as quiet as possible" must be eradicated.

The mother should be encouraged to treat the child as normally as

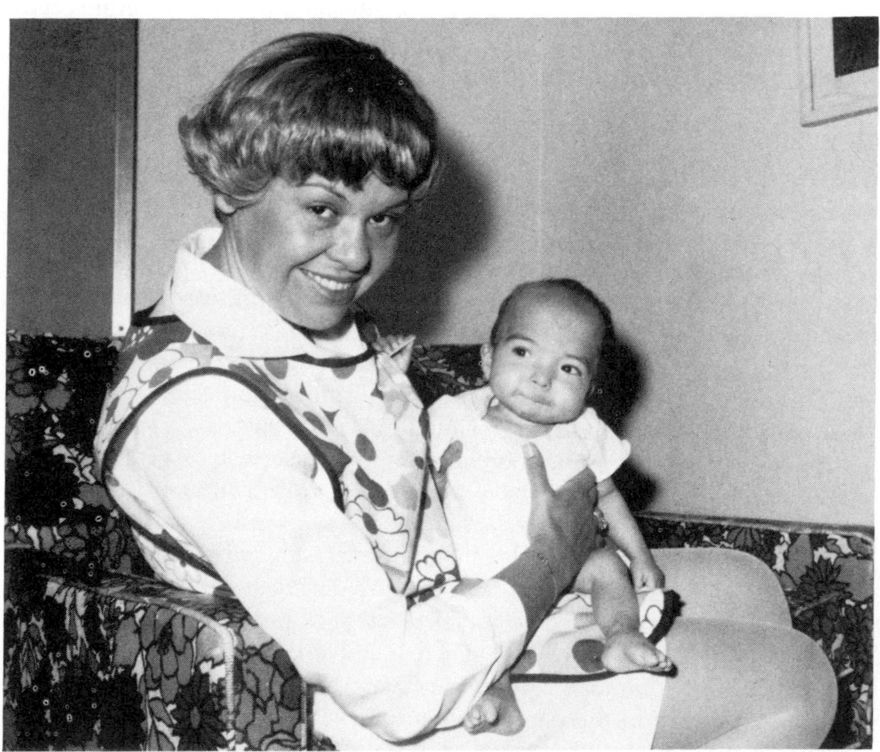

FIG. 1. Amy is 15 months of age. Developmentally she is closer to a nine-month-old infant due to the effects of her disability.

possible. She should be encouraged to set limits for this child just as she does for her other children. Many parents admit that it is very difficult to treat this child like their other children, and they feel the need to give this child special considerations.

ASSESSMENT OF DEVELOPMENT

Physical development is emphasized because it is less generally recognized that parents can have an influence on the physical development or physical retardation of their child. The child with congenital heart disease is frequently a smaller child than his normal peers and this may be secondary to his pathologic condition. In addition, the child who is not stimulated to be active and have the same routines and exercises of the normal child is less likely to mature physically. This lack of encouragement on the part of the parents may have an influence on the child's total development. The restrictions that the parent puts on the child may influence his self-image. Green and Levitt (1962) have studied this constriction of self-image in children with cardiac problems. They found that children with cardiac conditions draw themselves smaller than normal children. Also, when a normal child draws himself in relation to a peer, he always pictures himself as the larger. The child with a cardiac condition draws himself the same height as his peer.

As stated, the child with a cardiac condition is frequently smaller than the normal child in physical development. This may influence his drawing. However, the effects of social and perceptual experiences are also thought to influence his body image. The small size of his drawing may be the result of his feelings of needing continual help and being dependent on his parents. He views himself as small and insignificant as an individual.

In another study (Neuhaus 1958), the child with cardiac involvement was felt to have a much higher incidence of neurotic behavior and dependency feelings than the normal child. This tendency seemed to decrease as the child gets older. The higher incidence of neurosis in the young child may be explained on the basis of their shorter period of time living with a chronic disease. It may also be explained on the basis of parental anxiety and overprotection.

In both studies it is evident that the child with a cardiac condition needs a great deal of support and guidance to see himself as a significant person. The parents must be helped to avoid making the child so dependent on them that he cannot see himself as a significant being. The parents need guidance to give assistance only when necessary and to be able to relinquish the protective role as the child matures. Other siblings must also be included in this discussion as the situation of the child with the cardiac condition also affects them. A general rule of thumb is to let the child determine his own activity tolerance level. The child usually stops when he is tired. Very strenuous competitive sports may be excluded from his physical activity as a precautionary measure. However, the old idea of severe restriction of physical activity is now considered obsolete. These restrictions only lead to severe emotional and social deprivation that interfere with the child's future adjustments.

The infant with a congenital heart defect will be more prone to cyanosis of the extremities. All newly born infants have a tendency towards cyanosis as the blood does not circulate freely to the extremities. This immature pattern of circulation is complicated by a cardiac defect. The color of the extremities of a newborn without a cardiac anomaly will usually improve by adding warmth via blankets or clothing. When there is a lack of oxygenation due to cardiac involvement, the extremities will remain blue-tinged despite the application of warmth. The infant's color should also be assessed around the oral mucasa. The cyanosis will tend to worsen when the child cries. Older children may also have overt signs of poor oxygenation of their tissues and there may be clubbing of the fingers or toes.

CARDINAL SIGNS ASSESSMENT

The respiratory rate and pattern are good indicators of the amount of oxygenation and cardiac output available to the infant or child. The newborn has shallow rapid respirations. This irregular pattern is exaggerated when a child has a cardiac defect. The most dramatic response to the diminished oxygenation is the retracting chest. The retractions are often accompanied by grunting sounds and obvious laboring of respirations when there is a severe defect. This interference with respirations is exaggerated when attempts are made to feed the infant.

The nurse helps the parent to learn to feed the child, causing the least amount of fatigue. This can be done by making sure that the nipple holes are adequate, that the infant is held in a semiupright position, that the formula has the greatest amount of carbohydrate content in the least amount of fluid, that the child be bubbled frequently and gently, that he be allowed to rest more than the normal child, that he be given frequent small feedings, and that the mother be given adequate time to adjust to the feeding of this child while there is professional help available. It is impossible to set a time table suggesting when the mother will be able to assume the total responsibility for the feeding of the infant. Early initiation in a positive manner is essential as a beginning. Frequent problems with the feeding delay the mother's ability to assume the feeding role independently. A community health nurse referral is especially helpful to give the mother continued guidance with feeding at home. It is also helpful as the mother may not retain much of the information she has been given in the hospital.

If a referral is not made, the nurse should provide the mother with a telephone number to call for assistance. The number should be written down and clearly marked with the agency and persons to contact. Any clues as to how to "cut through the red tape" of the telephone system of the agency should be included. Every attempt should be made to make the utilization of the number free of anxiety. It is frequently difficult for the mother to seek assistance, so her attempts should be rewarded by a positive response. This will give her confidence to call again.

The preschooler with a congenital heart disease may need help from his mother to supplement his feedings because he may tire too soon and not complete an adequate nutritional intake. While we do not want to encourage the mother to take away the child's opportunity to feed himself, she must be aware of her responsibility to lend a hand, when necessary. The child with a congenital heart disease will still need to establish the same autonomy as any other child and his own self-limitations are the best guide in judging how much he is able to assume for himself. Helping the child when he is tired will give him a sense of trust in his adults. This sense of trust will be of utmost benefit when the child is subjected to periods of hospitalization and especially if the child is faced with surgical correction. If the child has had positive experiences with adults helping him when it is necessary, then he will trust them when he knows he is going to need help when hospitalized. The parents can be taught to assess the child's respiratory status during feeding periods. They can gauge the child's tolerance based on the changes they observe. If the respirations become greatly increased or more irregular they will know the feeding should be stopped to allow the infant or child to rest. In the same way, cyanosis can be assessed to determine the child's tolerance for feedings.

The blood pressure of children is being assessed more conscientiously to see if there is a correlation between elevated blood pressures in children and hypertension in adults. In a study by Lauer et al (1975) on school-age children they found virtually no hypertension in children ages six to nine years of age. However, in the 14 to 18 year olds there were 8.9 percent with systolic hypertension and 12.2 percent with elevated diastolic readings. Hypertension of both the systolic and diastolic recordings occurred in 4.4 percent of the adolescents. The criteria used to determine hypertension was a systolic pressure of 140 mm Hg or above or a diastolic pressure of 90 mm Hg or above. In addition to the children diagnosed as hypertensive, 16.7 percent were considered to have elevated blood pressure readings. The children with cardiac defects are in a higher risk group than the normal children screened in the Lauer study. Therefore, the blood pressure recordings are more significant.

The size of the cuff is very important. The cuff should not be less than half the length of the upper portion of the child's arm or greater than 2/3 of its length. In the newborn, the flush method is used. Children with cardiac defects often have blood pressures taken on all four extremities. Each recording should be clearly marked as to the extremity used.

The pulse rate can be taken radically or apically. The apical pulse is often the method of choice with children with cardiac problems. To evaluate the child's circulatory status, it is not unusual to have recordings also taken of the temporal, carotid, pedal, popliteal, and femoral pulses as well. It is important to note the quality of the pulse as well as the rate. The pulse should be counted for a full minute as these children frequently have irregular rhythms and counting for a full minute will give more accurate assessments.

With all of the findings it is valuable to compare them with tables which have norms for children of various age groups.

CARDIAC SURGERY

Despite the many daily anxieties created by having a child with congenital heart disease, the parents are not always willing or ready to accept cardiac surgery as therapy. It is the responsibility of the physician and also some of the other members of the health team such as the social worker or religious advisor to help the parents to understand the rationale for surgery and to help them make intelligent decisions regarding it. The parents frequently find it difficult to make the decision for the younger child as he is too small to help in the decision. The older child can be included in the discussion and his reaction can be evaluated as part of the decision-making process.

Many factors can influence the parents' decision regarding surgery. When the newborn is severely handicapped and gasping for breath the parent may be eager to have surgery as they see it as an only chance for the infant to survive. For a toddler or preschooler who has been severely incapacitated by the heart defect, the parent may look at the surgery as another stressful situation to which they would rather not subject the child. This is an especially common reaction when the child is hospitalized frequently and reacts poorly to hospitalization.

When the child's physical appearance mimics the severity of the defect, the rationale for surgery is more evident. However, when the child looks and acts "normal" it is more difficult to understand the necessity for the surgery.

Another factor which may influence the parents' attitude toward surgery is the medical information they have received regarding the defect. Due to the difficulty in making definite diagnoses in infants, the mother is frequently given conflicting or false information. If she has been told the child will "grow out of it" she may reject the surgery on this basis. She may also doubt the competence of the medical personnel who have not been able to give her an exact explanation of what is wrong with her child's heart.

Another realistic factor in the decision-making process is the financial strain the surgery might cause. A social worker or financial counselor can be helpful in dicussing this concern.

The availability of a facility equipped to do pediatric cardiac surgery is another factor. Traveling long distances may make the decision especially difficult, especially if it means separating the mother and child from the rest of the family for a long period of time. The risk which surrounds the surgery procedure as well as the projected life expectancy can also be relevant factors in the decision. Also the reactions of relatives and friends as well as the parents' experience with other families who had similar surgery cannot be underestimated.

In the study by Glaser (1964) it was also brought out that the parents had a great deal of anxiety about the cardiac catheterization preceding the surgery. The parents were very concerned that the child might die.

Preparation for Surgical Intervention

The age of the child is one of the primary factors in the preparation for cardiac surgery. The younger children do not seem to be as eager to participate in their preoperative teachings as the older children. It is most appropriate to identify the child's ability to understand the preoperative preparation and to adjust it accordingly. While I will make the assumption this will be done, the plan of care I will now describe will probably best fit the school-age and adolescent child.

The child should be made aware of the environment in which he will find himself immediately preoperatively, and during his convalescent period. Depending on the clinical facilities this may be two different places or it may be one and the same. The child who is admitted for cardiac surgery has usually been hospitalized previously because the child usually has a cardiac catheterization as part of his preoperative evaluation. This procedure is usually done in the same hospital as his cardiac surgery. However, the child may have been on a completely different unit than any of the ones he will be subjected to on this hospitalization. The preparation of the child is best done in small sessions and when the child is fairly well rested. Therefore, it is good to plan his sessions after the rest period that normally takes place on the hospital unit. The preparation should give the child an opportunity to ask questions, to act out his fears, and to digest new information. In keeping with normal developmental factors the teaching will best take place when accompanied by the use of toys or books appropriate to the age of the child. The child should be exposed to the same types of things that he will be exposed to postoperatively. He should be introduced to tourniquets, to syringes, to blood pressure cuffs, to oxygen equipment, to suction equipment, to blow bottles, and to the intensive care unit if it is to be utilized. The child will have previous experience with some of these things but reintroducing them will give the child an opportunity to express how he feels about them.

For instance, it would be quite rare for a child with a congenital heart disease not to have had his blood pressure taken. But this does not mean that a blood pressure cuff should be omitted from his preoperative teaching. A good way of seeing how he feels about the blood pressure cuff is to have him apply it to a doll and to see how he explains to the doll what he is going to do or how it is going to feel. This will give us valuable clues regarding how to introduce blood pressure taking to the child postoperatively. In the same manner each of the other items should be introduced to the child. In addition to this equipment, puppets can serve a valuable role in preoperative preparation. It is sometimes much easier for the child to express through a puppet on his hand how he feels than it is to express to a professional person, eye to eye, how he feels. With a puppet, he finds it perfectly legitimate to explain to you that he does not like being stuck with needles, or that he does not want to have his surgery done, or that he fears separation from his parent. Giving the child an opportunity to express these things makes it easier to give anticipatory guidance. It also suggests to us ways that the child may be able to express his anxiety postoperatively. For instance, if he used the puppet effectively preoperatively then why not give it to him postoperatively to see if he can again express his fears?

If the child was unable to utilize the puppets for self-expression preoperatively, then postoperatively we would know they were not the answer. If the child seemed to need a mode of expression and was not able to communicate verbally then we can be especially attuned to nonverbal clues. The nurse should record on her nursing notes the reaction of the child to the equipment so that the people caring for him immediately postoperatively will have the advantage of this information.

The child needs to be taught how to deep breathe and how he will be turned postoperatively. The degree to which he will participate postoperatively may be influenced by how creative the nurse is in introducing these activities to him. Postoperatively the nurse can then reap the benefits of this preoperative teaching. For instance, if the child was taught deep breathing by blowing plastic bubbles then this toy should be available postoperatively to achieve the same purpose. If the child was taught deep breathing by blowing up balloons, a good supply of balloons must be available postoperatively. If the blow bottles were utilized with a particular color water in them preoperatively, the same color water should be used postoperatively. If we expect the child to carry over his preoperative teaching to his postoperative period then the mechanism should be the same so the child recognizes what it is we are asking him to do.

When we are teaching turning as a preoperative exercise it is imperative to tell the child that postoperatively it may hurt to turn because of the chest tube(s). If we neglect to tell him about the chest tube(s) then postoperatively he may refuse to turn because he does not want to dislodge it (them) or he may quickly find that it hurts when he turns, concluding that it is best not to turn at all. Simple truth will aid in the postoperative period. The inclusion of the aspect of pain will help negate the child's using it as an excuse for not turning. The child is quick to point out the nurse's weaknesses and he may blame you, the nurse, for the pain, if he is not cautioned that it will be present. The child should also know he can receive medication to reduce the pain.

The child who is to be cared for in an intensive care unit deserves the right to be oriented to that unit preoperatively. The child will benefit from being introduced to his nurses and being called by name by them. This helps him to realize that they know him and that he will not get lost. This is especially important for the younger child who fears separation and fears the possibility of getting lost. The school-age child will also benefit from this because he appreciates people knowing who he is and respecting him as a person. The child is not accustomed to being called by his last name until he gets to high school, so it is a mistake for nurses to call him Jones or Smith or so forth. The child will respond best to that which he is used to, which may be a nickname or initials.

Plastic canopies distort the child's vision. It is helpful to have him get in a tent prior to surgery so he will be aware of these distortions. He is frequently better able to cope with this experience before he has the added stress of surgery. It is also possible to explain the pipes, machinery, and noise caused by the tent during this preoperative preparation (see Figures 2 and 3).

Sleep

Another valuable preoperative evaluation would be that of the child's sleep patterns. The nurse should keep a record of the child's sleep during the day as well as at night (see Table 1).

A preoperative sleep pattern would give clues as to how the child ordinarily sleeps. It would help in postoperative positionings for comfort. The comfort measures would also be altered by specific positioning in relation to the surgery.

The sleep pattern would also show how long the child ordinarily sleeps during a certain period. We could then plan our nursing care so it would not interrupt these normal sleep patterns. For example, if the child usually takes an hour afternoon nap then why wake him in 45 minutes to take his blood pressure? Why not let him complete his normal sleep and perhaps complete a satisfying dream?

One of the major nursing objectives should be to provide the child with adequate rest. This is achieved by planning treatments and medications to

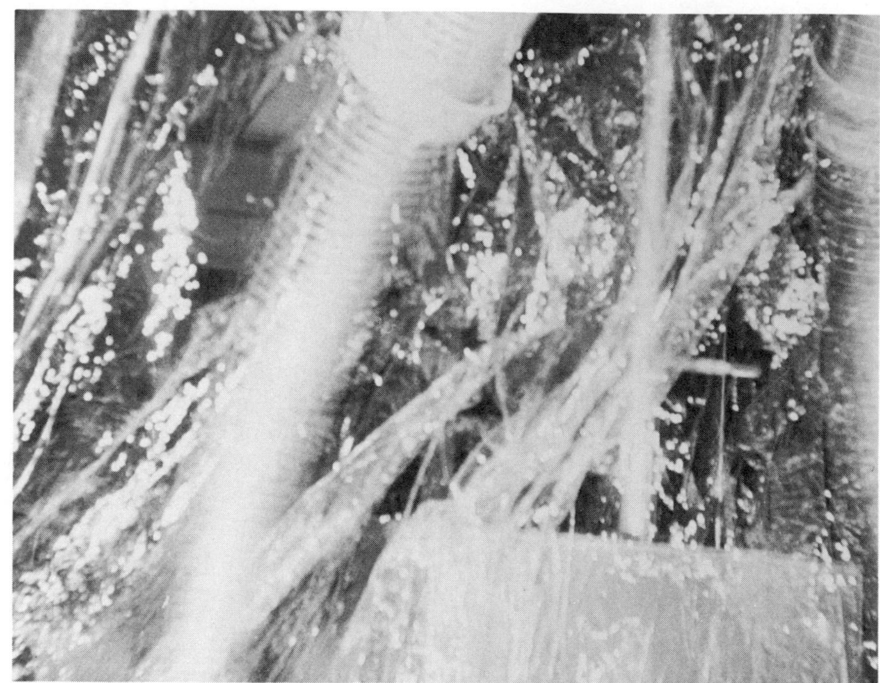

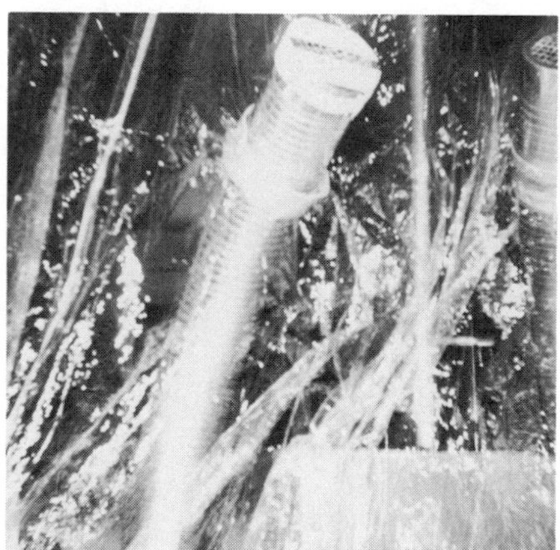

FIG. 2. Photos taken from inside an oxygen tent. Note the distorted image the child receives. Also try, with a child's sense of fantasy, to imagine what significance each of the parts play.

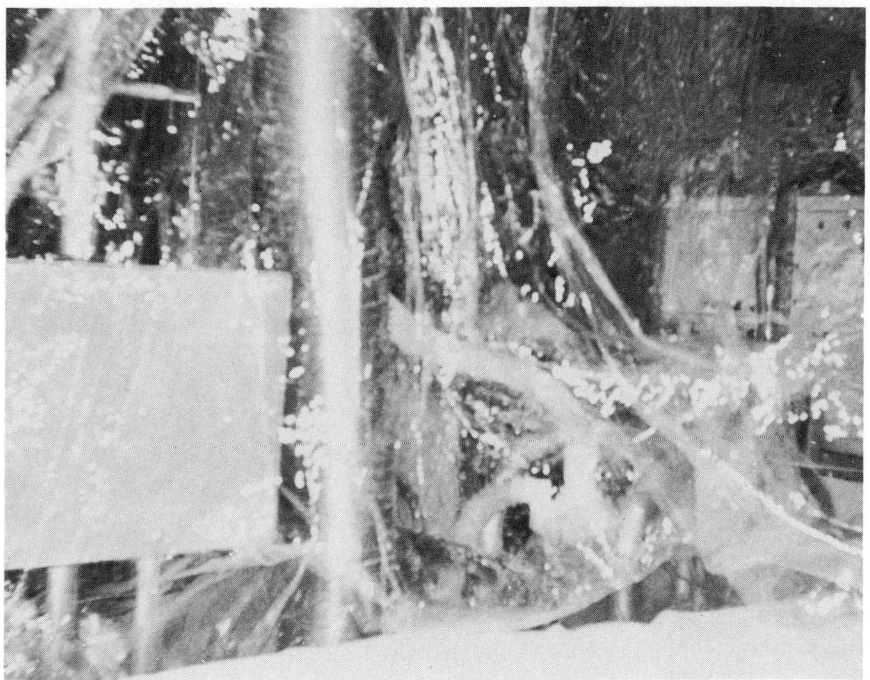

FIG. 3. Inside an oxygen tent, note the additional obstacles in this photo which interfere with the child's visual field.

TABLE 1

JOHN (Age 8)	**TIME**	**EXAMPLE**	**MEDICATIONS**
12/8/76	7:00 A.M.	Sleeping, left side, soundly	None
	7:15 A.M.	Beginning to awaken	
	7:20 A.M.	Fully awake & alert	
	2:00 P.M.	Took 15 min to fall asleep Brown teddy bear	Digitalis—10:00 A.M. Phenobarbital ¼ gr—10:00 A.M. and 2:00 P.M.
	3:00 P.M.	Awake & bright	
	9:00 P.M.	To bed at 8:00 P.M.—tossed, restless—asleep on left side 2 stuffed toys Prayers at bedtime	Phenobarbital ½ gr—8:00 P.M.
	11:00 P.M.	Very restless—awake	None

meet the child's individual needs as opposed to meeting the hospital routines. This will necessitate good organization so that the child will only be disturbed on a limited basis.

Elimination

Preoperatively the child is frequently up and around. After his initial urine specimen is collected, his elimination does not seem to be important unless he is on intake and output ordered by the physician. The child is free to go to the bathroom and does not get adequate practice using the bedpan. It is helpful to have him use it a couple times to familiarize him with how it feels and the adjustments needed to void or defecate in a less than adequate position.

It is also important to record the words used by the child to describe his need to eliminate. If new words are taught, they are frequently forgotten during periods of acute stress, and the child will revert to his familiar words. Foley catheters are frequently used postoperatively and they should be explained to the child during the preoperative preparation.

Constipation is guarded against both pre- and postoperatively as it is not favorable for the child to strain to defecate. If fluids cannot be forced to aid in this process, then the physician frequently orders a stool softener to be given.

Diagnostic Procedures and Preparation of the Child

There are a great number of diagnostic procedures which can be done to establish the diagnosis of heart disease and the child's readiness for surgery. Two of the more common ones are the electrocardiograph and the cardiac catheterization.

EKG (Electrocardiograph). The electrocardiogram records the activity of the heart. The electrical impulses of the heart result in contractions and relaxation of the heart. The EKG shows the cardiac cycle of the child. In a normal rhythm, the contraction of the atria is the first wave, the P wave. The contraction of the ventricles are related to the Q,R,S, and T waves. The tracing is obtained by having the child lie in a supine position in his bed or on the table in the treatment room. The child is prepared by explaining the reason for the recording. For example:

"John, the doctor wants a drawing of your heart action. This does not hurt and will not take long. We have a special machine to do this drawing. It looks like a brown box but when the cover is open you will see it is a very special box. It is equipped to draw lines. You might think it is scribbling or you might think it looks like the 'Etch-a-Sketch game.' (If you have an Etch-a-Sketch game this can be used to demonstrate to the child.) Special paper will come through the machine and it will be a very long line picture when we are through. To get this picture we must place special pieces of metal on your body. (Show the child an electrode.) Before we do this we put a special liquid, which comes from a tube and may feel cool, on several parts of you—like your arm. We will point out the areas as we go along. The liquid and the metal will be removed after we get the drawing. You can help by lying still while we make the drawing. Do you have any questions?"

After the procedure is completed the electrode compound is washed off and the child can resume his usual activity. More sophistocated recordings are available in some hospitals. The child may be scheduled for an echo cardiogram, vector cardiogram, or phono cardiogram. These cardiograms give more specific data regarding the defect. The phonocardiogram records the heart sounds more accurately than they can be assessed using a stethoscope. The vector cardiogram visualizes the heart more like its three-dimensional anatomy. The echo cardiogram utilizes ultrasound to record the echo of each portion of the heart. Coats (1976) states, "By tracking the same structure throughout several cardiac cycles, its *motion* as well as its configuration can be visualized" (p. 264).

Cardiac Catheterization The cardiac catheterization provides a much clearer picture of the specific defect than the electrocardiogram. This clearer picture is not obtained without an increased risk. The procedure is considered a surgical procedure requiring parental consent. A small, soft radiopaque catheter is inserted into the cardiac chambers and vessels. It is possible to establish a more definitive diagnosis by this technique. It may be done in a special cardiac catheterization laboratory or in the operating room. The parents must have a clear understanding of the procedure and be given sufficient time to ask questions. The thought of anything entering their child's heart can be an especially threatening situation. Their fear can be easily transmitted to the child.

The explanation given the child will, as always, depend on his age and level of understanding. The toddler or preschooler needs to know he will not be able to eat or drink the morning of the procedure. He will also be medicated as it is necessary for the child to be as relaxed as possible for the procedure. The school-age child and adolescent may enjoy seeing a diagram of the heart and the pathway the catheter will pass. They also need reassurance that the procedure will not cause undue pain or discomfort. The chief discomfort the child will experience is the local pain created by doing the cut-down. A common site for the cut-down is the groin in younger children or the arm in older children.

The nurse or technician accompanying the child doing the procedure should wear a lead apron to protect herself from the x-ray being used to follow the direction of the catheter. The nurse should stay at the head of the table and attempt to provide diversional activities during the catheterization. The time needed to complete the procedure varies greatly but the nurse should be prepared to entertain the child for as long as three hours. In the early periods, when the child is not yet bored, story telling or reading books will be effective. Later, the child gets tired of lying supine and more creative things such as magic tricks can be tried. During the procedure, the child needs assurance that things are progressing satisfactorily. If possible, he needs to know approximately how much longer it will take. Such an explanation follows.

"Henry, the catheter is now in your heart and they are beginning to get the answers they need to their questions. This part will take another twenty minutes. You are cooperating very nicely. Do you have any questions?"

If the child is of school age or adolescent he may also enjoy learning the names of the various equipment in the laboratory such as the flouroscope, the electrocardiogram (which is probably familiar to him), the pressure recorders, oscilloscopic apparatus, and blood analyzing equipment. It must also be understood that this equipment can be extremely frightening as its size is overwhelming and the space provided is usually minimal, making the room appear very "cluttered" and "official." The use of pictures, mobiles, brightly colored walls, and friendly personnel helps to lessen the negative impact of such an area.

After the catheterization is completed, the cut-down is removed and a dressing applied to the area. The child's vital signs continue to need monitoring for the next 24 hours. The dressing is observed for signs of bleeding. A drop in vital signs or bleeding at the site of the cut-down may indicate internal bleeding and necessitate prompt attention from the physician. It is not common, but it is entirely possible that, despite the most careful maneuvering, the catheter can rupture a vessel or cause phlebitis. The risks involved in left heart catheterization are higher than in right heart catheterization because of the increased difficulty in reaching the left side. It must also be remembered that the more serious and complicated heart conditions run a higher risk rate as the physicians cannot always predict the defects prior to catheterization. These defects may allow the catheter to pass in other areas than expected. Also, younger children run a higher risk due to the smaller size of the heart, which causes more difficulty in passing the catheter and in visualizing the parts. Children included in these categories will need more constant observations.

The child is usually permitted a regular diet and increased fluid intake after the catheterization. It is usually common to have the child remain quiet the day of the catheterization and then return to normal activity the day afterwards.

In addition to the visual observations made, the physician will obtain blood samples from the heart chambers for oxygen analysis and he will have pressure recordings within the chambers to help him identify the defect and its severity.

The parents and child, if he is old enough, both deserve an explanation of the findings as soon as possible after completion of the catheterization. If the catheterization is postponed for any reason, the parent and child should be told the reason so they will not worry unnecessarily. The stress related to this procedure should not be underestimated by the professional team.

The Intensive Care Unit

The intensive care unit has both positive and negative aspects in caring for the child undergoing cardiac surgery. Some of the positive aspects are that the nurses are usually more knowledgeable about the equipment and acute aspects of the postoperative period. The equipment is readily available for any emergency (Fig. 4). Medical personnel usually respond quicker to a call from this area. The unit usually is in closer proximity to the operating room if any emergency does arise and the child needs to return to surgery. The negative aspects are usually concerned with the fact that the nurses frequently are so overly involved in the physical care of the child that they relegate to lesser importance the emotional aspects. Also, the visiting per-

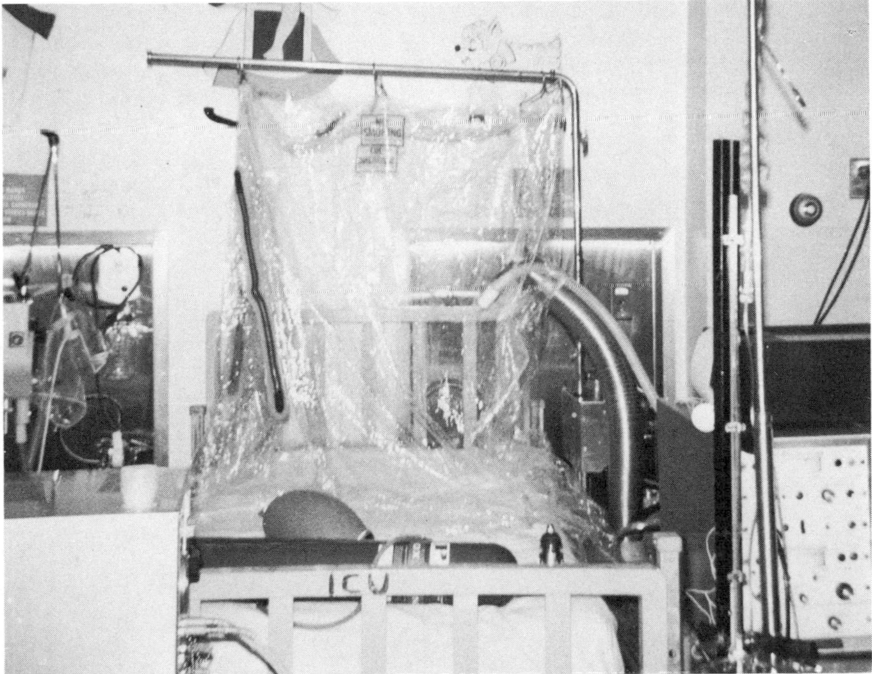

FIG. 4. An intensive care unit ready for a child returning from cardiac surgery. Emergency equipment is readily available.

mitted within this unit is usually very short and the parents are usually left out in another area where they receive little in the way of progress reports on their child. Another negative aspect is the fact that the child is in an area where all of the children are acutely ill and when he is awake he is repeatedly exposed to the seriousness of the condition of the other children. He seldom has the advantage of seeing some children up running around or hearing the cheerful laughter of children at play. He is frequently in an environment which is more sterile in nature than the rooms on the convalescent floors. This "sterility" can be somewhat alleviated by making the environment more conducive to the care of the children. For the child in an oxygen tent, this can be easily achieved by hanging mobiles inside the tent, by placing toys in the tent (ones that are appropriate, such as rubber or wooden ones), by adding musical toys to the tents to cut down on the amount of motors the child is exposed to, by making the child's visual field more colorful and less distorted (Figs. 5 and 6). The child who is somewhat immobilized should have some type of toy or book within his visual field so that he does not have to turn around to find it. When he wakes up he sees color or animals or things he is ordinarily exposed to in his immediate vicinity.

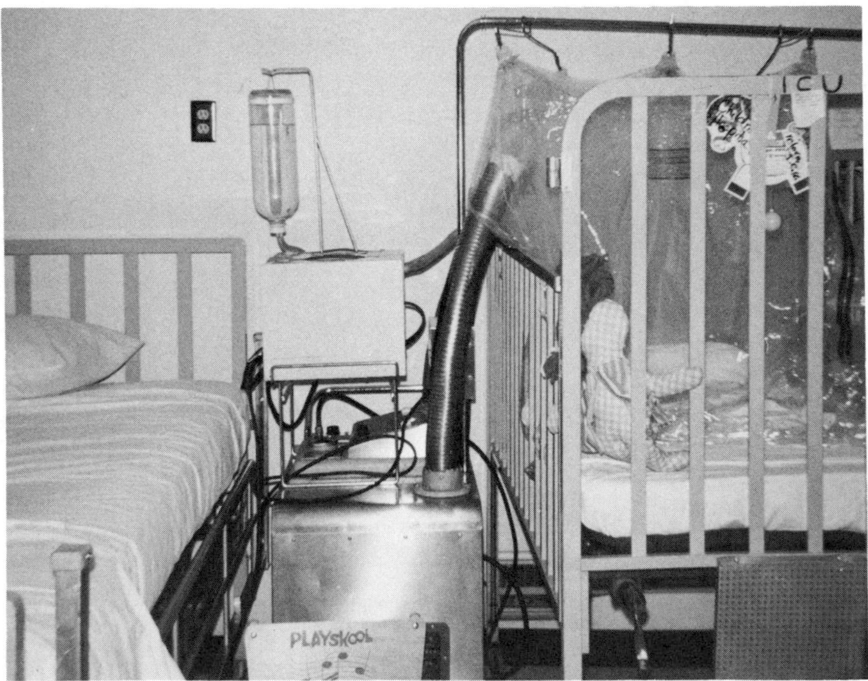

FIG. 5. Intensive care unit combining children's world and medical world.

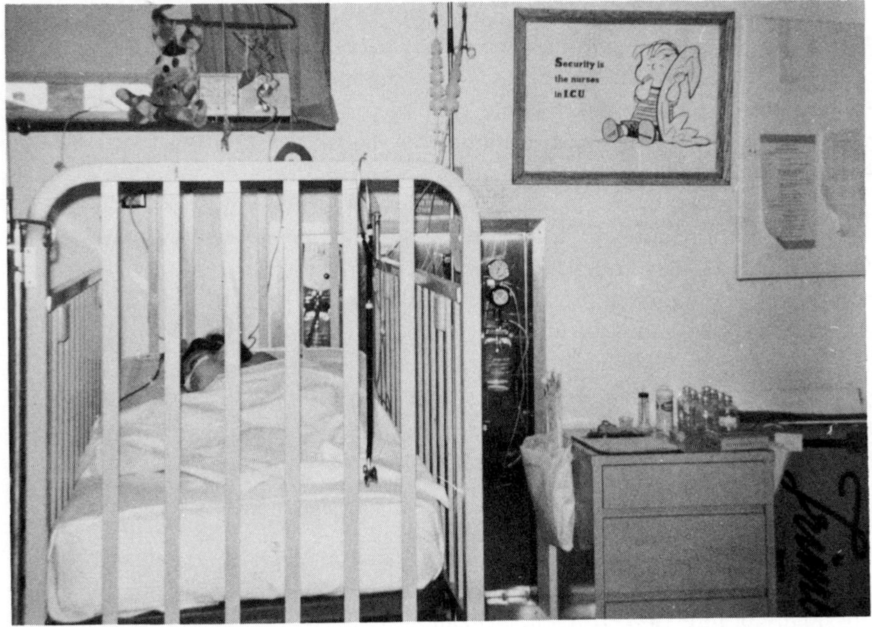

FIG. 6. Try to imagine what the child across the room thinks, when he wakes up and sees this acutely ill child. Note the attempts to brighten up the environment. What additional things can be done?

(Refer to Chapters 2 and 4 for a more complete discussion of toys and children's perceptions.)

The parents should also have the opportunity to be introduced to the intensive care unit, if they so desire. Some parents have stated that the visit to the intensive care unit has produced so much anxiety preoperatively that they felt less able to cope with their child's anxieties than if they had not visited it. Other parents have felt that it is a very important part of helping them to be more relaxed postoperatively. If they are not taken to the unit they should at least be told where it is and the easiest way of getting there. A small model of the unit can be used to orient the child and the parent. The use of the model allows you to point out equipment and activity areas without having them see the other postoperative children. They should also be well aware of the restricted visiting hours, if they exist. There is no easy answer as to what amount of time the parent should spend with the child postoperatively and many of the hospital policies seem particularly restricted in this aspect. We need to ask ourselves what reasons we have for restricting visiting hours and who benefits most by the restriction—the child and his family or the personnel responsible for his care. If it is honestly the child and family who are benefiting at a particular time it justifies the limited visiting. If it is the medical personnel who seem to be gaining the most then I think it behooves us to reevaluate the restrictions and to make necessary adjustments. In many hospitals visiting time is restricted to five minutes out of every hour. Following such regulations, a parent is asked to sit for a total of three hours in order to spend a mere 15 minutes with his child.

Parents are relieved to see that their child is receiving expert care. They also can ask more relevant questions if they can see actual care being given. Perhaps a viewing window would be more satisfactory than even entering the room, immediately postoperatively—especially if the child is dozing during the five-minute period that is allocated for visiting. A nurse, viewing with the parent, can then point out particular aspects about the child and his care. For instance, the parents may be so distracted by the equipment that is being used that they may benefit more by an explanation of this first. It takes time and courage for the parents to look past the equipment and to the child. Their five minutes may be up before this reaction takes place. If a viewing window is available, more time can be allocated without interfering with the ordinary activities of the unit. It would also conceivably cut down on the numbers of people in the area at any one time, and therefore, diminish the possibility of infection. It would also allow a discussion of equipment and the child's progress to take place away from the bedside of the children. This would be beneficial to both the child involved and the other children in the unit who may overhear conversations and think it is their progress being discussed.

Actual visiting in the unit would then have the specific purpose of communicating directly with the child. All communication with professional personnel could be done more effectively outside the intensive care unit. It is also difficult for the staff to establish any type of a meaningful relationship with the parents in a five-minute period. Meeting them outside would make it possible to spend a longer time with them (Fig. 7).

The viewing window should be accessible only with professional personnel available. If the parents were able to use this without supervision, it could heighten anxiety of both the parents and the professional staff.

Preparations

Is Preparation for the Emergency Situation Necessary? In the preoperative preparation of the child, I have not included the use of a doll with a tracheostomy. This decision is based on the assumption that it may cause unnecessary anxiety in the young child and even in the school-age child to expose them to the possibility of emergency situations. The tracheostomy is not a routine procedure and, therefore, it is not included in all preoperative preparation. If the physician has indicated that the child will

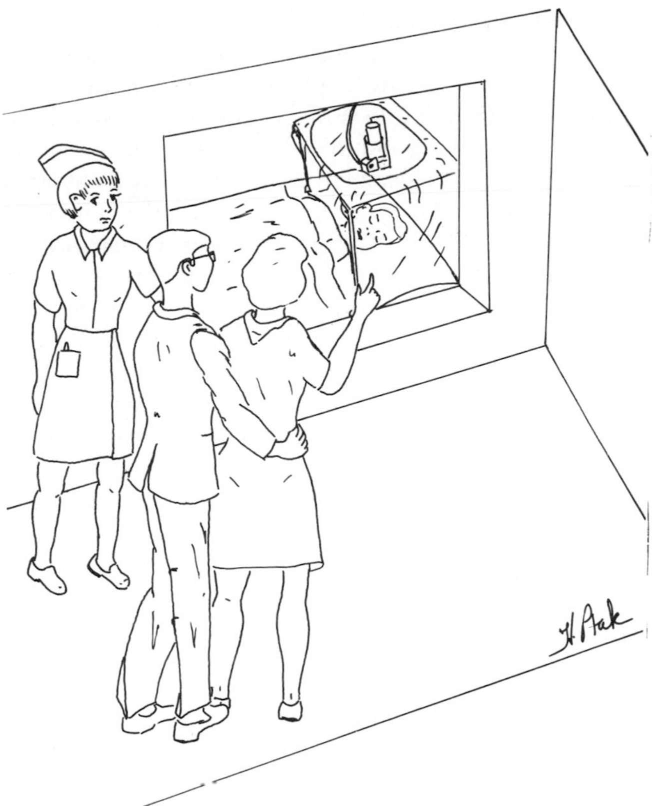

FIG. 7. A mother and father view their acutely ill child through the intensive care unit window. The nurse is available to answer their questions and give support.

absolutely have a tracheostomy, then utilization of a doll with a tracheostomy in place can be of benefit to the child. The child will have an opportunity to question why the tube is in place and should be introduced to the suctioning which will be done through the tracheostomy opening. In preparing the parents of the child, the procedure can be mentioned and explained and the rationale for not explaining it to the child should be included. The parents need specific information about where they should wait while the surgery is being performed. They should know who will talk to them after the surgery is completed. They should be treated with great respect and to do this adequately, sufficient time for asking questions and clarifying concerns must be provided.

The surgical procedure should be explained to the parents by the physician. The nurse is then in a position to explain the nursing intervention needed and to support the physician's explanation. She also uses this time to do significant teaching.

Preparation for Anesthesia. In many agencies the physician from the department of anesthesia will assume the role for preparing the child for anesthesia. In agencies where this is not done, the nurse can incorporate this into her preoperative plan. Models of the operating room or pictures are good visual aids for helping parents and children understand the complicated surgical unit. The use of small items to show and demonstrate are also included in the preoperative preparation. The mask that will be put over the child's face is an example of this. The mode by which the child will get to the operating room, the clothes that the people in the operating room will be wearing, a description of odors common in the operating unit, and a statement that the child will not be awake during the operation are all included in the discussion. An attempt should be made not to tell the child that he will be asleep but rather that it is a special type of a sleep that is induced by medication, so that the child will not fear going to sleep after the surgical procedure. The child should also be told that a doctor will watch him very closely during the entire time he is in this special sleep and will take responsibility for awakening him from his special sleep at the end of his surgery. The child should be told exactly when he will be separated from his parent. For instance, if the child can be accompanied to the operating room by the parent, he should know this. If the policies of the hospital do not permit a parent to accompany the child, then the child and parent should both know this. The child should know by what means he will be taken to the operating room, and who will take him there. For instance, if he is to go on an adult-type stretcher or if a small carriage will take him he needs to know (see Fig. 8). He should know if a person dressed in a green outfit will come to get him or if a nurse that he is very familiar with will take him. The child should also choose one or more toys which he would like to take to the operating room with him. A notation should be made on the Kardex regarding his choice so the toy or toys are included in the preoperative check list. This is all based on the idea that the more the child knows, the less fear there will be of the unknown and the less possibility there will be for misunderstanding.

The foregoing information can be applied to children undergoing any type of cardiac surgery. In addition, the nurse must be able to make additions or modifications to meet the special nursing responsibilities in relation to the child's specific diagnosis. For instance, there may be much more preparation needed for a child who is scheduled for open heart surgery with utilization of the heart lung machine than with a child who is having a closed cardiac procedure. A discussion of the many types of cardiac defects found in children is beyond the scope of this book. For this information, the student should refer to a book on pediatric surgery that explores the cardiac conditions and their respective intervention.

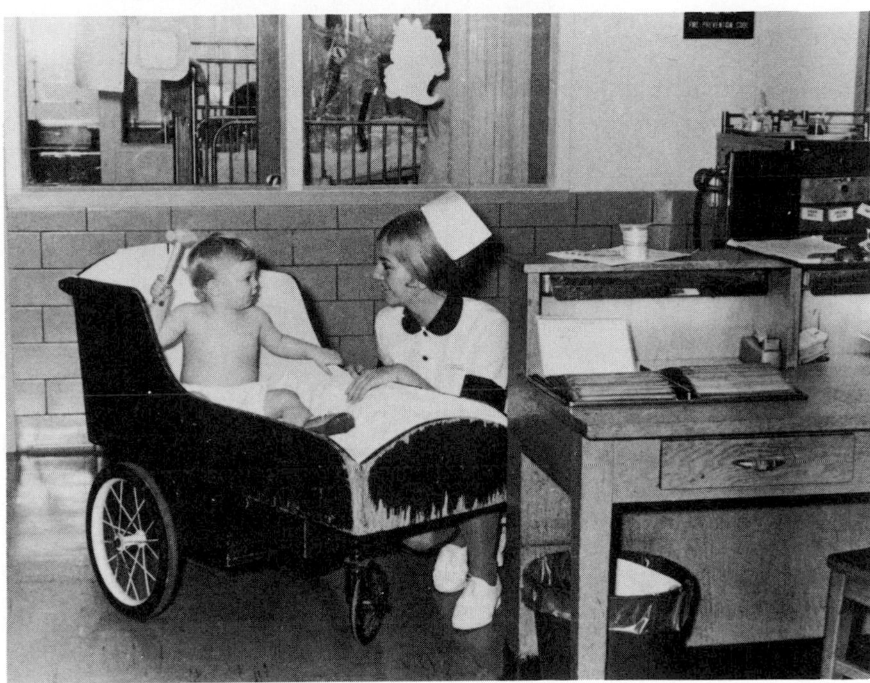

FIG. 8. Carts such as this one cut down on the fear of going to the x-ray, operating rooms, and to play activities. They allow the child to sit up and take favorite toys along.

POSTOPERATIVE CARE

In the postoperative period it is important to capitalize on the preoperative preparation of the child. For instance, as soon as he returns to the intensive care unit or area for his immediate postoperative care, he should be introduced to it in the following manner:

"Johnny, this is the intensive care unit you visited yesterday. I am your nurse, Miss Jones. Remember, I called you Johnny yesterday and said, 'See you tomorrow.' You are going into the oxygen tent that you saw yesterday. This oxygen tent may feel a little cool and may feel a little damp. That is to be expected. If you are cool, let me know so I can cover you, or wipe you off if you have moisture dripping on you. You now have the chest tubes you saw on the doll, Johnny, they are on your left side. Do not touch them. Soon I will ask you to breathe nice and deep. I will give you a balloon to blow, like you had upstairs. It will not be as easy to blow today as it was yesterday, but each day it will get easier."

In this way the child will be quickly reintroduced to his environment and to what has gone on prior to surgery. Consistent use of this technique will aid the child in his recovery and will aid the nurse in gaining the child's cooperation. The child should be repeatedly reminded that while he has pain now, each day he will have improvement and less pain. He needs more encouragement that he will get better than the adult patient does. He is usually more interested in himself and his immediate environment than he is in the future and, therefore, he needs more reassurance that this pain is transient in nature. The child will also want immediate gratification of his needs and he should know how to get gratification. If he must call for the nurse, then he should know the means of calling for the nurse. If a nurse will be with him continuously, then he should know there is a nurse by his side and a hand motion is needed to gain her attention.

During his immediate postoperative period, the child will derive a great deal of satisfaction from getting his physical needs met adequately. However, as he begins to progress in the convalescent period, he will need more and more attention given to his emotional needs. As he begins to improve, he will begin to question, verbally and nonverbally, reasons for the nurse's activity. A simple, truthful explanation is always the rule in guiding the explanations. The child who has undergone cardiac surgery frequently is exposed to a large number of people delivering care immediately postoperatively. Due to this, he is not always aware of who is directly responsible when he wants something. The nurse can play a key role in this by always identifying when she/he is responsible for his care and who is responsible when she/he is not available. In addition to meeting the emotional needs of the child, the nurse will be responsible for many of the other procedures which are done to and for the child during the immediate postoperative period.

Chest Tubes and Suction

The student will usually have had experience with chest tubes with adult patients prior to seeing them in the pediatric patient. The same principles apply to the pediatric patient as the adult patient. First, the tubes should be checked to make sure there is no kinking; second, the bandage around the tube should be free of drainage, and if drainage does appear, it should be encircled and watched for increase in drainage; third, a Kelly clamp should be available for each tube that is in place. In case of emergency, the student would clamp off the tube as close to the chest wall as possible. Fourth, the tube should be connected to some type of drainage. Frequently the three-bottle suction is utilized for drainage. One of these bottles is the drainage bottle, the second bottle the control bottle, and the third the safety bottle (Fig. 9).

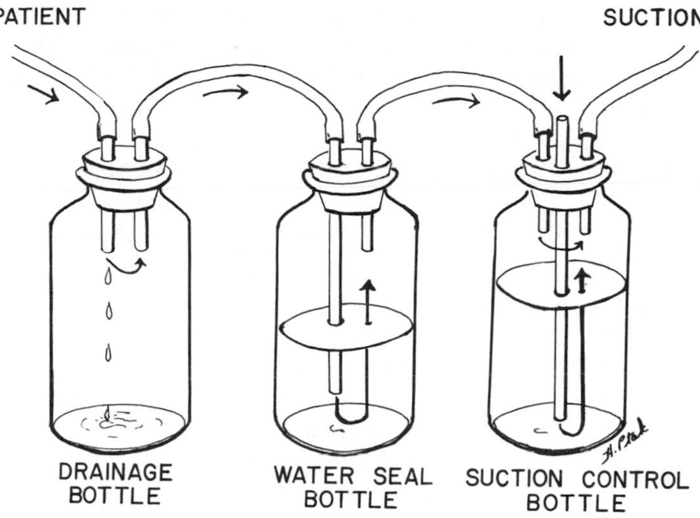

FIG. 9. Three-bottle system for closed chest drainage.

The tubes must also be securely anchored to the bed to help prevent undue tension on them. This can be achieved by placing adhesive tape around the tubes, without constricting them, and then using a safety pin to pin the adhesive to the sheet.

The tubes also need special attention when the patient is turned. Care must be taken not to have the patient's weight resting on the tubes. The tubes must also be replaced after turning to reestablish adequate draining. (For a detailed explanation of three-bottle suction, the student should refer to Dr. Jensen's textbook entitled *Introduction to Medical Physics.*)

The nurse must also know who is responsible for emptying and measuring the chest drainage. The procedure may vary from one institution to another. Some measure drainage after each tour of duty and others measure it daily.

Vital Signs

The immediate postoperative period will demand a great deal of the nurse's energy. She/he will be kept busy monitoring many things. Not the least of these is the child's vital signs. Vital signs are usually learned early by the beginning nurse and may seem "just old hat" after a period of practice. However, for the child who has undergone cardiac surgery, the vital signs may be more of a challenge.

Preoperatively, the vital signs were recorded by both physicians and nurses. Each had an opportunity to cross-check their results. In addition, vital signs could be obtained under differing sets of conditions. These results should be carefully recorded so they can be effectively utilized postoperatively (Table 2).

The variations in rates with activity can be used as gauges in planning postoperative activity. The use of varying areas for counting the pulse rate can also be useful postoperatively. If preoperatively all the pulse rates were taken on the left radial pulse, and postoperatively the child has a cut-down or intravenous infusion in that area, then the child's routine has to be disrupted. It is better to teach him that pulses may be obtained radially, apically, femorally, carotidly, or on the feet (dorsalis pedis). You can then explain to the child that any one of these areas may be used postoperatively to obtain his pulse. Letting the child count his own pulse or the nurse's pulse is also helpful in gaining his cooperation.

Pulse rates vary from one cardiac condition to another and from one age child to another age child. This creates problems in knowing what is "normal" for a certain child. The child's rate may also change due to the nature of the surgery. For instance, a child with coarctation of the aorta may lack pedal pulses. Postoperatively this rate is established by improvement in blood flow. The beginning student will need to read about pediatric surgery to become familiar with each cardiac anomaly and its particular influence on the child's vital signs.

The blood pressure is another invaluable monitor, if it is taken correctly. If possible, the child's pressure should always be taken with the same cuff. This is usually fairly easy to accomplish in a small well-equipped intensive care unit, but may be more difficult on a bigger patient unit, where only one or two cuffs are available for use with numerous children.

The limited distribution of the cuff also cuts down on the possibility of cross-contamination, which is so important both preoperatively and postoperatively with children having cardiac surgery. (The area of protection from infection is covered more thoroughly in a separate section.)

The cuff should be applied snugly and anchored securely before being inflated. This can be easily achieved if you have adequately prepared the

TABLE 2

JOHN (Age 8)	TIME	ACTIVITY	PULSE AREA	BP	R
	8:00 A.M.	Just awakened	100-Radial (lt)	100/62	16
	11:00 A.M.	Active play	110-Radial (lt) 122-Carotid (rt)	104/64	20
	12:30 P.M.	Following self-feeding	110-Radial (rt)	104/64	24

child and gained his cooperation. The child should know that it will feel tight on his arm when you pump up the cuff. The child may enjoy holding the dial so you can read it. This makes him feel a responsibility for helping with his own care. The acutely ill child may not be able to participate but may benefit from having a toy to hold during the procedure. If it is necessary to recheck the reading, be sure to tell the child you are inflating the cuff again. Frequent rechecking may cause anxiety to the child, so optimal conditions should be achieved prior to beginning. These optimal conditions include proper positioning of the child and the cuff, removal of clothing between cuff and arm, as much quiet as possible, and turning off any motors which may safely be eliminated during the short period of time needed.

When in doubt of a recording, ask another nurse to check it. No one should put her pride before the child's welfare. If a recording is not easily obtainable, it may very well be an early sign of distress.

The respiratory rate is probably more variable than either the pulse rate or the blood pressure. The respiratory rate can be significantly decreased during sleep or due to postoperative medication. Respiratory rate can be significantly increased by apprehension. It can be quite irregular when the trachea needs suctioning. Sternal retractions can develop when there is respiratory distress. Some of the variations obviously hold little significance while some of them are real clues for the nurse. A simple suctioning procedure may clear the passageway and reestablish a normal respiratory rate after rest. A rapid shallow rate may indicate more serious difficulty and coupled with other unfavorable vital signs, such as a decrease in blood pressure, may need immediate medical intervention. The child frequently returns from the operating room with an endotracheal tube. If the child does not have adequate respiratory ventilation, he will be placed on a monitor. The child is removed from the monitor as soon as adequate respiratory function is established. The endotracheal tube is removed when the child is fully conscious.

Other Recordings

The central venous pressure (CVP) is also monitored closely. This is done to be sure that the child is not receiving too much intravenous fluid or losing too much blood. The CVP is a recording of the amount of pressure in the right atrium. It is the reading used to evaluate the balance between the blood being pumped into the systemic circulation and the venous return to the heart. The CVP falls slightly with inspiration and it rises slightly with expiration. The nurse is responsible for taking the readings and monitoring the results. The readings should remain fairly stable if the child is progressing satisfactorily.

The child is on intake and output and may also be on urinary specific gravity recordings.

Each hospital has its own procedure for recording these nursing observations. In addition to those specifically ordered by the physician, the nurse has several more significant observations which will be useful in determining the child's progress or lack of progress.

NURSING OBSERVATIONS

One observation will be in relation to the warmth of the child's body. Is it only warm to touch on the trunk, despite a slight postoperative temperature elevation? What is needed to warm the child's cold extremities? Is a pair of cotton socks or mitts adequate? Does he need three cotton blankets inside the tent to rest comfortably? Or does he toss and turn and try curling up to get warm despite the use of three blankets?

In relation to medication for pain, does the child rest quietly after absorption or does he still have the look of anxiety in his eyes? Does he seem to need medication to achieve his much needed rest? Does he seem to need medication after visits from the physician or his parents, or the laboratory technician? Does he cough better if he receives his medication prior to coughing or should it be withheld for better results? Does any one procedure, such as suctioning, trigger his need for medication? Does his pain interrupt his sleep? Any of these recordings can be valuable guides to the physician responsible for ordering adequate doses of medication.

As a nurse, you should ask yourself what other observations are significant in caring for this child. Are vital signs, warmth, and pain the only indicators necessary to achieve effective nursing care? This necessitates an evaluation process which is extremely important. The evaluation process will include such factors, such as providing a safe environment, maintaining adequate fluid and electrolyte balance, and maintaining adequate oxygenation.

Providing a Safe Environment

In relation to meeting the objective of providing the child with a safe environment, we have already discussed the precautions in regard to chest tubes and the checking of vital signs by two competent persons when in doubt. As yet we have not included the use of side rails when the nurse is not at the bedside, the positioning of the oxygen tent for protection if the siderail cannot be pulled up, the precaution of not using woolen blankets in oxygen tents, and the correct positioning of electric equipment to avoid contact with the oxygen tent.

The child should be placed in an area where he will be exposed to the least amount of cross-contamination. This contamination may be the result of drafts due to opening doors, open windows, or other patients, staff, or family. His care should be limited to a few well-qualified professional personnel who are in optimum health.

The safe environment should also include a check of the child's toys. Toys with sharp edges should not be left in the crib as he might roll on them and hurt himself or puncture a tube.

Providing a safe environment also includes the use of restraints as a protection for the child. Younger children sometimes have mitts applied, rather than restraints, to protect them from pulling at the tubes.

Maintaining Fluid and Electrolyte Balance

The objective of maintaining adequate fluid and electrolyte balance has been partially covered in the discussion of CVP recordings and intake and output. The child will usually return from the operating room with parenteral fluids running. The physician's order sheet should be consulted for the proper amount and drops to be administered. The I.V. should be counted and regulated if the flow has been disturbed during transportation. In addition, depending on the postoperative course, it will soon be the nurse's responsibility to provide the child with adequate oral intake. This intake should be divided to allow for evening and night personnel to also offer the child fluids. Spacing of the allowed oral intake will decrease the child's possibility of extreme thirst on any one tour of duty. It will also diminish the possibility of the night nurse's feeling obliged to get the child to take all the remainder of the fluid intake for the 24-hour period.

Urinary output is usually not difficult to obtain from school-age children. Children who have not achieved continence provide more of a challenge. Depending on their age, they are used to voiding more frequently. However, many children will have indwelling catheters immediately postoperatively. This will necessitate additional care of the perineal area. The measuring of urinary output may be on an hourly basis during the immediate postoperative period. As the child progresses, it may be measured on each shift or daily. Again, it is the nurse's responsibility to be aware of the policy being followed as accurate reporting of intake and output is essential.

The reader is referred to Fig. 10 for a comparison of the adult and infant extracellular water turnover for a day. This will help to emphasize the extreme importance of keeping accurate account of all the fluid entering or leaving the child's body.

Normal individuals of all ages require 100 to 150 ml of maintenance water per 100 calories metabolized. Since the infant and child have higher metabolic rates per kilogram than does the adult, the younger patient needs more water per unit of weight than the older patient (Statland,1963). (Table 3.)

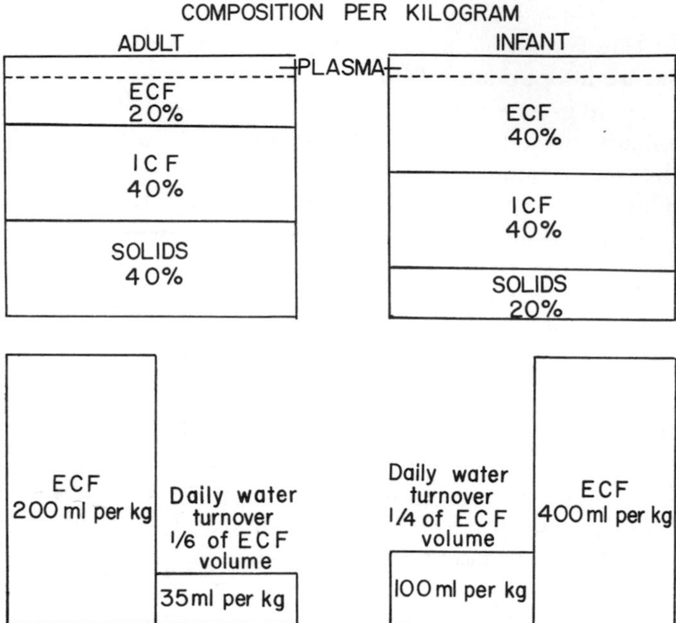

FIG. 10. Body water partition and comparison of daily water turnover to the extracellular fluid volume in the newborn and the adult (Courtesy of Statland, 1963).

In addition the nurse should be aware of the ordinary maintenance requirements of fluid. According to Statland, the amount of water given should approximate the fluid expended for ordinary physiologic activity. Studies in both infants and adults indicate that these losses are roughly proportional to energy expenditure (Table 4).

These are only maintenance requirements for the child. The intake will also include fluid to replace losses during the operative and postoperative period.

TABLE 3
Approximate Energy Expenditure During Parenteral Fluid Therapy*

AGE	WEIGHT (KG)	CALORIES EXPENDED TOTAL (PER 24 HR)	CALORIES EXPENDED PER KG (PER 24 HR)	MAINTENANCE WATER PER 100 CAL (ML)
4 Months	5	500	100	100
2 Years	15	1250	83	100
10 Years	30	1700	57	100
Adult	60	2300	38	100

*Adapted from Statland, 1963.

TABLE 4
Usual Expenditures of Water Per 100 Calories Metabolized*

EXPENDITURE	WATER (ml)
Insensible perspiration	45
lungs	15
skin	30
Sweat (sensible perspiration)	20
Stool	5
Urine	30 to 80
Total	100 to 150

*Adapted from Darrow and Pratt (Courtesy of Statland, 1963).

The nurse should also aid the physician in determining losses which are not easily measured—the loss by perspiration, drainage, or bed-wetting. The wet sheet may be a poor way to estimate loss as fluid quickly spreads in sheets and gives a false impression of a large loss. However, it is important to include this information in the nurse's notes. For example: "Sheet changed—moderate amount serosanguineous drainage in area of chest bandage. Drainage appeared between 8:00 and 10:00 A.M."

In addition, the nurse needs to observe the child for perspiration. It is not enough to assume that if his johnny shirt is dry, then he is not perspiring. The perspiration may show on his forehead or the palms of his hands. A flushing of the child's face is also significant, as it may be a clue to additional water losses.

For information about intravenous equipment, the reader is referred to a pediatric nursing textbook and to the company supplying the intravenous equipment in a particular hospital.

Maintaining Adequate Oxygenation

The child will usually receive oxygen immediately postoperatively. This can be achieved by using an isolette with an infant or an oxygen tent with an older child. Infrequently an adolescent may receive nasal oxygen. The nasal administration of oxygen dries the mucus membranes and is more irritating to the child. Oxygen administered by other methods is given with mist and this lubricates the mucus membranes. If for any reason, the child has to be transported to another area for x-ray, nasal oxygen or mask oxygen can be used during the transporting.

The administration of oxygen by isolette provides a fairly constant oxygen supply unless the top of the isolette is opened. Most nursing care can be effectively administered through the portholes. If the top is opened, the infant may become hypoxic. If so, the isolette should be closed and a high concentration of oxygen delivered to resaturate the isolette. The liter flow of oxygen should be prescribed by the physician. The 40 percent concentration may be in effect if it is a very small infant; however, it is not nearly so important if the child's blood supply to the eyes is mature.

The oxygen tent does not guarantee as good a supply of oxygen for the older child. There is a wider area involved, the light weight plastic canopy is less effective than the harder plastic, and there is more possibility for oxygen to escape because the tent is only tucked under the mattress or bed linens. For making an oxygen bed, the student should refer to a pediatric nursing textbook.

According to Crocker (1970), continuous ultrasonic nebulization should never be used in infants and probably not in older children either, as it may supply as much as 6 ml per minute of fluid to the child and particularly in intubated infants, water intoxication may occur. It is possible to supply the infant or child with his total daily water requirement by ultrasonic nebulization.

The nurse should observe the child for signs of cyanosis. Cyanosis usually appears first in the child's fingernails. For this reason, any nail polish should be removed prior to surgery and left off during the child's postoperative period. Another area to observe is the child's lips or around the oral orifice. Cyanosis may be an expected symptom due to the child's cardiac condition and it may not disappear as a result of a palliative cardiac procedure. The reader will familiarize herself/himself with the cardiac defects to know whether this cyanosis is expected.

Adequate suctioning is also necessary to provide an adequate oxygen supply. The nasal passages should be kept clean and mucus suctioned from the trachea. Sterile technique should be adhered to during suctioning to cut down on the possibility of infection. Deeper suctioning may be necessary, and this is again determined by the policies of the hospital and the nurse's training. In some hospitals only physicians do the deeper suctioning, but it is becoming more common for nurses to be taught this procedure.

Crocker (1970) recommends that assisted ventilation be performed prior to suctioning episodes when a tracheostomy is in place. This ventilation is done with a suitable bag and adaptor for three to five minutes prior to suctioning in order to prevent the rapid aspiration of oxygen from the airway with resultant hypoxia.

Coughing, Turning, Deep Breathing

It is known that the nurse caring for the child postoperatively reaps the benefits of the preoperative teaching. He/She utilizes the same techniques used preoperatively to get the child's cooperation. Coughing, encouraging deep breathing, and turning the child every 1 to 2 hours aids in the maintenance of oxygenation.

Intermittent positive-pressure therapy is frequently used in addition to the administration of oxygen. In the less serious cardiac conditions, the child may not receive continuous oxygen therapy but may receive IPPB to help loosen secretions and clear the bronchial tree. On occasion postural draining is also ordered. The complexity of this procedure when chest tubes, endotracheal tubes, and pain are present is obvious.

Pain must not be forgotten as a possibility of causing respiratory problems and diminishing oxygen supply. The child may intentionally choose not to breathe deeply in order to decrease the amount of pain. It is the nurse's responsibility to evaluate the child's pain and to administer narcotics to keep him comfortable. Narcotics can decrease the respiratory rate and this should be kept in mind.

It is quite evident that the independent nursing activities play a big role in the maintenance of adequate oxygenation.

Cardiopulmonary Resuscitation (CRP)

The ABCs of cardiopulmonary resuscitation are Airway, Breathing, and Circulation. The signs of cardiac arrest are the absence of a heartbeat and an absence of carotid pulse. The signs of respiratory arrest are apnea and cyanosis. The goal of CPR is to counter these symptoms by ventilating the lungs and compressing the heart by manual pressure. The airway must be clear of vomitus, mucus or obstructions. The child's head and neck are hyperextended to open the airway. The child's jaw is pulled forward and up, to prevent the tongue from falling backward and obstructing the passage. The child's nose is closed off and mouth to mouth resuscitation is begun. In smaller children the mouth and nose may be covered by the nurses mouth, the object being to assure a tight seal. The nurse repeats the mouth to mouth every five seconds. To compress the heart, the nurse uses the heel of her/his hand. She/he puts pressure over the chest wall 80 to 100 compressions per minute. This is continued until rhythmic heartbeat and pulse return.

Reorientation to Time and Place

The intensive care unit should be equipped with clocks and calendars to help reorient the child to time and place. The younger child will enjoy having a children's clock. The type wound by pulling chains can be fun. The older child will benefit by an ordinary clock. The clock should be close by the bedside, so the child can refer to it easily. For older children, the calendars can be of the conventional type, with scenes depicting areas of the child's interest. For the younger child a calendar can be made and large numbers used. The numbers can be added daily so he knows the last one up is the day's date. In addition, clouds, rain, sun, or snow pictures can be added so the child knows the weather. This is especially important if the child cannot see out of the window. Changes of the weather can be made during the day if changes occur outside. This is helpful too if the parents are unable to get to the hospital because of inclement weather, the child has already been oriented to that possibility.

Convalescence and Discharge

The convalescent period will depend on the surgery and its follow-up supervision. The degree of activity will be prescribed by the physician. The parents and child must be fully informed of the activity allowed as well as any restrictions. They should be fully aware of their follow-up appointments. They also need to know any adverse signs which necessitate immediate medical care.

The child who has received a significant improvement in his physical condition due to surgical repair may have a difficult time adjusting to his new status. Glaser et al (1964) notes that the child and the parent may have a difficult time adjusting to the more vigorous physical activity now possible for the child. The child will need time to adjust to the extended privileges of independence with his peers. He may also have difficulty adjusting to the more strenuous educational goals now open to him.

If the surgery has been less successful, the parents and child have to learn to cope with the permanency of the condition and to readjust their goals in relation to the limitations imposed by the cardiac condition.

RHEUMATIC FEVER

Rheumatic fever is a medical condition requiring long-term care. It was chosen because of its high incidence of related carditis and extended care is needed even when carditis is not present.

The length of the period needed for treating the disease as well as the fear generated by repeated susceptibility to the disease are factors contributing to the respect given the disease. Also, the knowledge that the disease is responsible for the majority of heart disease in persons under 40 years of age makes it a particularly dreaded disease. It is also responsible for a significant number of deaths in children.

Rheumatic fever is a long-term disease that illustrates the significance of the host factor in relation to disease. Two factors which play a part in the disease are economics and environment. The child from a lower socioeconomic family is more prone to the disease. This may be related to the child's physical environment. If the house is crowded or damp, which are frequently conditions of the lower socioeconomic housing, the child is more susceptible to rheumatic fever. After the child becomes infected by the streptococcus organism, he is less likely to be able to combat the attack, and rheumatic fever follows. The child from a crowded home is more likely to be exposed to more bacteria because of his close associations with other people in the household or building. Also, in conditions of overcrowding, minor infections such as pharyngitis are less likely to receive medical attention.

Age is another factor. Children between the ages of five and fifteen years are most commonly affected. The children in this age range are also more susceptible to streptococcal infections. Latitude and altitude are also considered to affect the incidence of rheumatic fever. The disease has a higher incidence in temperate zones and in seasons when respiratory infections reach their maximum peak—late winter and early spring. The age factor seems to also play a role in reinfection. As the child gets older, he is less likely to suffer rheumatic fever as a result of reinfection with the streptococcus organism.

Lastly, heredity may also play a role in the disease as there is a higher than usual incidence of the disease in more than one family member.

Rheumatic fever seems to be decreasing in incidence as the standards of living are improved. Another important factor in the apparent decrease is the use of antimicrobial therapy. Stronger statements regarding decrease cannot be made, as the disease is not always reported; therefore, its true incidence is really not known.

Another factor which makes reporting difficult is the problem of making a definite diagnosis. The Jones criteria have been developed as a guide for physicians (Table 5).

Presenting Symptoms

The child who has had a Group A hemolytic streptococcus infection may recover with little attention to the illness. Approximately four weeks later, the child may have any one of a number of symptoms. He may report to the school nurse with a headache, or a sudden sore throat, or he may develop abdominal pain with nausea and vomiting. The headache or sore throat may receive little attention as the school nurse or parent may not link them to the child's previous illness. The abdominal pain may get better attention as it closely resembles the pain of appendicitis. The child frequently has a temperature elevation of 101 to 104 F. On closer examination by a physician the child may show additional signs such as a reddened throat, a rash on the trunk, or subcutaneous nodules.

If a physician is not available at school, the parent should be instructed to seek a medical opinion. Treating the child at home with aspirin may only mask the symptoms and delay the therapeutic regime.

TABLE 5
Jones Criteria (Revised) for Guidance in the Diagnosis of Rheumatic Fever*

MAJOR MANIFESTATIONS	MINOR MANIFESTATIONS
Carditis	Clinical
Polyarthritis	Previous rheumatic fever or rheumatic heart disease
Chorea	Arthralgia
Erythema marginatum	Fever
Subcutaneous nodules	Laboratory
	Acute phase reactions
	Erythrocyte sedimentation rate, C-reactive protein leukocytosis
	Prolonged P-R interval

SUPPORTING EVIDENCE OF STREPTOCOCCAL INFECTION

Increased titer of streptococcal antibodies
- ASO (antistreptolysin O)
- Other Antibodies

Positive throat culture for Group A streptococcus
Recent scarlet fever

*The presence of two major criteria, or of one major and two minor criteria, indicates a high probability of the presence of rheumatic fever. Evidence of a preceding streptococcal infection greatly strengthens the possibility of acute rheumatic fever. Its absence should make the diagnosis doubtful (except in Syndenham's chorea or long-standing carditis). From Jones Criteria (revised) for guidance in the diagnosis of rheumatic fever, American Heart Association, 1967.

The Acute Phase

The nursing responsibilities during the acute phase center around astute observations of signs and symptoms and alleviation of pain. The child admitted without a previous history of rheumatic fever will have diagnostic tests prior to instituting medical therapy. During this period, the child may be extremely uncomfortable due to pain in the large joints. The mother may say to you, "Please give him an aspirin, it helped his pain at home." It is important to explain to his mother and to the child that proper use of drugs is dependent on the tests which are scheduled. In the interim, the physician has not prescribed aspirin. The mother and child may benefit further by talking with the physician. The arthritis is usually associated with the large joints such as the wrists, elbows, knees, or ankles. These parts are very tender and usually swollen. They are painful to move and painful to touch.

Nursing measures can help to make the child more comfortable. The affected joint or joints may feel more comfortable when supported on pillows. When the child turns he may appreciate support to the limb. The child will benefit by a properly fitted foot board, one that supports the feet and not merely the bed clothes. The foot board must be placed so the feet can easily reach it without effort on the child's part (Fig. 11). If the bedclothes seem to be causing pressure on the affected parts, a bed cradle may be used. If it is, the child might enjoy a small, lightweight receiving blanket next to his body (his "security blanket").

During the acute phase, the child will frequently have a temperature elevation. This makes him more prone to perspire. A comforting measure is to bathe the child more frequently with tepid water. He will also need more frequent changes of bed linen. Skin care is also important. The child may try to "overprotect" his involved arms by not moving them at all. This will increase the possibility of irritation under the axilla due to perspiration. Cleaning, drying thoroughly, and applying a light dusting of talcum powder will help to prevent skin breakdown and also odor. The older child may try to discourage the nurse from washing under the axilla. The child offers a can of spray deodorant and tries to have just this used. He needs to know that repeated application of deodorants, without washing, will only add to the irritation problem. An explanation that you will move the arm as gently as possible will usually win the child's approval or at least his cooperation.

The observation of signs and symptoms will aid the physician in his/her attempt to diagnose the illness adequately. One of the responsibilities of the nurse is the accurate taking of a pulse rate. This is counted for a full minute to get as accurate a count as possible. The pulse is usually taken every four hours. In addition a sleeping pulse is frequently ordered during the night. The nurse must be very gentle so she/he does not awaken the child. If the child does wake up, the pulse should be scheduled for a later hour and the actual time recorded. A change in the quality of the pulse is an indication that there may be cardiac involvement. Rheumatic fever is closely associated with mitral valve lesions.

Pericarditis may be present. If so, the child will have a friction rub. A variety of murmurs may also be detected. It is the carditis that severly complicates the course of the disease. Competent management will help to decrease the possibility of congestive heart failure.

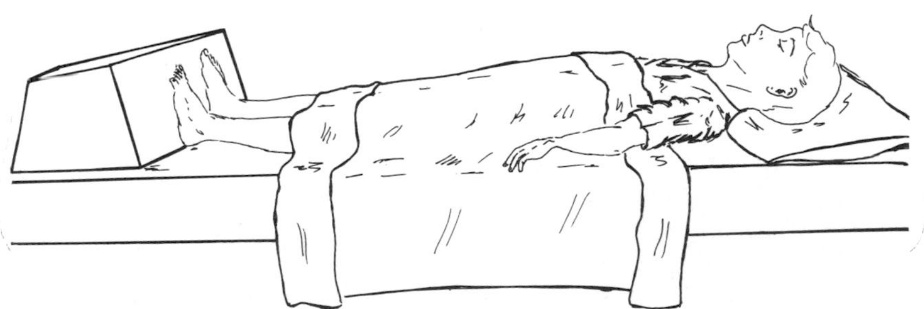

FIG. 11. Proper placement of footboard for maximum utilization.

Another observation the nurse can make is in relation to the rash that is sometimes present in children with rheumatic fever. It frequently appears during the child's bath and then disappears. The rash should be described and the areas involved clearly spelled out in the nurse's notes or progress record.

During the bath it is also possible to check for any nodules and describe their location. These subcutaneous nodules appear most commonly on tendon sheaths along the elbows, edge of the patella, scapula, vertebrae, and occiput. They are usually painless but their presence helps to establish the diagnosis. Any limitation of movement of extremities can also be evaluated during the bath. The bath is usually given by the nurse during the evaluation period, on the assumption that the child has the disease. After diagnosis the bath is usually given by the nurse until all signs of acute infection have subsided and the laboratory results are returning to normal or near normal ranges. Another less common condition associated with rheumatic fever is chorea. This is a twitching or involuntary movement of the body. This involvement of the nervous system is frightening to the child and the parents. The child must be protected from injury during this period. It may be necessary to pad siderails to decrease bruising if the child is thrashing too much.

Bed Rest

The child with acute rheumatic fever is usually placed on complete bed rest. This therapy is beginning to be questioned. Some physicians are now allowing the child out of bed after 48 hours on medication, while others still maintain bed rest for several weeks. The child with carditis is more likely to be kept in bed for extended periods. However, the physician will prescribe the activity restrictions for the individual child. The nurse will be responsible for trying to maintain this order. During the acute stage, the child is usually in pain and bed-rest is maintained easier than during the convalescent stage. During convalescent period, it becomes increasingly difficult to provide activities that will make him content, despite his restrictions. (This will be discussed in greater detail in relation to the convalescent period.)

Positioning of the child is extremely important because of the possible circulatory involvement and the effects of bed-rest. Rubber rings and donuts are not indicated. Careful attention to the bed linen to get rid of wrinkles is very important. Also, children are prone to drop crumbs, crayons, and other small objects, like paper clips in their beds. These items can cause pressure and lead to decubitus. The child will also benefit from having the head of the bed elevated. The degree of elevation needed for the child to be comfortable should be included in the observations. In the more acute circumstances, the child may be placed in an oxygen tent.

Mouth Care

The child who is having pain frequently breathes through his mouth. This will cause drying of the mucus membranes and perhaps cracking at the corners of the mouth. Mouth care should be given, using the child's toothbrush and paste from home. If these items are not available, a hospital mouthwash and cleaning with cotton tip applicators can be done until a toothbrush and paste are available. Some mineral oil or cold cream can be applied sparingly to the lips if they are cracking. Children are not usually receptive to the common lemon and glycerin offered adults for mouth care. A scientific rationale for selectively using lemon and glycerin is illustrated in a study by Van Drimmelen and Rollins (1969) on elderly people. Lemon and glycerin one-to-one dried the oral tissues at the first few days after instituting care. This drying can be very uncomfortable to a child who breathes through his mouth. It is also contraindicated in children immediately postoperatively when you are attempting to keep the mucus membranes moist. The lemon and glycerin tended to increase the moisture in the mouth after four or five days of use, but by this time the child is frequently well enough to resume brushing in the usual manner. The study did show, however, that cleansing with lemon and glycerin did improve the general condition of the mouth and the findings support the rationale for mouth care. (The prepared applicators for oral hygiene are saturated solutions of glycerin and lemon one-to-one.)

If the child uses an electric toothbrush at home, this may provide a nice link with home, if it can be brought in. It is necessary to make this judgment after exploring the type of electric toothbrush used. The battery-operated types can be used if oxygen is in use, but those that require electric cords should not be used when oxygen is in use.

Medication Therapy

After the preliminary laboratory tests are completed, the physician may begin a trial period with aspirin. Nursing responsibilities include administering the drug on a prescribed time schedule, noting relief of pain from the drug, noting the recurrence of pain if any, and noting side-effects such as ringing in the ears or nausea. In addition, the aspirin will aid in the comfort of the child by reducing the elevated temperatures.

This trial period is especially important as it may provide very essential information to the diagnosing physician. Very detailed nursing notes are essential during this period.

After the diagnosis has been established, the child is started on medication therapy. This may include a combination of salicylates, penicillin, and occasionally adrenal corticosteroids, and barbiturates. The steroids may be withheld to see if there is cardiac involvement and how severe it is. In approximately 50 to 70 percent of initial cases, cardiac involvement may not be an issue. The steroids have been found to be more effective than aspirin in combating the acute inflammation but they do not seem to cut down the cardiac scarring. For this reason, they are frequently omitted and aspirin given alone. The use of barbiturates is dependent on how anxious or active the child is during the acute phase. They are used more when carditis is present. Digitalis and diuretics may also be ordered for treatment of the heart failure during acute rheumatic fever. A course of penicillin is given to combat the Group A streptococci. The penicillin therapy is usually administered through adulthood on a prophylactic basis.

The length of time the aspirin or cortisone therapy is continued varies from six to twelve weeks, with the more involved forms lasting six months or more. The drugs are withdrawn on a gradual basis with close attention being given to the C-reactive protein and the sedimentation rate. The C-R protein gradually disappears from the blood and the sedimentation rate should decrease.

In long-term salicylate therapy, poisoning is a frequent occurrence. Toxic symptoms include nausea, vomiting, tinnitis, blurred vision, and headaches. Salicylates also interfere with prothrombin synthesis and signs of hemorrhage (such as ecchymoses) are common. The trend is away from massive doses of aspirin to more moderate therapy.

The nurse is responsible for checking with the child regarding any of these side-effects and notifying the physician before continuing therapy. Some children need enteric-coated aspirin to stop the nausea and vomiting due to irritation rather than poisoning.

The penicillin therapy is usually maintained on a long term basis. If carditis is present, it is not uncommon to have the penicillin continued throughout the child's lifetime.

Laboratory Tests

Sedimentation Rate and C-Reactive Protein The sedimentation rate and C-reactive protein are both blood tests. They usually necessitate a venous puncture and therefore can be a threat to the child. The sedimentation rate is also referred to as the ESR (erythrocyte sedimentation rate). The sedimentation rate is a nonspecific test, but it is frequently used when one is monitoring inflammatory processes. It is an estimate of the suspension stability of erythrocytes. In conditions such as rheumatic fever, tuberculosis, and cancer, there is an increased speed of sedimentation. The cause of this increase is not clear. However, sedimentation is known to be the result of the greater density of the erythrocytes than of plasma. The test has more value following the prognosis of the disease than in actual diagnosis.

The normal values vary according to the many different techniques available to the laboratory. The normal values are higher for females than males, and they also vary with age. For the normal values in a particular agency, the nurse should contact the laboratory. In some instances the normal values are printed on the lab sheet reporting the child's results.

The C-reactive protein or CRP is an indicator of inflammation or infection. Again, the change in the results is useful for prognosis and in evaluating the therapeutic plan of care, but the test is not specific for any disease entity. In some agencies a micro method has been devised for performing this test and a finger prick, earlobe prick, or heel prick will give the necessary blood. The child still needs adequate and honest preparation before the specimen is taken. The readings vary from 0 to +4. The +4 rating is given for maximum precipitation and the 0 reading for no precipitation. In persons free of disease there is no CRP in the blood serum: When there is an active inflammatory process the protein will be found. It can be found in the joint fluids as well as in the blood serum. The amount of the protein found is an indicator of the severity of the inflammatory process. Therefore, if a child had a +2 CRP, it indicates that his disease is presently less severe than the child who has a +4 CRP. When a child is first admitted with rheumatic fever, it is not uncommon for him to have a +4 CRP. After therapy is instituted, the CRP will decrease and eventually not be present.

Antistreptolysin 0 Titers The antistreptolysin 0 titers, also known as the ASO titer or ASTO titer or ASLO titer are agglutination tests again done from the venous blood sample or by the micro method. An elevated level is present when there has been a recent streptococcus infection. Usually a titer is considered significant if it remains elevated over a period of time. An elevated titer, according to Shaeffer and Goldin (1969), is 166 Todd units or higher. If the child has suspected rheumatic fever, a series of ASO titers will be drawn. If they produce low readings, the diagnosis of rheumatic fever will be ruled out. If the readings are elevated, they will be used along with the other clinical evidence to make a definitive diagnosis.

The Convalescent Phase

In most cases, the convalescent phase provides many more challenges to the nurse in providing care. The child is now usually free from pain and he no longer is content to remain in bed. Ideas for helping to pass the long hours can be found in Chapter 2.

During the convalescent phase it is necessary to make arrangements for the child's discharge. These arrangements may be complicated by the reluctance of the physician to return the child to living conditions which might predispose him to another attack. A medical social worker as well as a community health nurse can be valuable team members in preparing the child for the discharge and preparing the home for the child.

Sometimes the home is not the answer and other living arrangements have to be made. Foster home placement or convalescent hospitals have been effectively utilized when the child's home cannot meet his needs.

Basically, the home needs to be well heated and the child should have a bed of his own. Ideally he should have a room of his own. If he is discharged on bed-rest or modified activity, the bed is best placed on the first floor of the house. This will make it easier for the mother to grant his needs. The room should be equipped with the same type activities for occupying his time as were provided in the hospital. In addition, quiet times need to be provided for the child to do school work.

The mother will need assistance in understanding the child's impatience with his restricted activities. She will also need an explanation of the importance of follow-up for medical supervision and penicillin therapy. The mother can be supplied with a pamphlet, such as Home Care of the Child with Rheumatic Fever, for helpful hints about caring for the child.

It is not common for children to be placed outside of the home after hospital discharge. The usual plan is to return them to their place in their own family. The use of prophylactic penicillin helps to make this possible. Also, helping the family to understand the importance of protecting the child from exposure to illness is essential.

When the child is ready to return to school, the school nurse and teacher must be made fully aware of the child's limitations in activity, if any. The teacher should understand that the child should avoid exposure to infections and if he gets a minor cold he will be kept out of school as a precautionary measure.

The mother and teacher might appreciate reading the pamphlet entitled Heart Disease in Children to help them understand the disease process more fully.

Follow-up

In both the medical and surgical cardiac conditions, follow-up care is indicated. It is very easy for the mother to forget to continue the medication when the child appears well. The mother needs to know the reasons for the medication. She needs to develop an appreciation for a drug such as lanoxin, so she does not become lax in its administration. The financial strain of the illness needs to be periodically explored so that help can be sought if necessary. A social worker is usually well informed of the current funds available from local, state, and federal sources.

In both the medical and surgical cardiac conditions it will be necessary to help the child master the developmental tasks he has lost and to proceed to achieve new developmental tasks. If the child has relinquished trust as a result of hospitalization, he must be helped to master it again and move on to the next stage of development. The child who has been so restricted by disease that he did not have the opportunity to pass through the developmental stages at the expected time will need assistance to master them after his convalescent period.

As nurses we can begin this "restoration" of developmental achievement while the child is still hospitalized. There is reason to suspect that after a long hospitalization, with or without surgery, the child can begin to mistrust adults. This mistrust may just be caused by the child's feeling that his parents have deserted him. The nurse can begin to help the child to reestablish trust by emphasizing that the parents have him in the hospital because it is the best place for him to get well. The nurse emphasizes the fact that the parents want the very best for him and that they also want him back home as soon as possible. The child needs to know that, despite the many painful procedures he has had, the hospital personnel have helped to make him better. The parents should be encouraged to use a similar approach during their visits. If they come in and say, "I want to get you out of this terrible place as soon as possible," the child cannot help but mistrust adults. They all say different things.

Parents need guidance not to cast the medical personnel in a "poor light" hoping to win the child's approval. The child then wonders even more why the parents have "put him in the hospital."

One only has to ask a child, "Why are you here?" to appreciate how confused children really are about their hospitalization. Adults should not confuse them more.

The other factor which needs special emphasis is not to try to fool the child. Children deserve an honest and simple explanation so they can feel comfortable. As the child gets older he deserves an explanation of his cardiac status so he can make realistic vocational, educational, and social goals.

CASE PRESENTATION AND STUDY QUESTIONS

John is a three-year-old admitted for evaluation of a heart murmur discovered during routine physical examinations done on children of migrant farm workers. He has been in the area two weeks and is residing in a mobile home with his mother, father, and six other children. Both of John's parents work long hours and the length of their stay in the area is dependent on the crops. They estimate they will be here approximately one to two weeks before moving to another area.

John is being exposed to medical personnel and facilities for the first time. Despite his young age, he will be expected to cope with most of the experiences without the support of his family.

1. What types of things can you do for John to help overcome the effects of hospitalization?
2. Are there any past experiences which John has had which will help in his adjustment to the hospital?
3. What types of things might be done to help maintain contact with John's family?

John is scheduled for a cardiac catheterization on his third day of hospitalization. His parents have agreed to come to the hospital at 5:00 A.M. to sign the consent on the day of the catheterization. They have not visited John since admission.

1. What explanation do you have for the parents not visiting John?
2. Why would the parents arrive at the hospital at 5:00 A.M.?
3. Should a nurse be available to talk with the parents on their arrival?
4. Will the parents be able to see John at this hour? If so, what preparation will be necessary for the visit? Is preparation considered necessary?

The diagnostic workup is completed and John is found to have a ventricular septal defect. A telegram is sent to the parents requesting them to come for an appointment with the physician. Both parents come in for the interview. Despite a thorough and careful explanation, the parents deny their child has a heart defect.

1. Why do you think the parents denied the heart defect?
2. Was there anything the physician could do to change the parents' initial reaction?
3. What additional things are necessary, if any, to be done to help the parents understand?
4. What social problems do you think will be created by this diagnosis? (Include aspects in relation to the migrant family.)

The physicians have decided that John needs open heart surgery. They are aware of John's lack of previous medical attention. He has not even had beginning immunizations and his hemoglobin is low due to dietary deficiencies. The physicians feel pressured by time as they know the family, in their future work, will be located in rural areas without easy access to a large medical facility. They decide to ask the family to allow John to have his corrective surgery during this hospitalization. After a great deal of discussion, it is decided that John and his mother will remain for the surgery. The rest of the family will move southward for the next harvest.

1. What provisions will need to be made for John's mother? What other members of the team can be utilized in making these plans?
2. John's preparation will include emphasis on nutritional aspects. What information will you want to gather? What teaching will be included?
3. How will you prepare John for surgery? What aids can you use in this preparation? When will the preparation be done?
4. During the surgical procedure you spend some time talking to John's mother. You learn, for the first time, that she is pregnant and fears the expected baby will have a heart defect.
5. What immediate responses will you make?
6. What follow-up will you arrange?
7. Why do you think his mother revealed this information at this time? Will the added stress of pregnancy need to be considered when discussing John?

John returns from the intensive care unit on his fifth day postoperatively. He has been progressing adequately with only minor complications which responded readily to therapy. His mother will remain just three more days and then she will join her family. John will stay additional time in the hospital to compensate for the limited medical supervision he will receive at his next residence.

1. What preparations will need to be made before his mother leaves?
2. What suggestions should be made regarding John's future discharge?
3. How will John be prepared for his mother's departure? What changes can be expected in John's progress when he learns he will be left alone? How will you offset these changes?

BIBLIOGRAPHY

Barnes CM: Working with parents of children undergoing heart surgery. Nurs Clin North Am 4:11, March 1969

Blake FG: Open Heart Surgery in Children. Washington, DC, U.S. Department of Health, Education, and Welfare, Children's Bureau Pamphlet No. 418, 1964

Botwin ED: Should children be screened for hypertension? Mat Child Nurs 1:152, 1976

Coats K: Techniques in cardiac diagnosis. Nurs Clin North Am 11:259, 1976

Crocker D: The critically ill child: management of tracheostomy. Pediatrics 46:286, 1970

Darrow DC, Pratt EL: Fluid therapy: relation to tissue and the expenditure of water and electrolyte. JAMA 365, 432, 1950

Diagnosis, Therapy, and Prophylaxis of Streptococcal Pharyngitis in the Control of Rheumatic Fever. Wyeth Laboratories, May 1965

Doyle E: Congestive heart failure in infancy. Sanchez Panorama 5(3), 1968

Fink C et al: Differentiating rheumatic fever from juvenile rheumatoid arthritis. Patient Care, Nov 1968, p 71

Freidberg DZ, Litwin SB: The medical and surgical management of patients with congenital heart disease. Clin Pediatr 15:324, 1976

Glaser HH, Harrison GS, Lynn DB: Emotional implications of congenital heart disease in children. Pediatrics 33:367, 1964

Green J, Levitt EE: Constriction of body image in children with congenital heart disease. Pediatrics 29:438, 1962

———, Haggerty R: Ambulatory Pediatrics. Philadelphia, Saunders, 1968, pp 666–74

Heart disease in children. American Heart Association, 1956

Home care of the child with rheumatic fever. American Heart Association, New York, 1959

Jackson K: Psychological preparation as a method of reducing emotional trauma of anesthesia in children. Anesthesiology 12:293, 1951

Jensen J: Introduction to Medical Physics. Philadelphia, Lippincott, 1960, Chap 8

Kennaird DL: Oxygen consumption and evaporative water loss in infants with congenital heart disease. Arch Dis Child 51:34, 1976

Maxwell GM, Gane S: The impact of congenital heart disease on the family. Am Heart J 64:449, 1962

Neuhaus ED: A personality study of asthmatic and cardiac children. Psychosom Med 20:181, 1958

Owen SL: The Three R's & HBP: A unique approach to school health and high blood pressure education. Image 8:13, 1976

Pidgeon V: The infant with congenital heart disease. Am J Nurs 67:290, Feb 1967

Pitorak EF: Open-ended care for the open heart patient. Am J Nurs 67:1452, July 1967

Posey RA: Creative nursing care of babies with heart disease. Nursing '74 4:40, Oct 1974

Prevention of rheumatic fever. American Heart Association, New York, 1964

Raffensperger JG, Primrose RB (eds): Pediatric Surgery for Nurses. Boston, Little, Brown, 1968 Chap 3

Rogoz B: Nursing care of the cardiac surgery patient. Nurs Clin North Am 4:631, 1969

Ross J: The nurse and the patient with open-heart surgery. J Nurs Educ 1:25, Sept 1962

Shaffer J, Goldin M: Serodiagnostic tests in diseases other than syphilis. In Todd-Sanford Clinical Diagnosis, 14th ed. Philadelphia, Saunders, 1969

Statland H: Fluid and Electrolytes in Practice. Philadelphia, Lippincott, 1963, Chap 14, p 193

Stollerman GH: Connective tissue disease. In Barnett HL (ed): Pediatrics, 16th ed. New York, Appleton, 1977

Storlie F: Principles of Intensive Nursing Care. New York, Appleton, 1969

Swendsen L: Nursing care of the infant with congestive heart. Nurs Clin North Am 4:621, December 1969

Van Drimmelen J, Rollins HF: Evaluation of commonly used oral hygiene agents. Nurs Res 18:327, July–Aug 1969

SHIRLEY STEELE

13
Nursing Care of the Child with a Fatal Prognosis

The nurse caring for the child with a fatal prognosis needs to be ready to cope with many situations. He/she may be the person settling the ward after the death of a child. He/she may be called upon to give support to the grieving family. He/she may find herself/himself giving support to other staff or students.

To be able to meet these challenges effectively, the nurse should know the normal grieving process, should be aware of the many ways that adults view death, should know at what ages children understand death, and must have constructive means to cope with this knowledge.

The adult (and also the child) undergoes a predictable sequence of events when going through the grieving process. According to Engel (1964), the individual first goes through a stage of shock and disbelief, then through a stage of awareness, then through a restitution state, and finally resolves the loss. The reader is referred to the article for a more thorough explanation of this process.

The child with a fatal illness frequently evokes an immediate feeling of sympathy from the adults in his environment. After the initial reaction the adult gradually rearranges his feelings in accordance with other significant factors he learns about the child. Feelings of sympathy may change to impatience if the child's behavior is disruptive, or sympathy may change to overprotection if the child is afraid and insecure and so forth.

It is important to consider the conditions under which the adult is functioning in order to appreciate his reactions. The parent who has recently undergone other stressful situations may feel that he is being treated unfairly. He may become quite upset and shout obscenities at the physician giving the information. He may also be very hostile toward the nurse, who seems to support the physician's opinion. The parent who has recently gone through a similar grieving process may have that experience immediately revived, and begin crying hysterically.

REACTIONS TO CHILDREN WITH A FATAL PROGNOSIS

As nurses we need to examine our different reactions and the factors which influence these reactions. Certainly age is a major factor in influencing reactions to a fatal prognosis. When the child is a newborn, people frequently remark it is not so bad because the parents did not get a chance to know him. This is certainly far from the case because the parents have been planning for the child since they knew of the child's conception.

The healthy child is frequently considered the greatest loss. Statements such as, "He didn't have a chance to get started in life" are common. The adolescent who has entered college seems to have everything to live for. His shortened life is considered a tragedy. On the other hand, the adolescent who has "copped out" or was addicted to drugs is frequently written off as "no loss." The nature of the disease entity or other precursor of death are a factor. Adults often find it more acceptable for a child with a disability to die than they do for a normal child to die. There are also diseases which have particularly tragic connotations to the public at large. One of these diseases is cancer. Many people still view it as a brutal disease and sometimes even contagious or a cause for disgrace. People also think of cancer as a disease of "old age" and find it particularly difficult to accept in children.

Environmental conditions play a part. Why is it that when a child of a prominent family is fatally ill there is often more concern by the professional staff than when it is a child from a deprived family? There seems to be some misconception that children from "better" homes have more reason to be spared fatal illness. This may be partially based on the fact that these parents have supposedly given better medical supervision to their children and therefore the child should not be susceptible to serious life-threatening illness. It may also be partially based on the fact that the nurse is more closely associated with other professional people, and he/she therefore wants to believe that it cannot happen to professional people because that would include him/her in the potential parent category for having current or future children with premature susceptibility to death.

A person from a culture that permits its people to "act out" their grief is frequently less likely to be tolerated than people from cultures which are "stoic" and "quiet" about their grief. It is even possible to be more specific: on a busy, understaffed unit a child with a fatal illness may be resented because he demands so much additional and emotion-laden care. Or a terminally ill child may dampen the cheerful attitude of a small pediatric unit which prides itself on keeping the children happy and minimizing effects of hospitalization. In a well-equipped intensive care unit the child with a terminal illness may be taken so much as a part of the expected routine that the nurses become too impersonal and neglect his emotional needs which are heightened due to his fears of death as well as the effects of separation from his usual environment.

Particular seasons may influence people's reaction. People seem to be more involved if a child is very sick around a special holiday such as Christmas. If death occurs, the neighbors and friends are especially sympathetic: "What a shame to spoil their Christmas. Every Christmas they will remember this." People frequently tend to feel that the family who has only one child has a greater loss than families with more children. Or, the loss of a boy is more difficult than the loss of a girl. Or the child with a superior intelligence is a greater loss than one of lesser intellectual ability. Some feel that it is easier for a woman of childbearing years to have a child die than one who has completed her childbearing cycle, perhaps believing a future child can take the place of the dead child.

Availability of loved ones to be with the dying child is another factor. If a significant other is separated by a great geographic space and cannot be with his child, everyone feels quite sympathetic. If this person is on his way home, everyone seems to "hold their breath" hoping that he will arrive before the child's condition worsens or before death actually takes place. This list of reactions could be continued ad infinitum as the eminent loss of a child is usually viewed as a tragedy in American society. The list is incomplete but it reflects the wide diversity of reaction responses and helps to put the upcoming discussion into perspective.

The student of nursing who cares for the child will frequently have some of the same responses as the parents of the child. As the female student is frequently of child bearing age, she feels a real closeness to the situation. At first learning the diagnosis, the student may experience the same type of disbelief and denial that the parents have. Students may shy away because they are not able to cure the child. The student is in a period when having children is foremost in his or her mind. Their own close association makes it difficult for them to handle the situation from a professional vantage point rather than from the viewpoint of an involved parent. If the students have children of their own, they frequently see the patient as if he were their own child. Students will frequently wish or request not to be assigned a child with an illness with a fatal prognosis. They fear they will be incapable of handling the situation and unable to talk to the parents without showing overt affective responses such as tears, facial expressions of hopelessness, anxiety, and so forth. Students seem to be especially fearful that the child will die while they are caring for him and they will not be able to function effectively during this stressful period.

The student will frequently use his or her own faith as a means of coping with the situation. He or she will be influenced by recent experiences with other patients with a fatal prognosis or patients who have died. In addition they may have recently witnessed death in their personal lives. Some may never have had an experience with death and they fear the unknown.

For these reasons the student frequently needs a faculty member close by when he or she is caring for the child who has a fatal prognosis. It seems to help just to have moral support. Frequently conferences are also indicated to help the student express his or her anxiety and concerns. The student should also feel free to cry if he or she feels the need to do so. Again, they should be aware that the child will sense their emotions and they should try to use control in the child's presence. These periods of release usually make it easier for the student to continue to function effectively.

A frequent mistake in caring for the child with a fatal prognosis is to expect the child to act like he is terminally ill. Children usually do not want to be sick and they attempt to camouflage their illness. The adults in their lives need to keep this in mind. I have watched again and again children in for diagnostic workups who run and play in the play area, and their parents seem to be relatively relaxed prior to the time a diagnosis of a terminal disease is made. The parents frequently change their approach, the child is overprotected, the parents cry when they look at the child, they darken the rooms, turn off television or radios, and begin an oversolicitous role. Often the diagnosis is definitely determined at surgery and the child may be quite ill postoperatively, so that he does not immediately object to this restrictive changed environment. However, the child with a medical condition, such as leukemia, is greatly concerned by the new situation. It is difficult enough for the child to cope with the introduction of a large number of medications, painful diagnostic procedures, or irradiation therapy, without the additional changes in the environment and the way the adults in his life respond to him.

The first step in developing realistic goals will be to consider the developmental tasks for the age of the child, taking into account the regression which may accompany hospitalization. Another factor which weighs heavily on the nurses' decisions are the plans which are formulated by the rest of the professional team which includes the child's parents or significant others. Abrupt changes in the therapeutic plan are not wise. I have heard nurses dogmatically say, "I'll just go in and change that!" This type of change is rarely accepted by the child, the parents, or co-workers. Gradual changes which show results are much more readily accepted—such as suggesting the child have periodic play periods with the window shades raised, or periods to watch his favorite television programs. The child's enthusiasm during these trial periods will usually guarantee more of these sessions returning the environment to its normal state.

The parents of the child with an illness with a fatal prognosis usually play a big role in the hospitalization. Their role needs to be supported by making the hospital environment comfortable and humane. They must be helped to feel a part of the team so they feel a sense of belonging. The other relatives and siblings may not be as intimately included until the child is discharged, but they should not be excluded from the long-range plans. In fact, the child would greatly benefit during extended hospitalizations from visits from his siblings, friends, and pets. This is a two-way process. The other children also are aware of their hospitalized family member's condition and it helps to keep them reality-oriented. Too often, when a child dies the other children only remember the "well" sibling who went to the hospital, as they saw very little of the child as he progressed through his illness. The hospitalized child also feels very isolated by the hospitalization periods. He is not used to the individual attention of the parents and has learned to share them with his other siblings. A more natural state would be to continue this plan. If the hospital does not permit children to visit, then each time the child is discharged from the hospital the parents and children must make a readjustment to the usual family routine and this is often quite difficult. The other relatives should also be included as much as possible in the long-range plans. They often put pressure on the parents to change decisions which have been realistically made in the hospital. Many a well-meaning grandparent has forced the family to seek another medical decision in a far-off place that has publicized a "cure" or new method of care. This medical shopping can be expensive and disruptive to the child and the family as a whole. The shopping can have the positive effect of relieving some of the family's guilt feelings as they gain satisfaction from "knowing they have done all they can."

The diagnosis of a fatal illness is certain to have a disrupting effect on the family. The goal of intervention is clearly to help preserve the stability of the family unit.

If the extended family is unable to provide support for the family, then the family has to be helped to cope with that reality so they do not waste emotional energy being disappointed, disgruntled, or hostile toward their relatives. An excellent book for parents whose children have leukemia is *The Leukemia Child,* by Sherman written by a mother whose child experienced the medical regime and died. An early study by Bozeman et al (1955) of parents' reactions to their terminally ill child can help the reader to understand how parents progress through a series of reactions as they learn to cope with the threatened loss of their child. Such initial reactions as denial, self-injury, refusal to believe the diagnosis (or reversing it), and disbelief were common. Denial was used to try to blank out the diagnosis or to reverse the diagnosis. Most mothers were more concerned with improving the prognosis of the disease. Then feelings of guilt began to appear, with self-blame. Many felt if they had recognized signs earlier they could have prevented the disease.

Of particular significance to nursing personnel is the searching for any and all information on the disease that parents undertake. They seem to have to know all the current facts about the disease and its prognosis. The parents frequently present all this information to the nurse who then may become threatened. If the nurse reacts negatively the parent may become angered and resent the nurse. This creates a chain reaction which impedes care, unless ways are provided for the parents and nurse to utilize each other effectively. Parents should be given avenues for using their energies effectively, and while the child is hospitalized this may be accomplished by establishing a care plan that allows the parents to be with their child and help meet his emotional needs for love and comfort.

It is important during the early stages of the illness to help the parents to learn to cope with the diagnosis. At this stage the child is usually not incapacitated and the parent is certainly able to provide a great deal of his care. Parents must not be abruptly separated from the child. Helping them to feel they are an integral part of the care is an excellent way to help them to cope with the situation. Then, as the illness progresses, they will be better able to assist. They are introduced gradually to the progressive deterioration in the child's condition and see first hand the added responsibilities this deterioration will produce. The parents become increasingly willing to let the nurse take over as the child becomes increasingly difficult to manage.

It was also brought out in the studies that none of the mothers ever gave up hope until their child was actually moribund. This is especially essential to keep in mind when giving care to the child. Because the parents have a great deal of hope until very late in the child's illness, they will not understand a nurse's early pessimism. They do not want to realize that nurses have had more experience with the disease, either through the literature or experience, and may have more evidence to support an attitude of pessimism. The parents' attitude is based solely on their involvement with and their hope for their child.

It is important for the nurse to understand that what we consider to be an appropriately realistic attitude for the parents is not one that necessarily accepts the fatal prognosis. A realistic attitude may only be an acknowledgment that their child is seriously ill. Professional personnel should not attempt to deny the parents hope. As the illness progresses they become painfully aware of the irreversibility of the situation and their hope for recovery diminishes. It is not necessary to insist that the parent's relinquish all hope for research that will find a cure for the disease before their child's death. None of us is in a position to take such a negative position very strongly. The parents cannot help but have some appreciation of their child's serious illness as the medical intervention is instigated and implemented.

The Bozeman et al study brought out another point that may be more pertinent to some clinical areas than others. First, rivalry between the mothers and nurses took place for the possession of the child when areas such as feeding, affection, and disipline were taken over by the nurse. This factor may apply more readily where visiting hours are limited and parents take a very minor role in their child's hospitalization. In addition, the mothers were most upset when they were disturbed during visiting hours. They did not accept interruptions even when they were for the benefit of their child. In facilities where visiting hours are extended, this is less of a problem as the mother does not have to guard her limited time with the child.

The study also found that the parents received their greatest support from parents of other children with the same disease. Although it is seldom necessary to introduce these parents to one another, it might be relevant in an area in which the diagnosis of a fatal illness is rare. In an area that services many children with conditions having a fatal prognosis, parents seem to find one another very readily. Parents, especially mothers, have a need to be heard. They seem to derive some relief from their staggering news by being able to talk. As nurses, we must be willing to listen.

Another study (Geis, 1965) that should be helpful to the nurse is one in which mothers were interviewed, after the death of the child, about their impressions of the care their child received before death. All the mothers seemed most interested in the human element when asked what information nurses should have when caring for a child who is dying. They also wanted the truth and seemed to want more time to ask questions. One of the questions asked of these mothers was who they felt was the most helpful person after they learned their child would not recover. Of 21 parents interviewed, only one said the nurse was the most helpful. This information makes one wonder if the nurse can be more useful at this time. Thirty-three parents were asked who was the most helpful when the child died: five parents said it was the nurse. A mere five, despite the fact that eight mothers stated there was a nurse with their child at the time of his death.

This was a study done by a nurse to learn how we might improve services to the families of terminally ill children. Had the questions not been phrased "most helpful," the interviews might have been more positive for the nurses. However, from this admittedly small sampling, it is evident that nurses should try to improve nursing care by responding to the areas of the mothers' concern.

The mothers expressed their appreciation for talking to the nurse interviewer. One way of making ourselves more accessible to parents is to schedule short informal coffee breaks with them. If it is not possible to plan times away from the unit, at least include a few minutes of private interview or counseling time for the parents to vent their feelings. Remember that privacy is imperative as the child can easily grasp the tone of the conversation.

Another interesting finding was that little comment was made in relation to those technical skills that have been highly regarded by many nurses as their most significant contributions to patients. Technical skills are necessary to the nurse because she/he feels more comfortable if she/he can perform them well. However, the parent needs support during the crisis and technical skills, in and of themselves, do not fill the bill. The nurse who prides herself/himself on technical competence is frequently one who hurries in and out without giving herself time fully to evaluate the situation. She/he may set up a blood transfusion with great dexterity but forget to explain to the mother that John's blood count is down, but not dangerously low. Parents derive a great deal of support and satisfaction from explanations. Likewise, the child feels more secure when he receives explanations. The additional time spent is a source of great comfort to the parents and child. It indirectly aids the nurse also, as there is less parent anxiety and resulting questioning when this process is routinely carried out.

In another study by Meurer (1962), it was found that 22 of the 47 mothers interviewed said that the nurse helped them the most in the immediate adjustment to the hospital. This is a rewarding finding, but in reviewing the two studies it would seem that nurses realize their responsibility to the newly admitted patient but not to the child with a fatal prognosis if only five mothers felt the nurse played the most important role.

These are both small studies and Meurer's population was solely mothers of children with leukemia, while Geis' included mothers whose children died from other causes. Their major contributions are, however, in terms of looking at ways of improving nursing services through interviewing the consumers of the service.

A study by Friedman et al (1963) on a population similar to the Bozeman study brought out some other interesting facts. They found that parents seemed to accept the diagnosis intellectually rather than manifesting the great amount of denial described in the Bozeman study. The parents in this study expressed guilt for not reacting more quickly to the early signs of illness. The parental guilt seemed to be alleviated by learning that the long-term prognosis for children with leukemia was about the same regardless of when the diagnosis was made. It was also pointed out that parents did not seem to recall what they were told about the diagnosis, originally. They needed explanations later after the medical plan of care was decided. The parents seemed to need assistance in carrying out immediate details and appreciated the help of the physician with this aspect. This might also carry over to nursing in helping the family with such simple things as a telephone or a private area to discuss plans. Another point made in the study was that parents become confused and anxious if they receive varying reports about their child. This factor is a very good reason for team conferences, including all disciplines, to be held regularly on each child.

Another benefit derived from these team conferences is that the staff has an opportunity to undergo some of their grieving process during the child's course of illness. Then they are better able to help the parents cope when death actually occurs. Team members render essential support to one another. This is especially important for the young students of nursing as they need a great deal of support when dealing with the child with a fatal prognosis and knowing that persons in the field need the same support can be reassuring when coping with a stressful situation. It is helpful for team members to know that they can get support and even be relieved, if necessary, by other team members who understand the child and his parents.

Both the Bozeman et al (1955) and Friedman et al (1963) studies brought out the need for nurses to work with the parents rather than be in conflict with them. The child who is hospitalized readily transfers the change in authority from parent to hospital personnel and every attempt should be made to make this situation tolerable for the parents. Friedman et al also pointed out that when the child nears the terminal stage of his condition parents often begin to care for other children on the ward. This is important to keep in mind as nurses might misinterpret this as lack of interest in their own child because he is no longer providing the parent with the gratification he or she needs. Friedman sees this as a part of the grieving process just prior to the imminent death of the child. The nurse must be cautious not to make the parent feel any discomfort from their participation in these activities. It may be the only way they can cope with their child's death. It might be impossible for them to continue to enter their child's room when death is becoming a reality.

The role religion plays in the lives of the parents of children with an illness with a fatal prognosis is less well documented. In both the Bozeman et al and the Friedman et al studies only small sections are devoted to evaluating the role religion plays in the lives of parents with terminally ill children, and so it is difficult to evaluate the contributions of religion. This may be attributed to the fact that religion is frequently a private matter. It is less common for people openly to express their true feelings about spiritual matters. Members of certain religions are more likely to express their beliefs than others. Many hospitals and agencies have eliminated from their admission data the religious preference of the family, and this makes it even more difficult for the nurse to ascertain information about a family's religious background or current religious beliefs. Waechter and Blake (1976) suggest that parents find great emotional support in religious beliefs because they provide meaning for future events. They suggest that religion is a vehicle for the parents to obtain courage to live with the positive or negative outcomes which they must encounter. They see the parents' faith as aiding in their ability to bear the pain associated with their child's suffering.

The role religion plays in any family's life may vary greatly during certain periods. Even devout families may question their religious beliefs in the face of the impending death of their child. Other families may increase their reliance on religious rites as then they feel that their sorrow can be shared with others, and in this sharing they derive a sense of belonging or caring which is supportive during their persistently trying times.

The child facing death may well benefit from continuing fellowship with his clergyman. The younger child has a limited understanding of religion;

however, modalities which offer a continuance of his usual life pattern may give him additional and vital support. The older child and adolescent are better able to make their wants known regarding spiritual counselors. The nurse should be efficient in implementing the child's and parents' desires.

The following statements were made with regard to implications for physicians, but they are also extremely beneficial implications for nurses.

> Each parent of a child with a fatal disease reacts to the tragedy in a unique manner, consistent with his particular personality structure, past experiences, and the individualized meaning and specific circumstances associated with the threatened loss. In general, optimal medical management depends on the physician's awareness and evaluation of certain aspects of this specific background information. However, the parents of children with leukemia do share many similar problems that are inherent in the situation, and certain modes of adjustment commonly occur in a characteristic sequence. The parental behavior, though not stereotyped, is therefore predictable to some degree (Friedman et al, 1963).

CANCERS OF CHILDHOOD

According to a pamphlet prepared by the New York State Department of Health, the leading causes of death in childhood are: accidents 36 percent, cancer 12 percent, pneumonia 9 percent, diseases of the nervous system 6 percent, infectious diseases 5 percent, diseases of the digestive system 4 percent, and all other 25 percent. In studying this information it becomes apparent that many of the children with terminal illness will have a diagnosis of cancer of some type. The most common type of cancer in childhood is leukemia with an occurrence rate estimated between 30 and 40 percent. The next most common sites are the brain with 24.1 percent, and the kidney and lymph gland with 9.6 percent. Bone cancers account for 3.4 percent of childhood cancers, endocrine system 3.0 percent, digestive system 1.7 percent, and all others 11.4 percent *(The ABC's of Childhood Cancer).*

Meyers et al (1975) report on the survival rate of children under 15 years of age with a diagnosis of cancer. There were 8,282 children included in their sample population. The children lived in a variety of states in the United States. Forty-five percent of the children received their medical care at university medical centers. One year survival from all cancers rose from 50 percent in 1955 to 1959 to 65 percent in 1965 to 1969. The five year survival rate rose from 29 percent to 34 percent during the same time frame. Tumors of the brain and nervous system showed an improvement in five year survival from 34 percent to 45 percent. Leukemia five year survival rates increased from one to five percent. Children with retinoblastoma and thyroid cancer have achieved five year survival rates at the fantastic 90 percent level. Children with Wilms' tumor continue to have extended survival rates, as indicated in this comparison of 1955 to 59 to 1965 to 69, 41 percent to 60 percent. Hodgkins disease also showed dramatic improvement with five year survivals increasing from 42 to 66 percent. The childhood cancers which did not show significant gains were bone sarcoma, soft-tissue sarcoma, lymphoma and neuroblastoma.

In light of this information, the nurse will probably be exposed to children with leukemia, brain tumors, or Wilms's tumors in inpatient services. She/he will be formulating a plan of care focused around such medical orders as increased medications, control of temperature, relief of pain, diagnostic or therapeutic procedures, and surgery. In addition, she/he will be confronted with the reality that dealing with families during the crisis of impending death of a child is a sometimes draining personal experience. In some instances and with continual professional growth, she/he may find that this nursing intervention can be a fulfilling personal and professional experience.

LEUKEMIA

Focusing specifically on leukemia, the increased survival rates have been achieved because of the research efforts in this area. Future efforts of research will focus on continuing to discover the cause(s) of leukemia and finding effective agents to counteract the etiologic sources. In addition, research efforts will attempt to continue to evaluate the methods used to deliver the agents given to slow down the malignant process. As new discoveries are made, the overall management of these children becomes more complex rather than being simplified; and the role of the nurse also becomes more complicated.

By way of illustration, when the treatment of children with leukemia was started in 1948 by Farber, the child's survival time was so short that he frequently received a few medications and died within a short period of time. Contrast this therapy with the current management of a child with acute lymphoblastic leukemia (ALL). The child's management is likely to span a five-year period. During the course of his life he may receive several different combinations of oral, intramuscular, intrathecal, and intravenous medications. He may have lumbar punctures and bone marrow aspirations every month. He may develop meningeal leukemia. He may have internal and external hemorrhaging. He may have periods of extended hospitalizations alternating with periods at home. Instead of a few medications, he may receive a great variety of drugs that are prescribed at very specific times as they are given to coincide with definite cell division changes.

Stagner and Wood (1976) list the seven major classes of drugs which are presently being used with children with cancer: steroids, enzymes, plant alkaloids, purine antagonists, alkylating agents, folic acid antagonists, and antibiotics. As these drugs are intended to interfere with the proliferation of cells in the child's bone marrow, they will tend to decrease the child's immune responses. The depression of the bone marrow results in a leukopenic response. In addition, these drugs can also destroy lymphoid and phagocytic cells, and so further decrease the immunologic activity of the body. Lastly, the chemotherapeutic agents tend to alter the child's ability to produce antibodies. These anticipated side effects of therapy leave the child particularly vulnerable to infections.

The child health nurse often needs special skills to administer these medications. Depending on the age of the child even oral medications can be refused. Creativity—such as making a game of the task—is often wise. Bringing the known, such as a favorite television character, into the picture helps to make the unknown medication more acceptable. The added threat of injections increases the demands on the nurse. The best approach is to restrain the child as needed for his protection, be truthful that it will hurt, and then give the injection quickly and skillfully. Always allow ample time following the administration to comfort the child. Charting of reactions to the medications should be done and responses should be communicated to the physician. Side effects are frequent. Prolonged nausea and vomiting may necessitate cessation of a particular drug based on the physician's and nurses' assessment of the child.

Restraining the child for procedures such as lumbar punctures or bone marrows is often quite difficult. The child has a great ability to move even when he is very ill, and the nurse must use good body mechanics to be certain he/she does not unduly strain his/her own muscles during the procedure. In addition, he/she must of course concentrate on protecting the child from injury during the procedure. Some parents can offer consolation to their child and perhaps even diminish the need for restraining procedures by minimizing the child's fear. If the parents are not allowed in the room during the procedures then each time the child has the procedure done he should be given a simple, truthful explanation of it and told his parents will be waiting outside. It should not be assumed that the child remembers from the last time or that someone else has prepared him. The nurse in the immediate situation must do the preparation. Frequently medication is administered prior to these procedures.

Another area directly related to telling the child the truth is in relation to the diagnosis. This is frequently a highly charged subject. More consideration is being given to having professionals actually work with the child to face the problems of critical illness, hospitalization, and death (Vernick and Lunseford, 1967). The parents are encouraged to tell the child his diagnosis and then professional personnel are available to help the child work through his feelings. The real issue is probably not whether the child should know he is going to die, but rather how to support him so he does not have to feel the loneliness associated with not having people communicate openly with him.

While there is no simple answer to how this should be handled, the main considerations must be the age of the child, the wishes of the parents and the physician, and the past ways in which the child has been able to cope with stressful situations. Continual assessment is essential to be certain that the team members are sharing their observations of the child's behavior as well as his expressed awareness of what is happening to him.

An early study, which is frequently quoted, was done by Natterman and Knudson (1960) on 33 children with leukemia and related diseases, based only on the cognitive capabilities of children in various age categories. It was stated that in the age group zero to five years, separation was the most severe reaction observed; in the age group five to ten years, reactions to procedures were most intense; and in the group ten years and over, the reactions to death were the strongest. This agreed with findings reported by Nagy (1948) that children from three to five years of age did not understand, death and felt that it was not permanent, that it was only a change of some kind and could be temporary; children five to nine years old it was found, did recognize death but without exception regarded it as a person. At about the age of nine children achieve a realistic conception of death as a permanent biologic process. The realization that school-age children can and do understand death and its meaning supports the position for providing these children with more than empty excuses for the death of other children on the unit. It validates the idea of support for them during their illness. Adolescents are entitled to honest discussions and will need time to ask questions privately in addition to the times when discussions take place with parents present.

Numerous studies have been done based on the findings of early research that children under the age of ten years do not understand that they are going to die. Now, however, there are two studies, by Waechter (1968) and by Spinnetta, Rigler, and Kron (1973), that focus on the psychologic responses of children with fatal illness, and these provide evidence that, despite the child's cognitive incapability of fully understanding death, children with fatal illness have greater anxieties about death than children who have chronic illnesses that do not have fatal outcomes. These two studies shed valuable light on the topic as they document that children under six to ten years have anxiety greater than previously described. Waechter's study also showed that children who had a chance to talk about their illness had less anxiety than the children who were not given this opportunity. Of major importance in her findings is that the parent's perceptions of the degree of anxiety that their child possessed were not consistent with the child's expressed anxiety. These findings suggest that parents tend to deny that their child could have death anxiety. In a study by Ferguson (1976), it was concluded that children in the two-to-five–year range did not have late psychologic effects from their treatment of childhood cancer. Ferguson studied 18 children and concluded that only two of these children exhibited moderately severe adjustment problems. She attributed this to the flexible policies related to parent participation in the care of their children.

In relation to the overall nursing care, the parents' role has been well documented in the literature. When the mothers help to care for the child, the nurses serve as a teacher, counselor, friend, and stabilizer rather than a mother-substitute (Fig. 1). Therefore, the reactions nurses often feel at the death of a child may be minimized by the parent participation. The reactions nurses may have include sympathy, sense inadequacy, guilt, and repression. It seems beneficial not only from the parent's and child's standpoint but also from the nurse's standpoint to involve parents actively in the care.

One very important point to remember is to gauge parents' participation as carefully as possible, changing their participation readily if the situation warrants it. Many factors may influence the degree of participation the parent is able to give in any one day—such things as how well the mother was able to sleep the night before, whether she was able to eat enough to have the strength to be of help, and what reports she received from the physician. Mothers frequently can participate more when the reports are somewhat encouraging or at least do not seem too discouraging. Her partici-

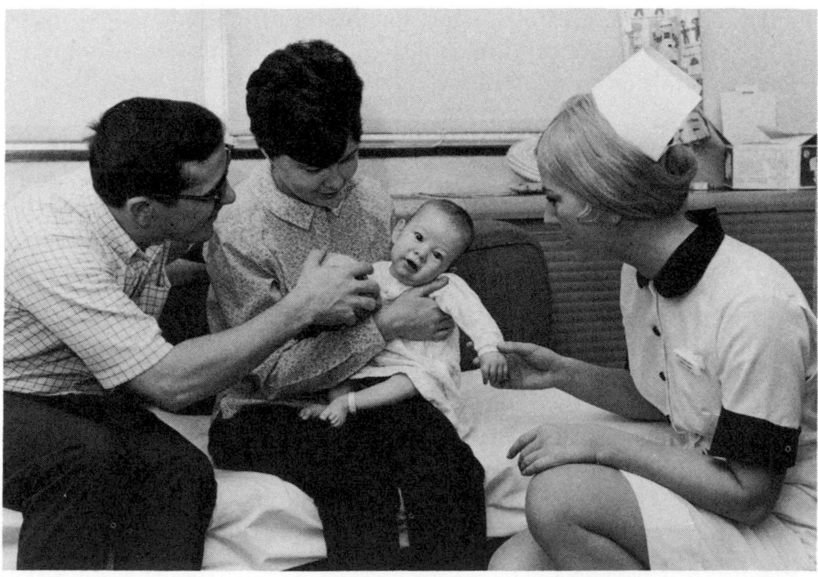

FIG. 1. Pediatric rooming-in provides an excellent opportunity for the family and nurse to learn from one another.

pation may also be influenced by what her responsibilities are at home. If she is expected to carry the full responsibility for the family, she may not feel up to any activity which involves physical effort. Her participation will best be utilized as emotional support for the child. The parent should be helped to participate in the role of a parent rather than trying to play the role of nurse. Too frequently nurses will ask the mother to monitor the intravenous flow. This is not an ordinary mothering task. It aligns her with a painful or tiresome procedure and may influence the child's perception of why she is visiting. He may feel that the mother is contributing to the punishment that he equates with painful or tiring procedures. If the nurse monitors the intravenous, then she/he helps to free the mother of the burden of bestowing the child's perceived punishment. The child-parent-nurse relationship is illustrated in Figure 2.

The roles the mother ordinarily has such as bathing, feeding, disciplining, and most important *loving* are her vital contributions. The mother is more comfortable assuming tasks she already knows. She has been perfecting these skills since the child was born and she is the expert in the area and can utilize her expertise to its fullest.

The nurse's expertise includes the technical skills of monitoring in-

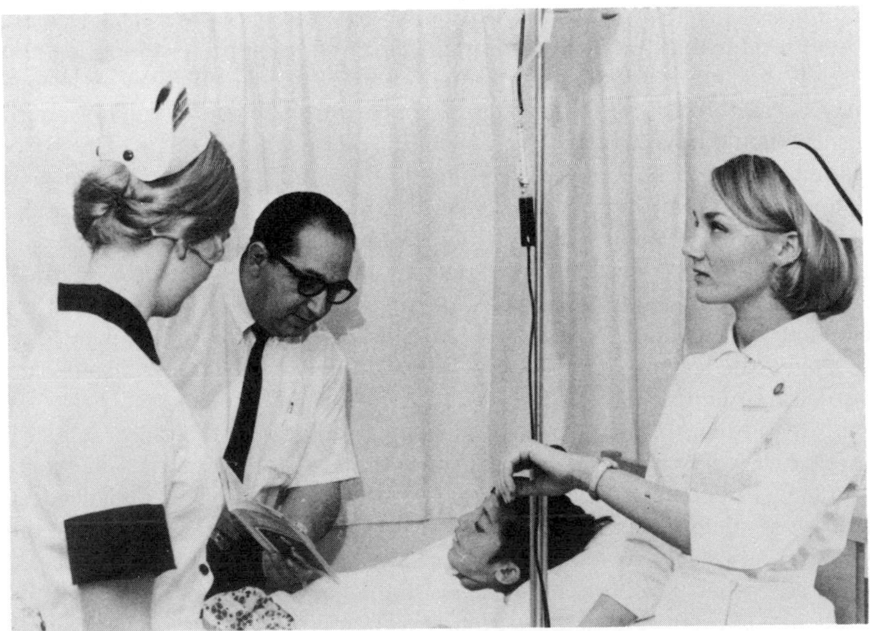

FIG. 2. This acutely ill boy benefits from the nurse's expertise in monitoring the blood transfusion. The father's expertise is used in providing diversional therapy.

travenous infusions, Foley catheters, and the maintenance of the suction equipment, as well as the vital communication skills that foster the child-parent-nurse relationship. However, the nurse is also able to do the mothering tasks in the absence of the mother. He/She should try to do them as consistently as possible within the pattern the mother has established. Mothers need to know that the nurse is willing and capable of being a mother-substitute when she is not able to be with the child.

The parents should also be aware of any changes that are made in the child's care so they can cooperate in following through on them. This is especially important if there are changes made in disciplining the child. In order for the child to benefit substantially, all the adults need to be aware of the program and carry through consistently.

Parents have a real need to be informed of changes in their child's condition. They are able to separate from the child more readily if they are certain they will be notified quickly if changes occur. A definite plan needs to be established to meet this objective. The Kardex needs to have emergency phone numbers, places where the parent will be, responsible adults who can receive messages, and the professional person who will assume the major responsibility for communicating this information.

Providing a safe environment for the child necessitates measures to protect him from infection and hemorrhage. The child is prone to develop mouth lesions, lesions around the finger- or toenails, and rectal lesions. These lesions of the mucus membrane can progress rapidly into a necrotic state if they are not found and treated quickly and effectively. The lesions may be cultured to determine appropriate antibiotic therapy. The mouth lesions should be treated with non-irritating mouthwash or rinses. The use of a toothbrush is frequently discontinued when the lesions are painful and extensive. Cotton tip applicators, mouth swabs, or a wet cotton cloth can be subsituted. The lesions will contribute to the child's anorexia. Liquids and foods should be altered to decrease irritation to the open lesions. Small amounts of mild fluids at room temperature will probably be the most acceptable to the child. Foods should be bland and soft to limit chewing that will open the lesions and cause bleeding. The feedings should be small and offered frequently so the child's intake is satisfactory.

In addition to lesions of the mucus membrane, these children are also prone to develop furuncles, herpes simplex and zoster, bacterial infections, and fungal infections. Early recognition of these conditions is enhanced by daily nursing observations. Bath time is an excellent period for assessing the young child's skin. The older child should be taught to assess his own skin for redness, rashes, swelling, tenderness, lumps, and lesions. He needs to be cautioned to report any of these symptoms immediately. The parents should know that these conditions can occur and not to treat them with home remedies as children on chemotherapy do not respond in the same way as children with normal immunologic systems. In addition to local therapy, it may be necessary to discontinue the chemotherapy if the secondary condition is severe.

The contagious diseases of childhood also pose problems for children on chemotherapy. The live virus vaccines are not given during the child's therapy. If the child is exposed to varicella or measles and develops the disease, he is likely to be acutely ill. Some physicians give zoster immune globulin to children exposed to varicella or gamma globulin to children exposed to measles.

These children also have a greater tendency to develop pneumonia, diarrhea, meningitis, peritonitis, osteomyelitis, vaginitis, and urinary tract infections. These infections severly complicate the treatment regime and usually necessitate hospitalizations to manage the acute phase. These hospitalizations tend to dissappoint the child and parents, which sometimes makes them reluctant to report the early symptoms of impending complicating illness.

Intravenous infusions with medications must be monitored closely so they can be discontinued if they infiltrate. The infiltration of some medications, such as vincristine and actinomycin D can result in sloughing of the tissue or chemical cellulitis. Soaks will usually be applied to the area as soon as the intravenous is discontinued.

To decrease the possibility of infection the child is sometimes placed on reversed isolation. In extreme circumstances, a child may be placed in a sterile environment. (See Chapter 10 for the implications of isolation to the child).

Hemorrhages will appear as petechiae or ecchymotic areas on the skin surface. More intensive internal bleeding may be evidenced by rectal bleeding, bloody vomitus, or changes in vital signs. The bleeding tendencies are due to the child's decrease in platelets. There is rarely any concrete evidence of trauma associated with the hemorrhage. Slight bumps can result in large bruised areas. Gentle handling is essential. This is a challenge when children must be restrained for lumbar punctures, infusions, intramuscular injections, and radiation therapy. Parents and children need to be alerted to this probability so they do not assume that someone has abused their child intentionally. Even the blood pressure cuff can cause bruising. The more frequent the vital signs have to be taken, the more likely is the possibility that bruising will occur.

The major reasons for the increased susceptibility to infection and hemorrhage are the immunologic depression and the decrease in platelets. However, the normal physiology of the child's skin also plays a part. The child's skin is less cornified and hairy than an adult's. The epithelial layer is thinner. The child's skin contains more water and electrolytes than the adult's and the sweat glands are underdeveloped.

The child's temperature regulation mechanisms are less stable than the adult's and they tend to have high temperature fluctuations. This is very common with acute infections and some hemorrhaging. The control of the temperature is attempted with medication such as aspirin. In addition, it may be necessary to give tepid sponge baths to help with evaporation. The child should be protected from unnecessary drafts and shivering during the treatment. The tepid water is applied using soft cloths and allowed to evaporate naturally. Clothing should be kept at a minimum. Sometimes the child is placed on a hypothermia mattress. He should be turned frequently and observed for pressure areas. Occasionally it is necessary to use a fan to help with the evaporation if the other techniques are not successful in lowering the temperature.

Stagner and Wood (1976) report the use of salt pork packs for the control of anterior nasal bleeding. The salt pork is cut into small portions. It is then used as an astringent pack which puts pressure on the bleeding point. They state that the salt pork stays moist and therefore is easier to remove than ordinary gauze or vaseline packing, which tends to irritate the mucus membrane when being removed. The pack is usually left in place for 12 to 24 hours and then removed. These authors also suggest the use of a dry tea bag to control gingival bleeding. The bag is applied to the bleeding site and aids in hemostasis.

Wherever bleeding occurs, it must be attended to immediately to cut down on odor, discomfort, and the possibility that bacteria will use the blood as a culture medium. If local measures do not result in control of the bleeding, transfusions of whole blood or one of its parts will be necessary. To decrease the possibility of infection at the site, the skin surface is usually prepared with Betadine.

During the long term course of the disease, the child will have periods of remission alternating with periods of relapse. Greene (1976) describes *complete remission* to be when the bone marrow is functioning adequately to produce adequate platelets and white and red blood cells. In addition, the marrow shows less than five percent blastocytes. *Relapse* is determined by the return of leukemia cells to the bone marrow, peripheral blood, or the central nervous system. The monitoring of the disease process in this manner is the reason for the frequent bone marrow and lumbar punctures done on these children.

In addition, lumbar punctures are done to give chemotherapy. This is necessitated because systemic chemotherapeutic agents do not enter the spinal column. In order to prevent or treat central nervous system infiltration, it is necessary to introduce the chemotherapy by the intrathecal method. In fact, Greene (1976) reports that Methotrexate is administered weekly or twice weekly for five or six doses early in the child's protocol. In addition to the intrathecal chemotherapy, cranial irradiation is also given.

The side effect of these therapies includes alopecia. Alopecia is a disturbing condition for the child and his parents. Often the hair falls out quickly and completely. The hair that grows back is usually finer than the child's original hair and it lacks lustre and the healthy appearance of normal hair. It is not unlike the fine hair of the newborn. Some children prefer to wear wigs during their long period without hair. Others find the wigs irritating, complaining of scalp itching, tightness, and general discomfort, which is probably not as great as described. The child should decide whether or not he wants to wear the wig without adult interference.

The use of prednisone is common in the treatment protocol. Prednisone causes weight gain and results in the round faces and abdomens common to these children. The weight gain is disturbing. The child's body image is affected. He may become quite uncomfortable due to the increased weight that interferes with his respiratory function. The child's appetite is increased dramatically during the early phase of the treatment. Later this increased appetite changes to a lack of appetite that is equally disturbing. Nausea is often responsible for the anorexic periods. The nausea is usually the result of medication. If the medication does not have to be given at a specific time, Greene (1976) suggests that the child might be given it during the evening so he can sleep through the hours of greatest nausea. The child must be observed frequently to be certain he does not vomit and aspirate. Severe vomiting can be exhausting to the child. Antiemetic drugs are sometimes necessary. Accurate recording of intake and output is essential to monitor the child's progress.

It is apparent from the foregoing discussion that these children will be seen during their long-term care in a variety of circumstances. Their long term course will include many painful experiences which are essential to prolong their lives. The trend is to have the children receive their care on an out-patient basis whenever possible. This trend fosters better family involvement, but also requires the parent to assume much greater responsibility for monitoring their child's progress.

ROLE OF THE NURSE AFTER THE DEATH OF A CHILD

Following the death of a child on a hospital unit, it is imperative to restore the unit to normality as quickly as possible. The school-age and adolescent children understand death and a simple explanation should be given to them. The parents of the children should know what has happened and how you explained it to the child. Frequently nurses try to make excuses to "cover-up" death on a unit. This violates the simple principle of telling children the truth. It also encourages the child to mistrust adults.

In a book by Bergmann (1965), it is brought out that although the nurses did their very best to protect the other children from the death of a child, the nurses themselves were so upset by the death that the children sensed it from the nurses' reactions. The other children then began to act out in accordance with what they felt their role was in relation to their dead peer. Although the acting out was not completely in tune with the situation, it pointed out that children can and do have a concept of death and are entitled to a simple explanation that will satisfy their curiosity.

The child who has an attachment to the dead peer may exhibit some of the following things during his mourning process. He may cling to an object from home so he feels more secure that he will not die. He may have periods of insomnia and need more support during bedtime hours. He may refuse to eat for a period of time. The child may go through a period of acting out and be quite obnoxious. His games and songs may center around the death of the child and he may seem quite callous in his approach.

It is important to keep in mind that children have less experience with death and therefore very little past experience to draw upon in resolving their grief. Mourning involves a departure from the ordinary, and a child may become so enveloped in mourning that he has very little energy left over for any other interests. It is best to tell the children straight forwardly that their friend or brother or sister has died soon after the death. This will usually give them an opportunity to ask questions. The child's questions may be related to their past experiences with death, such as, "We flushed my dead goldfish down the toilet, will you flush Mary down the toilet?"

The child with a long-term illness may have more reason than other children to fear that death will also claim him. He will probably need more time, on an individual basis, to express his anxiety. He may have the same physician as the deceased child and he begins to question the competency of his physician. He may question why the nurses let Mary die.

The child with a long-term illness may possibly have more experience with death because of his more frequent hospitalization and greater exposure to medical situations. But these experiences may not have helped him in learning to cope with death—they may only have served to make him feel less secure.

An example follows. Jim was ten years old when his hydronephrosis became extremely incapacitating. An ileoconduit was scheduled and the proposed surgery was explained to Jim. He had been hospitalized several times and was presently hospitalized three months because of problems with continuing his foster home placement. Jim's preoperative preparation was started and the thought of death became utmost in Jim's mind. One day he was overheard talking to another school-age child. Jim was relating all the deaths of children that had taken place on this busy hospital unit since his admission. At the end of the list he added his own name. Fortunately, this conversation took place in plenty of time to get professional help for Jim prior to surgery.

A factor which helps to restore the unit to normal is children's capacity to "forget" the death. They are quick to return to the ordinary daily activities and are thought to complete the grief process in much less time than adults. The children will, of course, be reminded of the death if the adults in their environment continue to show signs of unrest. This is another reason for professional personnel to be able to function under the stress created by death on the pediatric unit.

The child's misconceptions about death frequently revolve around the idea that death is a punishment for wrong doings. Therefore, the child who has been "bad" may fear death as his "punishment."

The child with a long-term illness may have secretly or openly wished the other child would die so he did not get so much of the staff's attention. This death wish is frequent in children, but the wished-for death rarely happens, so the child does not have to feel the guilt associated with having his wish granted. If the child does die, the child making the wish feels very guilty for his thoughts. The child will need help to understand that he did not really cause the child's death. He will also need assurance that children do sometimes wish people would die.

The death of another child, while it may be frightening, is usually less traumatic to the child than losing one of his parents or perhaps even a pet.

The reader is referred to the pamphlet entitled, "Helping Your Child to Understand Death" by Anna W. M. Wolf for answers to questions regarding death.

OUTPATIENT SERVICES

The intermittent nature of some of the illnesses with fatal prognosis such as leukemia necessitates attention to the care offered in the out-patient clinics, especially when the children are treated in a clinic which bears the name of the disease entity. Even children who previously received private medical supervision are frequently referred to the specialty clinic for their follow-up care. This often changes the whole pattern of care for this child and his parents. In one study (Bozeman et al, 1955), it was shown that parents were often quite hostile toward the clinic. The common complaints about clinic care include long waits, impersonal approaches, exposure to very sick children, lack of specific appointments, and lack of privacy, to mention but a few.

A concern by the professional staff in one clinic servicing children with leukemia was that the children get to know other children with the same disease and soon lose this attachment by the death of the other child. The appointment days were staggered so the child did not expect his friend to come on the same day, thus eliminating the possibility of strong peer relationships being formed. It was believed that the parent, rather than a peer, could better serve as the stable figure during clinic appointments.

It is important to remember that children with long-term illnesses learn to integrate their specialty clinic into their normal life style. For the school-age child his social groups then include his family, his community, his peers, his school, and his clinic. The way he perceives the clinic is largely dependent on interpersonal relationships. This places a great responsibility on the nurse in the clinic to become acquainted with the patients and to assume a major role in making the clinic experience as positive as possible. In addition to personal identity, the nurse should be sure that privacy is guaranteed each child, that he is accompanied for painful procedures, that he is prepared for all clinic procedures, and that his next clinic appointment is scheduled to least interfere with his personal plans. With pediatric care rapidly moving to the out-patient departments which are physically not ready to accept the large influx of patients, good interpersonal relationships can be a great compensation. Other nursing contributions to personalizing the out-patient care of children with a fatal prognosis might include the following techniques. The regularly scheduled visits to the clinic should be known in advance. All professional personnel should review the past records prior to visiting the child for his clinic examination. Children should be approached in the waiting area and addressed by name. Facts which are easily compiled, such as birthdate or upcoming special events, can further add to the individualizing of patient care. A comment such as, "Birthday wishes are in store for you this week!" can be helpful. A supply of children's birthday cards can be kept on hand to be signed by the child's physician and nurse. Other similar occasions can be acknowledged in the same manner. Children enjoy surprises, and small inexpensive gifts can be wrapped and put into a grab bag. This will further suggest to the child's significant others the professional personnel's interest in children. To any particular child it will signify a direct interest in him.

The waiting area should be well equipped with toys and activities to make the waiting period seem shorter. A donated supply of magazines can be useful for the parents (Figs. 3 and 4). Films, filmstrips, posters, and pamphlets can also be utilized in the waiting area. Some of this material can be geared to the children, while others may appeal to the parents and the children can utilize the time playing in another area (Fig. 5).

The waiting area should have comfortable seats for both the children and the parents. It should have a crib or play pen available for infants who could not be left at home. The waiting area should also be equipped with machines offering nutritious food items, such as fruit juice, milk, and crackers. Coffee is also considered a friendly offering and, if possible, it should be available for the adults.

It also helps to have the waiting area clean and aesthetically appealing. This will diminish the complaints of attending an outpatient service.

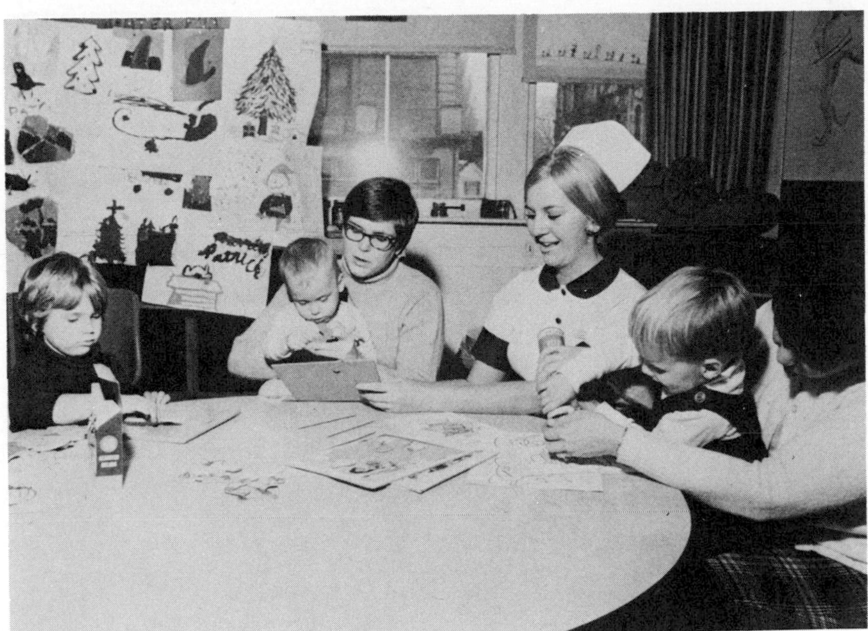

FIG. 3. Long waiting hours in the outpatient department can be fun when recreational therapy is provided. Student nurses can gain knowledge of normal growth and development from making observations about play activities.

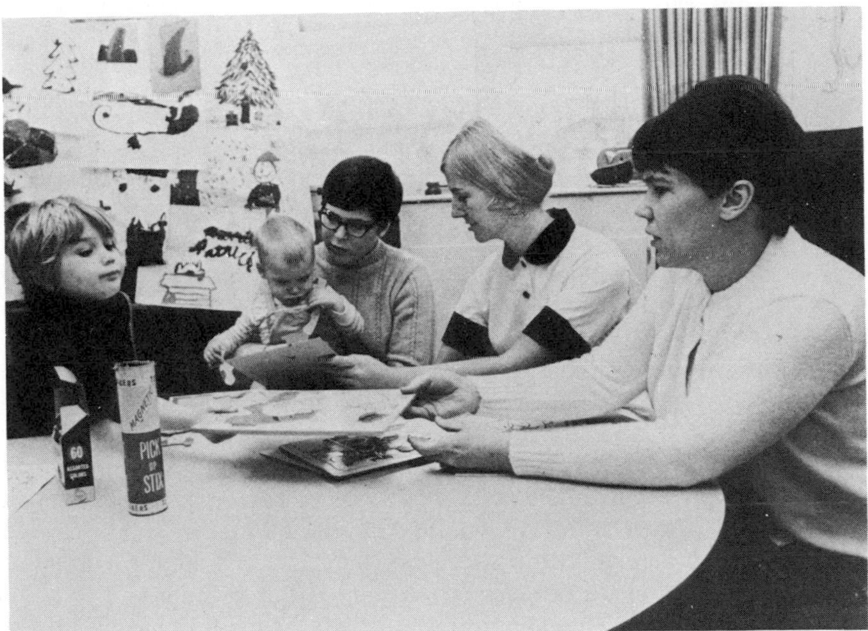

FIG. 4. The use of teenage volunteers in the outpatient department waiting room helps to increase interest in child care. It also frees the parents to talk privately to the professional personnel.

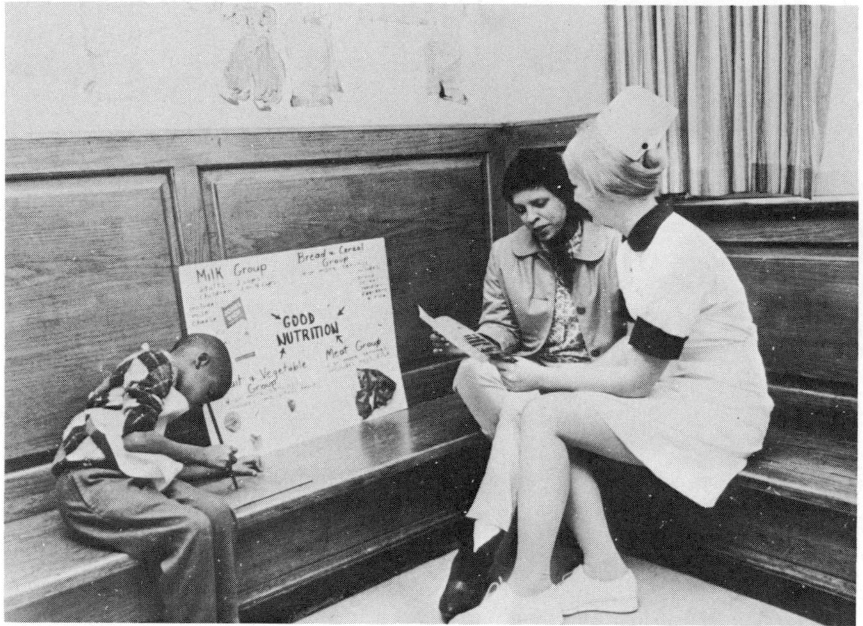

FIG. 5. Visual aids utilized in teaching during waiting time in outpatient department.

OUTPATIENT NURSING INTAKE INTERVIEWS

The nurse in the out-patient department should conduct an interview with the parent and child on each visit. It is important to know how the child is adjusting or coping between visits. The nurse is able to elicit this information by offering the child and parent an acceptable situation in which to verbalize. The parent should be taught to keep accurate records between visits, and her records are shared at this time. The records should indicate the medications the child has received between visits, with emphasis placed on identifying medications that were not given or tolerated. In addition, the record should contain estimates of vomiting or diarrhea to determine the hydration status of the child. If the child has an elevated temperature, it should also appear on the record. New areas of hemorrhage or infection should be recorded. The interview should provide for privacy and be carried out in a relaxed manner. If the interview seems hurried, appropriate information may be withheld or assessed inaccurately. It is important to know how much of a strain this long-term or terminal illness is having on the family. If it is reasonable, the whole family should come for visits rather than just the patient and parent. This can serve several purposes. One, the other children learn to appreciate some of the stress placed on their affected sibling. They also can see that the child is receiving excellent care and that everything possible is being done to prolong his life. Another important point is that the other children frequently suffer when there is a child in the family who needs a great deal of attention. Counseling may be indicated for the other children to help them understand what is taking place with their brother or sister. They may also need explanations for their parents' behavior. If possible, the interview should precede the physical examination so that the information gathered can be shared with the physician and other team members.

The following are examples of forms which can be utilized for outpatient nursing intake interviews. The first one is suggested when one is interviewing parent and child together on the initial visit. The second one is useful for follow-up visits. The third is for interviewing school-age and adolescent children without their parents. The fourth form is suggested for planning effective nursing care during the visit and also for determining needs for referral to other agencies. As the majority of these children return fre-

FORM 1.

UNIVERSITY HOSPITAL
U.S.A.

INITIAL NURSING INTAKE INTERVIEW (OUTPATIENT)

Name ______________________ **Age** ________ **Date** _____

I. Reason for appointment

II. Previous appointment or hospital admissions
(date, reason, action taken)

III. Family constellation

IV. Habits:
Eating (describe amount, how often, types of food, likes, and dislikes)
Elimination
Sleeping
Language development
Play—peer groups

V. Allergies

VI. Activities of daily living
Independent
Dependent
School
Social interests

VII. Special needs, fears, problems

FORM 2.

UNIVERSITY HOSPITAL
U.S.A.

FOLLOW-UP NURSING ASSESSMENT BASED ON PARENT RECORD—KEEPING AND INTERVIEW

Name ______________________________ **Age** ________ **Date** ______

I. Reason for appointment
(routinely scheduled or requested)

II. Hospital admissions or emergency treatment since last visit
(date, place, reason, actions taken)

III. Social behavior since last visit
(include school attendance, interactions with parents, siblings, peers)

IV. Medication regime
(include reactions to drugs, omissions, etc)

V. Vital signs
(include elevated temperatures and weight assessment)

VI. Blood tests
(include any results from blood work completed at other places and today's results)

VII. Changes in activity since last visit
(disabilities, regression in development)

VIII. Physiologic assessment
(estimates of vomiting, diarrhea, new bruises, petechiae, mouth lesions, etc)

IX. Changes in family status

FORM 3.

UNIVERSITY HOSPITAL
U.S.A.

NURSING INTERVIEW OF CHILD (OUT-PATIENT)

Name ______________________________ **Age** ________ **Date** ______

I. Reason for appointment

II. Preparation for visit

III. Habits:
Eating
Elimination
Sleeping
Play—peer groups

IV. Activities of daily living
Independent
Dependent
School
Social interests
Relationships with siblings

FORM 4.

UNIVERSITY HOSPITAL
U.S.A.
OUT-PATIENT NURSING INTERVENTION

Name ______________________________ **Age** ________ **Date** ______

I. In relation to child (incorporating principles of normal and development)

II. In relation to family

III. Community resources available to meet nursing objectives

IV. Follow-up plan of care

quently to the clinic, a Kardex is especially useful in compiling information. The simple guideline in utilizing these tools is to give as comprehensive a picture of this child and his family as possible.

Outpatient Examination

When the child's turn comes to go to the examining room, the nurse should greet the child and his parents (Fig. 6). The child will then be

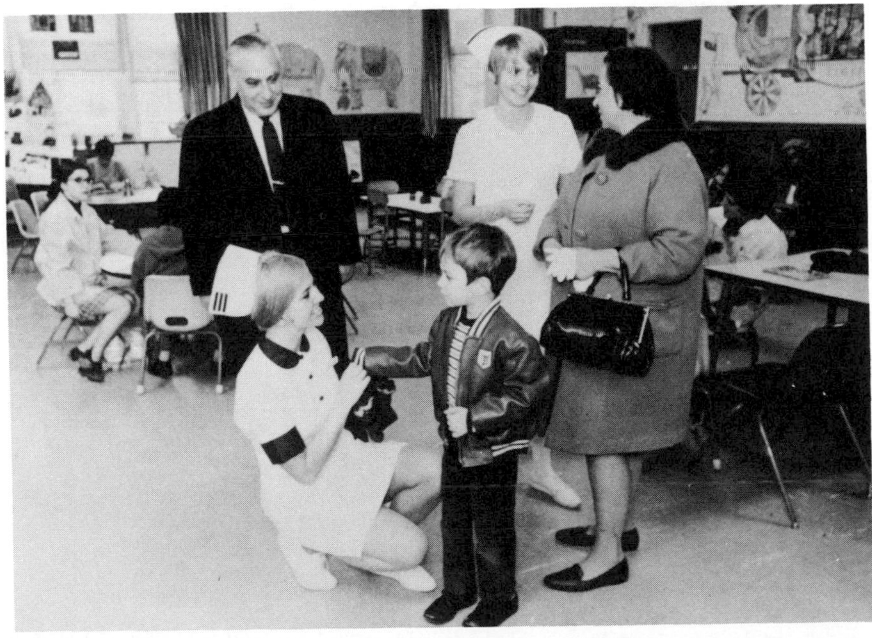

FIG. 6. The outpatient waiting room provides the nurse with an opportunity to meet the entire family.

encouraged to help in his preparation. He will be encouraged to guess how much he weighs, to take his own oral temperature, and to undress and get into the proper garb (Fig. 7). He will be offered all the privacy he desires during this procedure.

Questions that the child can adequately answer will be asked of him directly. An attempt should be made to have the child feel he is an integral part of the visit, not just an appendage. The child and parents should be introduced to the physician, if they have not previously met him or her. They are also introduced to students of any profession who may be present during the examination.

Many of the procedures which formerly necessitated hospitalization

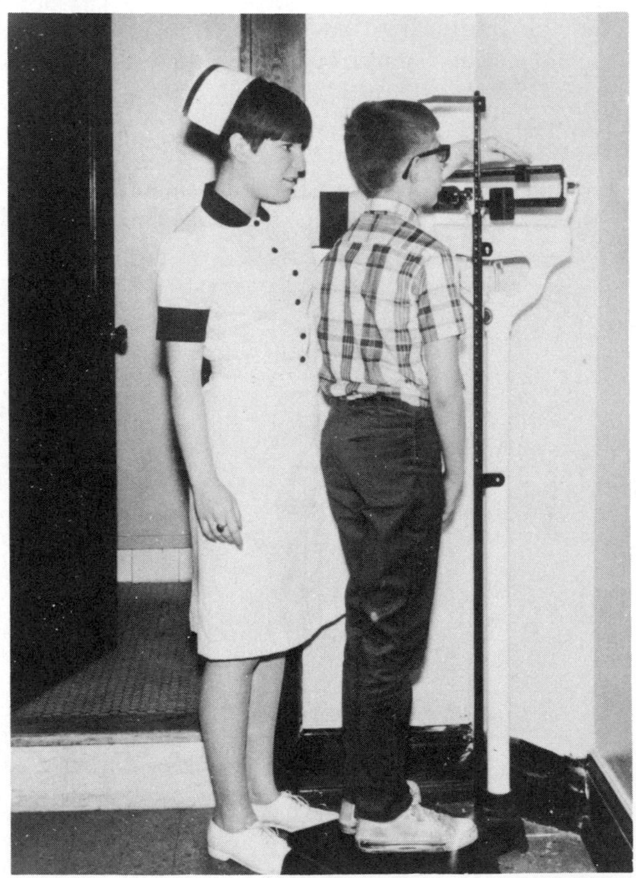

FIG. 7. John is a mentally retarded boy who enjoys having his height and weight monitored. (Courtesy of Cantalician Center, Buffalo, N.Y.)

now are done in the outpatient department. These include bone-marrow aspirations, blood counts, blood transfusions, and paracentesis. In a busy clinic the nurse must be able to teach the parent what signs to observe while the child is receiving a transfusion; be able to organize the work load to permit visitation with the child who is spending a period of time in the OPD, and offer support and a listening ear to the child and his significant others. If any of the procedures are done in a different area, the nurse should be very sure to give the parents and child adequate directions to the area. This will help to decrease the amount of anxious activity spent in finding unfamiliar areas.

Referrals to community health nursing can contribute effectively to help the family deal with grief, to help with treatment regimes or medications, and to encourage follow-up visits. The referral should try to indicate where in the grieving process the parent is at this time. If the parent is still in the period of denial, it is imperative for the community health nurse to know this. If the referral is sent after the death of the child, it is important for the nurse to know when the death occurred and also what the parents were told about the post-mortem, if one was performed. Home visits after death can be most helpful in identifying things that the parent felt were positive or negative about the care given their child. The community health nurse can also be an effective listener long after many of the family's friends and relatives have stopped permitting the parents to vent their feelings to them. The community health nurse is also in a position to evaluate how the family unit is beginning to function without the deceased member. He/she may be especially helpful with aiding the parents to cope with the fears the other children may develop in relation to death.

Group meetings of parents of children with long-term or terminal illness may be very beneficial. Parents can discuss their feelings as well as problems they are having caring for the child. Professional personnel should be a part of these groups so they can help the parents work through some of the difficult situations and also to help correct any false impressions the parents may have about the disease process. For a more thorough discussion of groups the reader is referred to the appropriate section in Chapter 11.

HOME CARE

As home care programs are expanded, the care of the child with a terminal illness has not created any great problems. Depending on the particular home care program, the child has received in the home the services of laboratory technicians, oxygen therapists, and medical, nursing, physical, and occupational therapists. The parents who have participated in the program seem to receive satisfaction from keeping their ill child at home as long as possible. The added security of knowing they can telephone a professional person any time during the day or night lessens their anxieties. The child benefits greatly by not being separated from his home and family for long periods. If more home care services are established, outpatient departments may begin to feel some relief from all of the additional services they now offer. With this added comprehensive home care, it becomes evident that the community health nurses in any area may be seeing a great many more patients with a fatal prognosis than they have in the past. Children may go to the hospital only for surgery or complicated therapies and immediately return home for their continuing care. This procedure necessitates better and faster communication between the hospital and home. An effective home care plan is based on the ability of the parent or family to assume a great deal of responsibility for the child's care. Parent education is esssential prior to placing the child on home care services. Some parents even learn to administer intravenous medications. An in-depth explanation of the treatment program is provided so the parent is able to cooperate fully. The parents' intellectual and emotional capabilities are assessed to determine when and how they will be started on the parent education program.

CASE PRESENTATION AND STUDY QUESTIONS

Susan is admitted to a four-bed unit on a busy medical floor. She is six years old and an only child. Her mother and father are both college educated. Her mother is a nurse and her father an engineer. Susan has received all her conscientious medical supervision from the same pediatrician. She has had one other hospitalization, for a fractured arm, approximately one year ago.

This admittance was precipitated by a series of minor symptoms which the pediatrician recognized as being consistent with lymphocytic leukemia. Susan has been bruising easily, has had numerous epistaxis without provocation, and is more irritable than ordinary. The pediatrician did a hemoglobin determination in his office and found it to be 8 g. The admitting diagnosis is anemia, unknown etiology.

1. What additional tests will be done to determine a more exact diagnosis?
2. Considering the host factors, is Susan a candidate for lymphocytic leukemia?
3. Are Susan's presenting symptoms congruous with other types of cancer? Are they related to conditions other than cancer?
4. Is Susan's room placement appropriate? Are there any changes you might suggest?
5. What factors will determine who prepares Susan for her diagnostic evaluation?

The bone marrow aspiration confirms the diagnosis of lymphocytic leukemia. The private pediatrician verifies the findings by additional consultation with the hematology department. He learns that the hospital laboratory is functioning at maximum capacity and that Susan's needs would better be met at a specialized hospital for the care of children with cancer. Susan's pediatrician is not affiliated with the other institution, so her care will have to be transferred if she is to go there.

1. What changes might be expected in the parents' attitude when they hear the diagnosis?
2. If Susan is transferred to the other hospital, what preparation needs to be done? How can you assist in the preparation?
3. How would you explain the transfer to Susan?

Susan is transferred to the other hospital and admitted to a four-bed unit not significantly different than her previous room. Susan's mother comes out to the desk and vehemently rejects the room placement. She wants Susan transferred to a private room immediately.

1. What do you think precipitated the mother's response?
2. What can be done to help the parents and child adjust to the new situation? Is a private room a good solution? Who can help to make this situation more tolerable? Will the "settling-in" situation be delayed under these conditions?
3. How will the mother's anxiety influence Susan? How can you give Susan additional support during this time?

During the nursing intake history Mrs. M. tells you Susan is here for treatment of her anemia. She further states that Susan will only be here two or three days so she will assume the responsibility for Susan's total care.

1. What information will you pass on to the physician from your interview?
2. Is it "normal" for a professionally educated parent to completely deny a diagnosis of leukemia? How soon do you think Mrs. M. will begin to be affected by the impact of her daughter's illness, or is she already affected?
3. What do you think Mrs. M. means when she states she will assume Susan's total care? What aspects of care should be delegated to the parent? How are these aspects altered because the mother is a nurse?

Susan is started on medication and begins to respond to therapy. For a period of time, Susan feels worse than she did on admission. Mrs. M. and Susan complain about many things during this time. Included in their complaints are alternating periods of being too hot or too cold, too much noise in the corridors, too little variation in the food, and too many visitors to the other children in the room.

1. What should you do about the complaints?
2. Why do you think they are being so hard to please? Are there ways of getting to the problems which are the root of the complaints?
3. Are these complaints very different from expected behaviors under similar conditions? Will some of the complaints resolve with the passage of time? If so, when can this be expected?
4. What anticipatory guidance should be given during this time? What is the rationale for providing anticipatory guidance?

Susan is now in remission and is ready for discharge. Mrs. M. and Susan present candy and thank-you's to the staff for their excellent care. You feel especially pleased as you recall the change in their attitudes since admission.

1. Do you feel Mrs. M. and Susan are sincere? If so, what factors influenced their "change in attitude"?
2. When Susan is admitted again, can you expect them to be as gracious as they are on this discharge?
3. What notations will you want to keep regarding this hospitalization experience? Why?

Two-and-a-half years elapse and Susan is hospitalized with severe hemorrhaging. She has been hospitalized for short periods on three other occasions and each time she has responded to therapy. This time it is evident that Susan will not respond. Mrs. M. has been very capably caring for Susan but now seems more interested in the other children and their parents than she is in Susan. Mrs. M. leaves the hospital for long periods and also spends extended time in the coffee shop. When she is on the unit she is usually found giving assistance and support to other parents.

1. How do you evaluate Mrs. M.'s behavior?
2. Is this behavior significantly different than other parents' reactions to their dying children?
3. What support can you offer Mrs. M? What other members of the medical team can give support?
4. How is Mrs. M.'s activity influencing the other parents?
5. Is Mrs. M.'s activity a part of her grieving process? How do you think this will contribute to Mrs. M.'s behavior when Susan dies?

BIBLIOGRAPHY

ABC's of Childhood Cancer. New York State Department of Health, 1959 (rev 1966)

Ariel IM, Park GT (eds): Cancer and Allied Disease of Infancy and Childhood. Boston, Little, Brown, 1960

Bergmann T: Children in the Hospital. New York, International Universities Press, 1965

Bivalec LM, Berkman J: Care by parent–a new trend. Nurs Clin North Am 11:109, March 1976

Bonine GN: Students' reactions to children's deaths. Am J Nurs 67:1439, July 1967

Bowlby J: Grief and mourning in infancy and early childhood. Psychoanal Study Child 15:9, 1960

Bozeman MF, Orbach CE, Sutherland AM: Psychological impact of cancer and its treatment. The adaptation of mothers to the threatened loss of their children through leukemia. Part 1. Cancer 8:1, 1955

Brauer PH, Cockerill E, Kutner BA: Constructive approach to terminal illness. New York, National Foundation, Inc.

Bright F, Luciana France M: The nurse and the terminally ill child. Nurs Outlook 15:39, Feb 1967

Carpenter KM: Parents take heart in the city of hope. Am J Nurs 62:82, Jan 1962

Clapp MJ: Psychosocial reactions of children with cancer: a program for rehabilitation. Nurse Clin North Am 11:73, March 1976

Crosby MH: Control systems and children with lymphoblastic leukemia. Nurs Clin North Am 6:407, June 1971

Dargeon H: Tumors of Childhood. New York, Hoeber, 1960

deBenneville AK: Nursing services in home care. In Schultz ED, Rudick E (eds): Nursing in Ambulatory Units. Dubuque, Iowa, Brown, 1966, pp 33–38

Easson WM: The Dying Child. Springfield, Ill, Thomas, 1970

Engel GL: Grief and grieving. Am J Nurs 64:93, Jan 1964

Evans A: Practical care for the family of a child with cancer. Cancer 35:871, 1975

Fagin C: Why not involve parents when children are hospitalized? Am J Nurs 62:78, Jan 1962

———: The effects of maternal attendance on the post hospital behavior of young children. Philadelphia, Davis, 1966

Family program in children's cancer unit. Hospitals 39:66, 1965

Ferguson JH: Late psychological effects of a serious illness in childhood. Nurs Clin North Am 11:83, March 1976

Fond KI: Dealing with death and dying through family-centered care. Nurs Clin North Am 7:53, March 1972

Ford, LC, Silver HK: The expanded role of the nurse in child care. Nurs Outlook 15:43, Sept 1967

Freidman SB, Chodoff P, Mason J, Hamburg D: Behavioral observations in parents anticipating the death of a child. Pediatrics 32:610, 1963

———, Karon M, Goldsmith G: Childhood leukemia: a pamphlet for parents. Washington, DC, U.S. Department of Health, Education, and Welfare, 1963

Futterman E, Hoffman I: Crises and Adaptation in Families of Fatally Ill Children. The Child In His Family. New York, Wiley, 1973

Gartner CR: Growing up dying: The child, the parents and the nurse. In Caughill RG: The Dying Patient. Boston, Little, Brown, 1976, pp 159–90

Geis DF: Mother's perceptions of care given their dying children. Am J Nurs 65:105, Jan 1965

Green WA, Jr, Miller G: Psychological factors and reticuloendothelial disease: observations on a group of children and adolescents with leukemia; an interpretation of disease development in terms of the mother-child unit. Psychosom Med 20:124, 1958

Greene P: The child with leukemia in the classroom. Am J Nurs 75:86, Jan 1975

Greene T: Current therapy for acute leukemia in childhood. Nurs Clin North Am 11:3, March 1976

Green-Epner CS: The dying child. In Caughill RE (ed): The Dying Patient. Boston, Little, Brown, 1976, pp 125–57

Gyuley J: Care of the dying child. Nurs Clin North Am 11:95, March 1976

Hamovich MB: Parent and the Fatally Ill Child. Duarte, Calif, City of Hope Medical Center, 1964

Harmon V, Steele S: Nursing Care of the Skin: A Developmental Approach. New York, Appleton, 1975

Hays JS: The night Neil died. Nurs Outlook 10:801, Dec 1962

Koocher GP: Talking with children about death. Am J Orthopsychiatry 44:404, 1974

Knudson AG, Natterson JM: Participation of parents in the hospital care of terminally ill children. Pediatrics 26:482, 1960

Lacasse CM: A dying adolescent. Am J Nurs 75:433, March 1975

Leventhal B, Hersh S: Modern treatment of childhood leukemia: the patient and his family, Nurs Digest 3:12, 1975

Mann S: Coping with a child's fatal illness. Nurs Clin North Am 9:81, March 1974

Meurer MC: Working with the mother to improve nursing care of the child with leukemia: nursing in relation to the impact of illness upon the family. New York, American Nurses Association Series No. 2, 1962, pp 14–21

Micheal P: Tumors of Infancy and Childhood. Philadelphia, Lippincott, 1964

Morrissey JR: Death anxiety in children with fatal illness. In Parad HJ (ed): Crisis Intervention. New York, Family Services Association of America, 1965, pp 324–38

Myers MH et al: Trends in cancer survival among U.S. white children, 1955–1971. J Pediatr 87:815, 1975

Nagy M: The child's theories concerning death. J Genet Psychol 73:3, 1948

Natterson JM, Knudson AG: Observations concerning fear of death in terminally ill children and their mothers. Psychosom Med 22:456, 1960

Ohman EW, Walans D: An approach to the nursing diagnosis of behavior in a pediatric speciality clinic. Nurs Science, April 1964

Quint JC: The threat of death: some consequences for patients and nurses. Nurs Forum 8:287, 1969

Rudick E: Nursing and the new pediatrics. Nurs Clin North Am 1:75, 1966

Scahill M: Preparing children for procedures and operations. Nurs Outlook 17:36, 1969

Sharp ES: Experiment in family-centered nursing in a pediatric out-patient service. The Alumnae Magazine 63:66, 1964

Sherman M: The Leukemic Child. Washington, DC, Department of Health, Education, and Welfare, Publications NIH 76–863 (no date)

Smith M: Ego support for the child patient. In Rudick E (ed): Pediatric Nursing. Dubuque, Iowa, Brown, 1966, pp 60–70

Solnit AJ, Green M: Psychological considerations in the management of deaths on pediatric services. Pediatrics 24:106, 1959

Spinetta JJ: The dying child's awareness of death: a review. In Chess S, Thomas A: Annual Progress in Child Psychiatry and Child Development. New York, Brunner/Mazel, 1975, pp 430–36

———, Rigler D, Karon M: Anxiety in the dying child. Pediatrics 52:841, 1973

———, Maloney LJ: Death anxiety in the outpatient leukemic child. Pediatrics 56:1034, 1975

Stagner SA, Wood A: The child with cancer on immunosuppressive therapy. Nurs Clin North Am 11:21, March 1976

Truth sustains leukemic children. Med World News, Sept 1964, p. 62

van Eys J: The Truly Cured Child. Baltimore, University Park Press, 1977

Vernick J, Lunceford JL: Milieu design for adolescents with leukemia. Am J Nurs 67:559, March 1967

Waechter E: Death anxiety in children with fatal illness. Unpublished doctoral dissertation, Stanford University, Ann Arbor, Mich Univ Microfilms, 1968

———, Blake FG: Nursing Care of Children, 9th ed. Philadelphia, Lippincott, 1976, pp 86–96

Wolf AW: Helping your child to understand death. New York, Child Study Association of America, 1958

Wollnick L: Management of the child with cancer on an outpatient basis. Nurs Clin North Am 11:35, March 1976

Wu R: Explaining treatments to young children. Am J Nurs 65:71, Jan 1965

Index